HEALTH PROMOTION
HANDBOOK

HEALTH PROMOTION HANDBOOK

SHERRI SHEINFELD GORIN, PhD

Senior Fellow in Cancer Epidemiology
School of Public Health and the Herbert I. Irving
  Comprehensive Cancer Center
Columbia University
New York, New York,
Associate Professor of Health Policy (Adjunct)
State University of New York at Stony Brook
Stony Brook, New York;
Senior Partner
Management Horizons
Setauket, New York

JOAN ARNOLD, PhD, RN

Associate Professor
School of Nursing
College of New Rochelle
New Rochelle, New York

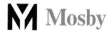 Mosby

St. Louis Baltimore Boston Carlsbad Chicago Minneapolis New York Philadelphia Portland
London Milan Sydney Tokyo Toronto

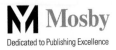

Mosby

Dedicated to Publishing Excellence

A Times Mirror
Company

Publisher: Nancy L. Coon
Editor: Loren S. Wilson
Developmental Editor: Brian Dennison
Project Manager: Deborah L. Vogel
Production Editor: Sarah E. Fike
Designer: Amy Buxton
Manufacturing Supervisor: Don Carlisle

Printed in the United States of America
Composition by The Clarinda Company
Lithography/color film by The Clarinda Company
Printing/binding by RR Donnelley & Sons

Mosby, Inc.
11830 Westline Industrial Drive
St. Louis, Missouri 63146

Library of Congress Cataloging in Publication Data

ISBN 0-8151-3611-0

98 99 00 01 02 / 9 8 7 6 5 4 3 2 1

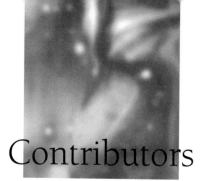

Contributors

Joan Arnold, PhD, RN
Associate Professor of Nursing,
School of Nursing,
College of New Rochelle,
New Rochelle, New York

Kristen Lawton Barry, PhD
Associate Research Scientist,
Department of Psychiatry,
University of Michigan;
Associate Director,
Serious Mental Illness Treatment Research
    and Evaluation Center,
Veterans Administration,
Ann Arbor, Michigan

Laurel Janssen Breen, RN, MA
Private Consultant,
Sea Cliff, New York

Karen J. Calfas, PhD
Director,
Department of Health Promotion,
Student Health Services,
San Diego State University;
Assistant Clinical Professor,
Department of Family and Preventive
    Medicine,
School of Medicine,
University of California-San Diego,
San Diego, California

Wendy Dahar, MPH
Health Outcomes Coordinator,
Division of Clinical Innovation and
    Preventive Services,
Kaiser Permanente,
Cleveland, Ohio

**Penelope R. Buschman Gemma, MS,
RN, CS, FAAN**
Assistant Professor of Clinical Nursing,
School of Nursing,
Columbia University,
New York, New York

Andrea C. Gielen, ScD
Associate Professor of Social and
    Behavioral Sciences,
Department of Health Policy and
    Management;
Deputy Director,
Center for Injury Research and Policy,
School of Hygiene and Public Health,
The Johns Hopkins University,
Baltimore, Maryland

Suzanne Kozich Giorgio, RDH
Clinical Faculty
Department of Dental Medicine,
Medical College Division,
Allegheny University of the Health
    Sciences,
Philadelphia, Pennsylvania

Joan I. Gluch, PhD, RDH
Director of Health Promotion,
Assistant Professor of Dental Care Systems,
School of Dental Medicine;
Senior Fellow,
Leonard Davis Institute,
University of Pennsylvania,
Philadelphia, Pennsylvania

Edith S. Lisansky Gomberg, PhD

Professor of Psychology,
Department of Psychiatry;
Adjunct Professor,
School of Social Work,
University of Michigan,
Ann Arbor, Michigan

Sherri Sheinfeld Gorin, PhD

Senior Fellow in Cancer Epidemiology,
School of Public Health and the Herbert I.
    Irving Comprehensive Cancer Center,
Columbia University,
New York, New York;
Associate Professor of Health Policy
    (Adjunct),
State University of New York at Stony
    Brook,
Stony Brook, New York;
Senior Partner,
Management Horizons,
Setauket, New York

Jacqueline Rose Hott, RN, CS, PhD, FAAN

Dean and Professor Emerita,
School of Nursing,
Adelphi University,
Garden City, New York;
Private Practice,
Great Neck, New York

Lorraine E. Matthews, MS, RD

Public Health Nutritionist,
Manager, Education, Nutrition, and
    Training,
Philadelphia Department of Public Health;
Adjunct Professor, Graduate Program in
    Nutrition Education,
Immaculta College;
Adjunct Professor, Department of
    Bioscience and Biotechnology,
Drexel University,
Philadelphia, Pennsylvania

Duncan Neuhauser, PhD

The Charles Eton Blanchard, MD Professor
    of Health Management,
Department of Epidemiology and
    Biostatistics,
School of Medicine,
Case Western Reserve University,
Cleveland, Ohio

Diane J. Powell, RN, MA, MBA

Principal,
Powell Associates Health Care Marketing,
Roslyn Heights, New York;
Adjunct Faculty,
School of Nursing,
Adelphi University,
Garden City, New York

David A. Sleet, PhD

Associate Director for Science,
Division of Unintentional Injury,
National Center for Injury Prevention and
    Control,
Centers for Disease Control and
    Prevention;
Professor of Behavioral Science and Health
    Education (Adjunct),
Rollins School of Public Health,
Emory University,
Atlanta, Georgia

Barbara J. Steinberg, DDS

Assistant Director of Dental Medicine and
    Surgery,
Allegheny University Hospitals MCP;
Professor of Surgery and Medicine,
Allegheny University of the Health
    Sciences;
Clinical Associate Professor of Oral
    Medicine,
School of Dental Medicine,
University of Pennsylvania,
Philadelphia, Pennsylvania

רפאנו ה' ונרפא

Heal us, O Lord, and we shall be healed.
(Daily Prayer, from Jeremiah 17:14)

מים רבים לא יוכלו לכבות את האהבה

Vast floods cannot quench love, no river can sweep it away.
(Song of Songs 8:7)

Health to my beloved family.
Sherri Sheinfeld Gorin

• • •

"But let there be no scales to weigh your unknown treasure;
And seek not the depths of your knowledge with staff or sounding line.
For self is a sea boundless and measureless."
(On Self-Knowledge from *The Prophet* by Kahlil Gibran)

For Rick, Michael, and Matthew, knowing of your love and support.
Joan Arnold

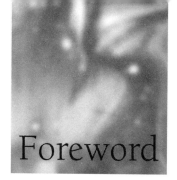

Foreword

The *Health Promotion Handbook* by Dr. Sherri Sheinfeld Gorin and Dr. Joan Arnold is a text that breaks new ground in several important areas, making it an especially admirable and valuable piece of work. First, it makes the reader think—not just incorporate useful information (with which this text happens to be filled), but really think, ponder, and reflect. The reader of this text will be challenged to be concerned not only with the body of knowledge, skills, and attitudes he or she is in the process of learning either as a first-time student or as a health care professional but also with renewing, sharpening, and expanding both understanding and clinical ability.

This text also makes the reader think about him*self* or her*self* and about his or her *own* attitudes toward health and health practices for *both* self and others in the context of doing clinical work that is health-oriented. Certainly in the practice of that function we call "health promotion," no one can be perfect—with only two general exceptions—in, for example, his/her own eating patterns, his/her own approach to exercise, and the way he/she manages stressors. The two exceptions to the nonperfectionism rule are, of course, not using tobacco products at all and not ever *ab*using any of the other recreational mood-altering drugs, such as alcohol.

Indeed, with few exceptions such as the two just mentioned, perfection in virtually anything is almost impossible to achieve. Therefore perfectio*nism* must by definition be destructive, for it must by definition lead to frustration, anger, feelings of guilt, and quitting the health practice for which one is trying to achieve perfection.

However, for the health care professional engaging in the work of health promotion, it is helpful to lead a *reasonably* healthy life oneself to enable one to show the flag, be personally knowledgeable about the content of the process, and be personally knowledgeable about the challenges one must meet on the road to becoming and being healthy. The personal, effective involvement of the health care professional in healthy living himself or herself is a recurring theme of this text (see especially Chapters 4 and 5). It is indeed a vital message that is given little emphasis elsewhere.

Second, in its ground-breaking endeavours, the approach to and program for clinical health promotion put forward in this text rests upon a theoretical base. That is unusual these days. So much of the work presently done in medicine, health promotion, and disease prevention lacks such a base, or at least lacks a conscious one. That is one reason why so many initiatives in these related fields ultimately fail over time. It is thus so good to see a work such as this one in which the several parts are tied together by common theory.

The theoretical base has several important components. First are the group of images set forth in Chapter 1: health as antithesis of disease, balance, growth, functionality, goodness of fit, wholeness, sense of well-being, transcendence of the potential for health, and empowerment. Second is the concept of collaboration between health care professional and patient/client as central to the effective practice of health promotion, whether in the clinical or the community setting. Third is the idea that for many health promotion practices there is a common approach to implementation that can be used across the board, an approach that always emerges within a dynamic political and economic context.

Fourth, among the ground-breaking elements of this text is the Health Promotion Matrix itself (see Chapter 5). It provides a standardized approach to health promotion interventions for individuals, groups, families, and communities, from small to large. The Health Promotion Matrix has several essential elements. It establishes what health and healthy behaviors are. It also integrates psychologic and social theory into the recommended behavioral change process toward health. Within the overall framework, the Health Promotion Matrix stresses the individualization of the approach to each patient/client.

It views the health care professional as a facilitator, not the director, of the behavior change process. It applies the classic planning model to the health promotion process, including the often-neglected step of needs assessment (termed by the authors: *image appraisal*). It offers literal "scripts" for the clinician-patient/client interaction that, with the obvious detail modifications for each specific intervention whether it be smoking cessation or weight management, provide guidelines for an effective interaction.

The *Health Promotion Handbook* is a thoughtful, useful, challenging approach to the subject that hopefully will help many students and professionals become and be highly effective promoters of health promotion.

Steven Jonas, MD, MPH, MS
Professor
Department of Preventive Medicine
School of Medicine, State University
of New York at Stony Brook

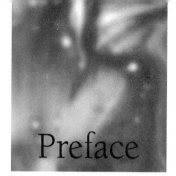

Preface

The *Health Promotion Handbook* is written to address the health promotion needs of individuals, families, groups, and communities. As a practice-driven handbook, this is designed to translate theories of health promotion into a step-by-step clinical approach for engaging with clients toward internalizing an idealized image of health, using the Health Promotion Matrix (HPM). The intended audience for this text includes practicing health care professionals and students in a variety of health-related fields, including nursing, public health, allied health, medicine, and social work.

ORGANIZATION
Part One

The five chapters in Part One, "Health, Health Promotion, and the Health Care Professional," describe the theoretical framework on which the text rests. Chapter 1, "Images of Health," begins with the various constructions of health characterized as themes, such as health as a balanced state, health as goodness of fit, health as transcendence, and health as power. These myriad images of health suggest how it is viewed by different clients and may explain some of the dynamics of change.

"Models of Health Promotion," Chapter 2, explores contemporary theoretical approaches to health promotion. It integrates the images of health with models of health promotion, from the macro-level, such as the social ecology model, to the micro-level, such as the health belief model. It highlights the moral underpinnings for these varied models of health promotion, as well as the cross-cutting constructs of empowerment and community. Approaches to the evaluation of health promotion programs founded on these contemporary models, and their consequent measures of change, are also discussed.

Within Chapter 3, "Contexts for Health Promotion," the myriad political and economic forces influencing health promotion are detailed. These factors range from the legislative (e.g., the National Consumer Health Information and Health Promotion Act of 1975, which has been amended by a number of subsequent acts) to the economic, from the perspective of major governmental programs and insurers.

"Agents for Health Promotion," Chapter 4, describes the processes health care professionals engage in with clients to promote health. Underlying these processes are the assumed values of collaboration, empowerment, and mutual participation.

Chapter 5, "The Health Promotion Matrix," is central to the unique thrust of this text as practice-oriented, yet grounded in both theory and the policy context. It describes the Health Promotion Matrix, a dynamic confluence of five dimensions, four client systems, and nine healthy behaviors that guide the health care professional's work with the client.

The HPM embodies five dimensions of the intervention process—image creation, image appraisal, minimize health depleting patterns, optimize health supportive patterns, and internalize idealized image—within the context of individual, family, group, and community client systems. The HPM defines nine healthy behaviors that together promote health. An abbreviated script reflecting the HPM acquaints the health care professional with the use of the dimensions. A more comprehensive script is found in the Appendix. Scripts specific to each healthy behavior are found in Part Two.

Part Two

Part Two of the text, "Practice Frameworks for Health Promotion," is organized around clinical approaches specific to the nine healthy behaviors: smoking cessation, eating well, physical activity, sexual awareness, injury prevention, substance safety, oral health, self-development, and productivity. An introduction to each chapter relates the healthy behavior to the Health Promotion Matrix. An up-to-date perspective on the healthy behavior follows, with case material integrated into the discussion. Finally, each chapter concludes with a practice-ready script for engaging clients in a dialogue about health promotion.

Chapter 6 explores smoking cessation, perhaps the key issue in health promotion. It begins by outlining the tobacco industry's influence on smoking and follows with descriptions of the major population subgroups who smoke, the causes of smoking, and the key interventions for smoking cessation. The chapter provides examples of techniques to help different target population groups quit smoking. A script contains the skills needed by the health care professional to serve as a counselor to different clients in tobacco control.

Chapter 7, "Eating Well," begins with a description of the role food plays in daily life. Unlike other behaviors, such as smoking, clients cannot simply stop eating. In changing eating behaviors, the health care professional must recognize that clients ingest food, not nutrients. Throughout the chapter, food is described as a promoter and sustainer of health—an image realized with the help of the health care professional's use of nutritional appraisals, reorientation of client choice in food selection, and the evaluation of programs designed to encourage healthy eating. The assessment of nutritional change strategies for an overweight woman who has high cholesterol is depicted. A script assists health care professionals to work alongside clients to imagine a healthy use of food and to alter their eating patterns.

Chapter 8 explores physical activity as a major contributor to risk reduction for multiple diseases, such as non–insulin-dependent diabetes mellitus, and as central to weight control and the maintenance of bone mass. Using transtheoretical theory, techniques for assisting sedentary clients are described, as well as mechanisms for engaging moderately or highly active clients. The Physician-based Assessment and Counseling for Exercise (PACE) program, an empirically tested program for systematic exercise development, is explored in depth. A script details a client-health care professional dialogue using the HPM that assists in creating positive, constructive images of fitness, as well as a realistic daily activity routine.

Chapter 9 looks at sexuality as a healthy dimension of being human. From a developmental perspective on human desire, the chapter examines the physiologic and psychosocial aspects of sexual coupling. Throughout, the chapter emphasizes the importance of health care professionals becoming comfortable with exploring the client's sexual history and status. The case found in this chapter lists ordered queries about sexual attitudes, beliefs, and behaviors that are suitable for use in an interchange between health care professionals and gay, lesbian, and bisexual teens.

Chapter 10 investigates injury prevention, whether to an individual in a motor vehicle, on a bicycle, in a pedestrian situation, in the home, at work, or during leisure activity. It begins with a description of the strategies for health promotion—education and behavior change, engineering and technology, and legislation and law enforcement—that target host, environment, and agent factors. Changing multiple settings, such as schools, worksites, communities, and health care sites is encouraged. The case in the chapter fosters injury prevention for children through the use of car seats. A script assists the health care professional in assessing the likelihood of unintentional injury from various threats, such as falls, fires, carbon monoxide and smoke, poisons and medications, home appliances, tools and equipment, and swimming pools. The chapter concludes with an HPM-based strategy to help clients acquire a safety consciousness and to implement a defense protocol.

Chapter 11 details the benefits of substance safety. It classifies several types of drugs, including prescribed, over-the-counter, and banned "street" drugs, such as marijuana, cocaine, and heroin; alternative medicines, such as herbs and vitamins; and "social drugs," such as nicotine, caffeine, and alcohol. Alcohol, the most widely used of the risky substances, is the focus of the remainder of the chapter. Differing rates and impacts of immoderate drinking by gender, age, and ethnic/racial groups may influence the strategies health care professionals adopt. Both the case and the script in the chapter encourage health care professionals to screen each client for at-risk alcohol use and to use direct feedback, goal-setting, and social reinforcement to change behavior.

In Chapter 12, oral health promotion is examined. The effects of common oral diseases and health conditions that place clients at risk for periodontal diseases, dental decay, and oral cancer are reviewed. The implications of community fluoridation efforts are detailed. For the individual client, proper toothbrushing and flossing techniques, as well as the use of sealants, are examined as preventive techniques. The interrelationship of oral health to general health promotion is emphasized throughout the chapter. An oral health promotion case involving a pregnant woman is followed by a more general script, using the HPM.

As Chapter 13, "Self-Development," unfolds, identity, self-esteem, and self-expression are discussed as the most persistent patterns that characterize individuals in relation to one another over time. Development is viewed from a lifespan perspective, with an orientation toward fostering healthy attitudes and behaviors about growth and the aging process. The importance of affiliative connections and social supports throughout development is explored. Enriching self-acceptance and cultural sensitivity is addressed. The importance of spirituality is detailed. A framework for fostering personal growth through an acceptance of life losses is found in a script at the conclusion of the chapter.

"Productivity," Chapter 14, focuses on the importance of worklife as a seminal force in health promotion. Human beings are goal-directed and derive satisfaction from the exchange of effort for the reward of money. Further, as explored in the chapter on self-development, work affects an individual's self-identity—while the work becomes the person, the person also tends to become what he/she does. The chapter begins with a discussion of the definitions of productivity within two models and the manifestations of the *gray zone,* which is a term that describes a state between maximal productivity and illness. An assessment package designed to examine health for its relationship to productivity is described. A case for a worker in the gray zone is presented, and an HPM-founded script designed to enrich the goodness of fit between worker and job is detailed.

Part Three

Part Three, "Political and Economic Considerations in Health Promotion," explores the factors shaping the present and the future of the field. Chapter 15, "Economic Considerations in Health Promotion," recognizes the pivotal role economics plays in directing health promotion practice at present. Classic tools of analyzing the financial advantages of health promotion practices are offered. A detailed example of a systematic cost and benefit analysis for a managed care organization ends the chapter.

The final chapter of the text, "Future Directions for Health Promotion," points to the larger influences on health promotion practice of the future, such as a growing aged population, the increased role of managed care, and the need for an ethical dialogue. Using the HPM as a conceptual framework, health care professionals, participating alongside the client system, can shape the future of health care.

ACKNOWLEDGMENTS

It is with deep appreciation that we thank the following individuals for their contributions to this text:

C. Darlene Como, for her encouragement and support of the proposal.

Brian Dennison, for his meticulous and insightful organizational suggestions.

Sarah Fike, for her impeccable and attentive copy editing.

Stephen L. Sheinfeld, J.D., for his knowledgeable guidance on the complexities of legal research and for his wise counsel.

Lois Stein, for her steadfast assistance in gathering library resources.

Charlotte Moslander and Shannon Weidemann, librarians, College of New Rochelle, for their helpful library research.

The outstanding contributors, each of whom greatly shaped this text and to whom we are indebted.

Finally, although this book is dedicated to our families, we wish to again acknowledge the special contributions our spouses, Brian Gorin and Rick Arnold, and children, Aaron and Evan Gorin and Michael and Matthew Arnold, as well as our parents, Al and Trudy Sheinfeld and Marjorie and Robert Hagan, made to our completion of this work.

Sherri Sheinfeld Gorin & Joan Arnold

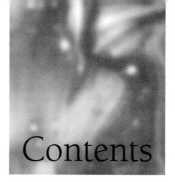

Contents

PART *three*
POLITICAL *and* ECONOMIC CONSIDERATIONS *in* HEALTH PROMOTION

HEALTH, HEALTH PROMOTION, and the HEALTH CARE PROFESSIONAL

CHAPTER

1

Images of Health

Joan Arnold and Laurel Janssen Breen

What do you imagine when you think about health—your health? What level of health do you think you possess now? What level of health would you like to achieve? How is health uniquely defined? These critical questions beckon examination by the health care professional and the client. Searching for their clarification provides a person the opportunity for self-discovery about one's personal image of health. Once conceptualized, this image of health provides a person direction for health promotion actions.

Health may be a baffling subject, yet it is a desired aspiration for all. Contemporary thinking about health emphasizes empowering community groups and individuals to realize their own health aims. Despite widespread interest directed toward defining health at a theoretical level, few frameworks are applicable to clinical practice. The Health Promotion Matrix (detailed in Chapter 5), however, embodies a theoretically grounded approach to health promotion that is designed to respond to practice realities. The Matrix is based on the idea that health is a resource for everyday living (World Health Organization, 1986; in press) and is defined by the individual, family, group, and community specific to its own image. Perhaps then, health is achievable as a person defines it within the parameters of his/her own being, family, and community. The various frameworks from which clients and health care providers develop their images of health are derived from an array of health models. The images of health, as described in this chapter, are organized into nine categories, each reflecting a unique view. These categories portray health as the antithesis of disease; a balanced state; a growth phenomenon; a functional capacity; goodness of fit; wholeness; well-being; transcendence; and finally, empowerment. A careful examination of the concept of health and its evolution will reveal the complexities of the image of health.

IMAGINING HEALTH

Health has been viewed from a multitude of perspectives. Health may be a reference for disease, defined by determining forces, or a panacea. Although an elusive term, health may be projected by the human system as autonomy and integrity. Health may be the uniquely characteristic strengths of a person, family, and community. It could also be a

3

capacity for sustaining itself through growth, development, and self-care. Curiously, health care professionals, regardless of discipline, know more about disease, pathology, and dysfunction than about health. Although valued and desired as a goal, the diagnostic precision found in conditions of illness, disease, and social problems is not evident in the study of health. Our clients look to us as providers of health care to assist them in their desire to be healthy. As clients strive to shape a personal picture of health, the health care professional witnesses the coalescing of different images of health into the client's own unique composite. This unique image may differ from the health care professional's image of health and expectations for the client's health. The health care professional must be able to recognize differences in views and enfold them into the therapeutic process and must discover a shared approach to working toward the client's goals. The health care professional also must accept the inherent challenge of accepting the client's right to self-determination and must commit to assist the client in achieving these health aims.

The images of health presented in this chapter reflect a clustering of a multitude of views on health. Inherently, there will be a merging of views across the images. This cluster of images is offered to stimulate a revisioning of health. Health cannot remain an enigma; it stands on its own as a life process, to be imagined and realized within the unique capacity of every person, family, group, and community.

Health as the Antithesis of Disease

In the image of health as the antithesis of disease, health and disease are viewed as opposite states, with health as the absence of disease. Dubos (1965, p. xvii) referred to "the states of health and disease (as) the expressions of the success or failure experienced by the organism in its efforts to respond adaptively to environmental changes." The conditions of health and disease are expressions of bipolar thinking. In this context, health is measured by morbidity and mortality statistics within a given population. These indexes of illness and death are used to appraise health and to direct interventions in specific aggregates. Persons suffering from disease were, and still are, ostracized from society. Social standards of health can lead to negative perceptions toward persons with diseases that are in contradiction to desirable social expectations of health. Consider the treatment of persons with leprosy, disabling conditions, acquired immunodeficiency syndrome (AIDS), and drug addiction; they are often feared and viewed as not socially acceptable. Their condition or illness is contradictory to what is defined as health by society, and their presence threatens perceived social order.

With health defined as the absence of disease, evaluative statements are made within the parameters of illness, using a system of signs and symptoms for disease. "This definition of health has been largely the result of the domination of the biomedical sciences by a mechanistic conception of man. Man is viewed by physicians primarily as a physico-chemical system" (Smith, 1983, p. 46-47). Health care professionals are trained to make evaluative statements of illness by formulating a diagnostic statement from symptomatology and objective data. An evaluation statement of this nature requires comparison to established norms. Illness becomes a deviation from the norm. Health then is a condition of the norm, whereas illness falls outside the range of normal. Rather than defining the components of health, the medical model, relying on illness identification, merely identifies health as the absence of disease. Thus parameters for being healthy are not identified, except for what falls within the range of normal. However, what falls within the norm may be suboptimal, and by establishing these narrow ranges of normal, mediocrity becomes an acceptable definition of health, and because of this, optimal conditions of normal may never be realized.

Health as a Balanced State

The image of health as a balanced state incorporates epidemiology, which provides an important framework for the clarification of the term health. *Epidemiology* is the study of patterns of health; the patterns of disease, disability, death; and other problems in populations of persons (Leavell & Clark, 1965). In a broad definition that has been widely accepted epidemiology is called "the study of the distribution and determinants of health-related states or events in specified populations and the application of this study to control of health problems" (Last, 1995, pp. 55-56). A major goal of epidemiology is to identify aggregates, or subpopulations, in the community at high risk for disease. The intent is to identify risk factors that put the aggregate at high risk and then to modify or reduce those risks. Once identified, preventive efforts are directed at the aggregate in the hope that these interventions will benefit the population. Efforts such as screening, case finding, and health education are geared toward populations who are most likely to gain from specific interventions developed for a particular disease (Gordis, 1996).

In the epidemiologic framework, health is identified along a continuum of health-illness-death. The origins of health and illness are indicative of other processes before the human being is affected. Key to these processes are the interactions of conditions in the environment, factors of the agent for disease, and predisposing genetic forces. "Heredity, social and economic factors, or physical environment may be creating a disease stimulus long before man and stimulus begin to interact to produce disease" (Leavell & Clark, 1965, p. 17). The preliminary interaction of the human host, potential disease agent, and environmental factors in disease production is referred to as the period of *prepathogenesis* (i.e., the period before disease). Prepathogenesis is the period of health. The balance between the host, potential agent, and environment is reflective of the equilibrium inherent in the condition of health. It is not until the disease-provoking stimuli produce changes in the human system that the period of *pathogenesis,* or disease, results. The prepathogenesis period can be thought of as the process in the environment, whereas the period of pathogenesis is the process in the human being, or human system.

Disease is a state of disequilibrium, or "dis-ease," and health is a state of balance, or equilibrium. Equilibrium is achieved through the interaction of the multiple factors and forces that influence and contribute to health. The balance of health is reflected in the nature and intensity of these interactions. Physical, physiologic, psychologic, social, cultural, spiritual, political, and economic forces interact and contribute to the unique picture of health for each individual, family, and community, as well as the image of health for populations of persons, families, groups, and communities. Health is both a singular condition and a condition of society, as well as a balance of these forces.

The earlier World Health Organization (WHO) (1947) definition of health stated: "Health is a state of complete physical, mental, and social well-being, and not merely the absence of disease and infirmity." Freedom from disease and illness implies a balance among three significant sources of well-being—physical well-being, mental well-being, and social well-being. Dunn (1961) uses the WHO definition to expand on the idea of complete well-being, in which well-being implies being well not only in the body and mind but also within the family and community and having a compatible work interest. Dunn was able to move beyond the interrelatedness of wellness of the body, mind, and environment to define high-level wellness. "High-level wellness for the individual is defined as an integrated method of functioning which is oriented toward maximizing the potential of which the individual is capable. It requires that the individual maintain a continuum of balance and purposeful direction within the environment where he is functioning" (Dunn, 1961, pp. 4-5). In effect, health is viewed as balance along a goal-directed continuum within the context of the environment. The dynamic nature of health is implied as health potential is maximized. In other words, rather than health being a complete static state, health means maintaining completeness on an ongoing basis. Balance and dynamism are combined, as balance is maintained while a person, family, group, or community moves purposefully toward a goal.

Cultural ideologies and tradition also influence the image of health as balance. The image of balance is a central tenet of Oriental medicine (U.S. Office of Alternative Medicine, National Institutes of Health, 1994). For example, balance is found through harmony of yin and yang. The forces of yin and yang are described as active/passive; masculine/feminine; stimulating/nurturing; and heavenly/earthly. Energy balance is possible through the interrelatedness of these seemingly opposite forces working together. Imbalances of yin and yang are believed to be manifested within the function of internal organs and can result in disturbances of vital energy represented on the body's acupuncture meridians.

Ayurveda, an ancient medical system that originated in India, defines the trinity of life as body, mind, and spiritual awareness (Fugh-Berman, 1996). To a practitioner of Ayurveda, imbalances in doshas—physiologic principles, or bodily humors—can cause specific diseases. Various foods and emotions are believed to cause imbalances.

Health care professionals can enhance congruity with their clients by blending an awareness of balance in culture and belief systems.

Health as Growth

The foundation of health as growth builds on the beliefs of noted developmental theorists (e.g., Dewey, 1963; Piaget, 1963; Elkind, 1981; Erikson, 1963; Duvall, 1985; Havighurst, 1972). This category of health is viewed as the successful fulfillment of certain tasks appropriate to particular life stages. Persons are seen as having a capacity for growth that can be enhanced and supported; this development is seen as an ongoing process that occurs continuously and systematically throughout the lifespan. Growth is viewed as progressive. "All people are growing and can grow, given the appropriate combination of support and challenge in the environment. Active involvement, ongoing investment in the person, characterizes the developmental perspective" (Hatfield & Hatfield, 1992, p. 164). Health is seen as being intimately determined by individual life-style and behavior choices. Interventions at critical life stages are believed to be the most effective and foster optimal growth. Through identification of certain "transition points," the unique needs, behaviors, and motivations of certain populations are targeted. "These transition points are circumstances or points in the life course when there are likely to be changes in behavior and when changes in behavior may have a higher probability of being induced" (Borgatta, Bulcroft, Montgomery, & Bulcroft, 1990, p. 385).

The concept that overall wellness in each particular life stage involves the achievement of certain cognitive, physiologic, and psychologic competencies is integral to a lifespan approach to health as growth. Established norms are used to measure growth at each stage. An established pattern of expected progression through the stages is viewed as both desirable and is anticipated. The movement from one stage of growth to another is predicated on some of the life skills and tasks accomplished in an earlier stage. The "failure" to achieve certain developmental skills during a particular stage may be viewed as retarding growth into the next stage.

Within this framework, there are risks of a fragmented approach to overall wellness if the attainment of certain competencies are seen as separate entities (Omizo, Omizo, & D'Andrea, 1992). Universally applied frames of reference may be seen as narrowing, or limiting, the health potential of certain individuals, families, groups, or communities. By emphasizing a prescribed framework for development, the unique trajectories found in human growth may not be appreciated. The forces that culture, age, and gender play when ignored or undeveloped in the establishment of these norms may result in a biased definition.

How the concept of aging is visualized within the framework of a life-span definition of health demands attention. In its narrow definition, old age is delineated as the final, end stage of life, a time of anticipated decline when dependency and helplessness are expected outcomes. It is viewed as a time of final goal attainment, thus abandoning a need for establishing health challenges for this population. From a broad viewpoint, aging is recognized as being a "complex cultural issue" that cannot be defined from biologic parameters alone. "The perception of aging for a given culture reflects what is individually and collectively needed, believed and valued within it at a given point in time" (Restrepo & Rozental, 1994, p. 1326). While there may be altered physical abilities and changing expectations, aging persons retain the capacity for full participation in life. Aging is an imprecise term that can be understood as both a loss and a goal, depending on the perspective. The process of aging is the process of life.

Health as Functionality

In the category of health as functionality, health is seen as the capacity to fulfill critical life functions. Functional health patterns for individuals include all activities that influence the person's relationship with the environment. Physiologic functions include digestion, hydration, sleep, elimination, and circulation. Psychologic functioning encompasses behavior, communication, and emotional development. Fulfillment of these functions define a healthy individual. Likewise, families have functions to fulfill, including the capacity to nurture their members through physical, emotional, educational, and social supportive activities. Further, communities function to provide their membership with resources to sustain themselves. A community is vital when members can meet their needs and in turn participate in the community's further development.

Functionality is viewed as the ability to carry out a given task. When a person's, family's, group's, or community's functioning capacity is limited, health is altered, and adaptation is necessary to adjust to the environment and to fulfill functions. "However, adaptive behavior has a wider scope. It may involve not only a modification of the individual organism but also a more or less extensive transformation of its environment" (Smith, 1983, p. 69). From this perspective, disability is viewed as a "different" ability that requires an altered environment so that a person can achieve vital life functions (i.e., the environment is made accessible and available to those with "different" abilities). Persons with disabling conditions become equally able.

Rehabilitation, a form of preventive intervention, focuses on recovering remaining capacity to maintain function. The strengths and capacities of the individual are realized differently to restore function, even if that function is modified. Recovering the capability to function as independently as possible enables the person, family, group, or community to depend less on other forms of support. Returning function, even if modified, enables social utility and a sense of purpose.

Health as Goodness of Fit

The image of health as goodness of fit rests on the meshing of the determining factors of health. Human biology, environment, health care, and life-style have been identified as the four major determinants of health (Lalonde, 1974). Despite the relative importance of each of these determinants, special attention has been directed at the significance of individual life-style in influencing personal health. This focus on life-style was inevitable as demographics have shifted, revealing an extended lifespan; as morbidity and mortality data have reflected a growing recognition of the replacement of communicable disease with chronic disease; and as the health care system has become increasingly focused on costs.

Life-style is about choosing. Individuals, families, groups, and communities choose options that set into motion the unique interaction of factors and forces that have the potential to produce health or illness. Much progress in the overall major decline in death rates for the three leading causes of death among Americans—heart disease, stroke, and unintentional injuries—has been traced to reduction in risk factors (i.e., life-style modifications) (U.S. Department of Health & Human Services, 1991). Despite these advances, resulting from preventive interventions, the United States continues to be burdened by preventable disease, injury, and disability. Focusing on life-style alone, however, rather than viewing health as an outcome of a multiplicity of determinants, can easily result in "blaming the victim."

One must remember, however, that life-style is only one of four factors that determine health. Life-style is about choosing, to whatever extent possible. However, certain biologic factors, although modifiable, are largely uncontrollable. In addition, environmental determinants of health are often negotiated at the public policy level, leaving individuals, families, groups, and communities without a sense of personal control. Other environmental factors such as poverty, racism, and resource allocation challenge the client's potential for health and limit choice. Also, the availability, accessibility, affordability, appropriateness, adequacy, and acceptability of health care (National Institute of Nursing Research, National Institutes of Health, 1995) enable or diminish health potential. No one factor alone determines a client's health, which is shaped by the interlocking of these forces. Yet, there is opportunity for change to occur at the point these factors interface.

Health as Wholeness

The holistic nature of health is central to healing and complementary health care delivery. Appreciating wholeness is enhanced by a framework that supports multiple interactions (Bertalanffy, 1968; Laszlo, 1972). The idea that every aspect of a human being, family, or community is linked and interacting is derived from a systems theory orientation. The human being is constructed of subsystems that work together, as well as a subsystem of the family and community, which also are interacting parts of each other.

Each system is a subsystem while simultaneously a suprasystem. Boundaries define each system and allow, through their regulation, the flow of input and output that maintain energy and enable growth. In this framework, health can be viewed as the integrity and unity of system function. Supporting the integrity of the human system is the focus for promoting and maintaining health.

Human beings are considered whole (i.e., more than and different from the sum of their parts). "The whole has a unity, organization, and individuality that is not not discoverable by means of the analysis of its parts. In fact, the analysis of the parts of the organism results in decreased perceptions of the qualities of the whole" (Blandino, 1969, in Smith, 1983, p. 77). Based on the framework of Maslow (1968), Smith (1983) considers health to be the complete development of the individual's potential. Smith's image of health, the eudaimonistic model, focuses on the entirety of the organism, including the physical, social, aesthetic, and moral—not just the behavioral and physiologic—aspects. In the eudaimonistic sense, health is wholeness. To be healthy is a goal toward which the human system strives.

Health as Sense of Well-Being

Much of what people describe as "feeling healthy" is a subjective sense of "well-being"—a subjective interpretation of personal indicators that produce a vague sense of everything being all right. While the actual structure of general well-being is not clearly understood, it is thought to include the following contributors: emotions, beliefs, temperaments, behaviors, situations, experiences, and health (Wheeler, 1991). Well-being is an imprecise term and is personally understood. It may include estimations of a level of happiness or the presence or absence of a mood related to a specific occasion. There is some consensus that "well-being," while mainly an elusive term, is constructed of three components (Seedhouse, 1995). They are life satisfaction, which is thought to be a cognitive function; positive affect; and negative affect, which as well as positive affect is experiential.

It is known that individuals experience the sense of "well-being" in very different ways. The pursuit of "well-being" includes no formal definition, no clear-cut guidelines. However, the individual does know and understand some means for attaining this state. Perhaps it is not necessary or even possible to have a precise and objective definition of certain human experiences.

For many persons, humor is an important aspect in achieving well-being. In attempting to comprehend and live through the myriad of life experiences, a person can shift his/her perception of reality through humor and its outward expressions. Humor is understood as a powerful tool, affecting both neurologic and physiologic transmissions in the body. It can reduce tension and frustration and startle a person out of complacency. "A life that has no humor or play is one in which insecurity, fear, defensiveness, rigidity and fanaticism have an advantage. These are all aspects of a local, limited sense of self, a personal ego that defines itself only in terms of limited space and time" (interview with Larry Dossey, in Lawlis, 1996, p. 190-191). Laughter and humor are powerful emotional expressions that add vitality and "joy" to the experience of health and life.

Health as Transcendence

Viewing health as transcendence is to see the human potential for growth and development as limitless. Any boundaries of mind and body are believed to be self-imposed. According to this framework human beings are constantly evolving, and new tools and modalities of treatment are evolving, also. Health is this process of self-discovery. Understanding on a cognitive level is not necessary for an intervention to be therapeutic. Some aspects of healing are experienced and understood by the client and health care professional at different levels of awareness. Persons are presented with a multitude of choices during their lifetimes. Moving outside of one's comfort zone and stretching the edges of one's self can promote insecurity. Therefore redefining health involves loosening boundaries and transformation. Support in this process is desirable and augmenting.

Health is seen as being interrelated with the larger universe, integrating emotional and spiritual factors. The "self" is experienced and explored based on a definition that transcends far beyond the ordinary definition to a "manifestation or expression of this much greater 'something' that is our deeper origin and destination" (Lawlis, 1996, p. 5). The process of "body-mind-spirit" is understood as a unified whole that has great potential for experiencing, altering, and expressing health.

The perceived meaning that one attaches to an experience or an event is recognized as having an integral connection to one's overall health experience. These perceived meanings affect both the choices and impact of health interventions. Spirituality generally can be defined as "one's inward sense of something greater than the individual self or the meaning one perceives that transcends the immediate circumstances" (U.S. Office of Alternative Medicine, National Institutes of Health, 1994, p. 8). This "spiritual" nature of health is experienced as fully as any of the "physical" components.

Health as Empowerment

A strong link between individuals' or communities' sense of power and the level of health they experience has been identified (Robertson & Minkler, 1994). This power has been closely associated with the perceived degree of life "control and mastery." Powerlessness has been identified as a broad-based risk factor for the development of disease. The empowerment process, as a health promotion intervention strategy, has been correlated with improving the health of populations (Wallerstein, 1992). Health professionals must respect and acknowledge the significance of their clients' right to "name their own experience" as an integral part of the empowerment process. Without this, there is the risk of subjectively overwhelming or affecting the lives of others by setting up a health agenda "for" clients that they "must" follow (Labonte, 1994).

Movement toward health evolves from a fully engaged sense of self. Definition and direction for health comes from this strength. In partnership with the health care professional and others in the community, change occurs as individuals and communities work toward the implementation of this personal vision of health.

Empowerment, in its fullest meaning, is context bound. It extends to include an awareness of all the forces that individuals, families, groups, and communities face as they attempt to transform their reality (Airhihenbuwa, 1994). Culture is one of these forces. Pender (1996) reminds us that cultural models need to be fully explored as future health conceptions are developed. This "communal life view" is seen as a functional component of the attainment of health. Health experiences and choices originate from within a cultural perspective. Cultural values, attitudes, and behaviors are seen as an integral part of a personal definition of health and disease. The empowerment process can be expanded through actions that focus on improving the health of communities. Targeting only individual change dilutes the process. "Hence the empowerment process is maximized when community residents at large become mobilized around health concerns and initiate collective actions for well-being of the entire community" (Braithwaite, Bianchi, & Taylor, 1994, p. 414). Because of the interrelatedness of all people, health is a universal experience. "Individual health is an illusion" (Dossey, 1982, p. 148).

Gender also influences the relationship of power and health. Differences in gender identity influence health behavior choices.

> "Women are the gatekeepers of their own health and the health of the family. Healthy families strengthen society. Self-care health-related behaviors conducted by the woman for herself, and her family through her care and teaching of family members, creates a potential for health that is powerful and possible" (Foster, 1994, pp. 79-80).

Feminist contributions toward changing the medical model of health have expanded the definition of health. Feminist health agendas include issues such as self-determination, the legitimization of personal experience, and the value of social support. The roles that freedom of choice and individual wellness have played in women's health have been incorporated into a restructured model of health and wellness for all individuals (Travis, Gressley, & Crumpler, 1991). Women's refusal to accept some of the physical and mental "diagnoses" of illness imposed on them has led to a reclaiming of power for themselves and their communities.

Empowered health is based on the belief that individuals possess numerous and diverse self-care abilities. Persons require certain skills of self-care to feel in control and to direct their own life course, and community change depends on the ability of its individuals' to self-direct. Self-care involves competency, which is achieved by professionals transferring necessary skills and knowledge to individuals and communities. Much of the provision of "health" can now be seen as within the grasp of the consumer. The actual ability to control and shape this vision is dependent on a redistribution of power within the health care system.

The Health Promotion Matrix, which is discussed in detail in Chapter 5, specifies nine health behaviors (Box 1-1), that when taken together, shape an image of health. As the client moves toward internalizing these behaviors through the discovery of self-care, power is realized. In this way, the actualization of the nine healthy behaviors not only empowers the client but also supports the image of health as power. Self-determination and self-care are the essence of health when health is viewed as power.

Box **1-1**

The nine healthy behaviors of the Health Promotion Matrix

1. Smoking cessation
2. Eating well
3. Physical activity
4. Sexual awareness
5. Injury prevention
6. Substance safety
7. Oral health
8. Self-development
9. Productivity

Summary

There are many ways to envision health. Each frame of reference creates a different image of health. Images of health influence personal decision-making as well as the establishment of health policies and programs. The health care system, from the smallest unit of service to the entire system, reflects a particular image of health. Health care professionals dedicate their interactions and interventions to the promotion, protection, and restoration of some image of health.

Health is dynamic. The possibility for blending and exploring new images of health is endless. As health is redefined there are greater opportunities to expand its meaning and significance. Once viewed as a narrow condition of not being ill, health is now viewed as a resource for everyday living—a source of power. Empowerment is generated by self-determination and self-care and allows individuals, families, groups, and communities to define health and act on their own definition.

Each client's right to his/her own image of health must be guarded. The health care professional supports the client's ability to enter and participate in the process of actualizing his/her defined image of health. The health care professional does not override or negate the capacity of clients to form their own images of health. Health care professionals must protect the client's entitlement to health. Building consensus through participation, collaboration, flexibility, and creativity fosters health.

References

Airhihenbuwa, C.O. (1994). Health promotion and the discourse on culture: Implications for empowerment. *Health Education Quarterly, 21*(3), 345-353.

Bertalanffy, L.V. (1968). General system theory. New York: George Braziller.

Borgatta, E.F., Bulcroft, K., Montgomery, R.J., & Bulcroft, R. (1990). Health promotion over the life course. *Research on Aging, 12*(3), 373-388.

Braithwaite, R.L., Bianchi, C., & Taylor, S.E. (1994). Ethnographic approach to community organization and health empowerment. *Health Education Quarterly, 21*(3), 407-416.

Dewey, J. (1963). *Experience and education.* New York: Collier Press.

Dossey, L. (1982). *Space, time and medicine.* Boulder, CO: Shambhala.

Dubos, R. (1965). *Man adapting.* New Haven, CT: Yale University Press.

Dunn, H. (1961). *High-level wellness.* Arlington, VA: Beatty.

Duvall, E.R.M. (1985). *Marriage and family development* (6th ed.). New York: Harper and Row.

Elkind, D. (1981). *Children and adolescents* (3rd ed.). New York: Oxford.

Erikson, E.H. (1963). *Childhood and society* (2nd ed.). New York: Norton.

Foster, J.C. (1994). A woman's health agenda. *Holistic Nursing Practice, 8*(4), 74-88.

Fugh-Berman, A. (1996). *Alternative medicine: What works.* Tucson, AZ: Odonian Press.

Gordis, L. (1996). *Epidemiology.* Philadelphia: W.B. Saunders.

Hatfield, T., & Hatfield, S.R. (1992 November/December). As if your life depended on it: Promoting cognitive development to promote wellness. *Journal of Counseling and Development, 71,* 164-167.

Havighurst, R.J. (1972). *Developmental tasks and education* (3rd ed.). New York: McKay.

Labonte, R. (1994). Health promotion and empowerment: Reflections on professional practice. *Health Education Quarterly, 21*(2), 253-268.

Lalonde, M. (1974). *A new perspective on the health of Canadians.* Ottawa: Government of Canada.

Last, J.M. (Ed.). (1995). *A dictionary of epidemiology* (3rd ed.). New York: Oxford University Press.

Laszlo, E. (1972). *The systems view of the world: The natural philosophy of the new developments in the sciences.* New York: George Braziller.

Lawlis, G.F. (1996). Transpersonal medicine: A new approach to healing the body-mind-spirit. Boston: Shambhala.

Leavell, H.R., & Clark, E.G. (1965). *Preventive medicine for the doctor in his community: An epidemiologic approach.* New York: McGraw-Hill.

Maslow, A.H. (1968). *Toward a psychology of being* (2nd ed.). New York: D. Van Nostrand.

National Institute of Nursing Research, National Institutes of Health. (1995). *Community-based health care: Nursing strategies. National nursing research agenda.* Bethesda, MD: Author.

Omizo, M.M., Omizo, S.A., & D'Andrea, M.J. (1992, November/December). Promoting wellness among elementary school children. *Journal of Counseling & Development, 71,* 194-199.

Pender, N.J. (1996). *Health promotion in nursing practice* (3rd ed.). Stamford, CT: Appleton & Lange.

Piaget, J. (1963). *The origins of intelligence in children.* New York: W.W. Norton.

Restrepo, H.E., & Rozental, M. (1994). The social impact of aging populations: Some major issues. *Social Science and Medicine, 39*(9), 1323-1338.

Robertson, A., & Minkler, M. (1994). New health promotion movement: A critical examination. *Health Education Quarterly, 21*(3), 295-312.

Seedhouse, D. (1995). 'Well-being:' Health promotion's red herring. *Health Promotion International, 10*(1), 61-67.

Smith, J.A. (1983). *The idea of health: Implications for the nursing professional.* New York: Teachers College.

Travis, C.B., Gressley, D.L., & Crumpler, C.A. (1991). Feminist contributions to health psychology. *Psychology of Women Quarterly, 15,* 557-566.

U.S. Department of Health and Human Services. (1991). *Healthy people 2000: National health promotion and disease prevention objectives.* (PHS No. 91-50213). Washington, DC: Superintendent of Documents.

U.S. Office of Alternative Medicine, National Institutes of Health. (1994). *Alternative medicine: Expanding medical horizons. A report to the National Institutes of Health on alternative medical systems and practices in the U.S.* Washington, DC: Author.

Wallerstein, N. (1992). Powerlessness, empowerment, and health: Implications for health promotion programs. *American Journal of Health Promotion, 6*(3), 197-205.

Wheeler, R.J. (1991). The theoretical and empirical structure of general well-being. *Social Indicators Research, 24,* 71-79.

World Health Organization. (1947). Constitution of the World Health Organization. *Chronicle of the World Health Organization, 1*(1-2), 29-43.

World Health Organization. (1986). Health promotion. A discussion document on the concept and principles. *Public Health Reviews, 14*(3-4), 245-254.

World Health Organization HED/HEP. (In press). *Health education and health promotion in developing countries* [on-line]. Available: http://www.who.org

CHAPTER

2

Models of Health Promotion

Sherri Sheinfeld Gorin

As discussed in Chapter 1, health is an evolving concept. Long focused on disease and the absence of ill health, health is now commonly recognized as a powerful state. Health is seen as multidimensional and denotes a sense of wholeness. The highly influential World Health Organization (WHO) definition (1984) of health reflects concern for the individual as a totality rather than a sum of parts, places health in the context of the environment, and equates health with productive and creative living (Pender, 1996).

This chapter expands on the multiple definitions of health. Further, it explains health promotion within the constraints of several different models (e.g., the global and national policies; the environmental approaches; the life cycle model; and the health attitude, belief and behavior change approaches) and details their implicit approach to health. Generally, the loci of change are both the classic micro- (individual) and macro- (societal) level (Zaltman, Kotler, & Kaufman, 1972). Micro includes the individual and family; macro refers to the group, community, and population levels.

The models present a simplified picture of part of the health promotion phenomenon. Several of the models could be characterized as theories of social relations. In general, a theory (1) contains constructs (i.e., mental images, such as "health") that it seeks to explain or account for in some way; (2) describes relationships, often causal, among constructs; and (3) incorporates hypothesized relationships between the constructs and observable variables that can be used to measure the constructs (i.e., "operationalized" constructs) (Judd, Smith, & Kidder, 1991). Several of these theories, such as that of social cognition, have been empirically verified and thus provide strong evidence for their veracity.

Each of the models discussed in this chapter (Table 2-1) addresses the constructs of empowerment and the importance of community participation. In particular, these crosscutting constructs highlight the importance of values in health promotion. Values are fundamental to the discussion of health; to value something is to choose it for its own sake in preference to other alternatives. Consonant with the empowerment construct, the health care professional is seen as a partner in the process of creating health; this role is examined more fully in Chapter 3.

While the health promotion models in themselves are not inclusive—and not fully discussed in this text—they reflect the dominant orientations to the study of change in the field of health promotion at present. Further, many of the concepts found in these models

Table **2-1**

Health promotion models and health themes

MODEL	PRIMARY HEALTH THEME	MACRO/MICRO FOCUS
GLOBAL POLICY	All themes but health as the antithesis of disease	Macro
NATIONAL POLICY		
Health promotion/disease prevention	Health as a balanced state	Macro/micro
	Health as sense of well-being	
Risk reduction	Health as the antithesis of disease	Macro/micro
ENVIRONMENTAL APPROACHES		
Ecological	Health as goodness of fit	Macro
	Health as wholeness	
Social marketing	Health as well-being	Macro
Political economy	Health as empowerment	Macro
PRECEDE-PROCEED	Health as functionality	Macro
Social responsibility	Health as empowerment	Macro
LIFE CYCLE MODELS		
Innovation diffusion theory	Health as growth	Macro/micro
Stages of change*	Health as growth	Micro
HEALTH ATTITUDE, BELIEF, AND BEHAVIOR CHANGE APPROACHES		
Health belief model*	Health as functionality	Micro
Health promotion model	Health as functionality	Micro
Protection motivation theory	Health as sense of well-being	Micro
Theory of reasoned action	Health as functionality	Micro
Prospect theory	Health as the antithesis of disease	Micro
Social learning theories		
Stimulus response theory	Health as functionality	Micro
Social cognitive theory†	Health as functionality	Micro
SPIRITUALITY AS A CONSTRUCT		
	Health as transcendence	Micro

*Also considered part of transtheoretical model
†Also considered part of transtheoretical and health belief models
PRECEDE, Predisposing, reinforcing, and enabling constructs in ecosystem diagnosis and evaluation;
PROCEED, Policy, regulating or resourcing, and organizing for (I) health education, media, and advocacy;
and (II) policy, regulation, resources, and organization; and (III) educational and environmental development
and evaluation.

undergird the foundation of the Health Promotion Matrix, which is explored more fully in Chapter 5. Additionally, even as these models are guiding research and intervention development at present, they are at the same time undergoing verification and modification through the use of approaches similar to those outlined in the last part of this chapter.

GLOBAL POLICY

The global policy is based on the WHO definition health, which is the broadest, most inclusive definition of health and is designed for citizens of the world:

> Health is a state of complete physical, mental, and social well-being, and not merely the absence of disease or infirmity.

In 1978, at Alma-Ata, Kazakhstan, representatives of nations throughout the world expressed the need to develop access to primary health care that would enable their citizens to lead socially and economically productive lives. This meeting was followed by one in 1988 in Riga, Latvia, to identify the remaining gaps in health care, particularly for infants, children, and women of childbearing age. Strategies to achieve health for all persons by the year 2000 were drafted. These included (1) empowering persons by providing information and decision-making opportunities; (2) strengthening local systems of primary health care; (3) improving education and training programs in health promotion and prevention for health care professionals; (4) applying science and technology to critical health problems; (5) using new approaches to health problems that have resisted solution; (6) providing special assistance to the least developed countries; and (7) establishing a process for examination of the long-term challenges that must be addressed beyond the year 2000 in achieving health for all (WHO, 1988). To implement the aim of the first conference and to develop the strategies of the second, WHO (1984) adopted the following five principles of health promotion:

1. Health promotion includes the population as a whole in the context of individuals' everyday lives, rather than focusing on persons at risk for specific diseases.
2. Health promotion is directed toward action on the causes or determinants of health.
3. Health promotion combines diverse but complementary methods or approaches, including communication, education, legislation, fiscal measures, organizational change, community development, and spontaneous local activities against health hazards.
4. Health promotion is particularly aimed at effective and concrete public participation.
5. While health promotion is basically an activity in the health and social fields and not a medical service, health care professionals—particularly in primary health care—have an important role in nurturing and enabling health promotion.

The WHO definition of health promotion assumes a multidimensional characterization of health and incorporates a multitude of strategies, including individual and community change and legislation, under its rubric. The WHO definition assumes a person does not have sole control over his/her health, thus does not "blame the victim" for the attainment of this resource. It does, however, allow people to take responsibility for their choices within a context of concomitant social responsibility for health. Further, on the philosophical level, it implies that health is a means to an end—"a resource"—and an instrumental value, or good for what it brings. Health, like power, is a resource differentially distributed in society (Gutiérrez, 1990). In the global policy model, health is not a good in and of itself or a value in its own right, but a resource for living.

NATIONAL POLICY

It is estimated that in the United States unhealthy life-styles are responsible for 54% of the years of life lost before age 65 years, environmental factors for 22%, and heredity for 16% (McGinnis & Foege, 1994). Further, population-wide approaches to reduce the effects of behavioral and environmental factors, such as tobacco use, diet, inactivity, sexual behavior, microbial agent use, firearm use, drug and alcohol use, toxic agents, and motor vehicles, could decrease the 70% of early deaths for which they account (McGinnis & Foege, 1994).

Attention to influential scientific articles regarding environmental and behavioral health dangers and federal interest in cost reduction for health care expenses led to the development of the *Healthy People 2000: National Health Promotion and Disease Prevention Objectives* (U.S. Department of Health and Human Services [USDHHS], 1991) document. This monograph is the most recent of several national initiatives to develop health objectives for the country and has spawned a number of similar state initiatives. Details of the plan are found in Chapter 3, but in general, it identifies three broad goals: increase the lifespan of healthy life for Americans, reduce health disparities among Americans, and provide access to preventive services for all Americans. The document organizes 22 priorities for action within the categories of health promotion, health protection, preventive services, and surveillance and data systems (USDHHS, 1990). The categorization of the objectives into the areas of health promotion, health protection, and preventive services follows an outline found in other parts of the health promotion literature.

The document mixes both a health promotion and a disease prevention approach, in that each of the categories includes objectives for wellness and risk reduction. In general, the concept of health promotion developed in these approaches emphasizes the role of individuals, groups, and organizations as active agents in shaping health practices and policies to optimize both individual wellness and collective well-being. For example, in the case of family planning, the objectives are stated in terms of avoiding behaviors, such as unprotected sexual activity, and encouraging positive views of sexual relations.

Health Promotion

Health promotion strategies are those related to individual life-style—personal choices made in a social context—that can have a powerful influence over one's health prospects. These priorities target issues, including physical activity and fitness; nutrition; tobacco, alcohol, and other drug use; family planning; mental health and mental disorders; and violent and abusive behavior. Educational and community-based programs can address life-style choices in a cross-cutting fashion.

Health Protection

Health protection strategies are those related to environmental or regulatory measures that confer protection on large population groups. These strategies address issues such as unintentional injuries, occupational safety and health, environmental health, food and drug safety, and oral health. Interventions applied to address these issues generally are not exclusively protective in nature—there may be a substantial health promotion element as well—and the principal approaches involve a community-wide, rather than individual, focus.

Disease Prevention

The disease prevention model focuses on the avoidance of illness and agents of illness, as well as the identification and minimization of risk. This approach is found throughout the health promotion literature, most particularly in the *Guide to Clinical Preventive Services: Report of the U.S. Preventive Services Task Force* (USPSTF, 1996) report and throughout a set of objectives in *Healthy People 2000*.

Epidemiologic data are the foundation for the development of this model. As discussed in Chapter 1, epidemiology focuses on how diseases originate and spread in populations (Lilienfeld, 1976).

In a preventive approach, the natural history of the disease is examined to identify the interrelationship between the outside etiologic, or causal, agents and the biologic response of the host, as well as the effects of environmental social, and physical factors; community patterns of medical care; and the social and intellectual response of the host (Leavell & Clark, 1953). The target of the preventive intervention is selected based on the prevalence (proportion of the population affected) and the incidence (number of new cases per year) of the condition. In the case of the USPSTF, the target conditions selected are relatively common in the United States and are of major clinical significance. The natural history of a disease may not always be the same. For instance, the natural history of asthma may be quite different in certain urban areas with excessive industrial air pollution as compared with its course in relatively unpolluted rural areas. Similarly, the natural history of disease in a highly literate and medically sophisticated area may be different from the sequence observed in a remote region with generally poor medical facilities and little education about health principles (Hutchison, 1969).

Preventive services for clients in clinical settings include counseling, screening, immunization, and chemoprophylactic interventions. Priority areas for these strategies include maternal and infant health, heart disease and stroke, cancer, diabetes, chronic disabling conditions, human immunodeficiency virus (HIV) infection, sexually transmitted diseases, and infectious diseases. The prevention model also addresses cross-cutting professional and access considerations in the delivery of clinical preventive services.

The triage of primary, secondary, and tertiary prevention is relevant to the objectives stated in the document. Primary preventive measures are those provided to individuals to prevent the onset of a targeted condition (e.g., routine immunization of healthy children). Secondary preventive measures identify and treat asymptomatic persons who have already developed risk factors or preclinical disease but in whom the condition has not become clinically apparent (e.g., a Papanicolaou smear to detect cervical dysplasia before the development of cancer or screening for high blood pressure). Tertiary preventive measures are those directed toward persons as part of the treatment and management of clinical illnesses (e.g., cholesterol reduction in clients with coronary heart disease or insulin therapy to prevent the complications of diabetes mellitus) (USPSTF, 1996). Tertiary prevention is devoted to the amelioration of disease among those already ill; even clients with disease may envision health and thus participate in health promotion.

Defining risk. In the disease prevention orientation, individuals and groups are characterized by their relative "risk" for various diseases and disorders. According to The

Royal Society (1983), "Risk is the probability that a particular adverse event occurs during a stated period of time, or results from a particular challenge." The determinants of reducing risk are seen from three general perspectives, from the micro- to the macro-level: (1) assisting the health care professional to modify individual behavior to reduce the risk of premature mortality (Health Risk Appraisal); (2) altering community health care resources to reduce the risk for individuals and groups at risk for disease (Risk Approach); and (3) increasing the awareness of external sources of risk, such as specific technologies, in societal goals of health, safety, and environmental protection (Risk Analysis/Assessment/Management) (summary in Hayes, 1992).

The definition of risk denotes that the outcome is negative. Further, each approach to reducing risk, from the individual (micro-level) to the societal (macro-level), implies an assessment by an outsider that the risk taker's behavior is harmful. For example, the real or perceived benefits of smoking, eating, and drinking are seen differently by the person engaging in the activity than by an outsider judging these actions. At the micro-level, the individual has the responsibility to change his/her own behavior; at the macro-level, the determinants of health are embedded within larger societal or technologic structures and thus are beyond the individual's control. This same criticism concerning the control one has over environmental elements has been leveled against other models of health promotion.

Community risk prevention. Community-based health promotion programs, which primarily emphasize the prevention of chronic diseases, are becoming increasingly common. While aimed at the community as a whole, most community health promotion/disease prevention programs include some individual interventions for people at high risk and are modeled after the Health Risk appraisals methods of the Framingham Heart Study (Becker & Janz, 1987).

Although these programs are characterized primarily as a disease prevention approach, each has relied on multiple models of client change (Fincham, 1992), especially the "3 A's": program affordability, acceptability, and adequacy (Elder, Schmid, Dower, & Hedlund, 1993). Two of the earliest examples of these were the North Karelia (Finland) Project to prevent coronary heart disease (CHD) and the Stanford Heart Disease Prevention Program. The classic North Karelia project, started in 1972, was a comprehensive community program for the control of cardiovascular disease aimed at the total population but with special focus on middle-age men, among whom rates were highest (Salonen, Tuomilehto, Nissinen, Kaplan, & Puska, 1989). The Stanford Heart Disease Prevention Program (now the Stanford Five City Project, funded by the National Heart, Lung, and Blood Institute [NHLBI]) began about the same time, initially including three communities and later expanding to five. The aims were to increase participants' knowledge of risk factors for cardiovascular disease, to decrease their cigarette smoking, and to favorably change their diets (Maccoby, Farquhar, Wood, & Alexander, 1977; Fortmann, et al., 1995). This program was followed by other large cardiovascular disease community demonstration programs funded by the NHLBI, including the Minnesota Heart Health Program (MHHP); the Pawtucket Heart Health Program [PHHP] (summary in Shea & Basch, 1990; Stone, 1991); and for children and adolescents, the Child and Adolescent Trial for Cardiovascular Health (CATCH) (McGraw et al., 1994). The Stanford Five City Project, the MHHP, the PHHP, and CATCH have dual aims: health promotion and disease prevention (risk reduction). Each is designed to produce a measurable amount of change in risk factors and eventually in illness and death from cardiovascular disease in the communities being studied. Concurrently, the aims are to help community members choose and practice healthier behaviors in the areas of smoking, cholesterol-elevating diets, high blood pressure, obesity, and sedentary life-style.

In 1972, the Multiple Risk Factor Intervention Trial (MRFIT) began and documented risk factors in men ages 35 to 57 years until 1974. This was a highly influential screening project, having enhanced the understanding, for example, of the relationship between tobacco and total mortality and the development of CHD, stoke, cancer, and chronic obstructive pulmonary disease (COPD) (Stamler, Wentworth & Neaton, 1986). It has been followed by other large epidemiologic projects, such as those to evaluate the risks of heart disease in women, as well as those more focused on health promotion "per se," such as the Henry J. Kaiser Family Foundations Community Health Promotion Grants (CHPGP) (Wagner et al., 1991).

The Epidemiologic Catchment Area studies are major National Institute of Mental Health-funded research efforts in the behavioral health area designed to examine the prevalence of mental disorders and risk factors for symptoms in cities across the United States (Regier et al., 1988).

Differences Among Health Promotion, Health Protection, and Disease Prevention

Considerable attention has been paid to the differences among health promotion, health protection, and disease prevention to assist health care professionals in individual behavior change. The critical difference among them is the underlying motivation for the behavior on the part of individuals and aggregates (Pender, 1996). Health promotion encourages well-being and is oriented toward the actualizing of human potential and thus is positive in valence, or attractive to the client. Health protection, however, is directed toward a desire to actively avoid illness, to detect it early, or to maintain function within the constraints of illness. Disease prevention is similar to health protection, in that one is taking action to thwart the disease process by finding ways to modify the environment, behavior, and bodily defenses so that disease processes are eliminated, slowed, or changed (Parse, 1987). Because health protection and disease prevention approaches are oriented toward avoidance, they hold a negative valence, or are repulsive to the client.

ENVIRONMENTAL APPROACHES

Five major environmental approaches to health promotion have gained credence within the field: the ecological, social marketing, political economy, PRECEDE*-PROCEED,† and social responsibility approaches. They are similar in that they highlight the role of the environment in optimizing states of well-being; further, they emphasize the connection between well-being and a strong commitment to one's social and physical milieu (Stokols, 1992). The ecological model focuses specifically on the components of health promotive environments.

In the environmental approaches, healthfulness is seen as a multifaceted phenomenon incorporating physical health, emotional well-being, and social cohesion. Health may result from concurrent interventions in transactions between persons and environments

---

PRECEDE, Predisposing, reinforcing, and enabling constructs in ecosystem diagnosis and evaluation.
†*PROCEED*, Policy, regulating or resourcing, and organizing for: (I) health education, media, and advocacy; and (II) policy, regulation, resources and organization; and (III) educational and environmental development and evaluation.

over time (Stokols, 1992) and reflects the outcomes of joint interventions at multiple levels.

The Ecological Model

Ecology pertains to the interrelationships between organisms and their environments (Hawley, 1950). The social ecology approach is grounded in a contextually oriented view of human health and well-being (Moos, 1979). It attends to the social, institutional, and cultural contexts of person-environment relations. The model assumes that the healthfulness of a situation and the well-being of its participants are influenced by multiple aspects of the environment—both physical (geography, architecture, and technology) and social (culture, economics, and politics). Characteristics of the environment interact with those of the person, such as one's genetic heritage, psychologic predispositions, and behavioral patterns; health is a result of that interplay. Environments may vary, for example, in their lighting, temperature, noise levels, and space arrangements; these are seen both as objective characteristics and as being perceived differently by each person (subjective characteristics). The meshing of a unique environment and a particular person differs from context to context.

The model incorporates components of systems theory, such as interdependence, homeostasis, negative feedback, and derivation amplification (Cannon, 1932; Emery & Trist, 1972; Katz & Kahn, 1966; Maruyama, 1963). These systems concepts are used to understand the dynamic interactions between persons and their environments. Person-environment interactions move through cycles of mutual influence, where each affects the other. The varied levels of human environments, such as worksites, are seen as complex systems, in which each level is nested in more complex and distant levels. For example, the occupational health and safety of community work settings are directly influenced by state and local ordinances aimed at protecting public health and environmental quality (Stokols, 1992).

Environments differ by their relative scale and complexity, and the participants in those contexts may be studied as individuals, small groups, organizations, and larger aggregates and populations. Interventions may be strengthened by the coordination of individuals and groups acting within different environments, such as family members who make efforts to improve their health practices, corporate managers who shape organizational health policies, and public health officials who supervise community health services (Green & Kreuter, 1990; Pelletier, 1984; Winett, King, & Altman, 1989). Further, individuals' physical and emotional well-being are enhanced when environments are personally controllable and predictable (Karasek & Theorell, 1990). Environments that are too predictable and controllable, however, can become so boring that they constrain opportunities for coping effectively with novel situations, thus impeding growth (Aldwin & Stokols, 1988; Schaefer & Moos, 1992).

The ecology model recognizes the often times contradictory influences of environments and persons. For example, a socially supportive family or organization may enable individuals to cope more effectively with physical constraints (e.g., overcrowding, drab surroundings). A well-designed physical environment may not, however, spur much health promotion if interpersonal or intergroup relations result in conflict and stress.

Research deriving from ecology models focuses on characteristics of the environment and differentiates health outcomes in terms of their severity, duration, and overall importance to members of the setting. Research designed to optimize or enhance environmental quality and human well-being is central to these approaches.

The Social Marketing Model

Social marketing is a framework frequently used in health promotion programs to help design, target, refine, and implement programs (Kotter & Roberto, 1989; Manoff, 1985). It adapts the approach used in commercial marketing to the arena of health behavior. The marketing framework revolves around the use of the four *P*'s: product, price, place, and promotion. The product generally refers to the program (e.g., weight reduction) and any attitudes, beliefs, ideas, additional behaviors, and practices connected with the program or the behavior (e.g., health as a value). Price refers to any psychologic or social effort, opportunity, or monetary cost associated with the adoption and use of the product. Place is the distribution point for the product (e.g., an HMO). Promotion refers to the means of informing a target audience about the product and persuading them to use it (e.g., videos, brochures, television spots). A fifth variable is positioning, which refers to the unique niche of the product (e.g., a weight reduction program for dieting seniors). Finally, a sixth variable, politics, describes the social and economic context that can facilitate or hinder the marketing process (e.g., the reimbursement policies for weight control counseling). According to Winett (1995), social marketing variables combine to create a context within which the components of a health promotive intervention may be placed.

Political Economy Approach

The assumption of the political economy model is that the activities of organizations (as well as communities, groups, families, and individuals) are accounted for by the political (a structure of rule) and economic (a system for producing and exchanging goods and services) contexts in which they are embedded (Sheinfeld Gorin & Weirich, 1995). Fundamental to the relationships between organizations and their contexts is an exchange of resources, such as money, persons, information, space, and/or social legitimacy (reputation). These exchanges create a set of political and economic interdependencies both within the organization (among staff and workgroups) and within its context (its funders, regulators, accreditors, clients). An organization tends to be influenced by those who hold the political and economic resources the organization needs. Thus the organization attempts to satisfy the demands of a given outside (or inside) group if that group holds a resource critical to its survival, has discretion over its use of the resource, and few alternative sources of that resource are available. For example, accreditors and the "stamp of approval" (social legitimation) they give to a health care facility are increasingly important to managed care companies as they compete for clients. As a result, major accrediting organizations such as the Joint Commission on the Accreditation of Health Care Organizations (JCAHO) can demand significant changes in an organization by withholding a desired recognition.

The PRECEDE-PROCEED Framework

The PRECEDE-PROCEED framework, developed by Lawrence Green (1979), has been particularly influential in the planning of health education programs—a critical component of the health care professional's work. Health education planning generally proceeds in phases (Green & Krueter, 1990). The health care professional begins by assessing the quality of life experienced by those whom the program might effect. For example, a program might focus on general social problems of concern to individuals or communities, such as alienation (social detachment or separation) among adolescents. The professional then evaluates specific health problems that appear to be contributing to the social problems (e.g., the incidence of substance abuse among adolescents). Specific behaviors that appear to be linked with the health problems are identified (e.g., the frequency, duration, and use of several kinds of drugs and alcohol).

The health care professional then identifies predisposing, enabling, and reinforcing factors that have the potential for influencing a behavior (e.g., substance abuse). Predisposing factors that affect an individual's willingness to change include knowledge, attitudes, values, and perceptions, such as those identified in the health belief model, which is discussed later in this chapter. Enabling factors that facilitate or present obstacles to change include the availability and accessibility of skills, resources, and barriers that help or hinder the desired behavior; the PRECEDE framework puts particular emphasis on barriers created by social forces or systems, such as insurance coverage, health care professional practices, and the location of or access to treatment resources. Reinforcing factors refer to rewards or feedback given to persons adopting a certain behavior, that influence continuing that behavior. The focus of the intervention is then described (e.g., linking community members with funding sources to establish a school-based brief treatment center). After that, a program to combat the problem is developed and implemented. Finally, the program is evaluated (e.g., by clients and community members, who are provided with technical assistance from a university) as an integral and continuing part of program planning (cf. Fawcet et al., 1995).

The Social Responsibility Model

The social responsibility model, so named because of the primacy attached to the value of government intervention on behalf of health and its focus on health as an end rather than as a means, is best expressed in the work of several British Commissions (e.g., the Black Report and the Acheson Report) and in the writings of Downie, Fyfe, and Tannahill (1990). The definition of health promotion is expansive and assumes that health is a value to be pursued in its own right:

> Health promotion comprises efforts to enhance positive health and prevent ill-health, through the overlapping spheres of health education, prevention, and health protection (Downie et al., 1990, p. 2).

Supporters of the social responsibility model see health as an end, to be valued in its own right. They are critical of both the classic liberal position on health, yet in agreement with the preamble to the Constitution of WHO. At the micro-level, they argue that health is a moral value, in that individuals have a moral duty to do what they can to improve their own health. Well-being is a value of its own; positive pleasures accrue to the healthy. At the macro-level, they contend that health is a value that governments should promote and that access to health is a fundamental right that government must implement. They argue that if health is an instrumental value (a means or resource to obtain an end), as WHO defines it, reasonable governmental interventions would be limited. Under these considerations, health promotion would fall under only two categories—preventing costly ill-health and promoting functional health to carry on a job and not simply drain society's resources.

LIFE CYCLE MODELS

Two general models are based on the concept of change over time: innovation diffusion and the stages of change. Life cycle is an appropriate metaphor for the patterns of change experienced by an individual, family, group, community, or larger social group over time. Populations ebb and flow, and organizations are created, grow, sometimes become stagnant, sometimes revitalize, and sometimes die. Individuals move through transition points at birth, school years, entry to the workforce, partnering, parenthood, retirement, and death. These transitions are met by social and cultural constructions around the meaning of health that change from one stage of life to another. For example, parenthood may be seen as a time when individuals become more aware of their health, become more conscious of trying to improve health behaviors, or recognize that they are growing older and that their bodies are aging. At this point in the life cycle, individuals often reflect on "having no time" to keep healthy or physically fit (Backett & Davison, 1995, p. 635). From the perspective of inducing change toward health promotion, these transition points are circumstances in the life course when changes in behavior are likely to occur (Borgatta, Bulcroft, Montgomery, & Bulcroft, 1990).

Demographics also are key to life cycle models. The relative proportion of particular groups in society has enormous effects on the societal definitions of health promotion and the value placed on them. This is evident by the demographic transition developed nations are experiencing in the increased number and proportion of elderly populations.

Innovation Diffusion Theory

The innovation diffusion theory addresses the contexts within which innovations are adopted and used. *Innovations*—defined as new and qualitatively different ideas over time—require some conceptual reorientation among participants (Delbecq, 1978). Innovation adoption and use are influenced by three major factors: (1) the innovation itself, (2) the environment, and (3) the client system. For example, some clients may feel that the PACE exercise program described in Chapter 8 is an innovation. The characteristics of the innovation itself (e.g., its triability, relative advantage, observeability, initial fit with the client's needs, ability to be reinvented to match or be adapted to changing needs, and simplicity) may affect its adoption and use. These features emphasize the importance of tailoring an innovation's attributes to achieve its objectives.

According to innovation diffusion theory, a particular health care environment may differ from another in its affluence, complexity, rate of change, extent of conflict, and degree of cooperation, which influence the adoption and use of new ideas and programs (e.g., local political support encourages the adoption of and use of health promotion programs, such as PACE). Finally, the client system itself (e.g., the HMO within which the PACE program operates) may differ from that of other primary care settings in affluence; governance; structure; age; size; complexity; mission; degree of vulnerability; orientation toward, support of, and rate of change; cooperativeness; power; and extent of control over its members. These too affect the extent of adoption and use of innovations (summary in Sheinfeld Gorin, 1982).

When new, a health promotion program may move through the stages of adoption (from evaluation of the idea, to initiation of the program, to implementation, and finally to routine use). Similarly, the use of a program may increase as it continues (or decrease as it fails) to influence understanding among clients. Furthermore, persons exposed to a health promotion program may be classified on the basis of their innovativeness as innovators, early adopters, early majority, late majority, or late adopters. In community-based health promotion programs, new ideas, which often are first reported by the mass media, are mediated and modified through opinion leaders, who are often early adopters. The majority of persons are then influenced through interpersonal contact with opinion leaders, who are seen as credible sources of information. Collaboration among these leaders assists in both interpreting the needs of communities exposed to health promotion programs and in encouraging the adoption of new ideas (Rogers, 1983). These leaders help to encourage adoption by eventually persuading the majority of persons, which may occur earlier or later in the process of adoption.

The introduction of new behaviors that diffuse through a client system is achieved by both mass and interpersonal communication. The success of mass communication depends on five areas: the credibility of the source, content and design of the message, delivery channel, target audience, and the target behavior (McGuire, 1981). *Persuasibility* refers to any type of social influence. For persuasion to take place, a message must be conveyed, the person(s) must receive and comprehend the message and be convinced by it, the message must be retained, and there must be behavioral manifestations that demonstrate change has taken place. The aim of persuasion is to introduce inconsistency in two related beliefs, that, according to social adaptation theory, will lead to a reinterpretation of social reality (Fincham, 1992).

Stages of Change

The stages of change model is based on the assumption that individuals move through a series of predictable stages when changing behavior, such as stopping smoking or beginning an exercise program. These changes include the following (DiClemente, 1991; Prochaska & DiClemente, 1983; Prochaska, Velicer, Guadagnoli, Rossi, & DiCelemente, 1991):

1. Precontemplation (i.e., considering the change)
2. Contemplation of change (i.e., starting to think about initiating change)
3. Contemplation without action
4. Preparation (i.e., seriously thinking about the change within a given time period [e.g., the next 6 months] or taking early steps to change)
5. Action (i.e., making change in or stopping the target behavior within a 6-month period
6. Maintenance of change (i.e., maintaining the target behavior change for more than 6 months)
7. In some cases, relapse

The stages are not necessarily linear. For example, the average smoker who quits reports several and often many relapses before achieving maintained abstinence (Fisher, Bishop, Goldmuntz, & Jacobs, 1988). The stages of change model may, however, suggest intervention points for different individuals at varied stages (Prochaska et al., 1991).

Because the stages of change model addresses individual change over time, it is considered a component of the life cycle model. It also has been called the *transtheoretical model*. The transtheoretical model of change encompasses the health belief model, social cognitive theory, and the stages of change propositions and is oriented toward behavioral change in individuals and groups. In particular, it has been used to explain smoking cessation and physical activity changes in individuals.

The transtheoretical model of change includes a framework for understanding the mechanisms that may drive movement through the stages. These mechanisms are called the *processes of change* and relate to the transitions between various stages of change

(Prochaska & DiClemente, 1983). These processes draw heavily on components of other models, such as the health belief model.

The transtheoretical model also addresses the general element of decision making regarding adoption of a behavior, using a decisional balance approach. Decisional balance compares the strength of the target behavior's perceived pros with that of the perceived cons. The relative weight persons assign to a behavior's pros and cons influences their decisions about behavior change (Janis & Mann, 1977), such as continuing or ceasing to smoke.

HEALTH ATTITUDE, BELIEF, AND BEHAVIOR CHANGE APPROACHES

The following three theories—the health belief model, the theory of reasoned action, and the social learning theory—and their corollaries and derivatives are models of health promotive paths for individuals or groups. These models emphasize alterations in attitudes, beliefs, and/or behaviors.

Health Belief Model

The intention of one of the most prominent of these theories, the health belief model (modified by Becker, 1986), was to determine why some persons who are illness-free take actions to avoid illness, whereas others fail to take protective actions. Another aim of the health belief model was to predict the conditions under which people would engage in simple preventive behaviors, such as immunizations. The model was founded on the work of Kurt Lewin, who understood that the life space in which individuals live is comprised of regions, some having negative valence (one would seek to avoid), some a positive valence (one would seek to approach), and some a neutral valence (one would neither seek to approach nor avoid) (Lewin, Dembo, & Festinger, 1944).

The health belief model suggests that before an individual takes action, he/she must decide that the behavior, whether it be smoking, eating fatty foods, or engaging in unprotected sexual activity, creates a serious health problem, that he/she is personally susceptible to its health harm, and that moderating or stopping the behavior will be beneficial. The perceived barriers to undertaking a behavior are considered most salient to health promotive efforts (Janz & Becker, 1984). Perceived susceptibility to and perceived severity of harm are based to a great extent on the person's knowledge of a disease and its potential outcome. The model addresses the "cues to action" that motivate the decision-making process and self-efficacy about executing the target behavior. Although the combination of perceived susceptibility to and severity of harm provides the force for action and the perception of high benefits and low barriers provides a course of action, it is the "cues to action" that start the process of change (Rosenstock, 1974).

In an expansion of the health belief model, a separate construct of general health motivation was added. Motives are viewed as dispositions within which individuals approach certain categories of positive incentives. For example, the desire to maintain a state of good health is a component of health motivation (Becker, Drachman, & Kirscht, 1974; Maiman & Becker, 1984; Curry & Emmons, 1994). Within the last 10 years, the health belief model has subsumed the self-efficacy construct of social cognitive theory to better explain health behaviors (Rosenstock, Strecher, & Becker, 1988).

Health promotion model. The health promotion model is a framework that explores the complex biopsychosocial processes that motivate individuals to engage in behaviors directed toward health enhancement. It is a competence- or an approach-oriented model and has encouraged considerable empirical testing in the field of nursing (Pender, 1996). Based primarily on the health belief model and social cognitive theory, it is mainly directed toward change in individuals. The health promotion model links individual characteristics and experiences and behavior-specific cognitions and affects—including benefits of and barriers to action, interpersonal and situational influences—to a commitment to a health promoting behavior. The final behavioral outcome is concomitantly influenced by the *immediate* competing demands and preferences, which can derail a health promoting action (such as selecting a meal with high, rather than low, fat content because of taste or flavor preferences) (summary in Pender, 1996).

Protection motivation theory. The protection motivation theory is founded in the field of social psychology. It uses health threats, or fear appeals, to change behavior by highlighting the harmful personal consequences of health damaging behaviors. For example, a program to encourage substance safety among teens would use pictures of dead addicts under white sheets in the morgue and explicit warnings against drug use. The theory currently incorporates four focal cognitive appraisal processes: perceived vulnerability to a health threat, perceived seriousness of the health threat, perceived effectiveness of responses directed toward preventing the threat (response efficacy), and perceived self-efficacy (beliefs about personal competence). The latter process is derived from Bandura's social cognitive theory, which is discussed later in this chapter. Generally, however, because of the difficulty of determining the appropriate timing and dose of fear, the promotion of healthy alternative behaviors is more effective (Job, 1988).

Theory of Reasoned Action

Ajzen and Fishbein (1980) developed the theory of reasoned action, which is a mathematical description of the relationship between beliefs (verbalized opinions), attitudes (the judgment that the behavior is good or bad and that a person is in favor of or against performing the behavior), and intentions in determining action. The theory postulates that most volitional behavior can be predicted by beliefs, attitudes, and intentions; therefore efforts to change behavior should be directed at an individual's belief system. By altering the beliefs underlying attitudes or norms, changes in behavioral intentions, and subsequently in behavior, also can be induced (Azjen & Fishbein, 1980).

The first step toward this aim is to identify and measure the behavior to be changed. Once defined, the determinants of the behavior may be specified. A person's intention to perform (or not perform) a behavior is the immediate determinant of the action. Secondly, the person's intention is a function of two other determinants: (1) one's attitude toward the behavior; and (2) the subjective norm, or the person's perception of the social pressures put on one to perform or not perform the behavior in question (Ajzen & Fishbein, 1980). Individuals will intend to perform a behavior, such as brush their teeth, when they evaluate it positively and when they believe that important others, such as parents, think they should perform it. The relative weights of the additudinal and normative factors may vary from one person to another; thus one person may attach more weight to attitude, another, to normative influences.

Further, attitudes are a function of behavioral and normative beliefs, perceived consequences of behavior, and the person's evaluation of these. The social/normative factor consists of the opinions of important referent individuals or groups (such as parents or peers). The person's motivation to comply with those opinions reflects a sense of the consequences of conforming (or not) and his/her attention to the referents.

Specificity of intentions are highlighted in the theory. An action, such as exercising, is always performed with respect to a given target (e.g., walking rather than running), in a particular context (e.g., at work), and at a given time (e.g., during lunch) (Ajzen & Fishbein, 1980). The theory also considers external variables (e.g., access to family planning services for women using birth control) as being influential on a person's beliefs or the relative importance he/she attaches to attitudinal and normative considerations. Finally, the individual controls the relationship between the intention to act and the behavior. If a female maintains a positive attitude toward using birth control pills, is supported by a set of family and community norms supporting the use of contraception, and intends to use birth control pills, she ultimately will use them (Fishbein, Jaccard, Davidson, Ajzen, & Loken, 1980).

Prospect Theory

The prospect theory is a descriptive model of risk-related decisions that have different specific probabilities and is used to explain attitudes toward risk and value (Kahneman & Tversky, 1984). It has been applied primarily to monetary gambling choices. The assumptions of the theory are threefold. First, risk decisions are influenced by the subjective evaluations of relative gains and losses, as opposed to objective evaluations of absolute outcomes. For example, the "perceived value" of breast cancer screening would determine compliance with screening recommendations. The choice of a healthy, asymptomatic woman who fears the possibility of finding an abnormality to not comply with screening recommendations would reflect "risk-averse" behavior. Second, persons tend to make risk-averse choices for sure "gain" and to make risk-seeking choices for a gamble over a sure "loss." Third, the theory states that the degree to which a choice (or behavior) is seen as a gain or a loss can vary depending on how the consequences of the behavior are presented, or "framed" (Curry & Emmons, 1994, p. 309).

The prospect theory has been used to develop materials to encourage screening for breast cancer. A loss-frame presentation emphasizes the failure to receive positive consequences by not doing a specific action. The following is a loss-frame statement: "By not doing breast self-exams (BSE) now, you will not learn what your normal, healthy breasts feel like . . ." A gain-frame is reflected in the following sentence and emphasizes the positive consequences of doing a particular action: "By doing BSE now, you can learn what your normal, healthy breasts feel like . . ." (Meyerowitz & Chaiken, 1987, p. 504). These approaches are distinguished from the "fear appeals" of protection motivation theory, that, in this example, would emphasize the negative consequences of not having a mammogram (Wilson, Purdon, & Wallston, 1988).

Social Learning Theories

Social learning theory holds that behavior is determined by expectancies and incentives. Two approaches reflect this general theory: stimulus response theory and social cognitive theory. Social cognitive theory shares a general approach with stimulus response theory, although the role of cognition separates the two models. In social cognitive theory, expectancies are cognitive, or developed in the mind of the individual. Cognitive expectations (e.g., feeling capable of stopping) influence the conduct of a behavior (e.g., stopping smoking). In stimulus response theory, cognitive mediators are not present.

Stimulus response theory. Stimulus response theory rests on the belief that learning results from events (called reinforcements, or consequences of behavior) that reduce physiologic drives (e.g., tension, anxiety) that then activate behavior. Behavior analysis relies on classic operant conditioning techniques, and, in the field of health promotion, is most often applied to individuals, families, and groups. Behavioral analysis involves objective definitions of the actions to be changed, measurable procedures for change, and an emphasis on antecedent and consequent events to change behavior. Over time, individuals may be conditioned to respond to cues in their environment by associating behaviors (e.g., associating smoking with stimuli such as a cup of coffee in the morning). To extinguish such conditioned responses, the individual must be exposed to the conditioned stimulus (e.g., the coffee) without presentation of the unconditioned stimulus (e.g., a cigarette) (Rachlin, 1991).

Similarly, several other principles of behavioral analysis (e.g., the use of contingency management, feedback and goal setting, sharing and successive approximation, modeling, and prompting) may be applied successfully to encourage healthy behaviors. Contingency management involves a system of attaching rewards (e.g., praise) to goal attainment (e.g., losing weight). The initiation and maintenance of behavior change may be accomplished by providing feedback and rewards so that the positive behavior itself becomes reinforcing. For example, healthy eating practices may be reinforced by teaching individuals to prepare appealing, simple, and quick meals (Kelly et al., 1992). The likelihood of the behavior itself becoming reinforcing is increased if successive approximations (intermediate goals) are used with shaping tactics (Kazdin, 1994). Through these procedures, individuals perform behavior that is only within their repertoire and is the next step on a goal attainment gradient, with that (subgoal) behavior having a high likelihood of being reinforced. Programs teaching dieters how to lose weight begin with a low-fat variation of a meal dieters usually enjoy (such as vegetarian, rather than cheese, pizza). Further, such programs use models, such as successful program graduates, strategically.

Social cognitive theory. Social cognitive theory developed from the stimulus response and earlier classical conditioning theories. The cornerstone of the model is the "reciprocal determinism" between cognition, behavior, and environment (Bandura, 1986, p. 22). Rather than focusing on the automatic shaping of behavior by environmental forces, social cognitive theory emphasizes the importance of intervening thought processes (e.g., information acquisition, storage, and retrieval) and self-control on the performance of behavior. Most learning occurs through modeling, such as watching others prepare and eat meals, rather than trial and error. These vicarious and symbolic learning processes are affected by social influences. Self-regulatory processes, including self-generated inducements and consequences (e.g., telling oneself to exercise daily so that one can climb a flight of stairs more easily) are highlighted in the theory. Behavior can be explained in terms of a continuous and reciprocal interaction between cognitive, behavioral, and environmental determinants that are governed by self-efficacy, which is a cognitive mechanism.

Self-efficacy is a central concept in the application of social cognitive theory to health promotion. According to social cognitive theory (Bandura, 1986), both outcome and efficacy expectations are critical to behavior change, such as modifying a diet. An outcome expectation concerns one's estimate that a given behavior can produce a given outcome, such as maintenance of smoking cessation. Self-efficacy is the conviction that one can execute this behavior successfully. Individuals high in self-efficacy, or more confident of their abilities to maintain behavioral changes (e.g., smoking cessation or ideal weight), will attempt to execute it more readily, with greater intensity, and with greater perseverance in response to initial failure than will individuals with comparatively weaker self-efficacy (Baer & Lichtenstein, 1988; Devins, 1992).

Social cognitive theory affects change through phases: (1) promotion and motivation of persons toward changing a target behavior; (2) skills training so that individuals can acquire specific behavioral change skills; (3) development of support networks so that new behavior can be maintained; (4) maintenance of the behavior through reinforcement; and (5) generalization to all levels of interaction, from the family to the community (Lefebvre, Lasater, Carleton, & Peterson, 1987).

Self-efficacy has been distinguished from locus of control, a similar concept. Locus of control is a generalized concept about the self, whereas self-efficacy is situation-specific (i.e., focused on one's beliefs about one's personal abilities in specific settings).

SPIRITUALITY AS A HEALTH PROMOTION CONSTRUCT

Many popular books, newspaper articles, and radio and television programs have been devoted to the concept of spirituality. Historically, spirituality, known as *spiritualism,* has been found within the purview of religion and has been fostered by religious groups and institutions. More recently, while some persons are returning to religious institutions to renew their spiritual sense, others are redefining their connections to traditional religions to create a spiritual dimension. Within the context of religion, spirituality may be defined as follows:

> The spiritual core is the deepest center of the person. It is here that the person is open to the transcendent dimension; it is here that the person experiences ultimate reality. [Spirituality] explores the discovery of this core, the dynamics of its development, and its journey to the ultimate goal. It deals with prayer, spiritual direction, the various maps of the spiritual journey, and the methods of advancement in the spiritual ascent (Cousins, 1987, p. x).

Spiritual support for health promotion may be defined as perceived support from higher powers, a sense of self-love, and a sense of connectedness to others in the experience of being human. Spirituality may be manifest in an individual's beliefs (e.g., in a higher power or in the power of self-love), rituals (e.g., setting out candles for dead relatives), and practices (e.g., attending a synagogue, church, or other religious institution; praying; meditating; and/or challenging injustice).

Several interventions that explicitly use spirituality to promote health are found in the health promotion field; these include therapeutic touch ("laying-on of hands"), directed healing (by healers), distant healing (intercessory prayer), and spiritism ("espiritismo," a healing system used alongside a spiritist). To bring the body, mind, and spirit together, meditation (the attempt to achieve awareness without thought) is often practiced.

Within the field of health promotion at present, spirituality is considered a construct, or a mental image, rather than a fully developed model. It has not yet been posited in relation to other constructs that together may predict or are outcomes of health promotion (such as social support, quality of life, and empowerment). Interventions designed to assess the construct have not yet been rigorously evaluated. More operational measures of spirituality are necessary to assist in the systemic testing of a model.

CROSS-CUTTING CONSTRUCTS

The concepts of empowerment and community-capacity building, as central foundations of the field of health promotion, transverse all the models. Each concept purports a set of moral values, on which an ethical practice of health promotion can be based. The implications of these two concepts in health promotion practice are detailed in Chapter 3.

Empowerment

Empowerment is a term with considerable weight and contested meanings. Health is significantly affected by the extent to which one feels control or mastery over one's life or by the amount of power or powerlessness one feels (Wallerstein, 1992). At the core of empowerment is power, which is found in the process of increasing personal, interpersonal, or political exchanges (Gutiérrez, 1990). Empowerment is thus a central component in the health promotion strategy. Its roots are in community psychology, feminist theory, liberation theology, and social activism.

A set of moral values underpins the empowerment construct in health promotion. Moral values may be defined as the "humanly caused benefits that human beings provide to others . . . By way of illustration, we may say that love and justice are moral goods" (Kekes, 1993, p. 44). Moral values founding the empowerment construct include promoting human diversity (promoting respect and appreciation for diverse social entities) and self-determination (promoting the ability of clients to pursue their chosen goals without excessive frustration and in consideration of other person's needs) for individuals and marginalized groups, especially communities.

The concept embodies the larger political aspects of power. "Empowerment theory is based on a conflict model that assumes that a society consists of separate groups possessing different levels of power and control over resources" (Gutiérrez, 1990, p. 150). Power is a nonmaterial resource differentially distributed in society. Questions of power are key to empowerment (e.g., Who has more power in a relationship? Are there attempts to share power?). Empowerment is thus attentive to rights and entitlements in relationships and to personal control over exchanges.

Power is the ability to predict, control, and participate in one's environment. Empowerment is then the process by which individuals and communities are enabled to take such power and act effectively in transforming their lives and their environments (Miller, 1985). In health promotion, empowerment exists along a continuum—from personal through community organization to political action (Labonte, 1986). Therefore it is as empowering for an individual to join a smoking cessation program and succeed at quitting smoking as it is for an organization taking action to prohibit cigarette advertising in its local community.

Within the empowerment model of health promotion, however, Becker (1986) cautions that health may become a moral imperative. The pursuit of health may become more important than the pursuit of any other values, including distributive justice. Pursuit of health alone can then encourage the growth of narcissistic, atomistic communities. As the dominant value, health may become more important, particularly to the individual, than seeking opportunities for more vulnerable members of society to attain it.

Community Participation

Community participation is also called public participation, and, while an evolving concept subject to numerous interpretations, it may be defined concretely as: "a group of people living in the same defined area sharing the same basic values and organization," or abstractly as "a group of people sharing the same basic interests" (Rifkin, Muller, & Bichman, 1988, p. 933).

McKnight (1986) highlights the sense of connectedness among members of a community in describing its characteristics: (1) capacity oriented, as opposed to the deficiency approach of traditional health care professionals; (2) informal, which often is perceived by professionals as being disordered, messy, and inefficient; (3) rich in stories that "allow people to reach back into their common history and their individual experience for knowledge about truth and direction for the future" (these stories are often ignored and even threatened by professionals who want "communities to count up things rather than communicate"); and (4) as having incorporated celebration, tragedy, and fallibility "into the life of the community" (p. 58).

The emphasis health promotion puts on the community is explicitly political, in that the community becomes a mediating structure between the domain of everyday life of individuals (micro-level) and the larger social/political/economic context within which individuals live (macro-level). Capacity is built as communities increase their abilities to participate in economic and political decisions, thereby enhancing the health of all communities (McKnight, 1990).

If one intervenes in the community to explicitly promote health as a common good, as envisioned by the emancipatory communitarian approach, the health care professional must balance the moral values of both self-determination and distributive justice (promoting the fair and equitable allocation of bargaining powers, resources, and obligations in society) (Bell, 1993; Prilleltensky, 1997). One must maintain the balance between individual rights and social responsibilities in the promotion of health for all of society's members. For, within a community-based model of health promotion, one must guard against a "tyranny of the community," in that not all communities are just and fair. In an oppressive community, such as in the early days of the United States or in the Middle Ages, large numbers of groups are excluded from shaping the social goods and values (Shapiro, 1995). Additionally, stronger communities may oppress weaker ones (Prilleltensky & Gonick, 1996). Health care professionals must consider under what conditions individuals should sacrifice their personal uniqueness for the good of the community, as well as how many resources the community should provide to promote the health of a few.

PROGRAM EVALUATION MODELS FOR HEALTH PROMOTION

Program evaluation, or evaluation research, is the systematic application of social research procedures for assessing the conceptualization, design, implementation, and utility of social intervention and human service programs (Rossi & Freeman, 1993). Program evaluation generally is used for assessing program effectiveness and efficiency, for improving programs and service delivery, and for guiding resource allocation and policy development.

The program evaluation process depends on a program's goals and is embedded in a definition of health promotion and a unique concept of health. To move from a concept of health to a theory of health promotion and finally to a test of one or more aspects of that model in an operating program, one must be able to measure key constructs.

Health may be measured subjectively (from the person's or community's own experience or sense of feeling "well," "in touch," or "empowered"). Yet, health also may be measured objectively (e.g., measuring resting heart rate or muscular strength). The data derived from interviews with clients or listening to their stories may be combined with data obtained from physical measures of client physiologic functioning, observations of client behavior, or psychometrically sound assessments of the client's attitudes, beliefs, and behaviors. These two types of measures may refine one another to create a more perfect picture of health.

The experience of health may vary both within and among clients. Yet, consensus has developed around the use of several general instruments to measure health among individual clients—conceptualized as a healthy quality of life. One of the more widely used and translated instruments, the Short Form Health Survey (SF-36), addresses six factors in measuring healthy quality of life: mental, physical, social, role, general health perceptions, and symptoms (Fylkesnes & Forde, 1992; McHorney, Ware, & Raczek, 1993; Ware & Sherbourne, 1992). The instrument is comprised of a series of questions, is easy to administer, and is comprehensible. Its psychometric, or measurement, properties are known and highly regarded.

Program evaluation, as an assessment of the processes and effects of a health promotion program and/or its components, begins with setting an evaluation agenda, including examining health promotion models and the program focus and design. The agenda generally is set in consideration of or in conjunction with those who will use the research and those who will be affected by it. Next, the research is formulated, planned, and implemented. As with other forms of social research, this process is systematic to ensure maximal construct validity (a strong relationship between the constructs and their measures) and/or reliability (constancy or consistency of measures over time, place, and person). Finally, the results are disseminated so that they may be used for program change. Generally, the findings are shared with key decision makers and/or client groups.

Within this general framework, the health care professional may adopt one of the following four main models of evaluation, each of which implies a different understanding of the relationship between the program and its stakeholders (those with interest in the program's processes and effects). The four models are (1) evaluation as synonymous with applied research; (2) evaluation as part of systems management, as an aid to program administration; (3) professional judgement; and (4) evaluation-as-politics (Smith & Glass, 1987). Each is discussed in turn.

Evaluation as Social Research

The first model considers evaluation as a form of social research, with the concommitant use of the scientific method, either from a positivist or a constructivist tradition. The positivist scientific tradition assumes relationships within causal models. For example, the impacts of an intervention to reduce smoking among adolescents ("the cause") are assessed relative to the "effects" on quit rates. Program goals are well-specified and measureable. Rigorously designed comparative studies, true field experiments, randomized clinical trials, and quasi-experiments are implemented. Methodologic rigor, including both internal validity—in testing for causality—and external validity—or the generalizeability of the evaluation—are critical. The evaluation is primarily summative (conducted at the outcome of the effort), comparative, and quantitative. Program success is judged relative to a comparison group in an experimentally controlled setting.

A constructivist tradition, as a part of ethnomethodology, focuses on person's lived experiences, with those experiences understood as being located in a particular sociohistorical context. In this methodology, the evaluator is a research instrument himself/herself and produces a type of narrative, text, or case report for the evaluation (Schwandt, 1990). For example, in a study of programs to increase community empowerment, the evaluator uses focus groups, intensive interviewing, and case studies. The evaluator is seeking to understand the multiple discourses on how people experience becoming healthy (Labonte & Robertson, 1996; Marlett, 1994). The evaluation may be either formative (provides information before the program is complete) or summative and qualitative. Program success is judged by criteria developed by the stakeholders and/or relative to other similar programs.

Evaluation as a Contributor to Systems Management

The second model incorporates evaluation into systems management, with the organization being an interrelated set of inputs, processes, and outputs. The evaluator describes these system parts and relates them to each other, relative to the stated goals. The program manager can then make decisions to regulate and improve the functions of the system. Research methods include program audits, performance appraisal, goal attainment, scaling, cost analyses, and client satisfaction surveys. The evaluator is interested in the level of attainment on performance indicators of the given goals and in discrepancies between the stated objectives and performance (Thompson, 1992). The evaluation tends to be formative, in that information is conveyed to program administrators during the assessment process and is produced in a technically proficient manner.

Evaluation by Professional Judgment

A third model, professional judgement, considers experts to be the appropriate persons to make judgements about the quality of a program. This model is found in accreditation approaches and assumes that peer review is objective, reliable, and valid. The experts' methods include direct observation, often using checklists and interviews with clients. The experts judge the program data against established standards, and program administrators and others in the profession generally are the audience for the evaluation. Other groups with an interest in the evaluation generally are not considered.

Evaluation-as-Politics

Evaluation-as-politics, the fourth general model, highlights the proposition that evaluation and politics are inextricably intertwined. Evaluation studies are not directed simply toward one decision-maker but at all major stakeholders who play a role in maintaining, modifying, or eliminating the program. In the evaluation-as-politics approach each program has stakeholders and active partisans competing with each other for a greater share of authority over resources and social affairs. "At every stage, evaluation is only one ingredient in an inherently political process" (Rossi & Freeman, 1993, p. 417). The model uses a variety of methodologic approaches, from controlled experiments to naturalistic case studies. Different reports or presentations are prepared for different audiences. The credible evaluation report is comprehensible, correct, complete, and reasonable to partisans on all sides (Cronbach, 1982).

Summary

The numerous health promotion models explored in this chapter differ in their view of health—the outcome they wish to describe or explain. Each varies in its intended target, whether micro (individuals, groups, families) or macro (communities or aggregates). Further, the moral values implied by the cross-cutting constructs of empowerment and community suggest different uses of these theoretical approaches. Each question asked about the process and outcome of health promotion calls for a different evaluation model and measurement approach.

As the health care professional works with the client to move from an image of health to its internalization, these models of how change occurs and how to assess these variations will guide the intervention.

References

Ajzen, I., & Fishbein, M. (1980). *Understanding attitudes and predicting social behavior.* Englewood Cliffs, NJ: Prentice Hall.

Aldwin, C., & Stokols, D. (1988). The effects of environmental change on individuals and groups: Some neglected issues in stress research. *Journal of Environmental Psychology, 8,* 57-75.

Backett, K.C., & Davison, C. (1995). Lifecourse and lifestyle: The social and cultural location of health behaviors. *Social Science and Medicine, 40*(5), 629-638.

Baer, J.S., & Lichtenstein, E. (1988). Cognitive assessment. In D.M. Donovan & G.A. Marlatt (Eds.), *Assessment of addictive behaviors* (pp. 189-213). New York: Guilford Press.

Bandura, A. (1986). *Social foundations of thoughts and actions.* Englewood Cliffs, NJ: Prentice Hall.

Becker, M. (1986). The tyranny of health promotion. *Public Health Review, 14,* 15-23.

Becker, M.H., Drachman, R.H., & Kirscht, J.P. (1974). A new approach to explaining sick-role behavior in low-income populations. *American Journal of Public Health, 64,* 205-216.

Becker, M.H., & Janz, N.K. (1987). On the effectiveness and utility of health hazard/ health risk appraisal in clinical and nonclinical settings. *Health Services Research, 22,* 532-551.

Bell, D. (1993). *Communitarianism and its critics.* Oxford, England: Clarendon.

Borgatta, E.F., Bulcroft, K., Montgomery, R.J.V., & Bulcroft, R. (1990). Health promotion over the life course: Strategies for effective action, I. The historical and social context. *Research on Aging, 12*(3), 373-388.

Cannon, W.B. (1932). The wisdom of the body. New York: Norton.

Cousins, E. (1987). Jewish spirituality: From the sixteenth-century revival to the present. In A. Green, (Ed.). *World spirituality: An encyclopedic history of the religious quest.* (Vol. 14). (pp. ix-x) New York: Crossroad.

Cronbach, L.J. (1982). *Designing evaluations of educational and social programs.* San Francisco: Jossey-Bass.

Curry, S.J., & Emmons, K.M. (1994). Theoretical models for predicting and improving compliance with breast cancer screening. *Annals of Behavioral Medicine, 16*(4), 302-316.

Delbecq, A.L. (1978). The social political process of introducing innovation in human services. In R. Sarri & Y. Hasenfeld (Eds.), *The management of human services* (pp. 309-39). New York: Columbia University Press.

Devins, G.M. (1992). Social cognitive analysis of recovery from a lapse after smoking cessation: Comment on Haaga and Stewart. *Journal of Consulting and Clinical Psychology, 60* (1), 29-31.

DiClemente, C.C. (1991). Motivational interviewing and the stages of change. In W. Miller & S. Rollnick (Eds.), *Motivational interviewing* (pp. 191-203). New York: Guilford Press.

Downie, R.S., Fyfe, C. & Tannahill, A. (1990). *Health promotion: models and values.* Oxford, England: Oxford University Press.

Elder, J.P., Schmid, T.L., Dower, P., & Hedlund, S. (1993). Community heart health programs: Components, rationale, and strategies for effective interventions. *Journal of Public Health Policy, 13*(4), 463-479.

Emery, F.E., & Trist, E.L. (1972). *Towards a social ecology: Contextual appreciations of the future in the present.* London: Plenum Press.

Fawcet, S.B., Paine-Andrews, A., Francisco, V.T., Schultz, J.A., Richter, K.B., Lewis, R.K., Williams, E.L., Harris, K.J., Berkley, J.Y., Fisher, J.L., & Lopez, C.M. (1995). Using empowerment theory in collaborative partnerships for community health and development. *American Journal of Community Psychology, 23*(5), 677-697.

Fincham, S. (1992). Community health promotion programs. *Social Science and Medicine, 35*(3), 239-249.

Fishbein, M., Jaccard, J.J., Davidson, A.R., Ajzen, I., & Loken, B. (1980). Predicting and understanding family planning behaviors: Beliefs, attitudes, and intentions. In I. Ajzen & M. Fishbein (Eds.), *Understanding attitudes and predicting social behavior* (pp. 131-147). Englewood Cliffs, NJ: Prentice Hall.

Fisher, E.B., Bishop, D.B., Goldmuntz, J., & Jacobs, A. (1988). Implications for the practicing physician of the psychosocial dimensions of smoking. *Chest, 38,* 194-212.

Fortmann, S.P., Flora, J.A., Winkleby, M.A., Schooler, C., Taylor, C.B., & Farquhar, J.W. (1995). Community intervention trials: Reflections on the Stanford Five-City Project experience. *American Journal of Epidemiology, 142,* 576-586.

Fylkesnes, K., & Forde, H. (1992). Determinants and dimensions involved in self-evaluation of health, *Social Science and Medicine, 35*(3), 271-279.

Green, L. (1979). *Health education today and the PRECEDE framework.* Palo Alto, CA: Mayfield Publishing Co.

Green, L., & Krueter, M.W. (1990). *Health promotion planning: An educational and environmental approach* (2nd ed.). Palo Alto, CA: Mayfield Publishing Co.

Gutiérrez, L. (1990). Working with women of color: An empowerment perspective. *Social Work, 35,* 149-154.

Hawley, A.H. (1950). *Human ecology: A theory of community structure.* New York: Ronald Press.

Hayes, M. (1992). On the epistemology of risk: Language, logic and social science. *Social Science in Medicine, 35*(4), 401-407.

Hutchison, G.B. (1969). Evaluation of preventive services. In H.C. Schulberg, A. Sheldon, & F. Baker (Eds.). *Program evaluation in the health fields* (Vol. 1, pp. 59-72). New York: Human Sciences Press.

Janis, I.L., & Mann, L. (1977). *Decision making: A psychological analysis of conflict, choice and commitment.* New York: The Free Press.

Janz, N.K., & Becker, M.H. (1984). The health belief model: A decade later. *Health Education Quarterly, 11,* 1-47.

Job, R.F.S. (1988). Effective and ineffective use of fear in health promotion campaigns. *American Journal of Public Health, 78,* 163-167.

Judd, C.M., Smith, E.K., & Kidder, L.H. (1991). *Research methods in social relations* (6th ed.). New York: Holt, Rinehart & Winston.

Kahneman, D., & Tversky, A. (1984). Choices, values, and frames. *American Psychologist, 39*(4), 341-350.

Karasek, R. & Thorell, T. (Eds.). (1990). *Healthy work: Stress, productivity, and the reconstruction of working life.* New York: Basic Books.

Katz, D., & Kahn, R.L. (1966). *The social psychology of organizations.* New York: Wiley.

Kazdin, A.E. (1994). *Behavior modification in applied settings.* (5th ed.). Pacific Grove, CA: Brooks/Cole.

Kekes, J. (1993). *The morality of pluralism.* Princeton, NJ: Princeton University Press.

Kelly, J.A., St. Lawrence, J.S., Stevenson, L.Y., Houth, A.C., Kuliehman, A.C., Diaz, Y.E., Brasfield, T.L., Koob, J.J., & Morgan, M.G. (1992). Community AIDS/HIV risk reduction: The effects of endorsements by popular people in three cities. *American Journal of Public Health, 2,* 1483-1489.

Kotler, P., & Roberto, E. (1989). *Social marketing: Strategies for changing public behavior.* New York: Free Press.

Kotter, P., & Roberts, E. (1989). *Social marketing: Strategies for changing public behavior.* New York: Free Press.

Labonte, R. (1986). Social inequality and healthy public policy. *Health Promotion, 1*(3), 341-351.

Labonte, R., & Robertson, A. (1996). Delivering our goods, showing our stuff: The case for a constructivist paradigm for health promotion research and practice. *Health Education Quarterly, 23*(4), 431-447.

Leavell, H.R., & Clark, E.G. (1953). *Textbook of preventive medicine,* New York: McGraw-Hill.

Lefebvre, R.C., Lasater, T.M., Carleton, R.A., & Peterson, G. (1987). Theory and delivery of health programming in the community: The Pawtucket Heart Health Program. *Preventive Medicine, 16,* 80-95.

Lewin, K., Dembo, T., Festinger, L et al. (1944) Level of aspiration. In J. Hunt (Ed.), *Personality and the behavioral disorders: A handbook based on experimental and clinical research* (pp. 333-78). New York: Ronald Press.

Lilienfeld, A.M. (1976). *Foundations of epidemiology.* New York: Oxford University Press.

Maccoby, N., Farquhar, J.W., Wood, P.D., & Alexander, J. (1977). Reducing the risk of cardiovascular disease: Effects of a community-based campaign on knowledge and behavior. *Journal of Community Health, 3,* 100-114.

Maiman, L.A., & Becker, M.H. (1984). The Health Belief Model: Origins and correlates in psychological theory. In M.H. Becker (Ed.). *The Health Belief Model and personal health behavior* (pp. 9-26). Thorofare, NJ: Charles B. Slack.

Manoff, R.K. (1985). *Social marketing: Imperative for public health*. New York: Praeger.

Marlett, N. (1994). *Partnerships and communication in health promotion research*. Paper presented at the Third Annual Health Promotion Research Conference, Calgary, Alberta, Canada.

Maruyama, M. (1963). The second cybernetics: Decision-amplifying mutual causal processes. *American Scientist, 51*, 164-179.

McGraw, S.A., Stone, E.J., Osganian, S.K., Elder, J.P., Perry, C.L., Johnson, C.C., Parcel, G.S., Webber, L.S. & Luepker, R.V. (1994). Design of process evaluation within the Child and Adolescent Trial for Cardiovascular Health (CATCH). *Health Education Quarterly*, (Suppl. 2), S5-26.

McGinnis, J.M., & Foege, W.H. (1994). Actual causes of death in the United States. *JAMA, 270*, 2207.

McGuire, W. (1981). Theoretical foundations of campaigns. In R.E. Rice & W.J. Paisley (Eds.), *Public communication campaigns* (pp. 41-70). Beverly Hills, CA: Sage.

McHorney, C.A., Ware, J.E., Raczek, A.E. (1993). The MOS 36-Item Short-Form health survey (SF-36): Psychometric and clinical tests of validity in measuring physical and mental constructs. *Medical Care, 31*, 247-263.

McKnight, J.L. (1986). Well-being: The new threshold of the old medicine. *Health Promotion, 1*, 77-80.

McKnight, J. (1990). Politicizing health care. In P. Conrad & R. Kern (Eds.), *The sociology of health and illness: Critical perspectives*. New York: St. Martins Press.

Meyerowitz, B.E., & Chaiken, S. (1987). The effect of message framing on breast self-examination attitudes, intentions, and behavior. *Journal of Personality and Social Psychology, 52*(3), 500-510.

Moos, R.H. (1979). Social ecological perspectives on health. In G.C. Stone, F. Cohen, & N.E. Adler (Eds.), *Health psychology: A handbook* (pp. 523-547). San Francisco: Jossey-Bass.

Miller, M. (1985). *Turning problems into actionable issues*. Organize Training Center. Unpublished report.

Parse, R. (1987). *Nursing science: Major paradigms, theories and critiques*. Philadelphia: WB Saunders.

Pelletier, K.R. (1984). *Healthy people in unhealthy places: Stress and fitness at work*. New York: Dell.

Pender, N. (1996). *Health promotion in nursing practice*. Stamford, CT: Appleton & Lange.

Prilleltensky, I. (1997). Values, assumptions, and practices: Assessing the moral implications of psychological discourse and action. *American Psychologist, 52*(5), 517-535.

Prilleltensky, I., & Gonick, L. (1996). Politics change, oppression remains: On the psychology and practice of oppression. *Political Psychology, 17*, 127-147.

Prochaska, J.O., & DiClemente, C.C. (1983). Stages and processes of self-change of smoking: Toward an integrative model. *Journal of Consulting and Clinical Psychology, 51*, 390-395.

Prochaska, J.O., Velicer, W.F., Gaudagnoli, E., Rossi, J.S., & DiClemente, C.C. (1991). Patterns of change: Dynamic typology applied to smoking cessation. *Multivariate Behavioral Research, 26*, 83-107.

Rachlin, H. (1991) *Introduction to modern behaviorism* (3rd ed.). San Francisco, CA: Freeman.

Regier, D.A., Boyd, J.H., Burke, J.D., Rae, D.S., Myers, J.K., Kramer, M., Robins, L.N., George, L.K., Karno, M., & Locke, B.Z. (1988). One-month prevalence of mental disorders in the United States: Based on five Epidemiologic Catchment Area Sites. *Archives of General Psychiatry, 45*, 977-985.

Rifken, S.B., Muller, F., & Bichman, W. (1988). Primary health care: On measuring participation. *Social Science in Medicine, 29*, 931-940.

Rogers, E. (1983). *Diffusion of innovation*. New York: Free Press.

Rosenstock, I.M. (1974). The Health Belief Model and preventive health behavior. In M.H. Becker (Ed.), *The Health Belief Model and personal health behavior* (pp. 27-59). Thorofare, NJ: Charles B. Slack.

Rosenstock, I.M., Strecher, V.J., & Becker, M.H. (1988). Social learning theory and the Health Belief Model. *Health Education Quarterly, 15*(2), 175-183.

Rossi, P.H., & Freeman, I.E. (1993). *Evaluation: A systematic approach* (5th ed.). Newbury Park, CA: Sage.

Salonen, J.T., Tuomilento, J., Nissenen, A., Kaplan, G.A., & Puska, P. (1989). Contributions of risk factor changes to the decline in coronary incidence during the North Karelia project: A within-community analysis. *International Journal of Epidemiology, 18*(3), 595-601.

Schaefer, J.A., & Moos, R.H. (1992). Life crises and personal growth. In B.N. Carpenter (Ed.), *Personal coping: Theory, research, and applications* (pp. 149-170). New York: Praeger.

Schwandt, T. (1990). Paths to inquiry in the social disciplines. In E. Guba (Ed.), *The paradigm dialog.* Newbury Park, CA: Sage.

Shapiro, D. (1995). Liberalism and communitarianism. *Philosophical Books, 36,* 145-155.

Shea, S., & Basch, C.E. (1990). A review of five major community-based cardiovascular disease prevention programs. I. Rationale, design and theoretical framework. *American Journal of Health Promotion, 4,* 203-213.

Sheinfeld Gorin, S. (1982). The adoption and use of performance assessment systems. *Social Work Research and Abstracts, 18*(3), 74-75.

Sheinfeld Gorin, S., & Weirich, T. (1995). Innovation use: Performance assessment in a Community Mental Health Center. *Human Relations, 48*(12), 1427-1453.

Smith, M.L., & Glass, G.V. (1987). *Research and evaluation in education and the social sciences.* Engelwood Cliffs, NJ: Prentice-Hall.

Stamler, J., Wentworth, D., & Neaton, J.D. (1986). Prevalence and prognostic significance of hypercholesterolemia in men with hypertension. Prospective data on the primary screenees of the Multiple Risk Factor Intervention Trial. *American Journal of Medicine, 80*(2A), 33-39.

Stone, E.J. (1991). Comparison of NHLBI community-based cardiovascular research studies. *Journal of Health Education, 22,* 134-136.

Stokols, D. (1992). Establishing and maintaining healthy environments: Toward a social ecology of health promotion. *American Psychologist, 47*(1), 6-22.

The Royal Society. (1983). *Risk assessment: Report of a Royal Society Study Group.* London: The Royal Society.

Thompson, J.C. (1992). Program evaluation within a health promotion framework. *Canadian Journal of Public Health, 83* (Suppl. 1), 567-571.

U.S. Department of Health and Human Services, Public Health Service. (1990). *Promoting health/preventing disease: Objectives for the nation.* Washington, DC: Government Printing Office.

U.S. Department of Health and Human Services, Public Health Service. (1991). *Healthy people 2000: National health promotion and disease prevention objectives* (USDHHS Publication (PHS) No. 91-50213). Washington, DC: Government.

U.S. Preventive Services Task Force. (1996). *Guide to clinical preventive services.* Baltimore, MD: Williams & Wilkins.

Wagner, E.H., Koepsell, T.D., Anderman, C., Cheadle, A., Curry, S.G., Psaty, B.M., Von Korff, M., Wickizer, T.M., Beery, W.L., Diehr, P.K., et al. (1991). The evaluation of the Henry J. Kaiser Family Foundation's Community Health Promotion Grant Program: Design. *Journal of Clinical Epidemiology, 44*(7), 685-699.

Wallerstein, N. (1992). Powerlessness, empowerment, and health: Implications for health promotion programs. *American Journal of Health Promotion, 6*(30), 197-205.

Ware, J.E., & Sherbourne, C.D. (1992). The MOS 36-Item Short Form health survey (SF-36): Conceptual framework and item selection. *Medical Care, 30,* 473-483.

Wilson, D.K., Purdon, S.E., & Wallston, K.A. (1988). Compliance to health recommendations: A theoretical overview of message framing. *Health Education Research, 3*(2), 161-171.

Winett, R.A. (1995). A framework for health promotion and disease prevention programs. *American Psychologist, 50*(5), 341-350.

Winett, R.A., King, A.C., Altman, D.G. (1989). *Health psychology and public health: An integrative approach.* New York: Pergamon Press.

World Health Organization (WHO). (1984). Health promotion: A discussion document on the concepts and principles. *Health Promotion, 1,* 73-76.

World Health Organization (WHO). (1988). *From Alma-Alta to the year 2000: Reflections at midpoint.* Geneva, Switzerland: Author.

Zaltman, G., Kotler, P., & Kaufman, I. (1972). *Creating social change.* New York: Holt, Rinehart & Winston.

Contexts for Health Promotion

Sherri Sheinfeld Gorin

Health promotion between the client and the health care professional emerges within a context of policies, influential groups, and monetary exchanges. Healthy public policy provides the overall framework for health promotion to occur. *Public policy* refers to a general statement by some governmental authority or particular social group that defines an intention to influence the behavior of citizens by the use of positive or negative sanctions (Lowi, 1972; Mayer & Greenwood, 1980). Policy provides both a framework to which practitioners react and a target for advocates to change. Ultimately, through its influence on community norms and values, policy may effect change in client behaviors. This chapter details both the political and economic contexts for health promotion and the unique steps practitioners may use to change these conditions.

THE POLITICAL ECONOMY FRAMEWORK

As introduced in Chapter 2, conceptually, health promotion may be characterized as a political economy (i.e., a political system [a structure of rule] and an economy [a system for producing and exchanging goods and services]) (cf. Wamsley & Zald, 1967; Gargiulo, 1993). In the United States, political support for health promotion is defined by the degree that important actors at the federal, state, and local levels take interest in it, have the power and resources to influence it, and communicate their expectations and demands about it to concerned communities, organizations, groups, health care professionals, families, and individuals.

Political support is often embodied in legislation, such as the Year 2000 Health Objectives Planning Act and regulations borne of that legislation. It may also be reflected in the statements and actions of influential actors, such as accreditors (e.g., the Joint Commission on Health Care Organizations) or important scientific groups (e.g., U.S. Preventive Services Task Force). Finally, policy exists at the organizational level (e.g., the behavior of Boards of Directors).

From the perspective of the health care professional, the major economic actors in the field of health promotion are the varied payers who reimburse for services and programs (e.g., commercial insurance companies) and the general types of health promotive activities they support (e.g., smoking cessation counseling). In Chapter 15, other aspects of the economy of health promotion are explored.

The political economy perspective limits both the contexts and targets for health promotion. Further, while one can separate these contexts conceptually by their major intent or strategy—health or cost reduction—their aims and tactics may overlap. For example, the Surgeon General's *Healthy People 2000* document, while oriented toward health promotive goals, is embedded in a legislative context that emphasizes cost reductions, which are implicit in the suggested preventive actions. Another example is managed care systems, which are designed to reduce costs, in part through the use of preventive services.

POLITICAL CONTEXTS FOR HEALTH PROMOTION

The primary political contexts for health promotion are characterized as legislative (federal, state, local, and international), influential actors, and organizational policy. See Table 3-1 for a summary of the major political influences on health promotion.

Federal Legislation

Traditionally, public health law has been concerned with the protection and preservation of the public health and the processes of administrative regulation and rule-making resulting from the implementation of these aims. Because of its broad statutes, the federal government possesses several powers regarding health care: individuals may be denied the right to decide whether to submit to a medical examination or treatment; the state may collect sensitive health care information about a person or his/her sexual associates; if a disease is contagious, compulsory hospitalization or segregation from the community may be imposed. The government's ability to exercise public health powers requires a delicate balancing of the state's power to act for the community's common good and the individual's rights to liberty, autonomy, and privacy (Gostin, 1986). The inherent tension between these rights and interests has become litigious—most recently in the case of persons with AIDS (acquired immunodeficiency syndrome).

Within the broad context of public health law, federal legislation concerning health promotion has reflected a more sophisticated legal understanding of the scientific bases for the transmission of disease. As such, this legislation has focused on the most efficacious and least intrusive intervention approaches, such as counseling for long-standing, relatively intractable behaviors, such as smoking. Nonetheless, comparatively little omnibus legislation concerned with health promotion (i.e., legislation that addresses health promotion explicitly and comprehensively) was found at either the state or federal levels through a search of the: Congressional Index; the THOMAS system; an Internet listing of recent federal legislative activity; the LEGALTRAK system and *Westlaw,* on-line legal research databases; and the *U.S. Code.* There has been a proliferation of more specific legislation and regulation in health promotive activities, however, such as the federal Nutrition Labeling and Education Act of 1990 and the New Jersey statute requiring every hospital service corporation in the state to provide health promotion programs (N.J. Stat. § 17:48-6i, 1996).

The Nixon Administration created the President's Committee on Health Education in response to decades-long struggles with "the fact (that) the nation does not have the resources, no matter how great a portion of the GNP is allocated to health, to provide sufficient services after the patient becomes ill" (Guinta & Allegrante, 1992). The Committee report recommended the creation of public and private organizations to stimulate, coordinate, and evaluate health education programs. The Administration believed it could preserve the health of Americans, control escalating health care costs, and present

Table **3-1**

Major political influences on health promotion

INFLUENCE	FOCUS	EXAMPLES
Omnibus federal legislation for health promotion	Defined health promotion (hp) Created federal agency Expanded to include recent additions to hp	PL 94-317, National Consumer Health Information and Health Promotion Act of 1976 PL 103-183, The Preventive Health Amendments of 1993
Other nations	Integrates hp into health care system Sets voluntary agreements with industry No omnibus legislation	SFS-1982-763, Swedish Health and Medical Services Act (effective 1/1/83)
State legislation	Specifies laws for tobacco control, safety, nutrition No omnibus legislation for hp	Nutrition, Smoking, and Substance Abuse Acts of 1987
Local legislation	Implements ordinances for protection of public health Specifies laws for tobacco control, food policies No omnibus legislation for hp	New York City Clean Indoor Act, 1988 Contra Costa County Food Policy, March 2, 1993
U.S. Preventive Services Task Force	Reviews evidence of effectiveness for clinical preventive services Issues clinical practice guidelines	*Guide to Clinical Preventive Services*
Federal agencies Department of Health and Human Services	Establishes goals for hp nationally Encourages the development of hp legislation, policies, and programs in the states	*Healthy People 2000* *Healthy People 2000: A Midcourse Review*
Federal Drug Administration	Monitors and assesses specific drugs (especially tobacco)	
U.S. Department of Agriculture	Monitors and assesses nutritional programs (e.g., in schools)	
World health organizations World Health Organization (WHO)	Develops hp policies and programs, especially in Europe Encourages development of national legislation for hp	*Health for All in the Year 2000* policy Healthy Cities Projects

Continued

Table **3-1**

INFLUENCE	FOCUS	EXAMPLES
First International Conference on Health Promotion	Defined aims of hp internationally	*Ottawa Charter for Health Promotion* *Achieving Health for All* (Canada)
Voluntary and professional organizations	Encourage inclusion of hp on national, state, local political agendas; research monies for hp Advocate for hp, hp professionals	American Public Health Association American Cancer Society
Accreditors	Establish standards for hp Monitor and assess compliance with standards	National Commission for Quality Assurance Joint Commission for the Accreditation of Health Care Facilities
Media	Report and examine emerging issues in hp Increase attention to hp	Specialized health columns in newspapers, television news and specials, radio news and talk shows, Internet sites for health
Community advocacy groups and coalitions	Advocate for legislation, policies, monies, political attention to specific hp issues	Mothers Against Drunk Driving Doctors Ought to Care (anti-smoking) Smoking or Health
School districts and schools	Develop, implement, evaluate educational hp programs for children and youth	25 state-required comprehensive school health education programs 75% of local school districts with anti-smoking education in elementary schools
Worksites	Develop, implement, evaluate, consult for cost-effective hp programs to enhance productivity	81% of worksites maintain varied hp activities
Public health departments and health care facilities	Implement public health laws and develop policies Develop, implement, evaluate clinical and population-based, cost-effective hp programs	One half of public health departments provide clinical preventive care Blood pressure measurements, screening tests performed in 75% of all emergency room visits

The table's title banner reads: *Major political influences on health promotion—cont'd* a less costly alternative to national health insurance than was being proposed at the time (Guinta & Allegrante, 1992).

As a result of this initial interest, under President Ford, the National Consumer Health Information and Health Promotion Act of 1976 was the first legislation passed to address health promotion comprehensively. As an amendment to the Public Health Service Act, it established the Office of Consumer Health Education and Promotion and the Center for Health Education and Promotion, and it set forth national goals for health information and promotion and developed a systematic strategy for goal achievement. It also established the federal Office of Disease Prevention and Health Promotion in the Office of the Assistant Secretary for Health to coordinate prevention-related activities of Health and Human Services, to serve as a liaison with the private sector, and to operate a national health information clearinghouse. The Act defined health education and promotion as follows:

> A process that favorably influences understandings, attitudes and conduct, including cultural awareness and sensitivity, in regard to individual and community health. Specifically, it affects and influences individual and community health behavior and attitudes in order to moderate self-imposed risks, maintain and promote physical and mental health and efficiency, and reduce preventable illness, disability, and death (National Consumer Health Information and Health Promotion Act of 1976, p. 15)

The Report of the Senate Committee on Labor and Public Welfare for this Act stressed the influence of "activated patients," who were more involved in decision making, and community programs, specifically in schools and, in conjunction with the Occupational Safety and Health Administration (OSHA), union, and industry initiatives, for worksites. Nutrition to educate the "misnourished"—those who lack the knowledge to choose which foods are best for them—was of particular import to the Committee, as were the role of the media and federal programs to monitor these efforts. The report addressed health education manpower (sic) and asserted the importance of specialists in this area and the critical role nurses, in particular, should continue to play. The report also stressed the need to evaluate the effectiveness of community programs.

This Act was amended by a number of subsequent acts, including most recently, the Preventive Health Amendments of 1993 (Table 3-2). These amendments address breast and cervical cancer screening, injury prevention, prevention and control of sexually transmitted diseases, and production of biennial reports on nutrition and health. The most current omnibus legislation reflects the enormous recent influence advocates for women's health—particularly in breast cancer prevention—and AIDS advocates have had on the legislative process, as well as continued congressional legislative interest in nutrition.

No omnibus health promotion legislation has been enacted recently, despite a flurry of health legislation introduced in the 103rd Congress during 1993 and 1994, including a campaign to pass The Health Security Act—a comprehensive proposal from the Clinton administration with prevention at its core. The most current legislation concerned with health promotion and disease prevention programs addresses the implementation of recommended preventive health care services contained in the *Guide to Clinical Preventive Services* (USPSF, 1996) and the Year 2000 objectives of the Public Health Service (i.e., H.R. 177, *Comprehensive Preventive Health and Promotion Act of 1997*).

State Legislation

Public health law consonant with the federal statutes, particularly to impede the spread of infectious and venereal diseases, is found in all states (Gostin, 1986). Further, State Year

Table 3-2

Selected health promotion legislation

COMMON NAME	PUBLIC LAW NUMBER	CODE AND SECTION NUMBERS
National Consumer Health Information and Health Promotion Act of 1976	PL 94-317, Title I	42 U.S.C. § 300u et seq.
The Disease Prevention and Health Promotion Act of 1978*	PL 95-626, Section I	42 U.S.C. § 201 note, 247 et seq.
Health Promotion and Disease Prevention Amendments of 1984	PL 98-551	21 U.S.C. § 360bb et seq.
Consolidated Omnibus Budget Reconciliation Act of 1985	PL 99-272, Title IX	42 U.S.C. § 210 et seq.
Public Health Service Amendments of 1987	PL 100-177 and	42 U.S.C. § 242a et seq.
	PL 101-239	42 U.S.C. § 11111 et seq.
The Year 2000 Health Objectives Planning Act, 1990	PL 101-582	42 U.S.C. § 246 note and Title I, § 105 et seq.
The Health Information, Health Promotion, and Vaccine Injury Compensation Amendments of 1991	PL 102-168	42 U.S.C. § 300aa et seq.
Preventive Health Amendments of 1992	PL 102-531	42 U.S.C. § 236 et seq.
Preventive Health Amendments of 1993	PL 103-183	42 U.S.C. § 233 et seq.

NOTE: The above legislation was published in the *U.S. Code* in 1994.
*Current version at 42 USC § 201 note, 247b, 247c, 300u-5 (1994).

2000 plans, which often provide frameworks for state health promotion programs and may include population-based data, health status objectives, outcomes measures, and public health strategies (e.g., Florida's Healthy Communities, Healthy People Act of 1996) exist in 41 states and 2 territories. Seventy percent of local health departments use the plan as a framework for other initiatives (U.S. Department of Health and Human Services [USDHHS], 1995). There is no omnibus state legislation comparable to that at the federal level concerning health promotion, perhaps, in part, because sections of federal legislation limit state actions. Specific state legislation that addresses aspects of health promotion, such as tobacco control, safety, (e.g., the use of seat belts in cars and bicycle helmets), and nutrition, has passed. Because state legislation focuses on specific aspects of health promotion, unique political contexts can be found among different constituencies, even though desired outcomes may be similar. For instance smoking control has emerged as important in both state and local legislation, and all 50 states now require safety restraints for young children (National Highway Traffic Safety Administration, 1988). In addition, nutrition counseling is found in numerous state statutes, particularly in programs for birth center clients or teenage mothers and their families (e.g., Iowa's Nutrition, Smoking and Substance Abuse Act of 1987; Rhode Island's Health Care Act for Children and Pregnant Women of 1993; and the Tennessee Resource Mother's Program Acts [1992]).

Local Legislation

Numerous city governments, including New York, Los Angeles, San Francisco, and Houston, have instituted legislation concerning the protection of public health, particularly laws dealing with infectious and venereal diseases (Gostin, 1986). More than 1238 cities, as well as numerous localities, have passed laws regarding tobacco control (Shelton, & Frank, 1995). For example, more than 150 cities have enacted legislation or regulations restricting smoking in public places (e.g., New York City Clean Indoor Air Act, 1988). Nutrition, too, has been a focus of local municipalities. For example, the Contra Costa County (Northern California) municipality adopted a food policy requiring that healthful food that conforms to the U.S. dietary guidelines (1992) be served at all government functions (Cortes, Steeples, & Stone, 1995).

Other Nations.

In other nations, too, specific legislation has been proposed to address health threats such as air pollution and smoking. Unlike the United States, however, many European countries have not regarded omnibus legislation on health promotion necessary because health promotion activities are integrated into the health care system and many general Health Acts already make health care professionals responsible for health promotion and health education (Leenen, Pinet, & Prims, 1985). The Swedish Health and Medical Services Act, for example, emphasizes preventive activities and states that all forms of health and medical care are expected to include information and health education. In other cases, the limited role of legislation in advancing health promotion is a result of ethical issues concerning the control of personal behavior and life-style. In the case of some eastern European countries, turbulent political changes have impeded any unified legislative movement on health promotion. Further, many countries rely on voluntary agreements with industry, thus limiting the role of national government (Roemer, 1982, 1986; World Health Organization, 1988).

Beyond Europe, countries have either focused on specific targets in legislation (e.g.,

Australia) or have supported policy documents similar to those of the World Health Organization (e.g., Singapore), without accompanying legislation. In Australia, tobacco has received considerable attention through statuatory and judicial edicts, such as restrictions and prohibitions in the marketing and advertising of the product (Reynolds, 1994). In Singapore, health promotion has been proposed as a solution to some of the major health problems and has been expressed in national health policy (Chern, 1996).

INFLUENTIAL ACTORS

The most influential actors in the health promotion field include the U.S. Preventive Services Task Force, selected federal agencies, world health agencies, voluntary and professional organizations, accreditors, the media, and community advocacy groups and coalitions.

U.S. Preventive Services Task Force

The U.S. Preventive Services Task Force (USPSTF) was established by the U.S. Public Health Service in 1984. It is an independent panel of mostly nonfederal experts and physicians that uses a systematic methodology to review the evidence for the effectiveness of clinical preventive services (e.g., screening tests, counseling interventions, immunizations, chemoprophylaxis); assigns ratings to the quality of the data; and issues clinical practice recommendations reflecting the strength of the supporting evidence (Woolf, Jonas, & Lawrence, 1996). The Task Force has collaborated with medical specialties, as well as with its Canadian counterparts, in its deliberations. The Task Force has assessed 60 topic areas and published the *Guide to Clinical Preventive Services* in 1989. Most recently, it published the *Guide to Clinical Preventive Services* (USPSTF, 1996). The 1996 guide accompanies the Centers for Disease Prevention and Control's (CDC) *Prevention Guidelines* (Friede, O'Carroll, Nicola, Oberle, & Teutsch, 1997).

According to the Task Force, the most effective interventions available are those that address the personal health practices of patients. Talking is emphasized over testing, and changing the self-efficacy (the client's perceived ability to undertake a behavior) is central. The group encourages health care professionals to adopt a risk assessment approach to clinical practice, including assessing the factors that predispose a client to disease. The approach includes using the history and physical and laboratory examinations in a risk factor–oriented, rather than an illness- or a symptom-focused, manner. The health care professional is encouraged to address the seriousness of the target condition; its relative frequency; the accuracy with which it may be detected; the effectiveness of current interventions with the target condition; and the relative priority the client places on the target condition, as compared to the client's other concerns.

In practice, health care professionals are varied in their use of counseling—one of the Task Force's major recommendations to change client behaviors. The use of counseling has varied from 53% of the time in one recent study of clients with chronic disease in primary care (Russell & Roter, 1993) to 90% in an effort by physicians to promote exercise among clients older than 40 years (Royals, Chitwood, Davis, & Cole, 1996). Many health care professionals are uncertain in general about the effectiveness of counseling to reduce risks and are unsure of how to counsel. In practice, the effectiveness of counseling varies widely, with health care professionals somewhat more successful with clients desiring smoking control and weight reduction and somewhat less successful with changing the behaviors of older clients. Additionally, although 14.9% of all visits to physician offices are primarily for diagnostic, screening, and preventive activities (USDHHS, National Center for Health Statistics, Advance Data, August 18, 1994, as cited in Health Insurance Association of America, 1996), physicians find counseling time-consuming and difficult to track and to charge; thus physician time for counseling clients about health promotion is relatively short, often from 2 to 6 minutes (Mullen & Holcomb, 1990; Kushner, 1995; Ockene, Ockene, Quirk, Hebert et al., 1995; Patton, Kolasa, West, & Irons, 1995; Burton, et al., 1995; Price, Clause, & Everett, 1995; Schectman, Stoy, & Elinsky, 1994; Thompson, Schwankovsky, & Pitts, 1993; Ammerman, DeVellis, Carey, Keyserling et al., 1993; Cushman, James, & Waclawik, 1991; Logsdon, Lazaro, & Meier, 1989). Given these "real world" considerations in practice settings, the influence of the Task Force on health care professionals may be enhanced through the implementation of its recommendations during their training.

Selected Federal Agencies

Although health promotion policies are housed in several federal agencies, only the actions of the Surgeon General and the Centers for Disease Control and Prevention, which are under the Department of Health and Human Services (DHHS) and the Public Health Service are described briefly in this text. Other federal agencies responsible for health promotion are the Food and Drug Administration (whose recent efforts to regulate tobacco as a drug have been highly influential); the U.S. Department of Labor, Occupational, Safety and Health Administration (whose guidelines on workplace violence and initiatives in ergonomics have been important recently); the U.S. Department of Agriculture (which is particularly influential through the food stamps program for low-income Americans, the Special Supplemental Nutrition Program for Women, Infants and Children [WIC], and child nutrition programs); and the Environmental Protection Agency (which is particularly influential on enforcing the removal of toxic wastes, including recent efforts regarding toxic air pollution and the monitoring of pesticide use). In the case of the Surgeon General, the *Healthy People 2000* document prepared under its auspices, has had an unprecedented influence on the health promotion field because of the extent of participation that the health care community had in its preparation, because of its credibility, and because of the form and the content of its text.

The Surgeon General's Reports, begun in 1979, grew out of a health strategy devoted to the prevention of unnecessary disease and disability and the achievement of a better quality of life for all. In that year, *Healthy People: The Surgeon General's Report on Health Promotion and Disease Prevention* (1979) was published. The document originally was heralded as part of the "second public health revolution."

The first public health revolution. The first "public health revolution" began with the watershed 1848 *Public Health Act* in Britain, and from that point forward, the principles of state intervention in the lives of individuals to promote an outcome deemed of primary social value were established. In particular, the nineteenth century revolution sought to improve the social and physical environment to decrease traditional health hazards.

The Act, as well as the two that preceded it (the English Towns Improvement Act of 1847 and the Liverpool Sanitary Act of 1846), provided a remedy for particular problems, designated "nuisances," and allowed public authorities to order their removal. These "nuisances" were largely seen as things that smelled offensively, imparting the "miasmatic" idea that bad smells were a sign of disease. The Act authorized the undertaking of public health works, such as controls over slaughter houses, common lodging houses, and offensive trades. It contained building requirements for all new houses to be built with drains that connected to sewage systems where possible or to a cesspit. It also created a public health structure: a General Board of Health, which functioned as a national public health authority, and Local Boards of Health, which consisted of supervisors of local surveyors and inspectors of nuisances. Responsibility for sewers was vested in the local boards, which had powers to control and cleanse (Reynolds, 1994).

The second public health revolution. The second public health revolution, reflected in the Surgeon General's 1979 document, heralded the importance of life-style changes to health promotion, as well as the importance of reducing chronic disease. Early criticisms of the 1979 document and the "second public health revolution" were myriad (Neubauer & Pratt, 1981; Tesh, 1981). These criticisms focused on the importance attached to individual life-style change rather than on alterations in the social and economic factors that determine health. While the 1979 document recognized social and economic conditions as significant factors in determining health, it failed to specify this recognition in its policy recommendations. Instead, it placed the burden of change on individual behavior, attributing as much as 70% of ill health to individual life-style (Neubauer & Pratt, 1981). The life-style hypothesis of the 1979 document approaches disease as though ill health is the result of personal failure—a "victim blaming" strategy—rather than placing the cause and "solution" to disease in larger social and economic contexts (Navarro, 1976). The community response to this strategy was considerable, and concommitant changes in the health promotion field led to changes in subsequent publications by the Surgeon General.

The document was expanded in 1980 with the *Promoting Health/Preventing Disease: Objectives for the Nation.* This document was followed by *Healthy People 2000* (USDHHS, 1991) and most recently, *Healthy People 2000: Midcourse Review and 1995 Revisions* (USDHHS, 1995).

The *Healthy People 2000* (USDHHS, 1991) document provides a plan of action for the nation's health, with strategies to increase the proportion of Americans who live long and healthy lives by increasing life spans, reducing health disparities, and expanding access to preventive services. As did its forerunners, it used a Management by Objectives approach, with federal agencies taking charge of each of the 22 priority areas and the goals, objectives, and strategies for change within each area. The 22 priority areas are grouped into three broad categories: health promotion, health protection, and preventive services. Health promotion strategies are those related to individual life-style—personal choices made in a social context—that can have a powerful influence over one's health prospects (USDHHS, 1991). Health protection strategies refer to environmental and regulatory measures conferring protection on large population groups. Preventive services include counseling, screening, immunization, and chemoprophylactic interventions for individuals in clinical settings. Surveillance and data systems, as well as recommendations for each of four age groups, are found throughout the priority areas. The recent changes in the document reflect somewhat less attention given to life-style changes, although they still predominate, particularly in some relatively narrow goals for health promotion.

The Centers for Disease Control and Prevention also is unique in the measure of its influence on the health promotion field because it is one of the few (and the oldest) agencies devoted to the singular mission of promoting health and quality of life, by preventing and controlling disease, injury, and disability (the Office of Disease Prevention and Health Promotion is another). Through its 11 centers, institutes, and offices, it holds stewardship for a wide range of activities, including environmental health; infectious disease (e.g., human immunodeficiency virus [HIV], sexually transmitted disease [STD], and tuberculosis [TB]) prevention; injury prevention and control; occupational safety and health; the national immunization program; epidemiology; and health statistics. Its scope is international and ranges from the review of privatization efforts to work with state and local health agencies. Few health promotion efforts fall outside its auspices.

World Health Organizations

A variety of health agencies, ministries, and municipalities—both international and country-specific—have addressed health promotion. In particular, however, the World Health Organization (WHO) has implemented the *Health For All* policy, which, for the first time, views health as a resource for living. Another document, *European Health for All,* which is similar in intent to *Healthy People 2000,* embodies 38 regional targets within six themes: (1) a focus on primary health care; (2) the emphasis of the health care system should be on the promotion of health and the prevention of disease; (3) effective cooperation should involve all sectors of government and society; (4) a well-informed, motivated, and actively participating community is a key element to attain common goals; (5) international cooperation should be strengthened as health problems transcend national frontiers; and (6) present health inequalities should be reduced as far as possible (WHO, 1985). Equity is a key concern of *European Health for All;* the principles assert that people must be given social and economic opportunities to maintain and develop their health. Unlike *Healthy People 2000,* which is primarily concerned with life-style changes, more than one half of the *Health for All* targets require changes in legislation (Pinet, 1986).

European member states of the World Health Organization, formed in 1948 as a part of the United Nations, collectively adopted the *Health for All for the Year 2000,* a major policy document in various WHO fora. These same member states agreed to be monitored on their progress toward attainment of the strategy. Some member states are strengthening their national laws to bring them into harmony with *Health for All for the Year 2000.*

In general, however, the member states' commitment to *Health for All* has been patchy, with only moderate success toward meeting the regional targets. Poor progress is attributed to changes in national and international political and economic circumstances and to limited resources, but perhaps most importantly to a lack of political will to take the strategy seriously (Rathwell, 1992). Further, the strategy pays little attention to China and other Asian Pacific countries, where smoking, in particular, has burgeoned.

Healthy cities. The WHO European Regional Office to the Healthy Cities Project has fostered the development of Healthy Cities Projects worldwide, particularly in Europe. The project stresses a municipal approach to health promotion through extensive community participation, intersectoral cooperation, and the implementation of comprehensive city plans for health promotion. The Healthy Cities Projects began in Canada in 1984, and the WHO European Healthy Cities Project was initiated in 1986. The project has expanded through Europe, as well as other French- and Spanish-speaking regions of the world and the Asian Pacific region (e.g., Australia, Japan, New Zealand) and in an increasing number of developing countries (e.g., Iran and Ghana). There are about 200 Healthy Cities and Communities in the United States. Many of these projects are still in the implementation phase. Internationally, the support of national funding sources (e.g., the Finnish National Development and Research Center) and municipal public health administrators (e.g., the Association of Municipalities in the Netherlands, VNG) has been critically important to the Healthy Cities undertakings. Internationally and in the United States, universities have served as important resources for the effort. Many of the projects have not yet begun the evaluation phase, by measuring either the disease-prevention endpoints of morbidity and mortality or the health-promoting behaviors, such as the quality of the physical and social environment and the amount of community empowerment and action, resulting from the projects.

Canadian leadership. Canada has been a leader in promoting health, both nationally and internationally. *A New Perspective on the Health of Canada* (1974), or the "Lalonde Report" (named after the Canadian Minister of Health at that time) assessed priorities for improving the health status of the Canadian population and was instrumental in bringing attention to the health promotion movement (Lalonde, 1974). The report describes the relationships between access to health care services, human biology, environment, and individual behaviors, and it estimates the relative contribution to outcomes that progress in each of these areas might make (USPSTF, 1996). In 1986, Canada's Public Health Association and Health and Welfare Canada played a significant role in the development of health promotion internationally through their co-sponsorship (with the World Health Organization) of the First International Conference on Health Promotion in 1986, where the *Ottawa Charter* was produced, and nationally through the release of *Achieving Health for All: A Framework for Health Promotion* (the EPP report) (Health and Welfare Canada, 1986). Recent analyses of the EPP report revealed its attention to individual responsibilities and rights, health promotion and broad health determinants, as well as with its consonante with a more cost-contained health care delivery system (Iannantuono & Eyles, 1997).

Similarly, the Canadian government undertook one of the first comprehensive efforts to examine the effectiveness of clinical preventive care when it convened the Canadian Task Force on the Periodic Health Examination (CTFPHE) in 1976. Using explicit criteria to judge empirical research on clinical preventive services, the CTFPHE examined preventive services for 78 target conditions, releasing its report in a monograph published in 1979 (USPSTF, 1996; Canadian Task Force on the Periodic Health Examination, 1994). This was updated in 1994 in the *Canadian Guide to Clinical Preventive Health Care,* (CTFPE, 1994).

Voluntary and Professional Organizations

Numerous voluntary organizations, such as the American Cancer Society and the American Heart Association, by focusing on a single cause, such as cancer or heart disease, have advanced the health promotion agenda nationally and internationally and have educated clients. Similarly, professional groups, such as the American Public Health Association and the American College of Preventive Medicine, in pursuing their members' interests have either directly influenced omnibus health promotion legislation or specific legislation (e.g., concerning nutrition) and have provided direct service to clients. The single-cause organizations, such as the American Cancer Society, have advocated for changes (e.g., tobacco control) through lobbying for the passage of legislation (e.g., laws restricting smoking), by forming coalitions with other community and professional groups, and by supporting research (e.g., studies on the epidemiology of smoking).

The more than 300 professional associations contributing to health promotion in this country have assisted in the development of a national agenda concerning health promotion, have influenced legislation; and have engaged in education, screening, and other preventive services for clients. These associations include the American Public Health Association, Society for Public Health Education, American Nurses Association, American Academy of Family Physicians, American College of Physicians, American College of Preventive Medicine, American College of Nutrition, American Dietetic Association, American Physical Therapy Association, American Dental Association, and National Association of Social Workers. As they have in the past, voluntary and professional organizations will continue to influence legislation; the agendas of federal, municipal, state and local agencies; accreditors; employers; schools; health care facilities; communities; families; groups; and individual clients toward the prevention of illness such as cancer and heart disease and will continue to strive toward the creation of a health-promotive society.

Accreditors

Two major accrediting groups—the National Commission for Quality Assurance (NCQA) and the Joint Commission on the Accreditation of Health Care Organizations (JCAHO)—maintain standards relevant to the quality of organizations' structured health promotion activities. Two other smaller accrediting organizations—the Utilization Review Accreditation Commission (URAC) and the National League for Nursing-sponsored Community Health Accreditation Program Inc. (CHAP)—have specific initiatives under way that are related to the accreditation of behavioral health management organizations (Freedman & Trabin, 1994) or home, community, and public health care (CHAP).

These accreditors use a combination of on-site expert surveys of an organization and a review of written materials to determine whether an organization has met preestablished guidelines for health care. Accreditation indicates that an entity has adopted a set of quality standards and that its performance is continually reviewed. Accreditation is critical to the health care center's continued receipt of insurance funds, competition for employer health care contracts, and licensure for Medicare certification through "deemed status" and thus service to clients. Often, accreditation by these bodies serves as an alternative to federal and/or state inspection of health care facilities. These external accreditations are important adjuncts to the Continuous Quality Improvement (CQI) systems that monitor, correct, and enhance the services of many agencies.

The NCQA standards, including the Health Plan Employer Data and Information Set (HEDIS) "report card" requirements, guide the managed care industry. Within the field of health promotion and disease prevention, NCQA prescribes guidelines entitled "Standards for Preventive Health Services" that include informing members about health promotion, health education, and preventive health services available to them, as appropriate to different age groups (PH 3.2). The NCQA requires an organization to evaluate the use of preventive services among those at risk, including cholesterol measurement; exercise; smoking cessation; and counseling for prevention of motor vehicle injury, sexually transmitted diseases, and alcohol and other drug abuse. The evaluation process includes looking at both the groups at risk and the population as a whole. Under the guidance of the NCQA, consumers, insurance purchasers, and health maintenance organizations (HMOs) developed HEDIS to provide a set of measurements for HMOs to use to evaluate the quality of services and care they provide. The indicators of quality of care are mainly preventive and include the incidence of low-birth weight infants among an HMO's enrolled members and members' use of vaccinations, mammography, screening for colorectal cancer and cholesterol, prenatal care, and retina examinations (for persons with diabetes) (Centers for Disease Control and Prevention [CDC], 1995). HEDIS 3.0 (the most recent NCQA data "report card") even requires the availability of standardized medical advice to quit smoking in its Member Satisfaction Survey.

The JCAHO accredits about 15,000 health care entities, including ambulatory care centers, home health care centers, behavioral health care organizations, health care networks, corporate health services, long-term care organizations, hospitals, and pathology and clinical laboratory services. Since 1994, JCAHO has specified health promotion and disease prevention guidelines for health care networks, including HMOs, preferred provider organizations [PPOs], and other managed care entities that are performance- or outcome-focused. For behavioral health care organizations, JCAHO has identified draft standards for behavioral health promotion and illness prevention among those organizations' members and their families.

The Media

The media provide illumination and a focus of attention that is enormously powerful, particularly when the spotlight can be held in place. Through the agenda-setting process, the mass media may provide the first step to public awareness and change, or by withholding attention, they can leave issues in the dark (Wallack, Dorfman, Jernigan, & Themba, 1993).

The American public depends on the news media for reliable health information (Gellert, Higgins, Lowery, & Maxwell, 1994; Nelkin, 1985; Singer & Endreny, 1987). The media, particularly print, exert an agenda-setting function, in that issues reported in the media are more likely to be regarded as important and to merit public discourse than those that are not reported (Meyer, 1990; Wallack & Dorfman, 1992; Weiner, 1986). Generally, increased air time or copy space is devoted to more newsworthy topics (McCombs & Shaw, 1972). The media recently has begun to expand its coverage of health promotive life-styles, with daily newspapers, women's magazines, radio and television programs, and the Internet increasing space and air time devoted to topics such as types of exercise and healthy, low-fat foods.

The media may not always report health threats accurately, however. These inaccuracies may contribute to the public's overestimation of infrequent causes of mortality (e.g., deaths resulting from illicit drugs) and its underestimation of frequent causes (e.g., heart disease) (Adams, 1992-1993; Frost, Frank, & Mailbach, 1997).

Several direct interventions to promote health through the media have been undertaken and are of great strategic interest to health care professionals. Both vast potential and limitations have been found in the use of the media, particularly television, for health promotion. The use of televised campaigns, especially public service announcements, can be advantageous if the target group is large because of its cost-effectiveness relative to one-to-one clinical interventions. Results of televised campaigns are varied. Several projects aimed at reducing smoking and alcohol dependencies, for instance, have had limited success thus far (McAlister, 1982; Wallack, 1981). Others, however, such as the Stanford Three Community Study (Maccoby, Farquhar, Wood, Alexander, 1977), that aimed to reduce risk factors for coronary heart disease, produced impressive results in the reduction of blood cholesterol levels and in improved eating habits.

Successful media interventions tend to share several characteristics: (1) they use a multimedia approach with ties to community interventions, such as support groups (Hastings, 1989; McAlister, 1982); (2) they concentrate on knowledge or awareness rather than attitude and behavior change (Hastings, 1989; Roberts & Maccoby, 1985); and (3) they attempt to change more tractable behaviors, such as understanding one's problems (Barker, Pistrang, Shapiro, Davies, & Shaw, 1993). To evaluate media interventions, one must specify the type of changes desired in which population subgroups and under what circumstances (Barker et al., 1993). Longer time frames, such as a period of years, are also recommended in the measurement of change (Lorion, 1983).

From an advocacy perspective (i.e., seeking to use the media to influence those who can change the social environment), several approaches appear important. Media advocates frame issues in terms of root causes and focus on policy concerns rather than personal behaviors. They use the dramatic story, with characters, plots, villains, and heroes. Advocates take advantage of opportunities to respond to breaking news, such as a decision in a tobacco company trial, to create news of their own. Media advocates know what their adversaries' reactions to a story will be, and they sustain controlled communication with the press. They seek to understand their topic, plan their goals, and understand how the media work (Wallack, Dorfman, Jernigan et al., 1993).

Community Advocacy Groups and Coalitions

Community groups, such as Mothers against Drunk Driving (MADD) and Doctors Ought to Care (DOC) have been effective advocates for change in laws concerning drinking and driving (MADD) and smoking (DOC).

Drinking and driving has been the focus of considerable attention: the Surgeon General has called for stricter regulation of the advertising of alcoholic beverages, citizen groups such as MADD have lobbied for and legislators have passed laws raising the legal drinking age and establishing stiffer penalties for driving while intoxicated, the news media have devoted much coverage to the problem, and even the entertainment media have incorporated messages about drinking and driving into television programs (Office of Disease Prevention and Health Promotion, 1990). This widespread public concern and the resulting programs have reduced the proportion of motor vehicle deaths related to alcohol, although the decline has slowed lately (National Center for Health Statistics, 1990).

In the case of tobacco use, DOC and coalitions, such as Smoking or Health, have effectively organized community and professional groups toward changing legislation to outlaw smoking in public buildings, workplaces, restaurants, schools, and sporting events across the country, and, in conjunction with international partners such as the World Health Organization, in many parts of the developed world. They have influenced schools of medicine to include the counseling of smokers in the curricula, they have provided consultation for clinical trials in community settings (e.g., COMMIT and ASSIST, as described in Chapter 6), and they have galvanized community attitudes toward smoking control.

ORGANIZATIONAL POLICY

Organizations such as schools, workplaces, public health departments, and health care facilities are central to the implementation of health promotion legislation, regulations, and policies, as well as to the formation of new initiatives. These organizations wield considerable influence on community, group, and individual behavior.

School Districts and Schools

Lifetime patterns of diet, exercise, smoking, and coping, in particular, may be established in childhood. Because the 48 million children and youth in America spend much of their days in school, efforts to change these life-style patterns through local legislation and regulation have been promoted within the school context. Children may learn about their bodies and the effects of different life-style behaviors in this context. Children also may be linked to necessary preventive services, such as age-appropriate immunizations, nutritious meals, and regular organized physical activity. The school also may connect families to health insurance programs, thus enriching a family's ability to continue to receive preventive services.

The School Enrollment-Based Health Insurance Program, for example, provides low-cost health insurance to families who are not eligible for Medicaid and who cannot afford private insurance. The program targets families with school-age children, who represent 66% of the uninsured nationally. It provides an alternative to employer-based health insurance by using schools as the grouping mechanism to negotiate health insurance policies and is more stable because coverage is not disrupted if the parent changes or loses his/her job. A recent demonstration of the program in Volusia County, Florida, that used an HMO with well care benefits in its coverage found that children who had to pay for health care under this program were less likely to use health care than those who received a partial subsidy. The findings suggest that other factors, such as provider characteristics, health care need, transportation, and geographic access, may also influence use of the program (Shenkman et al., 1996).

Twenty five states require comprehensive school health education programs, and nine states recommend that local school districts implement such programs (Division of Adolescent and School Health, 1995); these programs vary in their intents and contents. Nationally, 75% of local school districts have antismoking education in elementary schools (National School Boards Association, 1989). About 63% of public school districts and private schools provide some instruction concerning alcohol and other drug use, and about 39% provide related counseling services (U.S. Department of Education, 1987). Twelve states require nutrition education from preschool through grade 12 (American School Health Association, 1989). Only one state requires daily physical education from kindergarten through grade 12.

Worksites

Nearly 110 million persons go to work every day; individuals spend more than one third of their waking hours at work (Gomel, Oldenburg, Simpson, & Owen, 1993). As a result, worksites are important components of community-wide health promotion efforts. Further, health promotion programs are seen as an employee benefit that increases employee morale and helps attract and retain good workers at relatively little cost. As of 1992, about 81% of employers have maintained worksite health promotion activities of varied types (USDHHS, 1993). Workplace programs, oriented toward promoting good health for employees to decrease costs of absenteeism, increase productivity, and/or create more effective organizations may include multifaceted supportive programs (e.g., smoking cessation policies and clinics), exercise facilities, Employee Assistance Programs (EAPs) for behavioral health promotion, and health insurance. In addition, under OSHA regulation, worksites integrate the protection of employee health through setting and enforcing safety standards, worker training, and safety education.

Worksite weight reduction and smoking cessation intervention studies have shown that programs making use of behavioral change strategies and/or incentives have resulted in greater changes than less-intensive approaches (Gomel et al., 1993). Although there are considerable methodologic problems associated with much of the worksite research, such as failing to obtain objective validation of self-reported behavior change or less rigorous designs, such as quasi-experimental or case study research (USDHHS, 1988), some more rigorous worksite multiple risk factor interventions have been evaluated in a randomized controlled design. Two, in particular, evaluated the effectiveness of brief counseling and follow-up contact with a health professional. One of these, the World Health Organization trial, demonstrated a significant effect of the intervention on risk factor change. This finding was confirmed by another, more recent randomized trial of 28 worksites, with behavioral counseling demonstrating a significant effect on smoking cessation and smaller increases in body mass index and mean blood pressure (Gomel et al., 1993).

In general, worksite programs tend to attract individuals who are in better health, between ages 20 and 65 years, youthful, physically fit, middle-class, and who are generally aware of health risks. Access to such programs is limited for workers in smaller businesses, those who telecommute, transiently employed persons, and employee dependents.

Public Health Departments and Health Care Facilities

Public health departments and other health care facilities are influential contexts on the process of health promotion. Public health departments, oriented toward optimizing the health of the entire community, have traditionally been concerned with health through the control of communicable diseases; health education; environmental sanitation; consumer protection; and the provision of medical and nursing services for the diagnosis, treatment, and prevention of diseases in hard-to-reach populations (USDHHS, 1994). They are particularly concerned with access to care. Public health activities generally are coordinated by a network of municipal, state, and federal agencies and are quite diverse (CDC and the National Association of County Health Officials, 1994).

About 40 million Americans receive one or more clinical services through public health departments, and about one half of these agencies provide clinical preventive care (CDC and National Association of County Health Officials, 1994). In almost one half (47%) of these departments, services are offered in a "package," including immunizations, health education, tuberculosis screening and treatment, well-child visits, nutrition services for women and children, sexually transmitted disease screening, partner identification and treatment, and HIV testing and counseling. Often, preventive care is built into the medical protocols departments must follow; many of these protocols are derived from federal regulations. Health departments are, however, changing rapidly under the pressure for managed care; privatization has begun in the Delaware State Division of Public Health, for example, and will continue elsewhere as well.

Hospitals are another venue for preventive activities, such as smoking cessation counseling. When clients are suffering from acute illnesses, they are more likely to listen to and heed a health care professional's advice regarding preventive activities. In fact, a review of several studies of brief, multicomponent bedside treatment programs regarding smoking cessation for a general hospital population revealed that hospitals can produce 20% to 25% long-term quit rates, which are comparable to those of formal clinic programs, even among smokers who may not be highly motivated to quit (Orleans, Kristeller, & Gritz, 1993).

Hospital emergency rooms provide another context for health promotion. They are the primary sites for clinical care among vulnerable members of the population, such as the homeless, the uninsured, and the working poor. More than 120 million persons visit an emergency room each year, generally for the treatment of a presenting illness or injury. Nonetheless, because of the volume of clients, opportunities exist for the distribution of preventive services such as screening tests, education and counseling, the delivery of primary care services, and the updating of immunizations. Blood pressure measurements, which are screening tests, are performed in about 75% of all emergency room (ER) visits; recent legislation mandates a vital sign measurement for all ER patients (Frew, 1991). Emergency room staff have an opportunity to counsel in injury prevention for the 35% of all visits resulting from an injury (McCaig, 1994). Nonurgent problems account for 55% of all visits, often among the more vulnerable in the population, thus enabling health care professionals to screen for hypertension, hypercholesterolemia, cervical cancer, and syphillis and to conduct other forms of early detection (Chernow & Iserson, 1987; Burns, Stoy, Feied, Nash, & Smith, 1991; Hogness, Engelstad, Linck, & Schorr, 1992; Hibbs, Ceglowski, Goldberg, & Kauffman, 1993). Although preventive care is provided in this setting and it serves as the primary clinical site for many in the population, it is not without problems. The waits are often long; elevations in blood pressure may be a result of anxiety, thus leading to misdiagnoses; and follow-up—critical to prevention of sexually transmitted diseases, for example—is rare (Avner, 1992).

ECONOMIC INFLUENCES ON HEALTH PROMOTION

The nation spends about 3.4% of its total health care expenditures on prevention-related activities (Brown et al., 1991). About 84.7% of Americans are covered by health insurance through insurers that include commercial companies; Blue Cross/Blue Shield nonprofit membership plans; and employer self-insurance, including administrative service contracts. Importantly, however, about 40 million persons, including 12 million children, are without any health insurance because they are employed by firms that do not offer coverage or because they live below the poverty line and cannot afford it (American Public Health Association, 1997). Some 21% of all poor children younger than 18 years (3.1 million) have no health insurance coverage (Summer, Parrott, & Mann, 1996). About 22 million additional Americans are underinsured (Clinton, 1992).

More and better insurance coverage for health screening and counseling would encourage wider use of these services. Some of the barriers commercial insurers face in covering preventive services include developing a market for such products and ensuring that it would be viable financially. Public insurance is unlikely to offer more preventive benefits (e.g., smoking cessation counseling) until they can be shown to be medically necessary and cost-effective (G.R. Wilensky, memorandum, September 6, 1990). Further, because health insurance was initially developed to protect individuals from the largely unpredictably high costs of hospitalization and catastrophic illness, by definition, health insurance is generally limited to services that are deemed "medically necessary" to diagnose and treat illness (Starr, 1982, 1994). Health promotion programs (e.g., nutrition counseling) meet none of these criteria; they are predictable, based on the presence of specific risk factors; relatively low in cost; and as preventive services, they have never been considered medically necessary (Riedel, 1987). Although some change has begun to take place in the way preventive services and their effects on longer-term behavioral change are considered, coverage for them is still considered in terms of the discrete physician visit (Davis, Bialek, Parkinson, Smith, & Vellozzi, 1990).

Another barrier to the coverage of preventive benefits is that generally both policy makers and insurers have used a higher standard of evidence than they apply to medical treatments when deciding whether services should be covered by insurance (Schauffler & Parkinson, 1993). Nonetheless, the Office of Technology Assessment concluded that rather than lowering the evidence for the effectiveness of preventive services, policy makers should raise the level of evidence required for therapeutic and diagnostic services (U.S. Congress Office of Technology Assessment, 1990).

Commercial insurance companies, Blue Cross/Blue Shield, federal insurance programs, and managed care are the major sources of monies for health promotion services. The World Bank, another source of funds, has a significant influence on international economies so its recent inclusion of health as an indicator of development will affect the health promotion field. Although not a source of funds, the pharmacologic, botanical, and biotechnology industries are briefly discussed in this text as contributors to the economy of health promotion. See Table 3-3 for a summary of the components of the major economic programs for health promotion.

Commercial Insurance Companies

Since the 1930s, commercial insurance companies have reimbursed the insured patient, or beneficiary, with stipulated sums of money to be applied against expenditures for the insured risks. Subscribers bear sole responsibility for identifying their need for care, locating the providers of care, and paying for the care. The insurer reimburses them for their "reasonable and customary" expenses (Shouldice, 1991). About 80% of health insurance is sold to groups, primarily employers; in the face of escalating costs, employers have begun to shift costs to employees and to limit the number of health insurance plans offered. Many of these employer groups are self-insured (i.e., they bear the entire risk for their employees internally); commercial insurance companies may then simply administer the plans without the attribution of risk.

Health insurers are driven largely by concerns over rising health care costs. Among employer groups, any employee demand for preventive services encounters pressures to control costs. Employees, too, may tend to resist raising premiums to pay for additional benefits (Steckler, Dawson, Goodman, & Epstein, 1987). Faced with increasing competition for the business of healthy employer groups, insurers are less likely to add any benefits that increase their costs relative to their competitors, unless a clear demand exists. Insurers who elect to cover preventive services, such as smoking cessation programs, may put themselves at risk of adverse selection, relative to their competitors, by attracting smokers who are more likely to use proportionately more medical care (Milliman & Robertson, 1987). Little is known about the impact of health insurance coverage on outcomes of preventive interventions, such as smoking cessation programs; thus, it is difficult for insurers to price them and for employers to finance them. Finally, insurers tend to look at whether benefits of preventive care will be realized over the time period the insurer covers the policyholder. Many of the benefits that accrue after a person quits smoking, for example, may not be realized by the health insurer if the policyholder switches plans. As a result, most insurance companies limit their time frame for benefits realization of smoking cessation to 2 years; the reimburseable health care costs for the smoker receiving the benefits at the end of 2 years must be lower than for the smoker not receiving these benefits (Schauffler & Parkinson, 1993).

Recently, however, to maintain a competitive advantage and to reduce costs, particularly among self-insured employers, commercial insurance companies have begun to focus on health promotion. Health promotion programs tend to enhance enrollee retention through enriched satisfaction—an increasingly important concern in the brutally competitive health care insurance market. A recent study of employees enrolled in health

Table 3-3

Components of major economic programs for health promotion

PROGRAM	FOCUS	EXAMPLE COMPONENTS
Commercial insurance companies	Reimbursement of client with fixed sum for expenses of insured risks May manage self-insurance by companies	48% offer nutrition programs 82% offer AIDS education 91% offer exercise/fitness programs 97% offer stress management 98% offer smoking cessation
Blue Cross and Blue Shield	Nonprofit medical contracts for medical services to members, generally reimburse on pre-set schedule Insurers of last resort to many	Preventive screenings offered Smoking cessation 47% of enrollees in managed care such as HMOs, PPOs, POS, Medicare managed care, integrated delivery system
Federal insurance programs		
Medicaid	Health insurance to low-income population and/or a disabled population	35% of beneficiaries enrolled in managed care Mandated preventive services of periodic screening, family planning for children younger than 21 years
Medicare	Health insurance to those older than 65 years Part A (compulsory hospitalization insurance) Part B (supplementary medical insurance)	13% of population enrolled in managed care plans Covers pneumococcal vaccines, hepatitis A vaccine, PAP smears, mammography Risk plans generally cover eyeglasses
Medicare Supplemental Insurance	Supplement to basic Medicare coverage	Dental x-rays and cleaning often covered
Federal Employees Health Benefits Program (FEHBP)	Voluntary health insurance coverage for 88% of active and retired federal employees	May choose managed care plan for preventive care
Veterans' Medical Care	134 hospitals operated to care for individuals who served honorably in armed forces	May choose managed care for preventive care
Indian Health Service	Medical care and health services for 2 million Native Americans, including Alaskan natives	Smoking cessation policies and programs

Table 3-3

Components of major economic programs for health promotion—cont'd

PROGRAM	FOCUS	EXAMPLE COMPONENTS
TRICARE/ CHAMPUS (Civilian Health and Medical Program for the Uniformed Services)	Comprehensive managed health care delivery system for active members of the armed forces, their dependents, and retirees; coordinates care in military hospitals and clinics with services from civilian health care professionals	Extensive clinical health promotion and disease prevention examinations (e.g., health risk appraisals, laboratory tests) and counseling (e.g., tabacco, diet, physical activity, safe sex)
Managed care organizations (MCOs)	Integrates financing and delivery of appropriate medical services to covered individuals	
Health maintenance organizations (HMOs)	Prepaid health care arrangements Subject to capitation	Health promotion programs most likely to be offered are weight control, stress management, smoking cessation
Preferred provider organization (PPO)	Contracts with providers to deliver covered services for discounted fee	56% cover adult physical examinations
Exclusive provider organization (EPO)	Similar to the HMO, but members must remain within the network to receive services	Similar to HMOs
Point of service plans (POS)	Combine HMOs and PPOs, network of contracted MDs	82% cover physical examinations
Managed behavioral health care	Mental health and substance abuse benefit package	Individual health risk assessments, self-help groups, outreach programs
Worker's compensation	Health insurance coverage for employees injured or ill on the job	Safe environments, safety inspections, counseling
The World Bank	Development for international economies	World Development Report 1993 supports intersectoral actions for health
Pharmaceutical, botanical, and biotechnology industries	Gene mapping, manufacture and production of drugs and botanicals, recombinant DNA technology, and compounds acting in the cell	Anticholesterol drugs, vitamins, minerals

* Source: *TRICARE Standard Handbook* [On-line], by TRICARE Support Office, U.S. Department of Defense. Available:http://ww.tso.osd.mil

plans of various types found that those who have been offered programs to stop smoking, manage stress, and control weight, and cholesterol and blood pressure screening or any health promotion program by their plan or physician are more satisfied with their health plan than those who have not been offered such programs (Schauffler & Rodriguez, 1994). According to the Health Insurance Association of America (HIAA, 1995), major health insurers offered a range of health promotive programs, including nutrition programs (48%), AIDS education (82%), exercise/fitness programs (91%), stress management (97%), and smoking cessation activities (98%). The components of these programs vary, as do their effectiveness. Since the 1980s, many insurers have offered rate advantages for nonsmokers and individuals who maintain a healthy weight; many also include medical screening benefits as an integral part of their policies (HIAA, 1995). Overall, however, an insurance industry survey found that only 14% of commercial insurance carriers and Blue Cross and Blue Shield plans offered nonsmoking discounts on individual health insurance policies. The survey further found very few carriers that offer nonsmoking discounts to groups (Schauffler, 1993b).

This varies, however, by region. In California, for example, only 21.5% had implemented a risk-rating policy using smoking status, although subsidies or payment for smoking cessation outside the plan was provided by 37%, and 87% had adopted formal worksite smoking policies (Schauffler, 1993b).

With regard to complementary medical approaches, 85% of insurance companies now cover chiropractic, a complementary medical approach relying on the manipulation of the protruding parts of the spinal vertebrae (Fugh-Berman, 1996). Many also cover massage therapy or acupuncture (the insertion of hair-thin needles into specific points on the body to prevent or to treat disease) when prescribed by a physician.

Blue Cross and Blue Shield

Blue Cross and Blue Shield (the "Blues") are nonprofit service plans that have loosely affiliated with one another. The "Blues" govern a network of more than 60 chapters that provide health insurance to nearly 100 million subscribers (about 40% of the U.S. population). To many, the "Blues" are the insurers of last resort. Blue Cross contracts with local hospitals to cover members at a set reimbursement schedule. To the client, Blue Cross provides "first dollar, first day" coverage. Blue Shield plans are nonprofit medical contracts for physician services. Members are reimbursed for those services according to a preset schedule. The two plans complement each other.

Blue Cross and Blue Shield have formed HMOs, preferred provider organizations (PPOs), point of service (POS) plans, and government health care plans, including a Medicare managed care network, and offer free health care benefits to eligible uninsured children (Caring Program for Children, which is funded through matching funds from 25 Blue plans). Recently, they have developed an integrated delivery system to partner with hospitals and/or physicians so that clients may move more easily from one level of care to another. They claim that 25% of Americans receive managed care coverage from Blue Cross and Blue Shield plans. Blue plans operate a total of 84 separate HMOs in 43 states and the District of Columbia. PPOs are the most popular form of managed care in the "Blues," with service to more than 19 million Americans through 72 plans. Fifty three POS networks are found in 43 states and include the services of 260,000 physicians and 3200 hospitals. The "Blues'" federal health plan is the largest privately underwritten health insurance contract in the world, with more than 43% of all federal employees and retirees enrolled (Blue Cross and Blue Shield, 1997). Recently, Blue Cross/Blue Shield plans have begun to join together to form single corporations to pool resources, creating for-profit subsidiaries, forming alliances with for-profit enterprises, or dropping their nonprofit status altogether and going public (Hoover's Company Profile, 1997).

Blue Cross and Blue Shield have, in some cases, developed model benefits for preventive screenings. For example, the King County Medical Blue Shield in Washington state routinely covers 75% of the costs of smoking cessation programs per policyholder up to a $500 lifetime maximum benefit. All groups with five or more employees receive the smoking cessation benefits at no additional charge. Reimbursement is restricted to 13 participating program providers that have signed contracts with the insurer and have agreed to accept payment based on prevailing charges as payment in full (Schauffler & Parkinson, 1993).

Federal Insurance Programs

The federal government's health insurance programs include Medicare for persons older than 65 years, Medicaid for low-income persons, the Federal Employees Health Benefits Program, Veterans' Administration medical care, and the Indian Health Service. Medicare is a federally administered program that provides hospital and medical insurance protection to persons 65 years and older, disabled persons younger than 65 years who receive cash benefits under Social Security or Railroad Retirement programs, persons of all ages with chronic kidney disease, and some aliens and federal civil service employees who pay a monthly premium. For the portion of the working population covered by Social Security, Medicare provides compulsory hospitalization insurance (Part A), as well as voluntary supplementary medical insurance (Part B) to help pay for physicians' services, medical services, and supplies not covered by the hospitalization plan.

Since its inception in 1965, the Medicare program has prohibited reimbursement for preventive services because they are generally seen as predictable and do not lower reimbursement costs (Schauffler, 1993a). The Medicaid program also restricts preventive services. Health maintenance organizations that have risk contracts with the Health Care Financing Administration are required to provide Medicaid enrollees with those preventive services covered under Medicare only. Recently, however, Congress has begun to add preventive services, such as pneumococcal vaccine, hepatitis B vaccine, Papanicolaou smears and mammography, as well as preventive services demonstration projects under Medicare as exceptions (U.S. Congress Office of Technology Assessment, 1990). Medicare recently has begun to cover chiropractic services.

To fill the gaps in preventive services, nearly 29 million Medicare enrollees supplement their Medicare benefits with private insurance (usually known as MedSup or Medigap policies). Of the most common forms of Medicare supplemental insurance (Disability Income Insurance, Long Term Care and Dental Expense Insurance), only dental insurance supplies and encourages preventive care, such as x-rays and cleanings. A growing number of Medicare beneficiaries have, however, begun to use HMOs that offer a wide range of preventive services. As of January 1, 1997, 13% of the Medicare population (4.9 million beneficiaries) was enrolled in managed care plans (Health Care Financing Administration [HCFA], 1997).

Since 1993, the number of both Medicare and Medicaid beneficiaries enrolled in managed care plans has experienced unprecedented growth. Managed care plans can serve Medicare beneficiaries through three types of contracts: risk, cost, and Health Care Prepayment Plans (HCPPs). Risk plans are paid a per capita (per person) premium set at approximately 95% of the projected average expenses for fee-for-service beneficiaries in a given county. Risk plans must provide all Medicare-covered services, and most plans offer additional services, such as prescription drugs and eyeglasses. Risk plans have enrolled about 86% of managed care participants. Cost plans are paid a predetermined monthly amount per beneficiary based on a total estimated budget. Cost plans must provide all Medicare-covered services but do not provide the additional services that most risk plans offer. HCPPs are paid similarly to cost plans but cover only part of the Medicare benefit package, excluding inpatient hospital care, skilled nursing, hospice, and some home health care. Nationally, three fourths of all beneficiaries have a choice of at least one managed care plan. The recently introduced "Medicare Choices" demonstration project allows beneficiaries to join a wider variety of managed care plans and to extend managed care coverage to rural areas (HCFA, 1997).

Medicaid, administered by each state according to federal requirements and guidelines, is financed by both state and federal funds. It provides medical assistance to persons who are eligible for cash assistance programs, such as Aid to Families of Dependent Children (AFDC) and Supplemental Security Income (SSI). Medicaid benefits may also be available to persons who have enough income for basic living expenses but cannot afford to pay for their medical care. Mandated preventive services include periodic screening and family planning for children younger than 21 years. Further, about 35% (13 million) of Medicaid beneficiaries are enrolled in HMOs (HCFA, 1997).

Since the 1980s, Medicaid has been phasing in health insurance coverage to a broader group of poor children through expansions in eligibility; by the year 2000 all poor children younger than 19 years will be eligible for Medicaid. Eligibility, however, has not necessarily translated into enrollment, as one fifth of all poor and near-poor children younger than 11 years who were income-eligible for Medicaid in 1994 (nearly 2.7 million children) were neither enrolled in Medicaid nor covered by any other form of health insurance. Nearly 80% of these children lived in families with wage earners (Summer et al., 1996).

The Federal Employees Health Benefits Program (FEHBP) provides voluntary health insurance coverage for about 88% of all 8.6 million active and retired federal employees. Employees choose among three competing health plans: (1) government-wide plans, (2) employee organization plans sponsored by employee organizations or unions, and (3) comprehensive medical plans, or HMOs. The program is jointly financed by premiums paid by the government which pays about 75% of premium costs, and by enrollees, who pay the remaining 25%.

Veterans' Medical Care operates 134 medical centers for the care of individuals who served honorably in the armed forces. Under the recent Veterans' Health Care Eligibility Reform Act of 1996, Veterans Administration Medical Centers may negotiate with managed care entities to provide health services, thus increasing the options for preventive services.

The Indian Health Service includes medical care and health services for approximately 2 million American Indians, including Alaskan natives. The Indian Health Service was among the earliest entities to enact smoke-free health care settings. Its evaluation suggested that daily cigarette consumption among clients decreased after implementation of the smoke-free policy (Anonymous, 1987).

Managed Care

Managed care is a system that integrates the financing and delivery of appropriate health care services to covered individuals and has served as an important recent influence on the provision of preventive services. Generally, it includes four elements: (1) arrangements with selected providers to furnish a comprehensive set of health care services to members, (2) explicit standards for the selection of health care providers, (3) formal programs for ongoing quality assurance and utilization review, and (4) significant financial incentives for members to use providers and procedures covered by the plan (HIAA, 1995). The two broadest arrangements for financing and delivery are fee-for-service indemnity arrangements and prepaid health care. Under fee-for-service indemnity arrangements, the consumer incurs expenses for health care from providers whom he/she selects. The provider is reimbursed for covered services in part by the insurer and in part by the consumer, who is responsible for the balance unpaid by the insurer. Under indemnity arrangements, the provider and the insurer have no relationship beyond adjudication of the claim presented for payment, nor is there a mechanism for integrating the care the consumer may receive from multiple providers (CDC, 1995).

Overall, a recent study found that persons enrolled in staff-model health maintenance organizations are much more likely to be offered health promotion programs, such as cholesterol or blood pressure screening, weight control, stress management, and smoking control, by their plan or physician than persons enrolled in an independent practice association and indemnity plan (Schauffler & Parkinson, 1993).

Although the field is changing rapidly, four managed care forms predominate: (1) HMOs; (2) PPOs; (3) exclusive provider organizations (EPOs); and (4) POS plans. Managed care structures are financed under either "risk" or "capitation" approaches. A "risk" contract is generally negotiated between an HMO (or a competitive medical plan, a federal designation for a plan that operates similarly to an HMO) and the Health Care Financing Administration. The HMO agrees to provide all services to enrolled Medicare members on an "at-risk" basis for a fixed monthly fee. Capitation is a negotiated amount that an entity such as an HMO pays monthly to a provider whom the enrollee has selected as a primary care physician.

HMO. Within the current health care system, the HMO is the best structured insurance vehicle to encourage prevention. HMOs are prepaid health care arrangements. The Health Maintenance Organization Act of 1973 committed the federal government to a time-limited demonstration of effort and support of HMO development. In this context, HMOs were defined as entities that provide basic health services to their enrollees, using prepaid enrollment fees that are fixed uniformly under a community-rating system without regard to the medical history of any individual or family. Basic services included preventive health services and health education. Health education covered the use of health services and methods of personal health maintenance, such as proper diet, exercise, and medication use (Shouldice, 1991). The original Act further required most employers to offer an HMO option to employees where federally qualified HMOs were available. The original Act was amended in 1976, 1978, 1980, 1981, 1986, and 1988.

The HMO provides comprehensive and preventive health care benefits for a defined population, and the consumer of an HMO agrees to use its providers for all covered health care services. The HMO agrees to provide all covered health care services for a set price—the per-person premium fee. The consumer must pay any additional fees (co-payments) for office visits and other services used. The HMO also organizes the delivery of this care through the infrastructure it builds among its providers and the implementation of systems to monitor and influence the cost and quality of care. The risk for the cost of care for the enrolled population is assumed by the HMO.

HMOs generally also are subject to capitation. The provider is responsible for delivering or arranging for the delivery of health care services required by the enrollee. This capitation is paid regardless of whether the physician has provided services to the enrollee. In a capitation arrangement, the physician shares with the HMO a portion of the financial risk for the cost of care provided to enrollees (Centers for Disease Control and Prevention, 1995).

The HMO is generally arranged into one of five kinds of service structures: (1) staff (contract with solo salaried physician practice); (2) group (HMO pays per capita rate to physician group); (3) network (contract with two or more independent group practices with fixed monthly fee per enrollee); (4) independent practice association (IPA) (contract with individual physicians or associations of private physicians on per capita rate, flat retainer, or negotiated fee-for-service rate); or (5) mixed (combination of two or more models in one HMO).

At present, HMOs provide a comprehensive set of services to a voluntarily enrolled population within a specified geographic area; providers are typically reimbursed on a capitated basis or through another "at risk" arrangement. About 90% of HMOs cover health promotive services (HIAA, 1995).

PPO. The PPO is a variant of the fee-for-service indemnity arrangement, wherein the PPO contracts with providers in the community to deliver covered services for a discounted fee. Providers under contract are referred to as "preferred providers." The PPO gives consumers greater freedom in choosing providers, but, as with the HMO, it tries to achieve savings by directing clients to providers who are committed to cost-effective delivery of care. PPOs have contracts with networks or panels of providers who agree to provide medical services and to be paid according to a negotiated fee schedule. Enrollees generally experience a financial penalty if they choose to get care from a nonaffiliated provider, but that option is available. PPOs pay for some preventive services, with 56% covering adult physical examinations (KPMG Peat Marwick, LLP, 1994 as cited in HIAA, 1995).

EPO. The EPO, too, is similar to the HMO, but the member must remain within the network to receive benefits. It uses primary physicians as gatekeepers, often capitates providers, has a limited provider panel, and uses an authorization system and other features of the HMO. EPOs are regulated under insurance statutes, rather than HMO regulations, in states where they are allowed to operate (Kongstvedt, 1993).

POS. Point of service (POS) plans combine characteristics of both HMOs and PPOs, by using a network of contracted participating providers. Employees select a primary care physician, who controls referrals to medical specialists. If care is received from a plan provider, the employee pays little or nothing out of pocket; care provided by nonplan providers are reimbursed by fee-for-service or capitation arrangements, and employees pay higher co-payments and deductibles. Financial incentives are used to avoid provider overuse. About 82% of PPOs cover adult physical examinations (KPMG, 1994).

Managed behavioral health care. The mental health and substance abuse benefit packages that cover most privately insured Americans involve some form of managed care. Separate companies devoted to this area and insurers now offer "carve-out" behavioral health care insurance to their customers in addition to their regular insurance offerings. The client group served by these companies and insurers requires specialized knowledge and skills, distinct from those used for the delivery of medical care. The response to these "carve-outs" has been positive, leading to considerable growth in this field. Three core methods are used to manage behavioral health care. In principle, the three methods are similar to those used to manage medical care; however, because of the uniqueness of the client groups served, their implementation differs. The three methods are (1) managed benefits, which are designed to control use and expenditures through, for example, the use of gatekeepers who authorize care; (2) managed care, which limits the authorization of benefits for reimbursement to only necessary and appropriate care delivered in the least restrictive, least intrusive setting by a qualified provider; and (3) managed health, which offers the use of health advisers, individual health risk assessments, self-help groups, crisis debriefing services, and outreach programs to frequent users of health care services (Freedman & Trabin, 1994).

The early growth in the managed behavioral health care industry emerged in part from community mental health centers (CMHCs), which were initiated in 1963 and whose emphasis was on shifting the locus of care from institutions to the community and who provided services to a defined geographic area. Behavioral health care developed well-coordinated, easily accessible continuums of care in each community. Individual case management programs were implemented, and communities became responsible for the care of defined populations in a defined area.

Self-insured businesses, too, through their funding of employee assistance programs (EAPs), created early incentives for managed behavioral health plans to promote wellness, decrease absenteeism, improve worker productivity, and reduce health care costs. A majority of conventional PPO and HMO plans cover mental health and substance abuse treatment programs.

Worker's Compensation

All state legislatures have enacted worker's compensation, or statuary disability benefits, laws that provide for health insurance coverage for employees who are injured or become ill while "on the job" during the course of employment (Shouldice, 1991). Benefits are established by state laws and include all reasonable medical care, rehabilitation services necessary to return the injured employee to work, and partial repayment of lost wages. Funds for worker's compensation come from employers and state and local taxes. To promote health and therefore save money, safe environments, including those with educational programs, safety inspections, and counseling on safe work practices, are stressed. Worker's compensation stress claim prevention and management is another emerging area for managed behavioral health care.

The World Bank

The World Bank, which is a specialized agency of the United Nations and is also known as the International Bank for Reconstruction and Development, provides loans to countries for development projects. Its affiliate, the International Development Association, makes loans to less developed member countries on a long-term basis at no interest.

The World Bank, concerned with the worldwide increases in the cost of health care and the inequities in access, devoted its annual *World Development Report* (WDR, 1993) to health. This marked a major shift in the concept of investing in health as an essential component of economic development, rather than as a negative input (World Bank, 1993). The report highlighted the importance of intersectoral actions to improve the enabling environment for health (e.g., the educational system). The WDR stressed the need for greater efficiency in the distribution of resources within the health care sector, emphasizing the most cost-effective interventions for conditions responsible for the greatest burden of suffering in each country. The WDR also encouraged reform to improve the efficiency of interventions that had passed the test for effectiveness. For the poorest and middle-income countries of the developing world, the WDR proposed basic packages of primary and public health services that should be fully implemented before public funds are used for more "discretionary" clinical services or less cost-effective interventions (USPSTF, 1996, p. 571).

Pharmacologic, Botanical, and Biotechnologic Industries

The pharmacologic industry, part of a multibillion dollar international market (Decision Resources, Inc., 1997), is a major force in health care, with more than $138 billion in sales in 1997 at 342 American companies. The largest American firms include Merck and Company, Bristol-Myers Squibb Company, American Home Products, Pfizer Incorporated, and Abbott Laboratories (Gale Research Inc., 1997). Although mainly oriented toward tertiary prevention, the industry does contribute to primary prevention. An example of this is the development of drugs for hypercholesterolemia, weight reduction, and osteoporosis. This part of the industry is growing and is poised to expand further with ongoing developments such as chemoprevention for breast cancer.

Consumer sales have helped to boost the rapidly growing botanical industry. About one fourth of all pharmaceutical drugs are derived from herbs (soft-stemmed plants) (Foster, 1990). Medicinal herbs (plants used for their effects on the body) are central to many complementary medical approaches. Botanical manufacturers, including 76 American firms that produce herbal preparations, vitamins, and dietary supplements, have annual revenues of about $4 billion. (Gale Research Inc., 1997). Some medicinal herbs (defined here more generally as a useful plant) that have been assessed for their effects on health include chili peppers (*Capsicum*), cranberries (*Vaccinium macrocarpon*), evening primrose oil (*Oenothera biennis*), garlic (*Allium sativum*), onion (*Allium cepa*), ginger (*zingiber officinale*), licorice (*Glycyrrhiza glabra*), St.-John's-wort (*Hypericum perforatum*), and valerian (*Valeriana officinalis* and other species) (Fugh-Berman, 1996). Considerable controversy exists, however, about the methodologic strength of the evidence supporting the effects of herbal and other complementary medical approaches to health promotion (Joyce, 1994; Ernst, 1994; Sewing, 1994).

The estimated $83.1 billion drug and biotechnology industries and the $13 billion worldwide biotechnology market (Institute for Health Care Business Development, 1997), are also growing. Companies in these industries produce genetic screening (e.g., spotting mutations in the breast cancer susceptability genes BRCA1 and BRCA2); detection and diagnostic products (e.g., tests for detecting cervical cancer); and drugs (oftentimes using recombinant DNA technology or developing compounds that act within the cell). (Weber, 1997). Biotechnology companies are also discovering the functions of human genes, as is the National Institute of Health-funded Human Genome Project. The genetic testing products produced by this industry, in particular, pose ethical quandaries for health care professionals in health promotion field. Questions about the sharing of genetic information with health and life insurance companies and managed care companies are the most pressing at present. The optimal process a health care professional might use to share genetic information with clients, and how it might encourage behavior change, also remains uncertain.

STRATEGIES FOR HEALTH PROMOTION IN THE POLICY CONTEXT

Health care professionals may adopt a variety of strategies to promote the health of populations. A strategy for policy change, the context of which was explored in this chapter, may be pursued concommitantly or subsequently to other strategies discussed in Chapters 4 and 5.

In its most rational form, the policy-making process proceeds from goal determination, to needs assessment and the specification of objectives, to the design of alternative courses of action, to the estimation of consequences of alternative actions, to the selection of a course of action, to implementation and evaluation, with a feedback loop to the goal-setting stage (summary in Mayer & Greenwood, 1980). Concurrently, the policy process may be seen as a "general course of action or inaction rather than specific decisions" (Heclo, 1972, p. 85), ruled by forces that are fluid and unpredictable (Hacker, 1996). The strategies designed to influence policy, therefore, must consider both its rational and its emergent processes.

The various tactics the health care professional undertakes also are part of a dynamic process, both directive—in pursuit of a larger aim—and directed—by those affected or potentially affected by the policy change. The first step in this process is building agendas, identifying problems in terms of pressing social problems, and developing a solution that incorporates the interests of affected groups. Second, the problems are defined by their prevalence, location in society, and importance. Their causes are detailed, and appropriate interventions are developed to ameliorate them. In this context, the use of social scientific methodology is central. Policy options are selected, and proposals advocating particular choices are advanced to an involved policy leader. Methods of policy persuasion, which is critical to influencing a choice, include determining the objectives of the persuasion (in written or oral form), diagnosing the audience (particularly gauging the degree of hostility to the ideas), and tailoring the objectives to the audience. Concommitantly, health care professionals develop a political strategy grounded in current realities through contact with interest groups, legislators, and others who wield power over the decision-making process and who can assist in the successful development and implementation of policy and its evaluation.

The target of the health care professional's influence determines the role she/he chooses to play in effecting this change. These roles include indirect involvement, such as identifying and communicating information from different sources; consultation through advocacy roles, such as citizen participation and coalition organization; and direct involvement, such as passing referenda and citizen initiatives and seeking political appointment and public office (Mico, 1978; Simonds, 1978).

Summary

Given these varied contexts for health promotion—both political and economic—the health care professional has a number of avenues to press for change, particularly for policy change. Within this complex context, where interests and exchanges are multiple, the health care professional may seek to affect one or several interrelated levels.

She/he may seek to advocate for changes in federal, international, state, local, or international legislation; regulation or policy; or accreditation standards. She/he may consider organizing coalitions with other voluntary or professional groups to push for change in the definition and practice of health promotion or to increase its attention to underserved community groups. She/he may share information with others about strategies for implementing Healthy Cities. She/he may organize client groups to advocate for change in Medicare or Medicaid reimbursement policies for health promotive care. She/he may run for political office on a platform supporting both quality and cost outcomes in managed care or provisions to protect the findings of genetic testing. The context for health promotion is one rich with possibilities for change. Further discussion of these roles, particularly in organizational policy change, is found in the next chapter.

References

Adams, W.C. (1992-1993). The role of media relations in risk communication. *Public Relations Quarterly, 37,* 28-32.

American Public Health Association. (1997, May/June). APHA board adopts managed care plan, extends task force. *The Nation's Health, 27*(5), 1, 20.

American School Health Association, Association of the Advancement of Health Education and Society for Public Health Education. (1989). *National adolescent student health survey.* Oakland, CA: Third Party Press.

Ammerman, A.S., DeVellis, R.F., Carey, T.S., Keyserling, T.C. et al. (1993). Physician-based diet counseling for cholesterol reduction: Current practices, determinants and strategies for improvement. *Preventive Medicine An International Journal Devoted to Practice and Theory, 22*(1), 96-109.

Anonymous. (1987, July 10). Leads from the MMWR: Indian Health Service facilities become smoke-free *Journal of the American Medical* Association, *258*(2), 185.

Avner, J.R. (1992). The difficulties in providing primary care in the emergency department. *Pediatric Emergency Care, 8,* 101-102.

Barker, C., Pistrang, N., Shapiro, D.A., Davies, S., & Shaw, I. (1993). You in mind: A preventive mental health television series. *British Journal of Clinical Psychology, 32,* 281-293.

Blue Cross and Blue Shield. (1997). What's Blue? [On-line]. http://www.bluecares.com/blue/about

Brown, R.E. et al. (1991). *National expenditures for health promotion and disease prevention activities in the United States.* Washington, DC: Medical Technology Assessment and Policy Research Center, Battelle. (Available from Office of Program Planning and Evaluation, Centers for Disease Control, Atlanta, GA.)

Burns, R.B., Stoy, D.B., Feied, C.F., Nash, E., & Smith, M. (1991). Cholesterol screening in the emergency department. *Journal of General Internal Medicine, 6*(3), 210-215.

Burton, L.C., Paqlia, M.J., German, P.S., Shapiro, S., Damiano, A.M., & the Medicare Preventive Services Research Team. (1995). The effect among older persons of general preventive visits on three health behaviors: Smoking, excessive alcohol drinking, and sedentary lifestyle [Special issue]. *Preventive Medicine: An International Journal Devoted to Practice and Theory, 24*(5), 492-497.

Butterfoss, F.D., Goodman, R.M., & Wandersman, A. (1993). Community coalitions for prevention and health promotion. *Health Education Research, 8*(30), 315-330.

Canadian Public Health Association. (1986). Ottawa Charter for Health Promotion. *Health Promotion, 1*(4), iii-v.

Canadian Task Force on the Periodic Health Examination. (1994). *The Canadian guide to clinical preventive health care.* Ottawa: Canada Communication Group.

Centers for Disease Control and Prevention and the National Association of County Health Officials. (1994). *Blueprint for a healthy community: A guide for local health departments.* Washington, DC: National Association of County Health Officials.

Centers for Disease Control and Prevention. (1995, November 17). Prevention and managed care: Opportunities for managed care organizations, purchasers of health care, and public health agencies. *Morbidity and Mortality Weekly Reports, 44* (RR-14), 1-12.

Chern, A. Su Chung. (1996). Health promotion policies in Singapore: Meeting the challenge of the 1990s. *Health Promotion International, 11*(2), 127.

Chernow, S.M., & Iserson, K.V. (1987). Use of the emergency department for hypertension screening: A prospective study. *Annals of Emergency Medicine, 16,* 180-182.

Clinton, B. (1992). The Clinton health care plan. *New England Journal of Medicine, 327,* 904-907.

Clean Indoor Air Act. Administrative Code of the City of New York, Chapter 5, § 17-501 to § 17-514 (1988).

Comprehensive Preventive Health and Promotion Act of 1997. H.R. 177, 105th Congress (1997).

Cortes, F., Steeples, M., & Stone, M. (1995). Promoting healthy eating: Contra Costa County's food policy. *American Journal of Public Health, 85*(10), 1449-1450.

Cushman, R., James, W., & Waclawik, H. (1991). Physicians promoting bicycle helmets for children: A randomized trial. *American Journal of Public Health, 81*(8), 1044-1046.

Davis, K., Bialek, R., Parkinson, M., Smith, J., & Vellozzi, C. (1990). Reimbursement for preventive services: Can we construct an equitable system? *Journal of General Internal Medicine, 5* (Suppl 5), S93-S98.

Decision Resources, Inc., Institute for Health Care Business Development. (1997). *Health care acquisition, technology, transfer, licensing, and sources of capital directory.* Montvale, NJ: Medical Economics Co.

Division of Adolescent and School Health. (1995). Atlanta, GA. Center for Chronic Disease Prevention and Health Promotion, Centers for Disease Control and Prevention, U.S. Department of Health and Human Services, U.S. Public Health Service.

Ernst, E. (1994). Placebos in medicine: Comment. *The Lancet, 345,* 65.

Foster, S., & Duke, J.A. (1990). *Eastern/central medicinal plants.* (Peterson Field Gurdes). Boston: Houghton Mifflin.

Freedman, M.A., & Trabin, T. (1994). *Managed behavioral healthcare: History, models, key issues, and future course.* Washington, DC: U.S. Center for Mental Health Services.

Frew, S.A. (1991). *Patient transfers: How to comply with the law.* Dallas, TX: American College of Emergency Physicians.

Friede, A., O'Carroll, P.W., Nicola, R.M., Oberle, M.W., & Teutsch, S.M. (1997). CDC prevention guidelines: A Guide to action. Baltimore, MD: Williams & Wilkins.

Frost, K., Frank, E., & Mailbach, E. (1997). Relative risk in the news media: A quantification of misrepresentation. *American Journal of Public Health, 87,* 842-845.

Fugh-Berman, A. (1996). *Alternative medicine—What works. A comprehensive easy to read review of the scientific evidence, pro and con.* Tucson, AZ: Odion Press.

Gale Research Inc. (1997). *Ward's business directory* (pp. 218-222). Detroit: Author

Garguilo, M. (1993). Two-step leverage: Managing constraint in organizational politics. *Administrative Science Quarterly, 38*(1), 1-19.

Gellert, G.A., Higgins, K.V., Lowery, R.M., & Maxwell, R.M. (1994). A national survey of public health officers' interactions with the media. *Journal of the American Medical Association, 271,* 1285-1289.

Gomel, M., Oldenburg, B., Simpson, J., & Owen, N. (1993). Work-site cardiovascular risk reduction: A randomized trial of health risk assessment, education, counseling, and incentives. *American Journal of Public Health, 83*(9), 1231-1238.

Gostin, L.O. (1986). The future of public health law. (Public health and the law: A symposium dedicated to Professor William J. Curran). *American Journal of Law and Medicine, 12*(3 & 4), 461-490.

Guinta, M.A., & Allegrante, J.P. (1992). The President's Committee on Health Education: A 20-year retrospective on its politics and policy impact. *American Journal of Public Health, 82*(7), 1033-1041.

Hacker, J.S. (1996). National health care reform: An idea whose time came and went. *Journal of Health Politics, Policy, and Law, 21*(4), 647-696.

Hastings, G.B. (September, 1989). The mass media in health promotion: Ten golden rules. Paper presented at the BPS International Conference on Health Psychology. Cardiff, Wales.

Health Care Act for Children and Pregnant Women. R.I. Gen. Laws § 398-42-12.3-2, 3.3 (1993).

Health Care Financing Administration. (1997). Managed care in Medicare and Medicaid. [On-line]. http://www.hcfa.gov

Health Insurance Association of America. (1996). *Source book of health insurance data.* Washington, DC: Author.

Health Maintenance Organization Act of 1973, 42 U.S.C. § 201 notes *et seq.* (1994).

Healthy Communities, Healthy People Act. Fla. Stat. §§ 408-601, 602, 604 (1996).

Heclo, H. (1972). Policy analysis. *British Journal of Policy Sciences, 2,* 83-108.

Hibbs, J.R., Ceglowski, W.S., Goldberg, M., & Kauffman, F. (1993). Emergency department-based surveillance for syphillis during an outbreak in Philadelphia. *Annals of Emergency Medicine, 22*(8), 1286-1290.

Hogness, C.G., Engelstad, L.P., Linck, L.M., & Schorr, K.A. (1992). Cervical cancer screening in an urban emergency department. *Annals of Emergency Medicine, 21,* 933-39.

Hoover's Company Profile. *Company capsule: Blue Cross and Blue Shield Association.* [on-line]. http://www.infoseek.com

Iannantuono, A. & Eyles, J. (1997). Meanings in policy: A textual analysis of Canada's "Achieving Health for All" document. *Social Science in Medicine, 44*(11), 1611-1621.

Institute for Health Care Business Development. (1997). *Health Care Acquisition, Technology, Transfer, Licensing, and Sources of Capital Directory.* Montvale, NJ: Medical Economics Co.

Joyce, C.R.B. (1994). Placebo and complementary medicine. *The Lancet, 344,* 1279-1281.

Kongstvedt, P.R. (1993). *The managed health care handbook* (2nd ed.). Gaithersburg, MD: Aspen.

Kushner, R.F. (1995). Barriers to providing nutrition counseling by physicians: A survey of primary care practicioners. *Preventive Medicine: An International Journal Devoted to Practice and Theory, 24*(6), 546-552.

Lalonde, M. (1974). *A new perspective on the health of Canadians.* Ottawa: Information Canada.

Leenen, J.J., Pinet, G., & Prims, A.V. (1985). *Trends in health legislation in Europe.* (Unpublished manuscript, available from WHO Regional Office for Europe, Copenhagen). (EURO Doc. ICP/HLE 101 E.)

Logsdon, D.N., Lazaro, C.M., & Meier, R.V. (1989). The feasibility of behavioral risk reduction in primary medical care. *American Journal of Preventive Medicine, 5*(5), 249-256.

Lorion, R.P. (1983). Evaluating preventive interventions: Guidelines for the serious social change agent. In R.D. Felner, L.A. Jason, J.N. Moritsugu, & S.S. Farber (Eds.), *Preventive psychology: Theory, research and practice.* Oxford, England: Pergamon.

Lowi, T.J. (1972). Population policies and the American political system. In R.L. Clinton, W.S. Flash, & R.K. Godwin (Eds.), *Political science in population studies.* Lexington, MA: D.C. Heath.

Maccoby, N., Farquhar, J.W., Wood, P.D. & Alexander, J. (1977). Reducing the risk of cardiovascular disease: Effects of a community-based campaign on knowledge and behavior. *Journal of Community Health, 3,* 100-114.

Mayer, R.R., & Greenwood, E. (1980). *The design of social policy.* Englewood Cliffs, NJ: Prentice-Hall.

McAlister, A. (1982). Mass and community organization for prevention programs. In A.M. Jeger & R.S. Slotnick (Eds.), *Community mental health and behavioral ecology: A handbook of theory, research and practice.* New York: Plenum.

McCaig, L.F. (1994). *National ambulatory medical care survey: 1992 emergency department summary. Advance data from vital and health statistics,* (DHHS Publication No. 245). Hyattsville, MD: National Center for Health Statistics.

McCombs, M.E., & Shaw, D.L. (1972). The agenda setting function of mass media. *Public Opinion Quarterly, 36,* 176-187.

Meyer, P. (1990). News media responsiveness to public health. In C. Atkin, L. Wallack (Eds.), *Mass communication and public health* (pp. 52-59). Newbury Park, CA: Sage.

Mico, P.R. (1978). An introduction to policy for health educators. *Health Education Monographs 6* (Suppl. 1), 7-17.

Milliman and Robertson, Inc. (1987). *Health risks and behavior: The impact on medical costs.* Brookfield, WI: Milliman and Robertson.

Mullen, P.D., & Holcomb, J.D. (1990). Selected predictors of health promotion counseling by three groups of allied health professionals. *American Journal of Preventive Medicine, 6*(3), 153-160.

National Center for Health Statistics. (1990). *Health, United States, 1989 and prevention profile* (DHHS Publication No. [PHS] 90-1232). Hyattsville, MD: U.S. Department of Health and Human Services.

National Consumer Health Information and Health Promotion Act of 1976, 42 U.S.C. §301 *et seq.* (1994).

National Highway Traffic Safety Administration. (1988). *Fatal accident reporting system, 1987.* Washington, DC: U.S. Department of Transportation.

National School Boards Association. (1989). Smoke-free schools: A progress report. Alexandria, VA: Author.

Navarro, V. (1976). *Medicine under capitalism.* New York: Prodist.

Nelkin, D. (1985). Managing biomedical news. *Social Research, 52,* 625-646.

Neubauer, D., & Pratt, R. (1981). The second public health revolution: A critical appraisal. *Journal of Health Politics, Policy, and Law, 6*(2), 205-228.

N.J. Stat. Ann. § 17-48-6i (West, 1996).

Nutrition Labeling and Education Act of 1990, 21 U.S.C. § 301 *et seq.* (1994).

Nutrition, Smoking and Substance Abuse Acts of 1987, Iowa Code Ann. §200-9 (Westlaw, 1997).

Ockene, J.K., Ockene, I.S., Quirk, M.E., Hebert, J.R. et al. (1995). Physician training for patient-centered nutrition counseling in a lipid intervention trial. *Preventive Medicine An International Journal Devoted to Practice and Theory, 24*(6), 563-570.

Office of Disease Prevention and Health Promotion. (1990). *Mass communications and health.* Washington, DC: U.S. Department of Health and Human Services.

Orleans, C.T., Kristeller, J.L., & Gritz, E. (1993). Helping hospitalized smokers quit: New directions for treatment and research. *Journal of Consulting and Clinical Psychology, 61*(5), 778-89.

Patton, D., Kolasa, K., West, S., & Irons, T. (1995). Sexual abstinenece counseling of adolescents by physicians. *Adolescence, 30*(120), 963-969.

Pinet, G. (1986). The WHO European Program. *American Journal of Law and Medicine, 12*(3 & 4), 441-460.

Preventive Health Amendments of 1993, PL 103-183 (42 USC 233 et seq.)

Price, J.H., Clause, M., & Everett, S.A. (1995). Patients' attitudes about the role of physicians in counseling about firearms. *Patient Education and Counseling, 25*(2), 163-170.

Rathwell, T. (1992). Realities of Health for All by the Year 2000 (review). *Social Science and Medicine, 35*(4), 541-547.

Riedel, J.E. (1987). Employee health promotion: Blue Cross and Blue Shield plan activities. *American Journal of Health Promotion, 1*(4) 28-32.

Reynolds, C. (1994). The promise of public health law. *Journal of Law and Medicine, 1,* 212-222.

Roberts, D.F., & Maccoby, N. (1985). Effects of mass communication. In G. Lindzy & E. Aronson (Eds.), *Handbook of social psychology: Vol. 2. special fields and applications.* New York: Random House.

Roemer, M.I. (1982). Market failure and health care policy. *Journal of Public Health Policy, 3* (4), 419-431.

Roemer, M.I. (1986). *An introduction to the U.S. health care system.* New York: Springer.

Royals, G., Chitwood, L.F., Davis, L.A., & Cole, J. (1996). Healthy people 2000 goal 1.12: Primary care physicians and exercise counseling. *Journal of the Mississippi State Medical Association, 37*(6), 605-608.

Russell, N.K., & Roter, D.L. (1993). Health promotion counseling of chronic-disease patients during primary care visits. *American Journal of Public Health, 83*(7), 979-982.

S. 1643, 104th Cong. 2nd Sess. §§104-344 (1996).

Schauffler, H.H. (1993a). Disease prevention policy under Medicare: A historical and political analysis. *American Journal of Preventive Medicine, 9*(2), 71-77.

Schauffler, H.H. (1993b). Integrating smoking control policies into employee benefits: A survey of large California corporations. *American Journal of Public Health, 83*(9), 1226-1230.

Schauffler, H.H., & Parkinson, M.D. (1993). Health insurance coverage for smoking cessation services. *Health Education Quarterly, 20*(2), 185-206.

Schauffler, H.H., & Rodriguez, T. (1994). Satisfaction with health plans. *Medical Care, 32,* 1182-1196.

Schectman, J.M., Stoy, D.B., & Elinsky, E.G. (1994). Association between physician counseling for hypercholesterolemia and patient dietary knowledge. *American Journal of Preventive Medicine, 10*(3), 136-9.

Sewing, K-Fr. (1994). Placebos in medicine: Comment. *The Lancet, 345,* 65-66.

Shelton, D.A., & Frank, R. (1995). Rural mental health coverage under health care reform. *Community Mental Health Journal, 31*(6), 539-552.

Shenkman, E., Pendergast, J., Reiss, J., Walther, E., Bucciarelli, R., & Freedman, S. (1996). The school enrollment based health insurance program: Socioeconomic factors in enrollees' use of health services. *American Journal of Public Health, 86*(12), 1791-1793.

Shouldice, R.G. (1991). *Introduction to managed care: Health maintenance organizations, preferred provider organizations, and competitive medical plans.* Arlington, VA: Information Resources Press.

Simonds, S.K. (1978). Health education: Facing issues of policy, ethics, and social justice. *Health Education Monographs 6* (Suppl. 1), 17-27.

Singer, E., & Endreny, P. (1987). Reporting hazards: Their benefits and costs. *Journal of Communication, 37,* 10-26.

Starr, P. (1982). *The social transformation of American medicine.* New York: Basic Books.

Starr, P. (1994). *The logic of health-care reform: Why and how the president's plan will work* (revised and expanded ed.). rev. New York: Penguin Books.

Steckler, A., Dawson, L., Goodman, R.M., & Epstein, N. (1987). Policy advocacy: Three emerging roles for health education. *Advances in Health Education and Promotion, 2,* 5-27.

Summer, L., Parrott, S., & Mann, C. (1996). Millions of uninsured and underinsured children are eligible for Medicaid. Center on Budget and Policy Priorities. [On-line]. http://www.cbpp.org

Swedish Health and Medical Services Act. SFS (Svensk forfattningssamling)-1982-736 (Effective 1/1/83).

Tennessee Resource Mothers Program. Tenn. Code Ann. § 990-68-1-1401 to 68-1-1408 (MICHIE, 1996).

Tesh, S. (1981). Disease causality and politics. *Journal of Health Politics, 6*(3), 369-390.

Thompson, S.C., Schwankovsky, L., Pitts, J. (1993). Counseling patients to make lifestyle changes: The role of physician self-efficacy, training and beliefs about causes. *Family Practice, 10*(1), 70-75.

U.S. Congress, Office of Technology Assessment. (1990). *Preventive health services for Medicare beneficiaries: Policy and research issues* (OTA-H-416). Washington, DC: Government Printing Office.

U.S. Department of Education. (1987). *Report to Congress and the White House on the nature and effectiveness of federal, state, and local drug prevention/education programs.* Washington, DC: Author.

U.S. Department of Health and Human Services, U.S. Public Health Service. (1988). *The Surgeon General's report on nutrition and health.* Washington, DC: Author.

U.S. Department of Health and Human Services. (1991). *Healthy people 2000: National health promotion and disease prevention objectives.* (DHHS Publication No. PHS 91-50213). Washington, DC: U.S. Government Printing Office.

U.S. Department of Health and Human Services, U.S. Public Health Service. (1993). 1992 National survey of worksite health promotion activities: Summary. *American Journal of Health Promotion, 7*, 452-464.

U.S. Department of Health and Human Services, National Center for Health Statistics (1994). *Advance data.* Washington, DC: Author.

U.S. Department of Health and Human Services, U.S. Public Health Service. (1995). *Healthy people 2000: Midcourse review and 1995 revisions.* Washington, DC: U.S. Government Printing Office.

U.S. Preventive Services Task Force. (1996). *Guide to clinical preventive services* (2nd ed.). Baltimore, MD: Williams & Wilkins.

Veteran's Health Care Reform Eligibility Act of 1996, PL 104-262, 38 U.S.C.A. 101 note *et seq.* (1994).

Wallack, L.M. (1981). Mass media campaigns: The odds against finding behavior change [Review]. (1994). *Health Education Quarterly, 8* (3), 209-260.

Wallack, L., & Dorfman, L. (1992). Television news, hegemony, and health. *American Journal of Public Health, 82,* 125-126.

Wallack, L., Dorfman, L., Jernigan, D., & Themba, M. (1993). *Media advocacy and public health: Power for prevention.* Newbury Park, CA: Sage.

Wamsley, G., & Zald, M. (1967). *The political economy of public organizations: A critique and approach to the study of public administration.* Bloomington, IN: Indiana University Press.

Weber, J. (1997, January 13). Drugs and biotech. *Business Week, 3509,* 110.

Weiner, S.L. (1986). Tampons and toxic shock syndrome: Consumer protection or public confusion? In H.M. Sapolsky (Ed.), *Consuming fears* (pp. 141-158). New York: Basic Books.

Woolf, S.H., Jonas, S., & Lawrence, R.S. (Eds.). (1996). *Health promotion and disease prevention in clinical practice.* Baltimore, MD: Williams & Wilkins.

World Bank. (1993). *World development report 1993: Investing in health.* Washington, DC: Author.

World Health Organization. (1985). *Targets for health for all.* Copenhagen, Denmark: WHO Regional Office for Europe.

World Health Organization. (1988, April 5-9). Report on the Adelaide Conference: Healthy public policy. Second International Conference on Health Promotion. Adelaide, South Australia.

Year 2000 Health Objectives Planning Act, 42 U.S.C. 246 note, § 105 *et seq.* (1994).

CHAPTER

4

Agents for Health Promotion

Laurel Janssen Breen and Joan Arnold

We are at a turning point in the delivery of health care—a time of transition. As with all transitions, there are the challenges of new role developments, altered relationships, and changes in the power structure. The questions and the answers are getting more complex. Health care professionals are redefining themselves within a society where key phrases are *shared decision-making* and *consumer partnership.* To paraphrase C. Everett Koop, past U.S. Surgeon General, the most critical clinical skill for the twenty-first century may be learning how to answer the questions our clients are bringing to us (Woolf, Jonas, & Lawrence, 1996).

This "how" extends far beyond the responsibility of maintaining clinical excellence. The health revolution beckons us to examine our professional health behaviors, risk factors, support needs, and overall well-being. As a community of health care professionals, how well-equipped are we to personally and collectively participate in the process of our own professional behavior change? Are we capable of collaboratively approaching a realignment of power with our clients and with each other? If we are capable of moving away from the need for consensus in the definition of health, will we also be able to embrace our own diversity in approach to its promotion?

As health care professionals embedded in an illness-oriented system, the challenge to redefine ourselves within this environment remains an ominous task. Our history includes a varied relationship with the public. Despite our many successes, it is suggested that in some of our past attempts to affect the health behavior of others, we have ". . . created or exacerbated a number of undesirable developments . . ." (Becker, 1993, p. 5). The health promotion movement needs to lend a watchful eye to its recent past as we move toward a reconceptualization of ourselves. As we move toward incorporation of ideals and philosophies, we must also be mindful of avoiding a "change-for-the-better" mind-set. The implication that a future state is by its very nature inherently more desirable than the current one is a philosophy borne of a homeostatic model (Kelly, 1989). Change, by its complex nature, requires vigilance and expert use of self.

HEALTH CARE PROFESSIONALS AS AGENTS FOR HEALTH PROMOTION

Movement from an illness-oriented perspective of delivering care to one that supports wellness as an ideal is foundational for the shifting paradigm of health promotion. Each health care professional must reckon with the impact of having been reared in an educational framework supportive of illness and disease as the model from which to understand health. Health, the opposite of illness, was defined as the state that could be restored and maintained when illness was treated effectively by the intervention skills of providers. If it was not seen as the opposite of illness, then health was viewed as part of an illness continuum and defined by illness parameters. Shifting to a wellness continuum requires a new view of health and illness. The health care professional becomes a provider of *health* care, having synthesized health as the new framework for practice. The provider views client systems through the lens of health, allowing for a different interpretation of client patterns, needs, and system responses. Needs are interpreted from knowledge, skills, and standards that promote health.

Defining indicators of wellness necessitates an understanding of the complexity and diversity of the human condition. Research to define and substantiate indicators of wellness is in its infancy stage of development. Outcome measures are only beginning to be established (Gillis, 1995). The focus and philosophy underlying the use of skills learned in the disease framework will not support the provider in the delivery of health promotion care. Health promotion requires a belief in the strengths and capabilities of the client, who defines and determines health care decisions. The provider remains a resource and facilitator of this process. The client is the expert, and the provider offers useful and meaningful information and skills that aids the client in closing the gap between his/her ideal image of health and current condition.

Clients may experience frustration, confusion, alienation, and invalidation when they look toward health care professionals for help in using available services to optimize their health. Although some of these services may be unfamiliar to clients, they come to providers with an openness to learn and choose for themselves. Creating paths for direct access to health care professionals enables clients to truly be consumers of *health* care.

DEFINING HEALTH CARE AGENTS

Who are health care professionals? A list of health professionals compiled by the U.S. Department of Labor with the number of employed providers in each category based on 1994 statistics is given in Table 4-1.

The directory of occupational titles and included job descriptions in Table 4-1 is not sufficient to reflect the vast and diverse roles of health care professionals. The National Consumer Health Information Act of 1976 called for the formulation of national goals regarding health information and promotion, preventive health care services, and education in the appropriate use of health care. It referred to medicine, dentistry, nursing, pharmacy, and public health as health professions and provided funds to research methods of dissemination of health information to the public. There continues to be a need to define and develop new occupational categories, including community health education aides; advocates or facilitators to act as bridges in the community, especially in low income areas; and other health professionals. The Act referred to the quality and success of these

Table **4-1**

Health professions with numbers of employed providers	
PROFESSION	**NUMBER EMPLOYED**
PROFESSIONAL SPECIALTY OCCUPATIONS	
Health diagnosing practitioners	
Chiropractors	42,000
Dentists	164,000
Optometrists	37,000
Physicians (MD & DO)	539,000
Podiatrists	13,000
Health assessment and treating occupations	
Dietitians and Nutritionists	53,000
Occupational Therapists	54,000
Pharmacists	168,000
Physical Therapists	102,000
Physician Assistants	56,000
Recreational Therapists	31,000
Registered Nurses	1,906,000
Respiratory Therapists	73,000
Speech-Language Pathologists and Audiologists	85,000
EXECUTIVE, ADMINISTRATIVE, AND MANAGERIAL OCCUPATIONS	
Health Services Managers	315,000

Data from *Occupational Outlook Handbook* by U.S. Department of Labor, 1996-1997, Washington, DC: Author.

educational programs resting on the need for more precise definitions, more standardized training, and some form of academic certification.

Although a projected slowdown in employment growth is expected, health care services will account for almost 20% of all job growth between 1994 and 2005. Factors contributing to continued growth in this industry include an aging population that demands increased services; a shift from hospital-based care to community-based services; and the increased use of medical technology for the purposes of diagnosis and treatment (U.S. Department of Labor, 1996-97). Occupations within health services are expected to increase at twice the rate of the U.S. economy as a whole. This expected growth represents an opportunity for health care professionals, distinguished by their capabilities, to become instrumental in shaping the rapidly changing health care system. To be considered a vital contributing part of the transforming system, health care professionals must anticipate and address societal health care needs within a wellness framework.

The call to extend specific occupational categories must also be expanded to include providers of complementary health care, which is now being demanded by the public (Colt, 1996; *Time,* 1996; *Consumer Reports,* 1996). Complementary health care has been referred to as complementary and alternative medicine. In 1991, Congress established the Office of Alternative Medicine (OAM) under the direction of the National Institutes of Health (NIH) to link the alternative medical community with federally sponsored research and regulations and to reduce barriers for bringing alternative therapies to the public. A report entitled *Alternative Medicine: Expanding Medical Horizons* (U.S. Office of Alternative Medicine, National Institutes of Health, 1994) identifies seven fields of alternative medicine listed in Box 4-1. There is growing demand and use of these alternative health care fields (Fugh-Berman, 1996). The impact that unconventional therapy has on the health care system is often underestimated.

> Roughly one in four Americans who see their medical doctors for a serious health problem may be using unconventional therapy in addition to conventional medicine for that problem, and seven of 10 such encounters take place without patients' telling their medical doctors that they use unconventional therapy. Furthermore, use is distributed widely across all sociodemographic groups (Eisenberg et al., 1993, p. 251).

Box **4-1**

Fields of alternative medicine

1. *Mind-body interventions*—explore the integral relationship between mind and body, emphasizing their interconnectedness
   - Psychotherapy
   - Support groups
   - Meditation
   - Imagery
   - Hypnosis
   - Biofeedback
   - Yoga
   - Dance, music, and art therapy
   - Prayer and mental healing
2. *Bioelectromagnetics applications (BEM)*—the ways living organisms interact with electromagnetic (EM) fields
   - Thermal nonionizing radiation (includes radio frequency [RF], hyperthermia, laser and RF surgery, RF diathermy)
   - Nonthermal nonionizing radiation (includes bone repair, nerve stimulation, wound healing, osteoarthritis treatment, electroacupuncture, tissue regeneration, and immune system stimulation)
3. *Alternative systems of medical practice*—70% to 90% of health care worldwide ranges from self-care according to folk principles to care given in an organized health care system based on an alternative tradition or practice
   - Popular (informal practices in the home, such as using herbal teas for a cold)
   - Community based (care that reflects the health needs, beliefs, and natural environments of those who use it, such as nonprofessional practices occurring in many urban and rural communities)
   - Professionalized health care systems (a delivery system based on theories of health and disease, including traditional oriental medicine, acupuncture, Ayurvedic medicine,

Use patterns of this "invisible mainstream" (Eisenberg, 1996, p. 20) reflect public interest in complementary modalities, and reimbursement for these services is gaining support. To gain total integration, with full provider rights and privileges, complementary and traditional providers need to become interrelated parts of one system of health care. Further, the safety, efficacy, mechanism of action, and cost-effectiveness of individual alternative treatments must be more fully explored (Eisenberg, 1997).

EMPOWERMENT

Within the last decade, most definitions of health promotion have included the concept of empowerment. Central to all of these definitions is the direct relationship between an individual's level of health and the amount of control that is felt over his/her life. The scope of the use of *empowerment* has grown beyond individual power to include an understanding of empowerment as a multifaceted dynamic interchange occurring on many levels (Airhihenbuwa, 1994; Labonte, 1994; Wallerstein, 1992).

Box 4-1

Fields of alternative medicine—cont'd

homeopathy, anthroposophically extended medicine, naturopathy, and environmental medicine)

4. *Manual healing methods*—touch and manipulation of soft tissues or realignment of body parts to correct a dysfunction of a body part that affects the function of other discrete body parts
   - Osteopathic medicine
   - Chiropractic
   - Massage and other physical healing methods
   - Biofield therapeutics (laying on of hands)
5. *Pharmacological and biological treatments*—the use of drugs and vaccines not yet accepted by conventional medicine; clinical safety and effectiveness trials to meet Food and Drug Administration (FDA) approval for these treatments have not been fully investigated because of lack of sponsors and funding
6. *Herbal medicine*—the use of plants and plant products as remedies; these remedies are often self-administered and purchased through herbalists, health food stores, and certain practitioners. Because of the FDA's skepticism about herbal remedies, these products are marketed as food supplements without specific health claims.
7. *Diet and nutrition in the prevention and treatment of chronic disease*—dietary and nutritional interventions to affect biochemical and physiologic processes in the body. This field includes orthomolecular medicine—the use of high-dose vitamins in the treatment of chronic diseases such as AIDS, bronchial asthma, cancer, cardiovascular diseases, lymphedema, and mental and neurologic disorders. Alternative diets are believed to provide greater resistance to illness and treat allergies.

Modified from *Alternative Medicine: Expanding Medical Horizons* (pp. 3-206), 1994, by U.S. Office of Alternative Medicine, National Institutes of Health, Washington, DC.

In its broadest definition, empowerment is a multilevel construct that involves people assuming control and mastery over their lives in the context of their social and political environment; they gain a sense of control and purposefulness to exert political power as they participate in the democratic life of their community for social change (Wallerstein, 1992, p. 198).

The incorporation of ideas regarding the "multidimensionality of empowerment" has further led to the visualization of empowerment as being part of a continuum. This "empowerment continuum" acknowledges that interventions at every level (individual, family, group, community, organizational, or political) have the innate potential to be empowering (Robertson & Minkler, 1994, p. 302).

Empowerment is not limited or defined by the level at which it occurs. The visualization of empowerment as a continuum can be seen as both a validation and a focus for practitioners. It frees up an understanding of the boundless potential of health promotion work. It acknowledges the diversity of approaches that practitioners at all points in the health/illness continuum use. Interventions at both the micro- and macro-level have the capacity to promote system change and to affect the overall well-being and health of communities. Any level can be the starting point for this change process. At a time when the goal is collective action and community-based care delivery for the purpose of maximum impact and cost-effectiveness, it seems important to not diminish the empowering effects of individual-based care. The empowered teenager who seeks out and correctly uses birth control gains mastery and control over his/her destiny. At a different level on the empowerment continuum lie the community education and political action work needed to secure the clinic this teenager and other classmates may feel comfortable enough to visit.

In the attempt to incorporate an expanded notion of empowerment, the health care professional is struggling with the concept of reengineering the provider/client relationship. There is a recognition that this new definition of empowerment brings an entirely new set of expectations. Behaviors and terminologies from a past paradigm are no longer useful. Beyond the generalized discussions regarding the philosophy of a shared power base and community partnership comes the real task of operationalizing this new construct of empowerment.

Traditionally, health care professionals have been the acknowledged "gatekeepers" to the health care system. As identified experts they possess the necessary education, skills, and language to successfully negotiate the complexities of the system. This starting point from within the system offers what might be considered an insider's view. From this vantage point, health care professionals have become comfortable with a concept of empowerment in which they are the ones doing the empowering. The timing and conditions of sharing power remained within the active control of the provider. Past emphasis has fostered the continuation of this arrangement. "Professionals, as the empowering agent, the subject of the relationship, remain the controlling actor, defining the terms of the interaction" (Labonte, 1994, p. 255). The client remains the receiver of this act. Almost automatically, our language resonates this passive client role. When speaking of a community, we address its need to "be empowered." Yet, empowerment has been difficult to define in terms of outcomes, since it is most easily recognized in its absence as powerlessness (Wallerstein, 1992).

Moving beyond this provider-centered view of empowerment means refocusing. It means stretching beyond what may be professional validation to true acceptance of the client as the expert in his/her own experience. Thus it means a transfer of knowledge, skills, resources, access, and language, but it extends far beyond that. Empowerment can only occur in an environment that supports its existence. "Empowerment is not something that can be given; it must be taken" (Rappaport, 1985, p. 18). Health care professionals need to learn how to establish and maintain this empowering environment—an environment in which the client at all levels sees the potential and value in seizing power. It is only from within this core of empowerment that a community can begin to identify its own needs. Beyond the transfer of important resources emerges an empowered community that is able to fully participate in its own self-determination. It connotes a shift from bureaucratic control to community control (Hanson, 1989).

THE CHALLENGE OF CROSS-DISCIPLINARY PARTNERSHIP

Whereas the basic ideas and philosophy of cross-disciplinary work are nothing new, the acceptance of the goal as a shared challenge may be. Historically, an uneven distribution of power has existed among health care professionals. Community perception, reimbursement issues, and territoriality are some of the issues underlying the development and maintenance of this pattern.

The importance of community participation has been presented as both a means and an outcome in achieving community health. This two-pronged goal acknowledges the capacity and necessity for communities to be intimately involved at all levels of system change if success is to be achieved. To bring about a specific goal or objective, the need for collective community action that is both deliberate and formalized has been stressed. Is the loose network of community health care professionals supportive of collaboration as a mutual goal? What mandates to its members does this suggest? How will the "community" of health care professionals achieve full participation and act as collective to forge a model of effective professional collaboration? What type of identity must be internalized to function in this capacity?

In his discussion of "authentic" partnership within a framework of total community participation, Labonte (1994) outlined a series of guidelines that can serve as a basis for grounding a collaborative practice. Based on these guidelines, the characteristics of a collaborative partnership include legitimacy/power sharing, self-knowledge, respect, and commitment (Box 4-2). These characteristics reflect the necessity for each participating partner to explore, expand, and question his/her relationship to certain needs and responsibilities. For a list of self-directed questions that address the collaborative process, see Box 4-3.

THE HEALTH CARE SYSTEM AS CONTEXT FOR HEALTH PROMOTION

The term *health system* is a misnomer. The U.S. health care delivery system did not develop *systematically,* and it is not a system that addresses the *health* needs of the nation. There is no overarching framework or identification of values and assumptions that organizes the settings for care and the delivery of health services. The ability to pay has been a significant factor in the ability to secure care, leaving those without insurance or overqualified for publically funded programs out of the system. Health care is not for all. Special needs and categories dictate eligibility for care. Fragmentation is regarded as the "central feature of the U.S. health care system" (Shortell, Gillies, Anderson, Erickson, & Mitchell, 1996, p. 1). The dream of seamless care addressing the trajectory of human needs across

Box 4-2

Characteristics of a collaborative partnership

LEGITIMACY/POWER SHARING

Each partner brings an established identity and accountability that is recognized by all. All partners must know and acknowledge their relationship to overall power. Differences in power and status are noted and able to be discussed. Negotiating a transfer of power and resources takes skill and trust. Some conflict is inevitable and must be confronted. This redistribution of power is part of the process and a desired outcome.

SELF-KNOWLEDGE

Individual partners must know who they are and what they can provide independently and in partnership with others. This self-awareness can support the capacity for continued growth and expanded identity.

RESPECT

The individual autonomy of all partners is recognized. Differences are explored within an environment of support. Existing boundaries between partners are able to be examined. All partners value the benefits that can be derived from a cooperative relationship. Effective communication and negotiation can flow from this core of esteem.

COMMITMENT

There is inquiry into the objectives of all the partners, but a vision of a shared goal is able to replace independent goals. There is an investment in maximizing impact through joint efforts. From this position comes the motivation and ability to delineate responsibilities and to build in purposeful, ongoing evaluation. All persons feel responsible for goal attainment. One measure of success is the level of cooperation that is achieved.

Adapted from "Health promotion and empowerment: Reflections on professional practice" by R. Labonte, 1994 *Health Education Quarterly, 21*(2) pp. 264-265.

the lifespan is far from a reality because fragmentation and specialization force clients to direct their own care. Others are simply alienated from health care services. Health care, rather than being valued as a basic human right and fundamental entitlement, is episodically provided within a cost-conscious context. An illness-driven nonsystem reveals the serious contradictions in the term *health system* and begs rethinking. Rethinking health care means reformulating the focus of care toward health and transforming the organization of care delivery to a more integrated system of care.

The health care delivery system must be altered to provide the context for health promotive care. Health can not be a realistic goal without a system to support it. Health care for all will remain an unfulfilled dream unless the practice environment supports the providers of health care to deliver health promotive services. Collaboration is the key. Collaboration among health care professionals that emphasizes a client-centered plan of care and collaboration among providers and clients that emphasizes health care needs form the foundation for rebuilding a health care system.

System change is accomplished through individual efforts and social policy. The individual provider possesses power, and power is enhanced through an effective partnership

Box 4-3

Self-questions to support a collaborative partnership

- Am I able to take an objective inventory of the skills I possess?
- What specific advantages might I gain from entering a collaborative relationship?
- Do I consistently and nonjudgmentally ask my clients about their use of other therapies?
- Do I feel threatened at the prospect of collaborative work?
- At what point along the "power continuum" do I view my profession?
- Do I look toward collaboration as a means to increase legitimacy?
- Do I feel I would have more to give than to get from collaboration?
- Do I feel others have a good understanding of my capabilities?
- Is it difficult for me to participate in mutual goal setting?
- Do I enjoy the role of being a resource and consultant?
- When consulting with others, do I feel patronized or talked down to?
- How frequently am I asked to consult outside of my discipline?
- Have my past experiences with collaboration been positive?
- In which areas do I consider myself an expert?
- How consistently do I meet the expectations of my clients?
- Am I adaptable to changing circumstances?
- Do I seek out objective evaluations of my work?
- How capable am I of integrating the feedback obtained from these evaluations?
- Am I often impatient when working in a group?
- Do I frequently refer outside my discipline?
- Do I view myself as a risk taker?
- Am I comfortable with the role of advocacy?
- Which professions am I most comfortable using as resources?
- Am I constantly updating my referral resources?
- How do I view my responsibilities within the area of public policy formation surrounding health promotion?
- What are my concerns regarding co-managing a client who is using other therapies?

with clients. The health care system can be altered to become more humane, responsive to human needs, and supportive of health—the health of clients and providers. Creating a dignified environment to receive care that is free from smoke, radiation, asbestos, allergens, and other toxic agents is an important start. Assuring that health care is available, accessible, affordable, appropriate, adequate, and acceptable is a challenge for providers and recipients of care (National Institute of Nursing Research, 1995). The findings of the U.S. Preventive Services Task Force (1996) suggest that interventions must address clients' personal health practices and that providers and clients should share in decision-making. Further, the Task Force urges that every opportunity must be made to deliver preventive services, especially to persons with limited access to care, and recognizes that community-level interventions must take place. The health care delivery system can be altered to become the context for health promotion. A collaborative model for changing the health system is recommended.

The health care professional is at the heart of change; the health care professional is an agent for change. Health care professionals are ideally positioned to collaborate with each other and to form alliances with clients to make a positive impact on the delivery system and on the pressing health care issues of our time. Functioning as an advocate for health is assuming an empowering role. The health care advocate strives to improve and protect health care and to create an environment for the promotion of health. At the crossroads of quality and effective care management, the health care professional advocates efficiency in care management as well as responsiveness to human needs. The system for care must become a system for health care, emphasizing the value and necessity of promoting health, as well as representing health through its own image and actions.

Collaboration rests on the knowledge, skills, and capabilities of each discipline, and collaborators should be willing to combine efforts for the greater good of clients, whether they are individuals, families, groups, communities, or the nation. Reform of the health care system through collaboration requires steadfast determination and reexamination of the way disciplines relate, what each discipline values, and the expectations of the community.

In *Remaking Health Care in America,* the issue of reform is put forth as a challenge to values:

> Health care reform will not succeed until we seriously challenge some of these core values. To what degree should autonomy be pursued at the expense of solidarity? To what extent should individuality be upheld at the neglect of the common good? To what extent shall we cherish self-determination while ignoring the development of a sense of other-directedness? To what extent does an emphasis on diversity threaten a sense of community? To what extent do we continue to support fragmentation and specialization as opposed to integration and a sense of wholeness? (Shortell et al., 1996, p. 2)

This challenge is not denying the importance of autonomy and individuality, but rather it calls for an increase in solidarity, support for the common good, the fostering of other-directedness, and the development of community. Reform means the promotion and protection of health for all—a health care delivery system that enables health care professionals to become *health* care professionals and is in fact a system for *health* care. Central to this set of beliefs is the idea that the system is centered on persons and communities, not developed for providers and organizations. Clients are engaged as full partners with health care professionals in the mutual process of re-creating health care.

CHANGING SYSTEMS FOR HEALTH PROMOTION

Creating a health care system for health promotion requires collaboration among the disciplines and with clients. System change is a process. The process of change can include instituting policies for health. Developing a new policy, implementing that policy, and evaluating the impact of the policy are the phases of the process of system change (Box 4-4). The entire process rests on collaboration from all levels of the system—individuals working toward a common, beneficial goal. The expansion of the Health Promotion Matrix (discussed in Chapter 5) to encompass agency-level change reflects an understanding that change at the individual, family, group, and community levels will be supported if the larger health care system commits to change. Changes in the system for health care are made through policy alterations and agency development. For example, at the corporate level, health promotive change could include opportunities for regular physical activity, healthful food selections in the cafeteria, and a smoke-free environment. Change cannot be promoted unless the overall system is transformed to a system for health.

Box 4-4

Steps for system change for health promotion

1. Approach the problem
2. Develop new policy
   a. Encourage institutional participation
   b. Gather information
   c. Prepare a written policy
   d. Plan an implementation strategy
3. Implement policy
   a. Communicate the policy
   b. Carry out the policy
4. Evaluate the impact of the policy.

Adapted from *Stopping Smoking: A Nurse's Guide* (pp. 41-49), by S. Sheinfeld Gorin, 1989, New York: American Health Foundation.

Step One: Approach the Problem

The critical decision to adopt and support a health promotive environment is the first and most important hurdle. Since the underlying structure and values of an institution are being challenged, the change will take time. However, every effort toward a healthy system is significant. During this step, it is most important to become familiar with the facts about health promotion. Cost-saving studies that relate to the promotion of health are critical to approaching the problem. Summarizing findings, especially of evaluation studies on the significance of health promotive interventions, creates a body knowledge supportive of shifting an institution's mission to the value of health. The health care professional becomes a resource for health promotion and informs other providers at the institution about the efficacy of health promotive interventions and the significance of improved health for individuals, families, groups, and communities. It is helpful during this step to hold discussions and conferences on subjects such as smoking cessation, eating well, physical activity, sexual awareness, injury prevention, substance safety, oral health, self-development, and productivity. Health promotion may be the topic of grand rounds, the focus of an institution's newsletter, or the organizing theme for case conferencing. Every opportunity to bring health promotion to the forefront of systems thinking assists in creating excitement about shifting institutional emphasis and generating enthusiasm among health care professionals for becoming agents of health promotion.

Step Two: Develop New Policy

Developing a policy requires health care professionals to participate with the public and to move from receptivity to responsiveness. Those willing to appreciate the data generated through Step One of the process of system change now respond to the call to develop policy. Policy development focuses on altering the mission of the institution to support health promotive actions. The participants at conferences, rounds, and any other forum in which health promotion was discussed become the critical mass for a more action-oriented Step Two. Recruiting the support of key participants is critical to policy development.

Success during this step is contingent on the best possible representation of participants. Consumers and providers form an alliance that pressures the institution to realign its mission to support health promotion activities. During this step, it is important to determine whether representatives from all of the institution's key components are involved. The communication network of the institution is activated to link as many providers as possible, thereby connecting the divisions they represent. Change is an organic process; the whole institution must be considered. Leaving out a vital component will weaken the process of change.

Moving from receptivity to responsiveness requires that participants learn to value change. Key to valuing health promotion is the recognition that health promotive interventions really make a difference. The most significant differences are the decreased cost of providing services, the increased quality of life of the recipients, and their positive evaluation of rendered care. Highlighting the care-related costs of an illness by comparison with the health promotive perspective makes the case even more convincing. Savings in health care costs coupled with consumer satisfaction provide definitive arguments for the institutionalization of health promotion.

Encourage institutional participation. To involve those affected in the change process, a task force may be formed. If diverse aspects of the institution are represented and if the capability of participants to expedite decisions is recognized, the task force will manifest the possibility for change. Representatives from all levels of the organization should be included. The activities of the task force may include gathering information from those affected to identify behaviors and attitudes about health promotion; reviewing and revising any existing policies; compiling information into a list of recommendations or developing a single policy; designing a health promotion policy implementation plan; and developing a budget for the change efforts.

Ideally and by necessity, the task force should be given real authority by the top-level administration and should have public support. The groundwork for creating trust and meaningful responsibility is cultivated during this stage. A sense of responsibility reduces resistance to policy changes and promotes trust among those involved. Early involvement and an educational thrust prepare the organization for system change.

Gather information. The first activity of the task force is to gather information from those who would be affected by a change in the care system: providers, consumers, and other staff. The task force explores their attitudes toward change and commitment to health promotion.

The task force should complete the following activities:

1. Gather research on health promotion.
2. Contact other representatives from health promotive systems and review the strategies for change that were successful for their systems.
3. Survey all those who would be affected by a shift to a health promotive environment; a questionnaire or focus groups may be used with the goals of identifying support for the health promotive policy, identifying opposition, and determining issues that are of most concern to the organization.
4. Gather data on the impact of creating a health promotive environment; the patterns of morbidity, mortality, sick days, disability claims, medical leaves of absence, productivity, and efficiency should be examined.
5. Develop baseline measures of the organization's standing in the community (i.e., determine what kind of "health image" the institution has); consumers and visitors

may complete questionnaires, or a focus group or town hall meeting may be held to examine the organization's image in the community.

6. Evaluate union contracts related to health benefits and health insurance.

Prepare a written policy. After reviewing surveys and other data, the task force should prepare a written report as a background for system change. The governing board will review the policy for approval. The best policy is brief, specific, and simple. The component parts of a policy are the policy statement; the rationale for policy; the statement of who will be affected; an effective date of implementation; and any enforcement procedures, if applicable.

Plan an implementation strategy. The following activities should be part of implementing a strategy for a health promotive system:

1. Create an implementation timetable.
2. Decide on a promotional campaign for communicating the policy to staff, clients, and the community.
3. Plan an effective communication method.
4. Decide on enforcement procedures, if applicable.
5. Plan staff education sessions.
6. Develop a plan to evaluate the policy.

Step Three: Implement Policy

The task force and the organizational administration set a target date to implement a health promotion environment.

Communicate the policy. Clear presentation of a health promotion policy increases the likelihood of its reception, since uncertainty is a major source of resistance to change. To minimize uncertainty, all parties affected should be informed and provided with the reasons and intended benefits for the change. This kind of awareness building is part of every stage of the process of systems change. The amount of time it takes to change a policy should not be underestimated. Three months to 1 year or more may be required, depending on the institution's size and the effectiveness of the communication network.

A public relations campaign should emphasize ways the institution will be strengthened by becoming a health promotive environment. It is beneficial to develop a variety of approaches to communicate the new policy to the community, providers, and clients.

Carry out the policy. While the health promotion policy statement is being distributed, the task force may develop a timetable for implementation. Time is a critical element in allowing persons to prepare for change. The time buffer usually gives persons time to adjust.

A date for the policy to take effect is then set. It is important to consider a date that may be of significance to the institution or will correlate with the intended purpose of the policy change. If any restrictions will apply, they should be phased in gradually so that no person feels alienated. During the transition period, educational sessions about health promotion may be planned. Giving incentives helps ease the adjustment and compensates for any changes that are viewed as restrictive.

Since systems change takes time, it is unreasonable to expect that creating a health promotive environment will happen instantly. Although the goal should be clear from the outset, hasty implementation reduces the support of persons who believe their rights to smoke or remain physically inactive, for example, are being limited or taken away. Implementing the policy before there is sufficient readiness can result in frustration, discouragement, and failure. It is crucial to prepare adequately and realize that acceptance requires time.

If a step-by-step approach to phasing-in health promotion occurs, a commitment to the strategies with a defined timetable should be communicated so that people know when each change will occur.

Step Four: Evaluate the Impact of the Policy

In this stage the administration, working with the task force, makes minor adjustments to the policy for health promotion, firmly establishes the health promotive environment, and evaluates the results.

Persons tend to resist change, especially system change that affects personal behavior and choice. A carefully designed plan can reduce resistance while enhancing cooperation, acceptance, and support for health promotive change.

Individuals enforcing the health promotion policy should keep the message positive and focused. The position of the institution on health promotion should be clearly stated.

The task force should plan an evaluation to determine the effectiveness of a health promotion environment and to provide information about any problems. The evaluation can measure immediate changes in attitudes and behavior or long-term outcomes, such as statistics on the number of sick days, productivity measures, and patterns of morbidity and mortality.

Short-term assessments can be undertaken using surveys 3 to 6 months after the policy has been implemented. The initial survey may be used as a baseline. This follow-up survey will measure the impact of the policy. Measurements of short-term outcomes may answer the following questions:

- Are persons complying with the policy?
- What are their attitudes?
- Have those affected persons implemented health promotive strategies?

Long-term effects are more difficult to measure. Long-term changes require at least 1 year to stabilize. Examples of long-term outcomes include answers to the following questions:

- Have there been any changes in use of sick time, requests for medical leaves of absence, or disability claims?
- Have the morbidity and mortality patterns decreased?
- Is the institution known in the community as an agency for health promotion through its actions?

Critical to the success of systems change is this collaborative model for change. Changes require the support of an institution's top administration and governing board. Change agents help set the agenda for a health promotion environment. They educate top decision-makers about the positive impact of a health promotive environment on employee productivity, provider and client health, and the institution's public image.

HEALTH PROMOTION AGENTS AND THE HEALTH PROMOTION MATRIX

As an agent for health promotion, the health care professional uses the Health Promotion Matrix to guide care. The matrix embodies the notion that the client is viewed in the context of his/her world, including the family, groups, and community. No human system can be viewed in isolation because multiple factors and forces are in constant interaction with human systems. Individual health cannot be fully comprehended without the context of family health, the impact of values contributed by group affiliations, and the constellation of associations and resources represented by the community. Appreciating the multidimensional nature of interacting human systems and the impact of multiple forces influencing these interactions assists in clarifying the complexity of health.

Health promotion has always incorporated the central ideas of change, development, and improvement (Kelly, 1989). Within this environment, major issues arise regarding the process of planning and participating in change. As health professionals, we are faced with the responsibility of articulating a "comfort zone" from which a consistent philosophy of practice can evolve. Our relationships to ourselves, our peers, and our clients come under examination. The tools and approaches we use in our daily practice are explored and tested for their ongoing viability and inclusion.

Empowerment as an important concept in the development of individual, group, and community change has been introduced. However, the jump between philosophy and practice is often a large one. Holzemer (in press) points to three key issues of ongoing health care reform in the United States: "access to services, the ability of (clients) to participate fully in services, and the shifting role of the gatekeeper in the care delivery system." The gatekeeper function is now viewed as a shared responsibility of the multidisciplinary team of health care professionals and the client. A multidisciplinary approach to health education will foster the sharing of power and enhance the breaking down of barriers between varying professions and among professionals and clients.

The Pew Health Professions Commission (1991) calls for improvements in the education and training of health professionals in response to a charge to explore the attitudes and skills that health professionals ought to possess to be most responsive to the health needs of the public as the new century approaches. The Commission was inspired by the belief that "the education and training of health professionals is out of step with the evolving health needs of the American people" (p. 3). The traditional model based on illness is recognized as inadequate. Change to a new model is recognized as the single greatest challenge facing health professional schools. The Pew Report (1991) identifies competencies that future health professionals should possess. These competencies include the promotion of healthy life-styles, caring for the health of communities, expanding client access to effective care, and involving clients and families in the decision-making process. Box 4-5 identifies practitioner competencies for the year 2005. Health care professionals are forewarned to acquire these competencies to practice in a health care system with a mission that emphasizes health.

The health care professional shapes all interactions with client systems by viewing the self as a therapeutic agent for the promotion of health. The agent translates knowledge and skills into meaningful and useful resources that the client can then integrate for self use in health care. This function of translation points to the importance of the health care professional as an interpreter of health promotive strategies. The agent's role as interpreter is key in sharing the culture of health with the client while simultaneously valuing the client's views. The bridge to be created is the connection between the client and available information and the choices currently known in the field of health promotion. Once created, pathways for health become evident. The client and health care professional join in a partnership dedicated to the client's self-determination for health. The interactional therapeutic process between the health care professional and the client will shape knowl-

Box 4-5

Competencies for 2005

Practitioners for 2005 should:
- Care for the community's health
- Expand access to effective care
- Provide contemporary clinical care
- Emphasize primary care
- Participate in coordinated care
- Ensure cost-effective and appropriate care
- Practice prevention
- Involve patients and families in the decision-making process
- Promote healthy life-styles
- Assess and use technology appropriately
- Improve the health care system
- Manage information
- Understand the role of the physical environment
- Provide counseling on ethical issues
- Accommodate expanded accountability
- Participate in a racially and culturally diverse society
- Continue to learn

From *Healthy America: Practitioners for 2005. An Agenda for Actions for U.S. Health Professional Schools*, by The Pew Health Professions Commission, 1991, Durham, NC: Author.

edge and skills that are meaningful and useful to the client. This is the process of facilitating and supporting health promotive care.

HEALTH PROMOTION IN A REFORMED HEALTH CARE SYSTEM

Until care is driven by a skilled, collaborative assessment of need rather than by cost containment alone, the burden for care delivery will continue to be shifted from one setting to another. Will the movement toward community-based care be redirected once cost exceeds expectations? Will managed care extend its boundaries once report cards demonstrate gaps in services demanded by clients? These and other critical questions must be reconciled so that cost, efficiency, quality, and human needs do not have to be competing forces in a changing health care system. Blending need, cost, efficiency, quality and diversity will enable a more unified approach to service delivery. Health care services must emphasize the provision of health promotive care. Health care professionals must ready themselves for participating in this process of reform and direct the service system through their unique capabilities, knowledge, skills, and standards.

Summary

Redefining the health care professional as an intervention agent within a traditional illness-oriented, provider-driven health care system is not an easy task. Yet the future of health promotion in a reformed health care system relies on active participation of health care agents in this massive reorganizational process. Realignment of client/provider relationships, cross-disciplinary partnerships, and the impact of consumer demands are shaping health care reform. This reshaping has been thrust upon health care professionals and has been greeted with skepticism, but it also has presented health care professionals with new opportunities for redefinition never before possible. Health care reform presents challenges and opportunities. The skills of future health care professionals must be obtained *today*. Accepting, valuing, and understanding how to participate in change guarantees a role in shaping the future of health care. Change, from simple to complex, emerges through systematic collaborative planning. The steps for systems change and the characteristics of shared empowerment detailed in this chapter will inform health care agents concerned about health promotion. Health care agents must understand the past, thoughtfully examine the present, and acknowledge that the future is a shared one.

References

Airhihenbuwa, C.O. (1994). Health promotion and the discourse on culture: Implications for empowerment. *Health Education Quarterly, 21*(3), 345-353.

Becker, M.H. (1993). A medical sociologist looks at health promotion. *Journal of Health and Social Behavior, 34*, 1-6.

Colt, G.H. (1996, September). See me, feel me, touch me, heal me. *Life*, 35-50.

Eisenberg, D.M. (1996). The invisible mainstream. *Harvard Medical Alumni Bulletin, 70*, 20-25.

Eisenberg, D.M. (1997). Advising patients who seek alternative medical therapies. *Annals of Internal Medicine, 127*, 61-69.

Eisenberg, D.M., Kessler, R.C., Foster, C., Norlock, F.E., Calkins, D.R., & Delbanco, T.L. (1993). Unconventional medicine in the United States: Prevalence, costs, and patterns of use. *The New England Journal of Medicine, 328*(4), 246-252.

Fugh-Berman, A. (1996). *Alternative medicine: What works*. Tucson, AZ: Odonian Press.

Gillis, A. (1995). Exploring nursing outcomes for health promotion. *Nursing Forum, 30*(2), 5-12.

Hanson, P. (1989). Citizen involvement in community health promotion: A role application of CDC's patch model. *International Quarterly of Community Health Education, 9*(3), 177-186.

Holzemer, S.P. (in press). Concepts basic to health and illness. In J. Leahy & P. Kizilay (Eds.), *Foundations of nursing: A nursing process approach*. Philadelphia: W.B. Saunders.

How good is your health plan? (1996, August). *Consumer Reports, 61*(8), 28-42.

Kelly, M.P. (1989). Some problems in health promotion research. *Health Promotion, 4*(4), 317-330.

Labonte, R. (1994). Health promotion and empowerment: Reflections on professional practice. *Health Education Quarterly, 21*(2), 253-268.

National Consumer Health Information Act of 1976, 42 U.S.C. § 201 *et seq*. (1976).

National Institute of Nursing Research. (1995). *Community-based health care: Nursing strategies*. Washington DC: U.S. Department of Health and Human Services, U.S. Public Health Service, National Institutes of Health.

Rappaport, J. (1985, Fall). The power of empowerment language. *Social Policy, 16*, 15-21.

Robertson, A. & Minkler, M. (1994). New health promotion movement: A critical examination. *Health Education Quarterly, 21*(3), 295-312.

Sheinfeld Gorin, S. (1989). *Stopping smoking: A nurse's guide*. New York: American Health Foundation.

Shortell, S.M., Gillies, R.R., Anderson, D.A., Erickson, K.M., & Mitchell, J.B. (1996). *Remaking health care in America: Building organized delivery systems*. San Francisco: Jossey-Bass.

The frontiers of medicine (special issue). (1996). *Time, 148* (14),

The Pew Health Professions Commission. (1991). *Healthy America: Practitioners for 2005. An agenda for actions for U.S. health professional schools*. Durham, N.C.: Author.

U.S. Department of Labor. (1996-1997). *Occupational outlook handbook*. Washington DC: Author.

U.S. Office of Alternative Medicine, National Institutes of Health. (1994). *Alternative medicine: Expanding medical horizons. A report to the National Institutes of Health on alternative medical systems and practices in the U.S.* Washington, DC: Author.

U.S. Preventive Services Task Force. (1996). *Guide to clinical preventive services* (2nd ed.). Baltimore: Williams & Wilkins.

Wallerstein, N. (1992). Powerlessness, empowerment, and health: Implications for health promotion programs. *American Journal of Health Promotion, 6*(3), 197-205.

Woolf, S.H., Jonas, S., & Lawrence, R.S. (Eds.). (1996). *Health promotion and prevention in clinical practice.* Baltimore, MD: Williams & Wilkins.

CHAPTER 5

The Health Promotion Matrix

Sherri Sheinfeld Gorin and Joan Arnold

The Health Promotion Matrix (HPM or the Matrix) (Figure 5-1) is central to the clinical practice of health promotion. It provides an organizing framework for assessing client systems and guiding them toward health. The Matrix equips the health care professional with an understanding of the client's images of health, a means for working with those images, and specific behaviors with which the professional and client may work. It serves as a means for understanding the client's view of health and as a blueprint for maximizing health promotive behaviors within varied contexts. Through the use of the Matrix, the health care professional can assist the individual to modify his/her behavior, engage a group or family in altering a pattern of actions, or enlist the support of a community in changing health care policies.

At its core is the notion of a health image. A *health image* is a picture, or concept, of health in the client's mind. The image is the client's representation of health, and as such, serves as a motivating force for change. Health care professionals may examine the client's image of health from two perspectives: first, from the client's idealized picture of personal health and secondly, relative to the client's current health status. These two perspectives are juxtaposed in a dynamic comparison to reveal the discrepancies, or gaps, between them. Further, in partnership, the health care professional and the client explore the gap to formulate ways the client may integrate the idealized image into everyday living. Ultimately, the client's current health status will be altered through the adoption of health promotive activities necessary to better realize the idealized picture.

THEORETICAL MODEL OF CHANGE IN THE HEALTH PROMOTION MATRIX

The HPM is a multicomponent model, along whose dimensions, client systems, and nine positive, or healthy, behaviors each client may be located. To some extent, all of the models of change and their embedded constructs explored in Chapter 2 form the basis for the HPM. The most salient of these contributions, however—found in two environmental models and two health attitude, belief and behavior models—are summarized briefly.

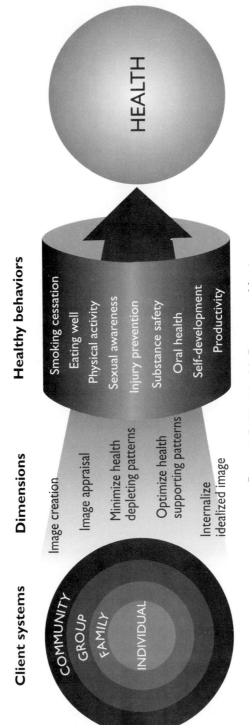

Figure 5-1 The Health Promotion Matrix.

The Ecological Model

The attention of the HPM to multiple client systems and levels of change—from the individual to the community—derives from an ecological model of health promotion. Within the ecological model, as in the HPM, healthy behavior is contextualized (i.e., it is grounded in the interrelationships between persons and their environments). These environments may be geophysical, policy, sociocultural, or may be composed of other client systems. The ecological model, as does the HPM, assumes that the healthfulness of a situation and the well-being of its participants is influenced by the interaction of multiple aspects of the environment with those of the person; health is a result of that interplay. The fit between a unique environment and a particular person differs from context to context. In the HPM, as a clinically oriented model, the appropriateness of both the client system and the selected intervention to achieve a healthy behavior depends on this fit.

Within the HPM, various levels of human environments are regarded as complex systems, and client systems are nested within one another. Interventions may be strengthened by the coordination of individual, family, group, and community clients acting to enrich health at different levels, or interventions may be weakened by contradictions among these levels. For example, as individuals make efforts to improve their health practices, family members who are supportive of these changes and public health officials who work to increase the accessibility and acceptability of health services can strengthen interventions. If any of these client systems, however, undermines the work of another, such as an overly critical family chiding a child's slow weight loss efforts, the efforts of one client system are sabotaged. Additionally, poverty itself may impede or delimit health promotion efforts through diminished resources and reduced social cohesion.

Innovation Diffusion Theory

Innovation diffusion theory addresses the contexts within which *innovations*, defined as new and qualitatively different ideas (e.g., the concept of imagining a health image), emerge (Delbecq, 1978). Clients may differ in their acceptance of the Matrix, and in particular, their abilities to imagine their own health. The relationship between the Matrix and the client system will be determined by the characteristics of both.

Social Cognitive Theory

In the social cognitive theory, as in the HPM, behavior can be explained in terms of a continuous and reciprocal interaction between cognitive, behavioral, and environmental determinants that are governed by self-efficacy, a cognitive mechanism. Social cognitive theory as a whole facilitates understanding of the means through which client change takes place.

Stages of Change

The stages of change model assumes that individuals move through a series of predictable stages in their behavioral change, such as stopping smoking or beginning an exercise program. The HPM proposes similar foci, from image creation to internalization of the idealized image of health. The stages are not necessarily linear, as client systems may reiterate stages before reaching the health goal. This model, as well as the HPM, may, however, suggest that different individuals rest at varied stages and implies varied intervention foci (Prochaska, DiClemente, & Norcross, 1992).

The Health Image

The concept of the health image, central to the Matrix and to the client's motivation for change, emerges from two main ideas: the authentic ideal, explored by early dynamic psychotherapists (Horney, 1936), and the image as metaphor, developed by organizational theorist Gareth Morgan (1986). Authentic ideals, including those for health, are dynamic; they arouse an incentive to approximate them, and they are an indispensible and invaluable force for growth and development. The image of the authentic self is always to a large degree removed from reality, differs from person to person, and is generally flattering. The impact it exerts on the client's life is strong. In general, authentic ideals make one humble, as they highlight one's unique growth paths.

Some people, however, craft a fictitious, or illusory, image of what they believe themselves to be, consciously or unconsciously. This image remains static and is an imaginative creation interwoven with and determined by very unrealistic factors (Horney, 1936). The ideal is worshipped; a move toward its attainment becomes a hindrance to growth because the individual either denies shortcomings in his/her pursuit of the ideal or merely condemns them. The greater it varies from reality, the more vulnerable the person is to outside affirmation and recognition or the more arrogant one becomes in the protection of the image (Horney, 1936). For these persons, the image includes few healthy components.

The image as a metaphor highlights the importance of "reading" organizational and other group activities through a deep appreciation of the situations being addressed. A metaphor is a device for embellishing discourse; yet it implies a way of thinking and a way of seeing that pervade how one generally understands one's world (Morgan, 1986). Metaphors, or our images of phenomena, bound our thinking and our language. Human behavior is complex and paradoxical; it can be understood in many different ways. For example, a health care professional may think about individual clients as if they are machines, with each body system and each selected intervention designed to achieve predetermined health goals and objectives. As a result, one would approach the client in a mechanistic way, forcing other qualities into the background. Instead, the health care professional may encourage the client to give shape to the fullness of his/her own image of health.

HEALTH PROMOTION MATRIX AS A CLINICAL TOOL

The Matrix, a clinical tool, is used by the health care professional and client as partners in health promotion. The client is classified within a system, along a dimension and in relation to the nine healthy behaviors. Further, the Matrix enables the professional and the client to devise and implement an intervention—from crafting the image to internalizing the idealized image—within each of nine healthy behaviors.

The Matrix offers a novel way of characterizing and intervening in patterns of behavior among clients as they seek a valued purpose—in this instance, health. Through the use of the HPM, the health care professional becomes aware of the multifaceted dimensions of the client's health and may compare a client's health to her/his image. In the case of an individual client, the Matrix lists the behaviors of an optimally healthy person, allowing the health care professional and the client to focus on specific actions, appropriate to the client's need. Thus, the Matrix directs the health care professional's thinking toward the optimal components of health promotion. As part of the clinical process, the Matrix assists health care professionals to individualize care with clients by identifying their unique health images, strengths, and capabilities, which allows the health care professional to focus on specific behaviors, appropriate to a client's need. Further, the Matrix assumes a reorientation of the health care professional's thinking toward the multiplicity of forces—biologic, psychologic, social, political, economic, cultural, and spiritual—impinging on clients as they begin the change process (Butterfield, 1990).

HEALTH CARE PROFESSIONAL AND CLIENT PARTNERSHIP

The client and the health care professional are involved in the change process through a partnership approach (Roter, 1987), with the client defining and engaging in the process of change and the health care professional functioning as the enabler or facilitator of that process.

As partners for health, the client and the health care professional work together to explore the client's desired image of health, conduct an assessment of health status, identify health depleting and supportive patterns, and facilitate internalization of the idealized image of health. Together, the health care professional and client explore actions that may move the client toward his/her own idealized images of health through the realization of each of the nine healthy behaviors. Within each positive health behavior, the client and health care professional engage with one another to move from image creation to the internalization of an image of health. A client may progress differently toward each of the nine behaviors; the composite of client movement depicts health for each client. Each client thus creates a unique picture of images and has specialized depleting and supporting patterns for every healthy behavior, as well as across these behaviors. A general guide to health care professional/client interaction, or script, based on the Health Promotion Matrix is found at the end of this chapter.

As previously stated, the health care professional is a facilitator of health promotion. The client directs the health agenda, which is a reflection of personalized health strengths, needs, and problems. The health care professional is careful not to undermine the client's right to self-determination. Rather, the role of the health care professional is to offer, or transfer, knowledge and skills that support the client in making an informed and deliberate decision about health and about taking those actions that may enhance health. The health care professional also assists the client in deciphering this information and translating it into meaningful and usable doses. The client gains power through this transfer of knowledge and skills. Further, with increased knowledge, the client is able to identify and to select preferred actions that foster movement along the HPM. Movement across the dimensions of the HPM may be slow as the client confronts difficult issues. For example, a client experiencing depletion and isolation may be unable to envision an image of idealized health or eliminate barriers that inhibit healthy change. The health care professional is accepting and supportive and does not pressure or try to influence the client. It is oftentimes difficult to restrain the tendency to encourage the client to select actions that support the professional vantage point and enhance the professional's expertise. Leadership in health promotion and consumer-directed actions hinges on the health care professional's ability to serve as facilitator for client-directed change and to validate the significance of decisions made by the client.

COMPONENTS OF THE HEALTH PROMOTION MATRIX

The Matrix delineates five dimensions for maximizing health promotive interventions and describes four client systems and nine positive health behaviors (see Figure 5-1 for a schematic summary of the Matrix). Each component of the typology is described in turn.

Foci of Intervention

Image creation. Entry into the Matrix begins with the client picturing an idealized image of health, a personally constructed vision that informs both the health care professional and client about how the client would like to see himself/herself in relation to health; it is the client's snapshot of the desired self. The ideal self is the "image of what we would like our self to be" (Erikson, 1968, p. 217; Sandler et al., 1963; Sandler, 1967). These images are often rich and varied and may emphasize the totality of being (Woods et al., 1988).

Creating an idealized image of one's personal health is difficult because many persons have learned to view health as the absence of disease and not necessarily something positive and achievable. Health becomes symptom reduction, rather than the promotion of positive patterns of change.

If asked to construct an idealized image of personal health, some would not be able to create such a vision. Some would pen an unrealistically thin woman or overdefined muscles on a man. Others would isolate a particular characteristic, a viewed weakness, and allow it to dominate their picture. Still others may merely see a disappearing self, being extinguished by disease.

Through the use of the HPM, then, the health care professional assists the client in clarifying or detailing his/her definition of health, as well as the relative value health holds for him/her. In conjunction with the client, the health care professional helps to crystallize a more positive and holistic image of health, one that is less encumbered by barriers and obstacles the client may have encountered in the past. This image is the aim of all subsequent intervention efforts; ultimately, the health care professional may work with the client in realizing his/her own idealized image of health.

For example, to assist the client in trying to create an image of himself/herself as a healthy person, the health care professional may ask the following: "What do you see if you try to picture yourself as healthy?" "What would you like to be?" or "How would you like to see yourself in relation to health?" Questions such as these assist the client in visualizing an image of himself/herself as healthy. The sketch of one's healthy self may be made on paper or described verbally and may require more than one session to complete. The health care professional may direct the client's attention to the multiplicity of healthy images: biologic, psychologic, social, political, economic, cultural, and spiritual. For example, the health care professional may begin with helping the client to imagine physical health. For the client, this may be viewed as optimal system function or a strong body that is "in shape," stress free, and impervious to stressors. This imagined picture may next include emotional stability (e.g., being calm and collected; "in touch" with one's feelings; and communicating happiness about oneself, others, and the larger world). A healthy image may be created by or include a family, group, or community of similar others, or it may belong to one individual. The image may involve communion with a higher being or be guided by a set of moral principles. The image of health may involve meaningful work, community change, intellectual accomplishments, economic success, or opportunities for leisure. Attempting to make the image of health tangible removes its obscure qualities and increases its power to motivate the client toward change. Further, the more specific and detailed the image, the more the health care professional can assist the client during image appraisal in recognizing what steps may be taken to achieve change.

At this point in the interchange, the health care professional and client move from forming a positive image—one that enables a client to align himself/herself with a motivating picture of himself/herself—to determining a more realistic picture of current health. Together, they move from the entry point (the client's idealized image) to the fuller picture of holistic health found in the Matrix (image appraisal). The HPM assists in enlarging the picture so as to reflect the totality of the client's health.

Image appraisal. During image appraisal, the health care professional and the client define the client's current health status. As the health care professional and the client begin to examine the client's idealized view of health, relative to the client's present state, a gap often emerges. This gap represents the difference between the client's visualized image of health and the actual patterns of behavior in which the client engages. In effect, the gap represents the divergence of the present behavioral patterns from the idealized image the client has now pictured. During the image appraisal process, the health care professional works with the client to recognize this gap. Various but futile attempts to achieve an ideal that may be unrealistic are not only frustrating but also nonproductive. Attempting to achieve an unrealistic ideal, even if desired and valued, may make change a near impossibility. Thus the health care professional and the client seek to determine the intervention strategies needed to attain the client's personal image of health and to recognize specific health goals that are desireable and achievable.

Image appraisal involves taking a full inventory of the client's health status (i.e., the actual state of health the client is experiencing at this time). This step requires a complete appraisal of the client's current health—the daily patterns of being and engaging in the world. Using the Matrix as a guide, the health care professional walks through a typical week, day-by-day, with the client, addressing each of the nine positive health behaviors—smoking cessation, eating well, physical activity, sexual awareness, injury prevention, substance safety, oral health, self-development, and productivity—and the contexts within which each behavior takes place (self, family, group, or community). The health care professional uses the Matrix to assist the client in painting the present health picture, identifying the patterns of practice that define the client's health. Once the picture is detailed, the health care professional assists the client in comparing the image of health with his/her present patterns of practice. The health care professional may start by discussing the healthy behavior with which the client seems to be struggling at present.

Beginning with an attempt to determine the client's motivation for change, the health care professional may then ask about any change attempts, with questions such as "Have you ever made any changes in yourself or your behavior?" "When did you make those changes?" and "Were you able to sustain those changes?" To assist the client in identifying the gap between the image and present health practices within the nine positive health behaviors, the health care professional may direct a series of queries to the client, starting with, for example: "How do you feel about being a cigarette smoker?" or, more specifically, "Do you have a car seat for your baby?" The image appraisal step often ends with the health care professional asking the client about changing present health practices to match those of the idealized image, with a question such as: "Would you like to stop smoking?" or "Are you interested in an educational program about taking care of your teeth during pregnancy?" Once the gap has been identified, and often, a commitment to change made, both begin the next steps in the process of change.

Minimize health depleting patterns. The health care professional now may assist the client in identifying depleting and supporting behaviors for one or more of the healthy behaviors. The Matrix enables the client, in conjunction with the health care professional, to analyze patterns that are either health depleting or health promotive and to begin to change them. Often, this proceeds in a problem-solving manner, from assessing the issues to developing choices, outlining alternatives, evaluating each, and then deciding on the optimal course of action.

With some behaviors, the two dimensions are addressed together. With other healthy behaviors, they are separated into two distinct areas. Sometimes, the health care professional works with the client to optimize supportive patterns first, then to minimize health depleting patterns. Depending on a client's concerns, he/she may express a concrete commitment to change, if this has not not already negotiated, during this step.

Because the client may need assistance in altering a number of behaviors to narrow the gap between the ideal and the actual state, this process may take place over an extended time period. Together, the health care professional and the client prioritize the intervention areas.

The HPM, particularly the nine positive health behaviors or their obverses, could be used as a starting point for isolating a set of depleting or supportive behavioral patterns. The health care professional, working with the client system, might start with any of the behaviors explored in Part Two, such as smoking, since tobacco is a major risk factor for morbidity and death. Interventions designed to assist clients to stop smoking have demonstrated some success (Royce, Sheinfeld Gorin, Edelman, Rendino-Perrone, & Orlandi, 1990; Sheinfeld Gorin, 1992); many of the scripts in Part Two are based on similar empirically tested approaches. Further, legislation and worksite policies have limited the places in which clients may smoke (Strasser, 1991; Hallett, 1986) and have made smoking illegal in many locales (Hirsch & Slama, 1992; Birnbach, 1990). Therefore the health care professional could work with any client system, in the area of smoking cessation, from an individual to change his or her behaviors to a community, for example, to stop tobacco sponsorship of sporting events.

Initially, the health care professional may develop an approach to assist the client in minimizing health depleting patterns, or barriers to change. To understand the depleting behaviors, the health care professional may ask the client to list behaviors that are damaging, such as cigarette or cigar smoking, or the absence of behaviors that are known to protect health, such as failing to wear a seat belt while driving. These barriers to behavior change may rest in physiologic forces, such as a craving; psychologic attitudes, beliefs, or intentions toward change; social and cultural norms or patterns supporting certain behaviors; or economic, political, or spiritual factors. Lack of accessibility, few community resources, limited motivation to change, family members who support less healthy eating patterns, or a stressful job are examples of barriers that may prevent the client from taking the first step toward change. The health care professional seeks to specify the techniques or tools that may assist the client to change. The health care professional, as a collaborator moving toward a common goal, negotiates these steps with the client.

Because health often is assumed until it is threatened, diminished, or depleted, specific strategies to bridge this gap and to address each barrier become the focus of an intervention. Depleting health behaviors may result from omitting an act that is health promotive or engaging in a behavior that is known to endanger or diminish health. The health care professional may begin dialogue to bridge the gap by asking, in the case of a smoker, for example, "What possible problems or barriers to stopping smoking do you see?" Oftentimes combining the use of the script with customized, culturally sensitive brochures, videotapes, and audiotapes, the health care professional works with the client to overcome each barrier. The health care professional also may suggest self-help groups to assist the client with change and/or pharmacologic aids (such as a nicotine patch).

Optimize health supportive patterns. Health supportive patterns are viewed as strengths because they support health, whereas health depleting behaviors are viewed as risks and problems because they undermine the process of becoming healthy. Optimizing supportive behaviors involves recognizing efforts toward undertaking healthy practices or those behaviors themselves.

Often, clients are given recognition only when a health goal is reached, as though health itself were a static and absolute state of being. A client who envisions a healthy ideal of being 50 pounds thinner than his/her present state could, however, receive praise and encouragement for every effort made toward altering eating patterns, in regularly monitoring his/her weight, or in altering the meaning and purpose food holds in his/her life. During this oftentimes slow but steady process, the health care professional would praise the client for engaging in the weight reduction process, as well as losing weight, despite any setbacks. Every instance of success is recognized as a gain, and the client is rewarded with support and encouragement by the health care professional. Similarly, the health care professional and the client may identify other health promotive beliefs, attitudes, and behaviors in which the client already engages. For example, a client may wear a seat belt on a regular basis, the family may join together for a balanced meal at least once a day, or a community may lobby for tobacco control legislation—all of which are health promotive and have the potential to optimize health. The health care professional may support and encourage clients to feel a sense of accomplishment for being successful in some of their present actions. These positive health actions provide the energy necessary to contend with depleting behaviors (i.e., to continue the process of change).

The health care professional relies on the strengths of the client and his/her support network to assist in the processes of change, keeping in mind that the health care professional is a critical participant in that support network. To optimize health supportive patterns, the health care professional may begin with the negotiated change, "Remember, you agreed to limit your drinking for the next month to one drink per day. Think of an activity you do frequently every day. Whenever you do that activity, think of your reasons to cut down on drinking." If the client agrees to reduce his/her drinking, for instance, the health care professional then works with the client to develop and monitor a strategy to implement the change, such as a signed Drinking Agreement.

In the case of smoking, the health care professional would obtain a commitment to a stop date or a plan to cut down. The health care professional would then provide materials to assist the client in stopping, including pamphlets, information on joining self-help groups, and literature on nicotine patches. The health care professional would review the factors that would support the plan and review the ways to overcome barriers to stopping. The health care professional tells the client when she/he will follow-up in person, by telephone, or through the mail. Generally, this follow-up should be soon.

Throughout, as the health care professional is guided by the Matrix, she/he would seek to understand the contextual influences on a healthy behavior, such as the environments within which an individual smokes or eats. She/he might move from the individual context of the smoker to that of the community, wherein the health care professional joins with others to advocate for legislation to restrict smoking.

As the client begins to cut down on cigarette, cigar, or smokeless tobacco use, or reaches a quit date and stops, for example, the health care professional supports these newly acquired behaviors and validates the client's accompanying attitude and belief structures. The health care professional supports health enhancing approaches by optimizing a client's health supportive patterns (e.g., stopping smoking, engaging in a regular pattern of walking 30 minutes a day, following a low-fat diet, using medication only if prescribed for a given malady, and finding creative and enjoyable hobbies). The health care professional assists the client toward further change by praising any movement toward narrowing the gap between the healthy ideal and the actual health status. For example, over time, a healthy family may begin to find an acceptable method for sharing household roles and responsibilities. During a period of years, a healthy community may provide for parks and recreational centers that enable members of the community to socialize and join with others in shared interests.

Internalize idealized image. At this point in the change process, the client has begun to close the gap between the idealized image and the real health status. The health care professional now assists the client to strive for greater consistency in daily actions relative to the created image of health. Health becomes less abstract and more tangible, as depleting patterns are ameliorated and supportive patterns are strengthened. The gap becomes narrower as life-style changes in a variety of areas become part of the client's new habits and routines. These new patterns no longer require constant surveillance. The no-longer-idealized-but-realized behaviors become part of the client's health status.

The health care professional continues to praise the client for the changed behaviors but also reviews the plan for further modifications so that the behaviors might be maintained indefinitely. Any problems with the intervention are noted, and supports are bolstered. The health care professional asks the client how she/he may be of further help and reaffirms the client's plan (e.g., to remain off cigarettes) for a specific length of time (e.g., 6 months). The health care professional's intent is to stabilize the altered health behaviors. As one set of behaviors is changed, the health care professional and the client may review the idealized image of health and the new present state, using the HPM, to determine the next starting point for change.

The process of moving from image creation and image appraisal, through minimizing depleting patterns and optimizing health supportive patterns, toward internalizing an idealized image of health is repetitive, involving reevaluations and reformulations of intervention foci. The intervention must be sustained to continue to support movement toward the aim. It is possible to achieve a health goal, then lose momentum and slide away from health promotive behaviors. With the continued support of the health care professional, the client would then need to formulate alternative strategies to move again toward an idealized image of health. It is possible for a client to enjoy having reached an idealized state. In addition, as a client grows and develops his/her ideals could change. It is also possible that a client might never reach the idealized state; nonetheless, the client may find success in the adoption of some health sustaining patterns. The health care professional encounters clients in a multitude of states and contexts; the potential for supporting, protecting, and enhancing health is always a challenge.

Positive Health Behaviors

Chapter 1 examines the multiplicity of images that comprise health. The HPM (see Figure 5-1) *operationalizes* health as the confluence of the nine healthy behaviors. These behaviors influence the internalization of the image of health for all clients: individuals, families, groups, and communities. All the behaviors are interconnected from both the client's and the health professional's unique perspectives. Each client brings a different vantage point to shaping a personalized image of health. Each behavior simultaneously influences every other health behavior, as well as the health of the whole client system. It is the interrelatedness of these behaviors that contribute to a fuller understanding of the client's image of health and appreciation of the obstacles and motivating forces that deplete or support movement toward the internalization of the idealized image. Movement toward internalization represents a unique composite of healthy behaviors for each client. The client may experience greater or lesser integration of each of the healthy behaviors at different points in time. A composite is formed by the individualized attention to each of these nine behaviors.

The nine behaviors were derived from the major national policy mandate in health promotion, *Healthy People 2000: National Health Promotion and Disease Prevention Objectives* (U.S. Department of Health and Human Services, 1991); evaluations of its success (e.g., Siegel, Frazier, Mariolis, Brackbill, & Smith, 1993); and a review of the status of health promotion research (summary in Redland & Stuifbergen, 1993). The healthy behaviors discussed in this text, such as physical activity and substance safety, are emphasized for several reasons: they represent common concerns for most clients, whether individuals, families, groups, or communities; feasible clinical interventions to change these behaviors have been developed and, in many cases, empirically tested for efficacy; the clinical interventions highlighted in this text (the script [see the abbreviated script at the end of this chapter and the comprehensive script in the Appendix]) use the social context and the psychologic processes for behavioral change; and finally, behaviors, although multidetermined and complex, are malleable for many clients.

As previously discussed, the client and the health care professional work together to explore the client's desired image of health and actions to realize the healthy behaviors and thus close the gap between the health image and the client's current health status. Viewing health as a process rather than a goal allows health to be envisioned as an evolving condition rather than an endpoint or perfect state. Attempting to comprehend the evolving complexity of health remains a challenge. Appreciating the complexity of health in a given human system means acknowledging the multitude of factors and forces that influence and determine it.

Clearly, heredity, or human biology, is a profound determinant of health, contributing predetermined risks, vulnerabilities, and strengths that shape health potential. The environment is similarly a powerful determinant of health. The environment comprises everything outside the human system and may include physical, social, cultural, political, and economic forces that are continuously interacting with the human system, shaping and reformulating health as the human system grows and changes through its life cycle. Health care is a major influencing force in health. The availability, accessibility, affordability, appropriateness, adequacy, and acceptability of health services determine, to a great extent, the capability of human systems to realize their health potential (National Institute of Nursing Research, 1995). Life-style is recognized as an enormous force in determining health. Patterns of decision-making and daily choices in living have a significant impact on health practices. Life-style choices directly influence the human system's potential for healthy living and longevity.

The factors and forces that determine health are not separate and distinct. These forces, including human biology, the environment, health care, and life-style, interact with each other (Lalonde, 1974). The human system cannot be separated from its history, the context within which it develops, the health care and treatment it is able to receive, and the multitude of life-style choices that are made each day. The health of the human system is a composite of these factors and forces, that, taken together and over time, begin to express the complexity of health for each individual, family, group, and community.

When seen as an absolute, the goal of health often seems unreachable to the average person and at best has to be modified or compromised. When viewed as a state of total well-being, the client may experience health as a perfection, which may lead to a sense of failure as the goal is not fully attained. Yet, when seen as part of a process unique to a particular client and subject to constant modification and revision, health becomes achievable. For, as the client changes through the process of self-identification and engagement with the health care professional, the image of health is created and re-created to fit the changing self. It is revisualized as individuals change their values and their behaviors. The potential to change the self in relation to health within the context of differing environments is facilitated through the use of the HPM.

While all desire health, some, perhaps because of poverty or alienation, are unempowered and denied access to society's valued resources. As a result, health becomes another resource denied. With the use of the HPM, the health care professional and the client may identify areas in which the client may increase his/her sense of control or mastery over his/her life, thus enhancing his/her power (Robertson & Minkler, 1994; Wallerstein, 1992; Caraher, 1994). Further, the HPM allows the health care professional to intervene with any client system, whether individual, family, group, or community.

Client Systems

Through its attention to varied client systems, the HPM addresses micro-level change within the individual client to macro-level change at the societal or multicommunity context. Throughout, the Matrix assists the health care professional in contextualizing the client's image of health within an environment that supports health promoting behaviors (Wallack & Winkleby, 1987).

The individual's rate and type of movement toward his/her own image of health is highly idiosyncratic and depends on the influences of genetic/intergenerational, developmental, contextual, and life-style patterns. Individuals may promote their health by following behaviors that are common within the family, by changing as a result of growth and development, and by choosing a deliberate course of action. Yet, this movement may be supported and/or hindered within the context of an intervention between health care professional and client or within the community. The individual may be influenced to engage in healthy behaviors as a result of a conscious decision; group norms, values and affiliations; or community-based mandates and policies.

Further, the health care professional is concerned with promoting health with all clients, regardless of current health status. Health care professionals care for individuals, families, groups, communities, and other aggregates within populations. In the case of tobacco use, for example, the health care professional could intervene with an individual who smokes through the use of individual cessation counseling, with a group through the formation of a nonsmoking support group, and with a community through the creation of smoke-free environments. These varying and diverse client groups each have the potential for health promotion, and each possesses an image of health that can be enhanced and actualized through health promotive interventions.

The most acutely ill adult, the neighborhood disrupted by community violence, the young child achieving normal milestones for growth and development, and the well-adjusted single-parent family are all potential clients for the health care professional as a caregiver dedicated to health promotion. The critically ill adult needs health restorative therapy but also health promotive interventions so that functional systems are protected and the overall health status is improved. The community suffering from random violence not only requires emergency strategies to curtail violence and prevent deaths but also interventions to promote the healing potential within the community and to eventually redefine power and protect vulnerable members. The child growing and developing normally can benefit from interventions that promote and protect healthy choices and decision-making and assist with sustaining those patterns over time. The functional single-parent family may benefit from recognition and support and assistance with uncovering resources that reinforce capabilities and allow for continued growth and role development. Each client, regardless of how well or how compromised, has the potential for health promotion. Minimizing health depleting patterns and optimizing health supportive patterns are continuing foci for the health care professional.

Health care professionals may adopt a variety of strategies to promote individual and collective well-being. Using the dimensions of the Matrix, several client-specific strategies (i.e., means for using a deliberately structured influence system to effect change through social interaction) may be undertaken.

The health care professional is a health promotion agent. Every interaction with clients is an opportunity for health promotive care. Regardless of the health situation the client faces, the professional in conjunction with the client can direct efforts toward health promotion. Each point of contact with the individual can be viewed from this vantage point. Individuals most often seek care when they are ill. The responsibility of the health care professional is to offer information and education to clients about the importance of promoting their health so that illness can be avoided or minimized, or at least diagnosed as early as possible. Treatment of disease is coupled with health promotive care. In addition to treating the identified problem, the health care professional uses this point of contact to inform about health risks that correspond to the particular developmental phase of individual clients according to their age, gender, race/ethnicity, culture, and socioeconomic status. Health risks differ according to developmental periods of the lifespan. Adolescents, for example, are at greater risk for accidents and suicide. Age also may impose health risks. Women older than 50 years are at greater risk for breast cancer. Gender clearly affects one's health potential. Heart disease is the No. 1 killer of American women, and lung cancer is the leading cause of cancer among women. Race/ethnicity and culture introduce other significant concerns about the health potential of clients. Heart disease affects African-American women, particularly those between the ages of 34 and 44 years, with greater severity. Poverty and low educational attainments are risk factors for *all* the major chronic diseases.

Strategies unique to the individual. In addition to using every point of contact with the client as an opportunity to discuss health promotion, the health care professional can discuss health promotion as a fit between the client and the environment. It is to the individual that so much of the health promotion field is directed, as he/she is a powerful locus of change both within himself/herself and through working with others. The environment may include resources such as medical insurance, transportation, and the willingness of family members to provide emotional support for change. The person's own resources may include his/her motivation, outlook on life, coping skills, and image of health.

In promoting health with individual clients, the health care professional may adopt several strategic skills that are closely linked to the educational process. The first of these is the discussion method, which is designed to teach the client more effective coping behaviors. The health care professional may enable the client to explore perceptions, rationales, and beliefs and to restructure unhelpful thought processes. The health care professional may pose questions to stimulate thinking, make comments to support and encourage self-examination, and provide "space" for the client to assess and try new behaviors.

The second strategy that is well-suited to the individual client system is one in which the health care professional teaches the client a brief and simple behavioral change. This didactic approach may include assertiveness training. An assertive behavior sequence contains four steps that help a client feel more empowered: (1) describe the behavior to be changed, (2) express the associated feeling, (3) request a specific change, and (4) identify the positive consequence. A didactic approach may also include steps in general problem-solving: (1) delay immediate, impulsive action—"stop," "think," "hold it;" (2) search for alternative definitions of the problem; (3) develop strategies to deal with the problem; (4) evaluate these strategies for feasibility and possible and expected outcomes; and (5) select and carry out specific actions. With increased information, clients may feel more empowered and thus more able to engage in their own health promotion (Gitterman, 1991, p. 22).

Visual methods are graphic presentations that allow the client to see patterns of relationships and behavior. For example, a genogram (a tracing of the family tree over several generations) may be used to identify intergenerational health risks. Charts and lists may be used to identify "pros" and "cons" for stopping smoking, for example. A hand-scored health risk appraisal to identify areas of risk can be added to the assessment database. Some health care professionals may include printouts of computer-generated health risk appraisals. Lists of lifetime screenings also can be shared with the individual. For clients who are visual learners, these graphic representations have powerful effects.

Action methods, including role-playing, modeling, and coaching, demonstrate effective communication skills and allow the client an opportunity to "try out" new skills. Clients may be helped to talk while doing, rather than to just talk. A client may role-play choosing healthy foods from the cafeteria. Another client may dramatize asking her partner to use a condom; the health care professional may give feedback on how she is perceived. The health care encounter with individual clients can include discussion of the nine healthy behaviors, which are identified in Part Two. (Each chapter includes specific suggestions for healthier behaviors.) Every encounter with the individual client provides an opportunity to ask about the individual's health goals and to engage the client in a discussion of personal health and self-perception of health.

These intervention strategies enable the client to actualize the HPM. Readiness and motivation to imagine a positive self-image rest on the client's willingness to work with the health care professional in the multidimensional process of health promotion. Offering information about health promotion; attempting to establish the personal meaning of health risks; and clarifying family, culture, socioeconomic, age, gender, and developmental contributions all influence the client's readiness and motivation to imagine positive health. These efforts not only serve to move the client close to the point of engaging in image creation but also position the health care professional appropriately to discuss image creation with the client. In this way, health promotion becomes a shared process. The client then directs the process as the idealized image is shaped and a more thorough assessment of health strengths, risks, and problems is mutually identified. The health care professional assumes the role of facilitator for health promotion. The professional informs, supports, and encourages the client as movement toward internalization of the idealized image is maximized.

The health care professional is mindful that many individuals do not seek care, even illness care. Many individuals ignore symptoms or treat health problems only when they become an emergency. The reasons for delayed, inadequate, or lack of treatment vary but are related to issues of access, broadly defined, that challenge community-based health care. Health care professionals identify individuals in the community who may be alienated or separated from the health care delivery system and try to find pathways that assist persons to secure health care. The health care professional responds to these challenges and attempts to ensure that all members of the community are linked to health services.

Strategies unique to the family. The health care professional also reaches out to families to address the mission of health promotion. Families provide the context in which individuals live and relate. They are a small group of persons who share love; intimacy; and often, responsibility for children. Connected by marriage, childbearing, and kinship, each family is self-defined and like no other (Reiss, 1980).

Individuals are born into a family that is called a *family of origin.* Families are influenced by their own intergenerational histories and cultures. Eventually, individuals may start a family of their own, which is called the *family of procreation,* with its own culture. The health care professional realizes that the individual members are greatly affected by the norms and values of the family. Many families evidence intergenerational themes (the same patterns repeated across generations), such as early or late marriage or childrearing, patterns of alcohol use, or an interest in sports.

Similarly, each family is a social system that serves and reflects the larger society. Each family has a communication style and a set of power relationships that reflect to some extent the surrounding society, thereby affecting the health and health potential of their members.

Strong families tend to produce competent children, to meet the emotional needs of the parents, and to serve as a viable social and economic unit (Garbarino et al., 1992). Families tend to work as a blending of different voices from three systems: the family unit (the family as a whole); the interpersonal subsystem (each of the two-person relationships, or dyads); and the personal subsystem (the individual). Each family member is an individual, a member of a dyad, and a part of the whole family group. Every family has boundaries that define who is a stranger. Those boundaries are challenged in adolescence, for example, as the youth begins to recede from familial authority and to seek important intimate relationships from outside.

The internal organization of the family creates expectations for how members are to act with one another, including the norms for intimacy, frequency of contact, and power assertion (Burgess, 1980). Families develop goals or themes—the priorities, values, and commitments the family sets for itself and for its members. Sometimes these goals differ within the family system, with one member wishing to pursue personal fulfillment at the expense of family business. In troubled families, problems exist with self-worth, communication, rules, and the link to society (Satir, 1972). The health care professional needs to identify with the family's own unique perspective on health (i.e., how the family defines health and the health practices in which the family engages). Similarly, the health care professional needs to recognize the differing interests of the family subsystems, particularly to mediate conflicts.

Strategically, the health care professional must acquire skills in working with small groups since the family is a group and the dynamics that characterize groups are characteristic of family functioning. Health care professionals may encourage family meetings to discuss health practices, such as smoking or eating, and may suggest documenting precursors to change, such as the number of cigarettes smoked or keeping a food diary. Concommitantly, communication patterns between several members of the family may become maladaptive; the health care professional may adopt visual methods, such as family sculpting, to dramatize the interpersonal relationships. With more vulnerable members, such as children, health care professionals may choose to play the role of internal advocate by offsetting power imbalances. Throughout, the health care professional is respectful of the family's dynamics and its representation of health.

Working with families as partners in health promotion requires skill in communicating with the family as a whole. Each member can contribute his/her unique understanding of the idealized image of the family's health. Joining with the family, the health care professional assists in the process of identifying an image of family health. Recognition that improved family health fosters improved individual health is often motivating and assists in image creation.

Next, the health care professional collects with the family a detailed assessment of health patterns and practices (Arnold, 1998). The assessment includes an understanding of the family constellation, using the genogram as the guide. Information about all members of the family is critical, not only over a three-generational span but also including members not living in the household. The assessment also includes family patterns of daily living, including nutrition, sleep/wake/rest, work/leisure, physical activity and fitness, sexuality, and education. Also explored with the family are intrafamily dynamics, including patterns of communication; role functions; patterns of decision-making; norms and values; the distribution of power among members; patterns of conflict management; the energy available to accomplish family tasks and goals; the capacity of the family to change and grow over time; the environment; the impact of illness on the family; and finally, the family's capacity for self-care. Together the family members and the health care professional define the health issues and problems the family will work on to address gaps between the idealized image of health and current health. The health care professional and the family analyze the patterns of the family that deplete support as well as family health. The health care professional facilitates the family's capacity to actualize its idealized image of health by offering knowledge and skills and translating these into meaningful resources for the particular family.

Strategies unique to the group. Groups are ubiquitous in health promotion. Efficient in the use of time and space, they enable the health care professional to affect a larger number of persons in one session than she/he might otherwise through individual sessions. Potentially a strong agent of change, the group may affect its participants indirectly through its own processes or structures. Directly, the health care professional may use the group to influence its members or the system toward change. The group also may be used to alter the behaviors and attitudes of others toward members of the group (Vinter, 1974). These effects may be both short term (i.e., within one interchange in the group) or longer term (i.e., over the life of the group).

In general, groups may vary by type, size, composition, structure, phase, and leadership characteristics. Types of groups may include the following:

1. Psychotherapeutic—small and with a focus on the intrapsychic processes of change

2. Support—may be somewhat larger and enable group members' use of one other as resources and models for coping
3. Task—goal-driven and devoted to accomplishing identified work
4. Educational—focused on training or the teaching and learning processes among its members

In health promotion, support groups, such as those for women who are dieting or adolescents at high risk for sexually transmitted diseases, are common. Task groups, such as those dedicated to developing a policy statement to reduce injuries on the job, and educational groups, such as a group of 50 who gather to hear a single lecture on enhancing self-esteem, are also common. Psychotherapeutic groups are less common in health promotion. Variants of these general types of groups (e.g., supportive-expressive groups [Classen et al., 1993]) are also found. Supportive-expressive groups combine therapeutic and support group concepts, often using alternative healing techniques, such as hypnosis. Another example would be a psychoeducational group formed by the health care professional to work on weight reduction, for example. Herein, the processes include concomitant transmission of information, exploration of problem-solving approaches, and expression of feelings. Another variant combines the psychoeducational group with outreach to the members of a client's social network. This type of group, developed to increase screening among women at high risk for breast cancer, seeks to change the client by increasing the health promotive norms and values among influential friends, family members, and others (Sheinfeld Gorin, 1995, 1997). Generally, depending on the type of group, effectiveness is enhanced by increasing client morale and cohesion. The dimensions of the HPM can help guide group processes toward promotive actions.

In effecting group change over time, the health care professional is concerned with three major dimensions of development. First, groups differ in their social organization, including the sociometric, role, communication, and power processes. Sociometrically, members vary in their affections for one another. Over time, an individual may be liked more or less by others in the group. The roles participants play in the creation and maintenance of the group reflects the establishment of new positions and the changing of positions within the group. Communication patterns change, reflecting who talks to whom and about what. Power processes, which describe patterns of control, as well as reactions to deviance and scapegoating, also will change at different stages of group development. These sociometric characteristics of the group are forces that shape the group's creation of a health image and the process the members will use to appraise member and group health behaviors.

Second, the group's activities, tasks, and operative processes, such as its modes of decision-making, will vary over time. Group tasks relate to the sequence of behaviors activated in response to the goals of the group. Problem-solving behaviors, dominant in psychoeducational groups, describe the processes occurring as problems are identified and solutions attempted; conflict resolution is one component of problem-solving in a group. As the group problem-solves, it will mobilize its health strengths and identify barriers that impede its health promotion.

Third, groups differ in their cultures, including their norms, values, and shared purposes. Changes may occur in the content and structure of norms and values. Client goals may change, both individually and collectively. Each of these are characteristics of a group over time and are amenable to the health care professional's strategic interventions. Further, each of these characteristics, as well as size and client composition, vary from group to group, thereby leading the health care professional to adopt alternative approaches to change.

Groups tend to move through predictable phases over time. The first of these is the formative phase, wherein individuals are located and prepared to become members of the group. The initial session is particularly important in group formation, as it sets the stage for what is to come. As such, generally, health care professionals facilitate introductions and goal-setting, as well as an initial exploration of the topics the group will begin to explore. At this initial phase, members seek similarity and mutuality of interests, as well as a commitment to group purpose. Generally, an emergent structure, with individuals playing particular task, socioemotional, and participative roles, such as the "silent member" or the "monopolizer," is evident (Classen et al., 1993).

The intermediate phase of the group, or the middle sessions, is characterized by a moderate level of group cohesion, clarification of purposes, and the involvement of members in goal-directed activities. During this phase, oftentimes the prevailing group structure may be challenged, with a consequent modification of the group's purposes and operating procedures. At this point, the health care professional may introduce topics that elaborate the HPM and that might not yet have been discussed by the group. After this phase, many groups may mature and thus enter the next phase. Others may continue to revise the group's structure, purposes, and operating procedures, although they continue to emerge with a higher level of integration and stability than in the earlier phases.

The next phase, maturation, is distinguished by a stabilization of group structure and purposes and operating and governing procedures, expansion of the group culture, and establishment of a set of effective responses to internal and external stresses. If the group's longevity is short term or has a predefined number of sessions, the health care professional would discuss the number of sessions remaining until termination. As the image of group health is internalized, health emerges as a collective value.

The final phase, termination, describes the dissolution of the group. The ending of the group may result from goal attainment, maladaptation, lack of integration, or previous planning to end the group (cf. Sarri & Galinsky, 1974; Yalom, 1985).

Group leadership is often the task of the health care professional. As leader, she/he maintains an awareness of the group's purposes and works to enhance its accomplishment. The leader's role is to facilitate the group's movement along the dimensions toward internalizing its image of health. She/he is aware of her/his own emotional responses that emerge in the group and may reveal them if they enrich the group's processes. If the health care professional co-leads a group, establishing ground rules, frequent feedback, and debriefing (reviewing what has transpired in each group) leads to more positive group experiences. An effective group is characterized by an optimal relationship among members; the leader's primary style, whether instrumental or task-oriented or socioemotional and/or participative; and the phase of the group. The health care professional's role is to negotiate this fit with the client system.

Strategies for the community. Intervention efforts directed at communities and their power to encourage change are emerging as critical to the growth of health promotion. Community strategies may be particularly salient for the empowerment of women and vulnerable groups at the grassroots level. Coalitions among organizations, community groups, and interested community members are prominent in contemporary strategies because of their strength in developing widespread public support for issues, actions, and unmet needs. Community coalitions (e.g., against breast cancer and AIDS) have become astute in their understanding and use of the political process in its broadest sense, including judicial, legislative, and regulatory structures and processes, for change. Coalitions, as other community strategies, have provided creative means for the involvement and retention of consumers and citizens in political advocacy and service planning. Communities continue to rely on the skills of the health care professional in resource development, including resource mobilization (especially in fund-raising) and management for the continued growth of health-related organizations based in their midst (Mizrahi & Morrison, 1993).

For health care professionals who want to adopt community organization approaches, some general guidelines may be followed (Cox, Erlich, Rothman, & Tropman, 1974; Mizrahi & Morrison, 1993; Klainberg, Holzemer, Leonard, & Arnold, 1998). These suggestions are founded on an empowering approach to the community.

Assessing the need for health promotion in the community enhances its experience and competence by identifying its needs, resources, barriers and alternatives, potential targets, and agents of change. The community's image of itself as healthy is discussed. The health care professional assists the community in listing the kinds of services and programs that are needed, through surveys, an inventory of community assets and resources, and focus groups. The health care professional provides technical assistance so that existing or emerging health problems may be analyzed by their nature, location, scope, and degree. Data regarding past change efforts and the perception of the problem by others involved with it may be collected. The health care professional may also identify community subgroups that possess characteristics or exhibit behaviors that place them at increased risk of developing diseases or disorders.

The health care professional would then seek to understand the social context of the subgroups in the community at risk as well as broader community problems, looking at their origins and the social, political, and economic structures that maintain them. The health care professional needs to understand how existing risk factors may be modified, and, if so, what the most cost-effective intervention might be.

The client is then further described by a physical location; by social, political, economic, and demographic characteristics; and by any divisions, cleavages, and coordinated parts so that a comprehensive health promotive intervention may be devised. Client changes over time and client relationships with other parts of the social context, such as coalitions with others in the municipality or state, are reviewed. Interventions may be extended beyond geographic boundaries if such networks already exist or could be facilitated. The health care professional may provide consultation in how to develop these intercommunity partnerships as catalysts for change.

Community structure and capacity are enhanced thereby minimizing health depleting patterns and optimizing health supportive patterns through the provision of technical assistance in strategic planning and resource acquisition. The health care professional may broker access to additional financial resources and provide technical assistance in developing and securing funds. She/he may assist in recruiting, developing, and supporting members and volunteers for community efforts. The health care professional may assist in defining the community's goals for action from its varied perspectives and prioritizing them, with processes and outcomes specified. She/he may assist in devising a strategic plan, while assessing the relative resources required to carry it out; sources of resistance and inertia also may be located and assessed. The health care professional may also assist in assessing the feasibility of the strategy.

Social and environmental barriers to the implementation of the plan are examined. Social marketing techniques, including the use of media campaigns, are undertaken to promote the adoption of innovative ideas. The health care professional promotes coordina-

THE HEALTH PROMOTION MATRIX: *An Abbreviated Script*

The following script, focusing on the individual, may be used with any client system and for every healthy behavior.

Image Creation	Imagine yourself as a healthy person. What do you see if you try to picture yourself as healthy?
	Have you considered the many ways health can be imagined (physical, emotional, intellectual, spiritual, social, cultural, political, economic)?
	Would you like to become more of the healthy person you imagine?
Image Appraisal	In what ways are you different as the healthy person you imagine than you are now?
	Are you be interested in working together to examine in more detail the patterns of behaviors that currently affect your health?

	Can we discuss your current behavior in relation to ....?
	  Smoking cessation
	  Eating well
	  Physical activity
	  Sexual awareness
	  Injury prevention
	  Substance safety
	  Oral health
	  Self-development
	  Productivity

	Have you ever made changes in yourself or your behavior that promote your health?
	When did you make those changes?
	Were you able to sustain those changes?
	What behaviors would you like to change now?
Minimize Health Depleting Patterns	In analyzing your current behavior in relation to your desired image of health, what limits you from getting there?
	If we called these depleting behaviors because they limit your ability to be the healthy person you imagine, could we make them into a list?
	Once these depleting behaviors are listed, can we look at them together and try to make sense of them?
	Why do you think it is so hard for you to change your behavior and sustain that change?
	Do you think there is anything that can be done to take away some of these road blocks so that you can be more of what you want to be?

THE HEALTH PROMOTION MATRIX: *An Abbreviated Script—cont'd*

Optimize Health Supportive Patterns	Can you think of ways that you have been successful in taking care of your health?
	How have these behaviors worked for you?
	Is there something to be learned from your success that can help you now to change other behaviors?
	Where do you find support when you need it?
	Can you ask for support to help you in your desire to be healthy?
	What kind of support would you ask for?
	Who would you ask? When would you ask? How would you ask for support?
Internalize Idealized Image	In what ways is your health more real to you now?
	Do you feel comfortable with yourself as a healthier person?
	How has your health become more important to you?
	Do you think you have the support you need in place right now?
	What will you do if this support changes? How will you adjust?
	Since you are always changing and so is your health, what modifications can you anticipate in order to sustain your healthy self?
	I'm very proud of you and the changes you have made to improve your health.

tion to gain and to increase community support through use of clients, client families, community members, local organizations or businesses, interest groups, and legislators, for example. Potential opponents and allies are involved. Conflict resolution training is provided. The action is implemented over time, using a schedule of resource commitments.

To internalize an idealized image of health, environmental support and resources are enhanced through the provision of ongoing information and feedback about community change, community satisfaction, and other processes and outcomes. Innovative ideas are reinvented to fit local needs, resources, and cultural traditions. Community changes are celebrated and recognized. The health care professional continues to advocate for policies and resource allocations consonant with the goals of the community. Using the results of evaluation, new goals, strategies, and tactics are developed.

Summary

Health care professionals occupy a pivotal role in the modification of the client system (whether individual, family, group, or community) by assisting the client to alter patterns of behavior. And, through the use of the Matrix, the health care professional may work with client systems to create an image of health by helping them to envision themselves as healthy. This is followed by image appraisal, in which the health care professional works alongside a client to assess the client's present health status. The gap between the client's idealized image and his/her present behaviors is uncovered through this dimension. Narrowing that gap is the task of the partnership between health care professional and client as they work to minimize health depleting behaviors. A commitment to change is developed and obtained after the client and health care professional design a strategy to address unique barriers to modifying unhealthy behaviors. Supportive behaviors are subsequently optimized, oftentimes through aligning the client with a helpful family member, friend, or colleague. The last dimension, internalizing an idealized image of health, reinforces the positive changes over time. The Matrix assists clients to become what they imagine.

References

Arnold, J. (1998). Family health assessment. In M. Klainberg, S. Holzemer, M. Leonard, & J. Arnold, *Community health nursing: An alliance for health* (pp. 239-268). New York: McGraw-Hill.

Birnbach, N. (1990). The battle against smoking. *Journal of the New York State Health Care Professionals Association, 21*(1), 14.

Burgess, R.L. (1980). Relationships in marriage and the family. In S. Duck & R. Gilmour (Eds.), *Personal relationships*. London: Academic Press.

Butterfield, P.G. (1990). Thinking upstream: Nurturing a conceptual understanding of the societal context of health behavior. *Advances in Nursing Science, 12*(2), 1-8.

Caraher, M. (1994). A sociological approach to health promotion for health care professionals in an institutional setting. *Journal of Advanced Nursing, 20*, 544-551.

Classen, C., Diamond, S., Soleman, A., Fobair, P., Spira, J., & Spiegel, D. (1993). *Brief supportive-expressive group therapy for women with primary breast cancer: A treatment manual*. Stanford, CA: Stanford University School of Medicine, Department of Psychiatry and Behavioral Sciences.

Cox, F.M., Ehrlich, J.L., Rothman, J., & Tropman, J.E. (1974). *Strategies of community organization: A book of readings.* (2nd ed.). Itasca, IL: FE Peacock.

Delbecq, A.L. (1978). The social political process of introducing innovation in human services. In R. Sarri & Y. Hasenfeld (Eds.), *The management of human services* (pp. 309-339). New York: Columbia University Press.

Erikson, E.H. (1968). *Identity: Youth and crisis*. New York: WW Norton & Co.

Garbarino, J., Abramowitz, R.H., Benn, J.L., Gaboury, M.T., Galambos, N.L., Garbarino, A.C., Kostelny, K., Long, F.N., & Plantz, M.C. (1992). *Children and families in the social environment* (2nd ed.). New York: Aldine de Gruyter.

Gitterman, A. (1991). Introduction: Social work practice with vulnerable populations. In A. Gitterman (Ed.), *Handbook of social work practice with vulnerable populations* (pp. 1-32). New York: Columbia University Press.

Hallett, R. (1986). Smoking intervention in the workplace: Review and recommendations. *Preventive Medicine, 15*, 213-231.

Hirsch, A., & Slama, K. (1992). Anti-tobacco measures in the world: The French case. *Tubercule and Lung Disease, 73*, 184-186.

Horney, K. (1936). *The collected works of Karen Horney: Vol. 1. The neurotic personality of our time, new ways in psychoanalysis, our inner conflicts*. New York: WW Norton and Co.

Klainberg, M., Holzemer, S., Leonard, M., & Arnold, J. (1998). *Community health nursing: An alliance for health*. New York: McGraw-Hill.

Lalonde, M. (1974). *A new perspective on the health of Canadians*. Ottawa: Information Canada.

Mizrahi, T., & Morrison, J.D. (1993). Introduction. In T. Mizrahi, & J.D. Morrison (Eds.), *Community organization and social administration*. New York: Haworth Press.

Morgan, G. (1986). *Images of organization*. Newbury Park, CA: Sage.

National Institute of Nursing Research. (1995). *Community-based health care: Nursing strategies. A report of an NINR priority expert panel*. Bethesda, MD: U.S. Department of Health and Human Services, U.S. Public Health Service, National Institutes of Health.

Prochaska, J.O., DiClemente, C.C., & Norcross, J.C. (1992). In search of how people can change: Applications to addictive behaviors. *American Psychologist, 47,* 1102-1114.

Redland, A.R., & Stuifbergen, A.K. (1993). Strategies for maintenance of health-promoting behaviors. *Advances in Clinical Nursing Research, 28*(2), 427-442.

Reiss, I. (1980). *Family systems in America.* (3rd ed.). New York: Holt, Rinehart & Winston.

Robertson, A., & Minkler, M. (1994). New health promotion movement: A critical examination. *Health Education Quarterly, 21*(3), 295-312.

Roter, D. (1987). An exploration of health education's responsibility for a partnership model of client-provider relations. *Patient Education and Counseling, 9,* 25-31.

Royce, J., Sheinfeld Gorin, S., Edelman, B., Rendino-Perrone, R., & Orlandi, M. (1990). Student health care professionals and smoking cessation. In P.F. Engstrom (Ed.), *Advances in cancer control* (Vol. 7). New York: Liss.

Sandler, J. (1967). Ideals, the ego ideal, and the ideal self. *Psychological Issues, 18,* 129-174.

Sandler, J et al. (1963). The ego ideal and the ideal self. *Psychoanalytic Study of the Child, 18,* 139-158.

Sarri, R.C., & Galinsky, M.J. (1974). A conceptual framework for group development. In P. Glasser, R. Sarri, & R. Vinter (Eds.), *Individual change through small groups* (pp. 71-88). New York: The Free Press.

Satir, V. (1972). *Peoplemaking.* Palo Alto, CA: Science and Behavior Books.

Sheinfeld Gorin, S. (1992). Student health care professional opinions about the importance of health promotion practices. *Journal of Community Health, 17*(6), 367-375.

Sheinfeld Gorin, S. (1995). Relationship enhancement intervention: Social support program for women survivors of breast cancer. 1995 program. *Proceedings of the American Society of Clinical Oncology,* 236.

Sheinfeld Gorin, S. (1997). The social support process for women survivors of breast cancer: Outcomes in quality of life and survival. In E.J. Mullen & J.L. Magnabosco (Eds.), *Outcomes measurement in the human services: Cross-cutting issues and methods* (pp. 276-289). Washington, DC: NASW Press.

Siegel, P.Z., Frazier, E.L., Mariolis, P. Brackbill, R.M., & Smith, C. (1993). Behavioral risk factor surveillance, 1991: Monitoring the progress toward the nation's Year 2000 health objectives. *MMWR, 42*(Suppl. 4), 1-21.

Strasser, P.B. (1991). Smoking cessation programs in the workplace: Review and recommendations for occupational health care professionals. *AAOHN Journal, 39*(9), 432-438.

U.S. Department of Health and Human Services, U.S. Public Health Service. (1991). *Healthy people 2000: National health promotion and disease prevention objectives* (DHHS Publication No. PHS-91-50213). Washington, DC: Government Printing Office.

Vinter, R. (1974). The essential components of social group work practice. In P. Glasser, R. Sarri, & R. Vinter (Eds.), *Individual change through small groups.* (pp. 9-33). New York: The Free Press.

Wallack, L., & Winkleby, M. (1987). Primary prevention: A new look at basic concepts. *Social Science in Medicine, 25,* 923.

Wallerstein, N. (1992). Powerlessness, empowerment & health: Implications for health promotion programs. *American Journal of Health Promotion, 6,* 197-205.

Woods, N.E., Laffrey, S., Duffy, M., Lentz, M.J., Mitchell, E.S., Taylor, D., & Cowan, K.A. (1988). Being healthy: Women's images. *Advanced Nursing Science, 11*(1), 36-46.

Yalom, I.D. (1985). *Theory and practice of group psychotherapy.* (3rd ed.). New York: Basic Books.

PART two

PRACTICE FRAMEWORKS *for* HEALTH PROMOTION

6

Smoking Cessation

Sherri Sheinfeld Gorin

EDITORS' NOTE

Smoking Cessation and the Individual Client System.   Although smoking is recognized as an unhealthy behavior and tobacco an agent of addiction, individuals continue to smoke. Communities, coalitions, and policymakers have developed programs, policies, and legislation to sensitize individuals to the health risks and dangers associated with tobacco and to prohibit smoking in worksites, schools, and other communal environments. Cigarette manufacturers have been required to place warnings on all packaging and advertisements for cigarettes. Courts have deliberated about the liability cigarette manufacturers must assume relative to the health outcomes of smokers. Public places, including restaurants and airplanes, have become smoke-free. Convincing research has also alerted the public to the effects of environmental tobacco smoke and its particular threat to infants, children, the elderly, and individuals who experience respiratory compromise. Regardless of the enormous changes that have been made on the community, agency, and policy levels to reduce tobacco use, many individuals continue to smoke. Additionally, the media still promotes tobacco use through magazine covers displaying cigar-puffing business moguls and through film, where brave protagonists break the newest taboo: smoking.

Smoking Cessation and Minimizing Health Depleting Patterns/Optimizing Health Supportive Patterns.   Editor Sherri Sheinfeld Gorin, PhD, describes groups of tobacco users—longtime smokers, those less-educated, and young women—who pose particular challenges to the health care professional's smoking cessation efforts. While most smokers quit on their own, these clients pose particular challenges. The health care professional's efforts to minimize the client's health depleting patterns by linking daily smoking cues (e.g., drinking a cup of coffee) to other, healthy behaviors (e.g., walking) and to monitor his/her own smoking are thus critical. The health care professional may further help the client to optimize health supportive patterns by enhancing the support network of family members, friends, and others toward cessation. The health care professional's advice, even if brief, can be highly influential toward change.

Script for a Brief Intervention   Sheinfeld Gorin has developed a brief script that may be used by a variety of health care professionals in any "teachable" moment with an individual client.

117

Adopted by the COMMIT (Community Intervention Trial for Smoking Cessation) program across North America and tested for use by nurses in a rigorous clinical trial, the script has demonstrated its adaptability, ease of understanding, and use.

It is estimated that about 200 million of the 1.2 billion persons living in developed countries will eventually be killed by tobacco (World Health Organization [WHO], 1997). In the United States alone, smoking results in 435,000 deaths (1 in every 5 persons) and billions of dollars in health care costs (Centers for Disease Control and Prevention [CDC], 1994c). Cigarette smoking is the most important single preventable cause of death in human society.

While per capita consumption of tobacco is decreasing in developed countries at about 1.5% per year, tobacco use is rising in developing countries at about 1.7% per year (World Health Organization, 1997). In China, for example, one third of all adults smoke, which amounts to one fourth of the world's smokers (Anonymous, 1996). Cigarette consumption in the developing world will exceed consumption in developed countries within the next decade (World Health Organization, 1997).

Extensive research links cigarette smoking to disability and premature death. Tobacco is responsible for more cancers and more cancer deaths than any other known agent. Of late, a *direct* etiologic link (on the P53 gene) has been found between benzo[a]pyrene, one of the many carcinogenic components of cigarette smoke, and lung cancer (Denissenko, Pao, Tang, & Pfeifer, 1996). Smoking is a prime risk factor for heart and blood vessel disease, chronic bronchitis, and emphysema (Newcomb & Carbone, 1992; Sherman, 1992).

Worldwide, the World Health Organization (WHO) has encouraged tobacco control through the development of national programs, support of advocacy, and information dissemination (Chollat-Traquet, 1992). In the United States, policy initiatives designed to inform the public about the hazards of tobacco use, create economic incentives to discourage smoking, and provide restrictions on the use or purchase of tobacco support a smoke-free environment (Bierer & Rigotti, 1992). Most recently, President Clinton approved rules subjecting regulations regarding the distribution of cigarettes and smokeless tobacco to children and adolescents to the authority of the Food and Drug Administration (FDA) (FDA, 1996). At the state level, legislative approaches have increased—through 1238 laws—to limit the use of tobacco (Shelton, Alciati, Chang, Fishman, & Fues et al., 1995). Further, myriad private companies have established formal policies to protect workers from environmental tobacco smoke (Shelton et al., 1995).

Groups such as the Coalition on Smoking OR Health, which includes the American Cancer Society (ACS), the American Heart Association (AHA), and the American Lung Association (ALA), have been active in lobbying the FDA to promote new regulations regarding children and smoking, and state attorneys general have joined to sue the tobacco companies for smoking-related costs. Similar coalitions exist in most states and many communities. Health care professionals have joined such groups to increase public awareness about the effects of tobacco and have advocated for legislative and regulatory action against this lethal product.

Many individuals support the idea of limiting smoking (Chapman, 1996), and recent

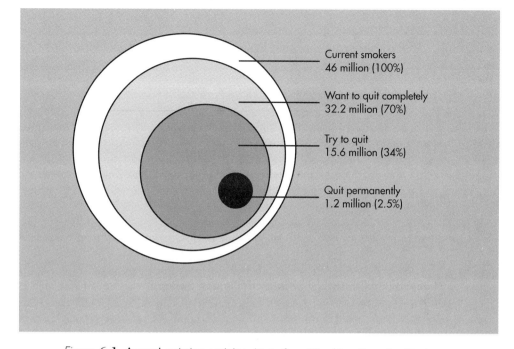

Current smokers
46 million (100%)

Want to quit completely
32.2 million (70%)

Try to quit
15.6 million (34%)

Quit permanently
1.2 million (2.5%)

Figure **6-1** **Annual quitting activity.** *(Data from "Smoking Cessation During Previous Year Among Adults—United States, 1990 and 1991," by CDC, 1993,* Morbidity and Mortality Weekly Report, 42 (26), 501-502; *"Cigarette Smoking Among Adults—United States, 1993," by CDC, 1994,* Morbidity and Mortality Weekly Report, 43 (50), 925-930; *and "National Age and Sex Differences in Quitting Smoking," by J. Pierce, G. Giovino, E. Hatziandreu, & D. Shopland, 1989,* Journal of Psychoactive Drugs, 21(3), 293-298.)

surveys reveal an encouraging decline in smoking prevalence in the United States (CDC, 1994c; CDC, 1996; Pierce et al., 1996). Most smokers want to quit, and more than one half have shown serious involvement in the quitting process, either by having quit for at least 24 hours in the past year or by intending to quit in the next 6 months (U.S. Department of Health and Human Services [USDHHS], 1990b; Curry, 1993) (Figure 6-1).

The combined effect of these efforts has been remarkable. Between 1965 and 1987, the prevalence of smoking dropped from 42.4% to 25.5%, but was virtually unchanged from 1990-92 (CDC, 1994c). Although some of this decline is attributable to the prevention of initiation, much of it reflects cessation. The "quit ratio," the percentage of persons who have ever smoked who have quit, has risen from 30% to 45% (USDHHS, 1990b). The proportion of those who have quit through formal programs is thought to be small, probably about 10% of former smokers (Fiore et al., 1990). Despite the drop in overall prevalence of smoking, since 1992, the smoking rate has risen by more than 20% among high school students (CDC, 1994a, 1994b).

THE TOBACCO INDUSTRY

The tobacco industry, through its enormous economic power, influences the promotion and sale of cigarettes worldwide. The tobacco industry is among the top U.S. industries, with 45 million customers spending about $55 billion per year on its products (Kluger, 1996). It is the primary source of agricultural income in North Carolina and Kentucky and a major contributor to income in five other states (Congressional Research Service Report and United States Department of Agriculture, as cited in Tinn, 1995). Although the major tobacco companies have diversified and also produce food items, soft drinks, beer, and other commodities, cigarettes are among their most profitable products. To promote cigarettes, tobacco companies spend more than $4.6 billion annually, $12.6 million a day (Lynch & Bonnie, 1994), on advertising, which is more than they pay for wages and salaries and nearly as much as they pay for tobacco (The Tobacco Institute, 1988). Tobacco companies are the largest national advertisers in print media.

Federal and State Government Involvement

Tobacco is one of the crops grown under a federal price support and production control program that was initiated during the Great Depression. In this program, farmers agree to limit production in return for a guaranteed buyer and a minimum price. The price of tobacco therefore is kept at an artificially high level. Despite some criticism, lawmakers have largely exempted tobacco from both spending cuts and a recent budget reconciliation provision that would have done away with the program (Tinn, 1995).

The federal government, all 50 states, the District of Columbia, and several hundred local governments tax cigarettes. Taxes increase prices, which in turn reduce purchases of cigarettes. Some research suggests that for every 10-cent price increase, 4% fewer persons will purchase cigarettes (Warner, 1981).

The World Market for Tobacco

Cigarettes are produced, promoted, and sold everywhere in the world. Although cigarette consumption is highest in developed countries, it is beginning to decline. As a result, tobacco companies are aggressively promoting their products in developing countries, which are reaping great economic rewards through hefty excise taxes, retail sales, and rural employment. The results of tobacco promotion have been disastrous, with 70% to 75% of the 1.1 billion smokers worldwide living in developing countries (WHO, 1997). In 1978, WHO stated, "Failing immediate action, smoking diseases will appear in developing countries before communicable diseases and malnutrition have been controlled, and the gap between rich and poor countries will thus be further expanded" (WHO Expert Committee on Smoking Control, 1979).

EPIDEMIOLOGY OF SMOKING

Smoking is influenced by powerful biologic, psychologic, social, and economic factors. The 1993 National Health Interview Survey shows that 46 million Americans older than 17 years are daily smokers (CDC, 1994c). Further, in 1996, total cigar consumption was 4.5 billion cigars; from 1993 to 1996, the consumption of larger cigars increased by 44.5% (CDC, 1997a). Approximately 23% of females and 28% of males older than 18 years are regular cigarette smokers (CDC, 1994c). About 19% of male and 18% of female high school seniors are daily smokers (CDC, 1994a). See Table 6-1 for smoking issues related to the populations described in the following sections.

Women

Since the late 1950s, tobacco companies have directed a concerted marketing effort at women. The percentage of women who smoke about equals that of men because women are abandoning the habit more slowly (CDC, 1997b) and taking it up more rapidly than men. Among employed women, blue-collar workers are more likely to smoke than those in other types of occupations (USDHHS, 1985); those with less education are more likely to smoke than the better educated. Further, although a number of studies suggest that fear of weight gain, dual-role stress, and withdrawal symptoms may make it more difficult for women than for men to break the smoking habit, most of the more recent studies have reported comparable relapse rates (Fant, Everson, Dayton, Pickworth, & Henningfield, 1996; USDHHS, 1980).

The probability for a woman who smokes to develop lung cancer, once primarily a male disease, is 2 to 3 times greater than that of a nonsmoking woman (USDHHS, 1979). Further, among certain women, smoking is a critical risk factor for breast cancer (Ambrosone et al., 1996).

Clinical evidence suggests that women who smoke cigarettes have greater difficulty becoming pregnant and have fewer reproductive years (USDHHS, 1980). The death rate of women who smoke and use birth-control pills is higher than that of nonsmoking birth-control pill users (Willett et al., 1987). Women who smoke have increased rates of vaginal bleeding, hysterectomies, and irregular periods, and their bodies require more menstrual cycles to become pregnant after oral contraception use is discontinued (Thomford & Mattison, 1986). In addition, long-term smoking may lead to early menopause (Baron, Bulbrook, & Wang, 1986).

Pregnant women. In 1994, about 15% of birth certificates revealed that mothers smoked during pregnancy; postpartum relapse is the norm among those who do quit before or during pregnancy (McBride & Pirie, 1989).

Infants in utero are at heightened risk from tobacco smoke and other environmental toxicants because their physiologic defense mechanisms are immature (Whyatt & Perera, 1995). Smoking reduces the supply of nutrients and oxygen to the fetus, which can retard growth and maturation and lead to long-term deficits in children's cognitive and physical functioning. Women who stop smoking during the last 6 months of pregnancy—when appropriate oxygen levels are crucial to growth—improve their chance of having a normal-size healthy baby. Women who continue to smoke, however, double their chance of having a low-birth weight infant and increase the risk of stillbirth and premature delivery (USDHHS, 1980). Smoking among low-income minority women is of particular concern because their babies are already at greater risk of having a low birth weight and other poor birth outcomes, compared with Caucasian infants.

Smoking during pregnancy can lead to abnormalities in the placenta, which contribute to congenital malformations of the baby, such as anencephaly, spina bifida, congenital heart disease, cleft palate and lip, inguinal hernia, strabismus and urogenital anomalies, respiratory and inner ear infections, decreased lung function, pulmonary hypertension in infancy, and heightened risk of childhood cancer and cancer later in life (Friesen & Fox, 1986). Additionally, the incidence of sudden infant death syndrome (SIDS) is higher among infants whose mothers smoke while pregnant (USDHHS, 1980).

Table **6-1**

	PRIMARY SMOKING ISSUES	**SPECIFIC CESSATION APPROACHES**
Intervention approaches particular to selected groups by gender, age, and status		
Women	Targeted marketing efforts	Emphasize self-control, illogic in advertisements; develop counteradvertising
	Less education, lower socioeconomic class	Target interventions to high-risk groups
		Advocate for changed legislation, policies for tobacco control
Pregnant women	Smoking by others in the home (environmental tobacco smoke [ETS])	Develop plan to reduce smoking in various settings (see Chapter 4)
Infants	Smoking by mother during pregnancy, and/or while nursing	Emphasize effects on child from mother's smoke (e.g., by measuring cotinine in breast milk)
Children	Smoking by others in the home (modeling and ETS)	Develop "no smoking" times, days at home
	Peer group influence	Cessation as an affirmative response
Adolescents	Process of separation and individuation	Not smoking is one's own decision; challenge them to stop
	Peer group influence	Peer pressure as self-pressure, cessation as an affirmative response
	Egocentricity and increased self-concern	Emphasize effects on appearance (e.g., smelly hair, yellow teeth)
	Feelings of invulnerability	Focus on relevant effects (e.g., shortness of breath)
	Present-orientation	Emphasize short-term effects (e.g., cost, bad breath)
	Smoking by others in the home	Explore smoking as a family problem
Adolescent women	Targeted marketing efforts	Analyze advertisements for illogic; develop counteradvertising

Both cotinine (a by-product of nicotine) and nicotine are found in the breast milk of smoking mothers, and these toxins may be transmitted to the infant. Even a mother who does not smoke but lives in an environment where she is exposed to smoke, transmits low levels of nicotine to her infant through breast milk (Axelrad, Sepkovic, Colosimo, & Haley, 1987; Perera, personal communication, November 28, 1997).

Table **6-1**

Intervention approaches particular to selected groups by gender, age, and status—cont'd		
	PRIMARY SMOKING ISSUES	**SPECIFIC CESSATION APPROACHES**
Adolescent men	Interest in portraying a "macho" image	Portray smokers as weak and babyish
	Marketing of smokeless tobacco	Analyze advertisements for illogic; encourage client to make his/her own choice
Elderly	Exacerbates conditions more common among elderly, such as heart disease, high blood pressure, circulatory and vascular conditions, duodenal ulcers, reductions in smell and taste, osteoporosis, diabetes	Emphasize short-term health benefits of stopping
	Drug dose alterations	Highlight increased efficacy of medications
Vulnerable populations	Divorced or separated men	Target intervention efforts to these high-risk groups
	Those with lower levels of education and income	
Minorities	Higher prevalence among African-Americans	Use culturally sensitive messages and community leaders (e.g., church leaders)
	Hispanic males have higher prevalence, women have lower rates	Use culturally sensitive messages; emphasize the impact on the family
	American Indians have higher rates of smokeless tobacco use	Use culturally sensitive messages; work with Indian Health Service and/or spiritual healers
		Advocate for changes in advertising, promotion practices targeted to high-risk groups
Persons experiencing psychologic distress	Depression and anxiety are risk factors	Focus on link between symptoms and smoking
	Psychiatric inpatients have higher rates	Make nicotine addiction part of treatment process

Children and Adolescents

The decisions children and adolescents make about smoking are critical because 90% of smokers begin smoking in their teen-age years (Kirn, 1987; Kandel & Yamaguchi, 1985). About 91% of adult smokers tried their first cigarette before age 20 years, and 77% became daily smokers before age 20 years (CDC, 1995). The 1994 Monitoring the Future Survey indicated that there has been no decline in smoking prevalence among high school seniors during the last decade; just less than 20% of seniors report daily smoking. Meanwhile, adolescent smoking rates among 9th- to 12th-graders have progressively increased (USDHHS, 1995; Nelson et al., 1995; CDC, 1994a). Teenage girls, in particular, are taking up smoking at younger ages.

High-school dropouts smoke at an extraordinarily high rate (an estimated 68% to 77% of dropouts reportedly smoke). When high school senior tobacco use prevalence rates are combined with those for dropouts, the smoking prevalence rate among U.S. adolescents nearly equals that among adults—about 25% (O'Malley, Johnston, & Bachman, 1995; Pirie, Murray, & Leupker, 1988; Flay, 1993).

Several developmental characteristics that occur during adolescence influence the decision to smoke, including the processes of separating from parents, acquiring adult skills, and gaining independence (Ericson, 1950). Adolescents experiment with a wide range of behaviors and life-styles, and they may view smoking as a badge of freedom, especially when the behavior is admired by other teenagers. Further, young persons are oriented to the present (Mittelmark, Murray, & Luepker, 1987), so they have difficulty envisioning the health effects of early smoking.

The influence of the peer group peaks during adolescence, and in most cases, perceptions of smoking and refusing to smoke play the most important role in adolescents' decisions whether to adopt the habit. A majority of teenagers, however, grossly overestimate the percentage of peers who smoke (Duryea & Martin, 1981).

Other traits of adolescence, such as egocentricity and increased self-concern, tend to make teenagers exaggerate their own importance. Thus they become more concerned about their appearances and self-images (Wong-McCarthy & Gritz, 1982). The concerns of teenagers make them susceptible to cigarette advertising claims that promise beauty, intelligence, and sexual attractiveness (e.g., in 1993, the three most heavily advertised brands, Marlboro, Camel and Newport, were the three most commonly purchased brands).

Adolescents also feel invulnerable. Though most adolescents believe that smoking endangers their physical health, their feelings of vulnerability to the negative consequences of smoking have been found to decrease rapidly from the 6th to 8th grade and to increase only slowly during the next 20 years (Urberg & Robbins, 1984). Their confidence in their own immunity leads them to let the perceived positive benefits associated with smoking outweigh the potential, but in their minds remote, long-term negative health effects (Killen, 1985).

Often, children and adolescents live in homes where one or both parents smoke, and this environment increases the likelihood that a child will smoke (Severson & Lichtenstein, 1986). If a teenager has both a parent and an older sibling who smoke, the likelihood of becoming a smoker is further amplified. In fact, teenagers are 4 times as likely to smoke if they have a sibling who models this behavior (Green, 1979).

Adolescent women. Twenty-eight percent of female high school seniors are currently past month smokers, a prevalence that is comparable to that for adolescent boys. The highest rates are among Caucasian girls (15.3% among 12- to 18-year olds), the lowest rates are among African-American girls (4.6%), and intermediate rates are among Hispanic girls (10.8%) (Huston, Chrismon & Reddy, 1996). Caucasian adolescent girls and girls of lower socioeconomic status appear to be at highest risk for smoking (French & Perry, 1996).

The reasons adolescent girls begin to smoke are varied and differ somewhat from those for boys. Comparisons of adolescent girl and boy smokers suggest that adolescent girl smokers are self-confident, outgoing, rebellious, and socially skilled, in contrast to the social insecurity characteristic of adolescent boy smokers (Clayton, 1991). For girls, participation in sports or in individual leisure activities seems protective against smoking initiation (Swan, Creeser, & Murray, 1990). Further, girls and women who smoke are not likely to encounter messages that encourage them to stop.

Adolescent men. Among adolescent boys, the use of smokeless tobacco such as snuff (shredded tobacco that is sucked not chewed) and chewing tobacco increased during the early 1980s, and state surveys have found little change since (Nelson, Tomar, Mowery, & Siegel, 1996). A 1994 report by the Surgeon General found that 20% of all high school boys were current users of smokeless tobacco (USDHHS, 1994); one third to one half of these used it at least once a week (USDHHS, 1986b). Production of smokeless tobacco has increased 45% since 1970, and between 1988 and 1991, advertising and promotional expenses increased 75% (USDHHS, 1986b; Nelson et al., 1996). Some adolescent males view smokeless tobacco use as a less serious health risk and a more socially acceptable behavior than cigarette smoking (Chassin, Presson, & Sherman, 1985). The tobacco companies, meanwhile, portray dipping snuff as fun, a sign of virility, and as American as baseball and country music (Koop, 1986).

The health hazards of smokeless tobacco are myriad. Long-term snuff dippers have 50 times the risk of cancers of the cheek and gum as nontobacco users (USDHHS, 1986b). Linkage has also been suggested for cancers of the esophagus, larynx, and pancreas. Other related health problems include periodontal disease, elevated blood pressure, and physical dependence (Connolly, Winn, & Hecht, 1986).

Smoking, drinking, drug use, and other risk-taking behaviors are often regarded by young men as necessary to demonstrate their masculinity and as symbols that they are approaching adulthood (Robb, 1986). Further, among some young men, these behaviors are considered to be part of a "macho" image. Smoking fills a need for excitement and may help a young man form a group of friends (Mosbach & Leventhal, 1988).

The Elderly

Smoking is the eighth of the top 16 causes of death for persons age 65 years and older (Rimer, Orleans, Keintz, Cristinzio, & Fleisher, 1990). About 41% of cancer deaths in men 65 years and older and 15 percent of cancer deaths in women 65 years and older are smoking-related (Rimer et al., 1990). These types of deaths are expected to rise as the effects of increases in smoking among women are realized. Smoking also complicates illnesses and conditions that are more common among older persons, notably heart disease, high blood pressure, circulatory and vascular conditions, duodenal ulcers, reductions in smell and taste, osteoporosis, and diabetes. In addition prevalence rates of cough, phlegm, and chronic bronchitis among smokers increase with advancing age. Also, drug dosages for the older person who smokes may be subtherapeutic or ineffective because of the interaction of nicotine and average drug levels (Rimer et al., 1990).

Vulnerable Populations

Smoking is particularly common among persons who experience difficulty in American society. For example 76% of male frequenters of a church-sponsored soup kitchen in Charleston, S.C., reported smoking cigarettes (McDade & Keil, 1988). Divorced or separated men have the highest prevalence of smoking—48.2%—among the general population (USDHHS, 1988). In addition, in the United States, smoking is more prevalent among the poor and less-educated (USDHHS, 1988); in Europe, however, smoking is more prevalent among the affluent (Onis & Villar, 1991).

Minorities. According to the 1993 National Health Interview Survey (CDC, 1994c), relatively more African-American men smoke than do Caucasian and Hispanic men, and relatively more African-American women smoke than do Caucasian and Hispanic women but smoke somewhat less than Caucasian women. African-American men have a 20% higher mortality rate from heart disease and a 58% higher incidence of lung cancer than do Caucasian men. African-American women have a 50% higher mortality rate from heart disease and higher incidences of fetal deaths, low-birth weight infants, and infant mortality than do Caucasian women (Ramirez & Gallion, 1993). In some minority communities, the adverse biologic effects of smoking are compounded by poverty, poor nutrition, and increased background exposure to environmental pollution (Freeman, 1989).

Because smoking is more prevalent among African-Americans than other groups, they develop a greater number of smoking-related cancers. Although African-Americans are more likely to be smokers and they smoke cigarettes with high tar and menthol levels, research indicates that they smoke fewer cigarettes per day than do Caucasians (Becker et al., 1992). Economic and educational differences account for observed gaps between African-Americans and Caucasians in knowledge of smoking risks (Brownson et al., 1992).

Although Hispanics have a lower rate of lung cancer and are generally believed to have lower rates of smoking than African-Americans or nonminorities, the smoking prevalence among Hispanic males is very similar to that among nonminority males. The smoking rates among Hispanic females are considerably lower than that of Caucasian females (CDC, 1987).

Tobacco use among American Indians seems to vary by tribe or reservation (USDHHS, 1989b). Often, the primary health risk is not from cigarettes but from smokeless tobacco. According to one regional survey, smokeless tobacco use is higher among American Indians than among any other segment of the population (Schinke, Schilling, & Gilchrest, 1987). American Indian children are frequent snuff dippers (Hall & Dexter, 1988; CDC, 1988). Most American Indians begin using tobacco at an early age. Usage declines after adolescence but remains significantly higher than the average for the United States (CDC, 1994a, 1994c).

The diverse Asian and Pacific Islander population is at particular risk for smoking-related diseases. Among California immigrant groups, smoking rates among men are 92% for Laotians, 71% for Cambodians, and 65% for Vietnamese, compared with 30% for the overall American population (Asian American Health Forum, 1989).

Persons experiencing psychologic distress. The link between poor mental health and regular tobacco use has been suggested by the high levels of depressive and anxiety symptoms reported by adult smokers and by teenagers initiating smoking (Patton et al., 1996), as well as high lifetime rates of major depression among adult smokers (Waal-Manning & de Hamel, 1980; Winefield, Winefield, Tiggeman, & Goldney, 1989; Glassman et al., 1990; Romans, McNoe, Herbison, Walton, & Mullen, 1993). Among inpatients of a psychiatric hospital, the rate of smoking may be more than twice that of the general population (O'Farrell, Connors & Upper, 1983; Gopalaswamy & Morgan, 1986; Gralnick, 1988). Further, one of the most common reasons given for relapses or near relapses is emotional upset (Shiffman, 1986).

Environmental Tobacco Smoke

Continuing research has demonstrated that environmental tobacco smoke (ETS) affects nonsmokers. Sidestream smoke from burning cigarettes has much higher concentrations of tar, nicotine, and carbon monoxide than exhaled (mainstream) smoke because it has not been filtered through the cigarette or the smoker's lungs (USDHHS, 1986a). A study that measured nicotine concentrations in nonsmoking workers exposed to cigarette smoke in a typical work environment found that the amount of nicotine absorbed by passive smokers during 4 hours was similar to that absorbed by light smokers (1 to 10 cigarettes a day) (Feyerabend, Higginbottam, & Russell, 1982). Inhaling the smoke from others' cigarettes can trigger severe allergic reactions (Speer, 1986). Given that Americans spend more than 80% of their time indoors, the potential influence of this type of smoking is immense (Ware, Dockery, Spiro, Speizer, & Ferris, 1984).

Epidemiologic evidence suggests that passive smoking is responsible for increased risk of lung cancer (U.S. Environmental Protection Agency [EPA], 1994). Among women, the excess risk is 24% for spousal exposure to tobacco smoke, 39% for workplace exposure, and 50% for exposure in social settings (Fontham et al., 1994). Women with highest level of exposure—those exposed during adulthood and childhood—have more than 3 times the risk of cancer than nonexposed women (adjusted odds ratio, 3.25). Among 13 studies evaluated by the National Research Council (NRC), (Committee on Passive Smoking of the National Research Council, 1986), the overall risk of lung cancer associated with ETS for men was 1.62 higher than that for nonexposed men.

As many as 9 million American children younger than 5 years may be exposed to ETS. Smokers' children suffer from passive smoking, with more respiratory symptoms and acute lower respiratory tract infections and reduced lung function (Expert Committee on Passive Smoking, 1986; Byrd, 1992). In homes where at least one adult smokes, babies are more likely to suffer acute respiratory disease (USDHHS, 1986a). Studies are remarkably consistent in showing an increased risk of respiratory infections among children younger than 2 years who live in homes where parents smoke (USDHHS, 1986a). The incidence of sudden infant death syndrome (SIDS) is also greater when parents smoke (EPA, 1994). Further, children may be at heightened risk of cancer later in life as a result of exposure to ETS (Crawford et al., 1994).

Why Do People Smoke?

More than 10 years of study attests to the multidetermined nature of smoking (Lichtenstein & Glasgow, 1992). Several theoretical approaches to understanding smoking behavior have been proposed. For example, the transtheoretical model of change, which encompasses the health belief model and social learning theory propositions, defines smoking as a process, in which a series of stages may be identified in the initiation of the smoking: initial use, experimentation, and transition to habitual use. Similarly, a set of stages has been associated with cessation: precontemplation; contemplation of quitting; action; maintenance; and relapse (DiClemente, 1991; Prochaska & DiClemente, 1983; Prochaska, Velicer, Guadagnoli, Rossi, & DiClemente, 1991). The stages are not necessarily linear; the average successful quitter reports several and often many relapses before achieving maintained abstinence (Fisher, Bishop, Goldmunz, & Jacobs, 1988).

Tobacco addiction is comprised of biologic, biobehavioral, psychologic, and sociocultural processes that evolve differentially over time, akin to a "career" (Fisher et al., 1988). (See Box 6-1 for a summary of the biologic processes.) As a "career," smoking is directed

Box 6-1

The physiology of smoking

With the first inhalation of a cigarette, the cilia lining the bronchial tubes of the lungs become paralyzed (i.e., they cease to flutter). With paralyzed cilia, mucus accumulates inside the bronchial tubes, causing the development of mucus plugs. Dried mucus plugs clog the bronchial tubes so that oxygen is unable to move through the lungs as readily. When this occurs, less oxygen gets to the alveoli, thereby reducing the amount of oxygen reaching the extremities of the lungs and stressing the other body systems—in particular, the heart.

In addition to paralyzing the cilia, the various chemicals and particles in cigarette smoke irritate the delicate cells lining the air passages. The mucus glands therefore continue to produce more mucus to try to protect the lungs. The extra mucus cannot be removed from the lungs, so more mucus plugs form. The mucus becomes a breeding ground for viruses and bacteria within the lungs, thus increasing one's susceptibility to respiratory ailments. "Smoker's cough" is an artificial way of clearing mucus from the lungs when it is not being moved by the cilia.

When the heart lacks oxygen because of decreased oxygen in the blood and the coronary arteries are narrowed by atherosclerosis and nicotine constriction, heart cells may die, leading to a myocardial infarction. Lack of oxygen to the heart itself causes destruction of a part of the muscular wall of the heart. The amount of damage done and the chance for ventricular fibrillation to occur determines the likelihood of survival.

Carbon monoxide found in smoke is carried by the blood instead of oxygen, thus causing the heart to pump harder to compensate. The nicotine causes blood vessels to constrict, resulting in increased blood pressure and the consequent strain on the heart. Cigarette smoke has been associated with a build-up of cholesterol in the arteries, which further restricts blood flow and increases the burden on the heart. The clinging of tar to the lungs, the entrapment of air in the weakened airways, and the loss of normal elasticity of the lung tissue cause elongation of the lungs, which subsequently contributes to emphysema. With emphysema, the oxygen demands of the body cannot be satisfied.

Finally, cigarette smoke contains carcinogens that lodge in certain areas of the body, causing the cells around them to become abnormal and to metastasize, or spread. The lung is one of the first organs in which the carcinogenic elements of cigarette smoke have a chance to lodge, thus serving as a primary site for the development of cancer.

In individuals who quit smoking, many of the disease processes reverse themselves, to some extent, with the notable exceptions of emphysema and cancer. After quitting, ex-smokers' bodies can begin to function normally again, and their chances of heart and lung disease decrease.

by an interplay of intrinsic and social, or environmental, factors. Smoking is also something the person pursues, akin to a vocational career. Smokers may be influenced by important others who smoke, such as a parent, teacher, or boss, or peers who smoke and are more accepting of other smokers. Individuals also smoke because it makes them feel like the "fantasy" smoker in cigarette advertisements: a macho male, an independent woman, sexy, thin, happy, beautiful, and rich. Many feel that cigarettes enhance the pleasures and diminish the unpleasant events of daily life.

Nicotine Addiction

Central to the maintenance of the smoking "career" is the biologic potency of nicotine, which makes the patterns of the smoking habit stronger and thus more resistant to change. Nicotine is considered by the U.S. Surgeon General to be an addictive substance, possibly the most addictive drug known (USDHHS, 1988). The current view of drug dependence, when applied to nicotine, suggests that over several years after initiation, smoking behavior increases and reaches a point at which plasma nicotine levels are maintained, or "regulated," within characteristic limits (Russell, 1978). Once engaged, these processes result in characteristic patterns of smoking that are highly resistant to change and that, when interrupted, result in a strong desire to smoke (craving) and then withdrawal (Killen, Fortmann, Telch, & Newman, 1988; Pomerleau, Fertig, & Shanahan, 1983). Almost all smokers meet the diagnostic criteria for tobacco dependence (Hughes, Gust, & Pechacek, 1988). Physiologic addiction to nicotine causes persons to smoke continuously while they are awake; they cannot stop smoking without craving more cigarettes and experiencing withdrawal symptoms.

Constitutional differences in sensitivity to nicotine may separate smokers and nonsmokers. These initial sensitivities may lay in families, as in the case of alcohol (Pomerleau, Collins, Shiffman, & Pomerleau, 1993). Smokers may originate from a population of persons who are constitutionally sensitive to nicotine (i.e., initial smoking leads to a rapid decrease in sensitivity, or increase in tolerance. Individuals who never smoke may originate from a population of persons who are relatively insensitive to nicotine and probably have limited capability to develop tolerance (i.e., they are not highly susceptible to its attractions, rather than deterred by its aversive effects) (Pomerleau, Collins et al., 1993).

Interaction of Nicotine and Conditioning

Intense, unconditioned stimuli, such as nicotine, lead to more rapid conditioning, stronger conditioned responses, and greater resistance to extinction (Rachlin, 1991). Nicotine's biologic potency and speed of action interact with the cues surrounding its use to strengthen the conditioning of those cues.

Short durations between a behavior and its reinforcers enhance the effects of those stimuli (Rachlin, 1991). The delivery of nicotine into the bloodstream takes about 7 seconds after inhalation and thus quickly reinforces the behaviors that lead to smoking. In contrast, most disincentives, such as foul-smelling breath or public disapproval, are subtle and gradual, which reduces their ability to discourage smoking (Fisher, Lichtenstein, Haire-Joshu, Morgan et al., 1993).

The conditioning to smoke is further complicated by nicotine's varied effects—reduced arousal, diminished anxiety, or increased stimulation—so that arousal, anxiety, or lethargy may serve as both a discriminate stimulus for smoking and as a conditioned stimulus for withdrawal symptoms and cravings after cessation (Leventhal & Cleary, 1980). Many smokers rely on nicotine's ability to control arousal level (i.e., they feel that cigarettes provide a boost when they feel mentally or physically down or calm them if they are upset or overaroused). In addition, the conditions that accompany those emotions or moods may themselves signal smoking or elicit conditioned withdrawal symptoms (Niaura et al., 1988).

The average pack-a-day smoker of 20 years has generally inhaled on cigarettes more than 1 million times (Fisher & Rost, 1986). This repetition also strengthens "the thorough interweaving of the smoking habit in the fabric of daily life" (Pomerleau & Pomerleau, 1987, p. 119).

FACTORS INFLUENCING SMOKING CESSATION

Smoking versus quitting is determined by the relative strengths of motivations to continue or stop. The motivations to continue smoking include the pleasure and other perceived cognitive benefits of smoking, body weight control, the avoidance of craving and withdrawal symptoms, social or peer pressures, and environmental cues (conditioning). Motives to quit may include concern for one's health, social pressures, or economic factors (e.g., the cost of cigarettes) (Benowitz, 1992). The health belief model (Rosenstock, 1991) suggests that before taking action to quit using tobacco, a smoker must consider smoking a serious health problem, feel personally susceptible to its health harm, and perceive that stopping smoking will be beneficial.

Avoiding Temptations

Before quitting, the smoker can make plans to avoid circumstances likely to prompt relapse, including plans for coping with personal and interpersonal stress as well as individuals who offer cigarettes or otherwise encourage relapse. Self-control research suggests success will be more likely if plans are executed far in advance of the temptation and if they minimize exposure to the temptation (McReynolds, Green, & Fisher, 1983). Caution is urged, however, because avoiding temptation is contradictory to the requirement of exposure to conditioned stimuli to extinguish conditioned urges.

Extinguishing Conditioned Responses

Smoking is conditioned by the cues, such as an early morning cup of coffee or a ride in the car. In a study by Abrams, Monti, Carey, Pinto, and Jacobus (1988), reactivity to smoking-related cues predicted long-term success of cessation efforts. Smokers may diminish their conditioned cravings for cigarettes after cessation through "cue extinction" before they quit by systematically avoiding smoking in response to the individual' own dominant smoking cues (Lowe, Green, Kurtz, Ashenberg, & Fisher, 1980). Former smokers should be encouraged to re-enter smoking-related circumstances when they are able to tolerate them without strong urges to relapse.

Abrupt Quitting

As the number of cigarettes is reduced, their salience and the desire for nicotine that they provide may *increase*. This may cause cues associated with the last few cigarettes to elicit especially strong or persistent conditioned urges to smoke (Fisher, Lichtenstein & Haire-Joshu, 1993). Survey data support the conventional wisdom that abrupt or "cold turkey" quitting is more advantageous than gradual withdrawal (Fiore et al., 1990). Abrupt cessation is not necessarily quitting impulsively or without planning. Planned quitting from the usual number of cigarettes per day to zero has been found to be more effective than gradual withdrawal, particularly in reducing relapse urges (Flaxman, 1978; Jarvik & Henninfield, 1988).

Self-Monitoring

Self-monitoring (e.g., keeping track of the number of cigarettes smoked per day) is critical to almost any cessation effort. Self-monitoring itself may institute behavioral change by breaking up habitual chains of behavior, thus making them easier to alter. Newer approaches, such as using hand-held computers to monitor cues to smoke, have reliably assisted in identifying predictors of smoking, especially idle time (Shiffman, 1993).

Social Support

Much research has been conducted on the role of social support in smoking cessation (review in Cohen et al., 1988). The smoking habits of family and friends are among the best predictors of whether a person continues or stops smoking (Eisinger, 1971; Graham & Gibson, 1971). Long-term abstinence of 1 year or more may be tied to the number of friends and relatives who smoke in a person's social network (Mermelstein, Cohen, Lichtenstein, Baer, & Kamarck, 1986; Cohen et al., 1988; Gottlieb & Baker, 1986). Additionally the amount of perceived support for cessation among friends and spouses and other family members is related to cessation (Mermelstein et al., 1986; Morgan, Ashenberg, & Fisher, 1988). Long-term cessation norms among family members and within worksites and communities are thus key to the maintenance of cessation (Fisher, Lichtenstein, & Haire-Joshu, 1993). The influence of others can also be negative, in that individuals who offer cigarettes to or smoke in front of those who have quit may contribute to subsequent relapse (Morgan et al., 1988).

Self-Help

The majority of smokers prefer less-intensive, self-help approaches (Fiore et al., 1990). Further, of the 44 million Americans who have quit smoking, 90% report that they have stopped without professional assistance (Fiore et al., 1990). Self-quitting means that smokers quit on their own without professional assistance, although they may have been prompted to stop by an external source or program (review in Glynn, Boyd, & Gruman, 1990). Self-help approaches may take several forms, ranging from completely unaided efforts to more elaborate, but self-administered programs (cf. Lichtenstein & Cohen, 1990). These cost-effective approaches generally include the use of self-help manuals (Altman, Flora, Fortmann, & Farquhar, 1987; Windsor et al., 1993; Hodgson, 1992; Wagner et al., 1990).

Unaided quitting results in somewhat lower quit rates compared with clinical interventions. Longitudinal data reveal that 1 in 5 smokers can be expected to be abstinent 1 year after going through a self-help program, and 1 in 20 smokers can be expected to achieve long-term abstinence (i.e., at least 6 consecutive months) (summary in Curry, 1993). One study found no differences at 12-month follow-up between quitters who received self-help booklets and those who quit without any assistance. Self-help studies have found that heavy smokers are less likely to succeed at quitting on their own than are lighter smokers (Cohen et al., 1989), a similar finding to that in the clinical literature. Additional support, particularly in the form of follow-up calls, appears to increase cessation (Orleans et al., 1991). Further state-of-the-art self-help materials, which are conceptually driven, do not appear to be superior to minimal pamphlets (Cummings, Emont, Jaen, & Sciandra, 1988).

INTERVENTION APPROACHES FOR SMOKING CESSATION

Quitting smoking is not usually an event; it is a process. Many individuals must try several times before they succeed. Deciding on one of many special techniques to use is related to which treatment is available, client interest, and financial resources. Stop-smoking programs vary from minimally intrusive (e.g., cessation pamphlets) to moderately intrusive (e.g., individual or group sessions) to quite intrusive (e.g., medication).

There is little consensus among health care professionals regarding the best smoking cessation program, since some programs work well for certain individuals but not for others. See Table 6-1 on p. 122 for intervention approaches for specific populations. A variety of problems, including reporting bias, differing measures of success, and alternative measurement points, make it difficult to compare the success rates of varied smoking cessation methods. A thorough review of cessation methods revealed the highest 1-year abstinence rates resulted from physician interventions with cardiac patients, (median quit rate, 43%) and by multiple programs (median, 40%) (Schwartz, 1987). Most quit rates did not vary markedly among programs, however, with most cessation methods resulting in a median success rate of 15% to 40% (Schwartz, 1992).

The best way to determine which program to select is to start with the simplest program first; evaluate its success; and if necessary, increase treatment intensity, first through one of the self-help programs and subsequently through more intrusive clinic-based approaches. Many of the clinic-based approaches use aversion therapy or other powerful change techniques. The last resort, most experts agree, is pharmacologic treatment.

The basic components of effective brief primary care interventions include (1) a strong quit-smoking message; (2) state-of-the-art self-help motivational or quitting and relapse prevention materials; (3) brief cessation counseling, which includes setting a quit date; (4) the use of pharmacologic adjuncts when indicated (e.g., nicotine replacement); and (5) follow-up support (Orleans, Kristeller & Gritz, 1993; Cummings, Giovino, Emont, Sciandra, & Koenigsberg, 1986; Glynn et al., 1990; Glynn & Manley, 1989; Ockene, 1987; Orleans, 1985). Since smoking is both an addiction and a learned, or habitual, behavior, almost all programs use some types of behavioral procedures to disrupt long-established patterns associated with smoking.

As a result of five National Cancer Institute-funded clinical trials with physicians (Glynn & Manley, 1991), cessation interventions have been summarized into a four-step program, or the four *A's:* (1) *ask* all patients about their smoking status; (2) *advise* smokers clearly to stop smoking; (3) *assist* their efforts with self-help materials; a quit date; and possibly nicotine gum or the transdermal patch, particularly with smokers who are not yet ready to quit; and (4) *arrange* follow-up support. A fifth step has been added for children and adolescents: *anticipate* guiding smoking cessation with each client.

Physicians' and Other Health Care Professionals' Support

Physicians' advice has a significant impact on helping clients stop smoking. Despite the growing evidence of the effectiveness of their counseling, physicians tend to concentrate only on clients with smoking-related illnesses (Jelley & Prochazka, 1991; Cummings et al., 1989; Kenney et al., 1988; Ockene, Aney, Goldberg, Klar, & Williams, 1988). Some physicians may feel that they do not have the right to advise others to stop smoking (Mochizuki, 1996). According to the Teenage Attitudes and Practices Survey (TAPS II), 25% of respondents 10 to 22 years old reported that a health care professional had said something to them about cigarette smoking, and 12% said the same about smokeless tobacco (CDC, 1995).

The primary care setting is one where "more" is better, in that more contacts and treatment elements lead to better outcomes (Fagerstrom, 1988; Baille, Mattick, & Webster,

1990; Kottke, Battista, DeFriese, & Brekke, 1988). A few studies have shown that when physicians are trained in patient-centered counseling techniques, their effectiveness increases, as compared with brief advice or usual care (Ockene, 1987; Wilson et al., 1988). For example, a cessation rate of 62% has been reported for COPD clients who received physician advice, compared with a 26% rate among clients with bronchitis and asthma who also received physician counseling (Pederson, Williams, & Lefcoe, 1980). Novel approaches to cessation, including using respiratory therapists and the National Cancer Institute (NCI) four-step model with feedback of pulmonary function tests and alveolar CO levels, have been proposed by the American Association for Respiratory Care (USDHHS, 1989a). To be effective, a system is necessary to identify smokers (e.g., through chart stickers), and nurses and nurse practitioners can be counselors (Sheinfeld Gorin, 1989). In managed care settings, a team approach of several health care professionals may be the most efficient (Hollis, Lichtenstein, Mount, Vogt, & Stevens, 1991).

Pharmacologic Interventions

The main effect of nicotine gum (nicotine polacrilex) or the patch (transdermal nicotine) is the relief of nicotine withdrawal symptoms and the prevention of short-term relapse. Behavioral skills training is most useful in warding off longer-term relapse (Lichtenstein & Glasgow, 1992). Pharmacologic agents, therefore, are best used as adjuncts to behavioral counseling (Covey & Glassman, 1991). Nicotine gum has been found most effective when used alongside intensive cessation strategies—either long or short term—or as an assist to short-term, less-intensive treatment approaches (Cepeda-Benito, 1993). The nicotine patch, too, is an effective aid to smoking cessation, doubling or tripling quit rates (summary in Fiscella & Franks, 1996). Higher-dose nicotine replacement (44 mg) is generally not warranted alongside more intensive treatment, although it may provide short-term benefit to some smokers trying to quit with minimal adjuvant treatment. Nicotine inhalers and nasal sprays may improve the efficacy of a replacement therapy and may be used as transitions to, or adjuncts with, the patch (Hajek, Jarvis, Belcher, Sutherland, & Feyerabend, 1989; Jarvis, Hajek, Russell, & West, 1987; Perkins, Grobe, Stiller, Fonte, & Goettler, 1992; Sutherland, Russell, Stapleton, Feyerabend, & Ferno, 1992; Hughes, 1993). Other drugs, such as clonidine, have demonstrated enhanced abstinence in the short term, although enduring effects are illusory (Covey & Glassman, 1991).

Acupuncture and Hypnosis

Some smokers find cessation success by using hypnosis, meditation, or acupuncture. Acupuncture may help smokers deal with the addictive component of smoking by focusing attention on, and appearing to treat, the problem. Acupuncture thus seems to have a placebo effect, similar to that of pills containing sugar but no medication (Schwartz, 1988). Hypnosis may be an effective adjunct to a smoking cessation program; it is of little value as a one-shot, single-session, "magic" cure (Kottke et al., 1988).

Aversive Conditioning

Aversive conditioning approaches may diminish the attractiveness of smoking or may result in the cigarette itself becoming aversive. One such approach is rapid smoking, in which a client puffs a cigarette every 6 to 8 seconds until the client senses that he/she will become nauseated. This is repeated several times in sessions that accompany quit dates and are continued until urges to smoke are reduced (Lichtenstein, Harris, Birchler, Wahl, & Schmahl, 1973; Danaher, Jeffery, Zimmerman, & Nelson, 1980). Despite its relative effectiveness in conjunction with cessation counseling and abstinence rates of 50%, acceptance of this approach is limited (Glasgow, Lichtenstein, Beaver, & O'Neill, 1981). Normally paced aversive smoking, which involves conventional smoking without distraction so that the smoking itself becomes aversive or distasteful, is sometimes combined with satiation procedures and group treatment and results in abstinence rates from 40% to 70% (Danaher et al., 1980). Other components of aversive conditioning, such as a butt jar, are often used in conjunction with other approaches.

Intensive Cessation Clinics

Often, clients need more intensive treatment to quit, such as an intensive cessation clinic. A state-of-the-art clinic for smoking cessation tends to use approaches that include (1) setting a quit date; (2) interrupting conditioned responses that support smoking; (3) identifying and preparing plans for coping with temptations after cessation; (4) attending to relapse episodes and encouraging the continuation of cessation; and (5) providing follow-up contact and social support for quitting and abstinence (Lowe et al., 1980; Lando, 1977; Lichtenstein, 1982; Hall, Rugg, Tunstall, & Jones, 1984). The American Lung Association's "Freedom from Smoking" clinics have demonstrated a long-term abstinence rate of 29% (Rosenbaum & O'Shea, 1992). These clinics, which can be located through the ALA, hospitals, Health Maintenance Organizations (HMOs), and other centers, serve a small percentage of all quitters, which may number as many as 2 million each year in the United States (Lichtenstein & Hollis, 1992; Fiore et al., 1990). The health care professional's support is critical to these clients' follow-through.

Relapse Prevention

Relapses are common in smoking treatment. An average of two to three relapses is common for successful abstainers (Fisher, Haire-Joshu, Morgan, Rehberg, & Rost, 1990; Fisher, Lichtenstein, Haire-Joshu, Morgan et al., 1993). In treatment, emphasizing the importance of renewed effort after relapse is warranted.

Explanations for relapse. At least two explanations have been offered for relapse: reversal theory and the abstinence-violation effect. Reversal theory (Apter, 1982; O'Connell, Gerkovich, & Cook, 1995), which holds that human beings are inherently inconsistent and reverse back and forth between opposing metamotivational states (i.e., states that pertain to how certain motivational variables are interpreted by the individual, such as playful versus serious minded or negativistic versus conformist) has explained smoker relapse during tempting situations. Relapse has also been explained by an abstinence-violation effect (Marlatt & Gordon, 1985), wherein a person who attributes a minor slip to his/her relatively unchangeable personal characteristics may in turn experience lowered expectations of success and consequently abandon cessation efforts (Curry, Marlatt, & Gordon, 1987).

Self-efficacy. According to social cognitive theory (Bandura, 1986) (see Chapter 2), both outcome and efficacy expectations are central to behavior change, such as smoking cessation in general or recovery from an initial lapse after one has stopped smoking. Smokers high in self-efficacy, or more confident of their abilities to maintain cessation after treatment, will attempt to execute it more readily, with greater intensity, and with greater perseverance in response to initial failure than will individuals with comparatively weaker self-efficacy (Baer & Lichtenstein, 1988; Devins, 1992). After an initial lapse, individuals with moderate levels of self-efficacy—those neither too optimistic nor too pessimistic concerning the adequacy of their skills for coping with difficult situations (such as a first lapse)—are also more successful at sustained smoking cessation. When one has experienced a relapse, confidence is good, but too much is not (G. Olson, in Boswell, 1990).

Smoking and body weight. The belief that cigarette smoking reduces body weight and that cessation produces a marked weight gain is an incentive for clients, particularly women, to both continue to smoke and to relapse (Gritz, Klesges, & Meyers, 1989; Gritz & Jeor, 1992; Klesges & Klesges, 1988; Pirie, Murray, & Leupker, 1991). The 1990 U.S. Surgeon General's report stated that smoking cessation could be followed by a mean weight gain of 5 pounds (2 to 3 kilograms); smoking seems to lower the body weight "set point," and cessation raises the set point (Perkins, 1993). More positively, however, even with weight gain, the pattern of fat deposition (e.g., waist-to-hip ratio) improves after cessation (Shimokata, Muller, & Andres, 1989). Further, levels of high-density lipoproteins increase with no change in total cholesterol of low-density lipoprotein levels after an individual quits (Gerace, Hollis, Ockene, & Svendsen, 1991).

SMOKING IN SPECIAL ORGANIZATIONAL SETTINGS

Health care professionals may join others to advocate for changes in the context of smoking. Within institutions, for example, they may act as agents of change to create smoke-free health facilities through the use of the techniques discussed in Chapter 4. Particular settings, such as hospitals, substance abuse treatment or cancer treatment facilities, or worksites or schools, may offer unique opportunities for intervention.

Hospitals and Other Health Care Settings

The numbers of clients who abstain from smoking in the hospital is growing rapidly in response to hospital bans, including the recent Joint Commission on the Accreditation of Healthcare Organization's (JCAHO) requirement that hospitals implement a policy to prohibit smoking unless countered by written medical orders (JCAHO, 1997; Longo et al., 1996; Brehm, 1966). The hospital provides an important opportunity for targeted discussions of cessation. When clients are suffering from acute illnesses, they are more likely to listen to and heed a health care professional's advice. Therefore, health care professionals should mention that smoking can worsen their conditions and impair healing. In fact, a review of several studies of brief, multicomponent bedside treatment programs for a general hospital population revealed that these programs can produce 20% to 25% long-term quit rates comparable to those of formal clinic programs, even among smokers who may not be highly motivated to quit (Orleans et al., 1993).

Studies of hospitalized clients with cardiovascular disease (including acute myocardial infarction and coronary artery disease) reveal that brief inpatient advice to stop smoking followed by telephone counseling yields high, sustained quit rates after discharge (Sachs, 1986; Emmons & Goldstein, 1992). Clients in the critical care setting are vulnerable, motivated to quit (Emmons & Goldstein, 1992), and therefore receptive to advice and support from a trusted health care professional. Those with less serious diseases or at the precontemplation stage may benefit from "motivational interviewing" techniques (directive, client-centered counseling approaches for initiating behavior change by helping clients to resolve ambivalence) like those used with unmotivated problem drinkers (Miller & Rollnick, 1991).

Smoking accounts for about 90% of the attributable risk for the chronic obstructive pulmonary diseases (COPDs) (USDHHS, 1984). Studies of cardiopulmonary inpatient and outpatient populations support the influence of the severity of the illness and symptoms on motivation for quitting (Foxman, Sloss, Lohr, & Brook, 1986) and the importance of physician advice to cessation (Pederson, 1982; Pederson & Baskerville, 1983; Tashkin et al., 1984).

Prenatal clinics. Clinical sites developed to serve pregnant women offer distinctive occasions for intervening in tobacco control. Because ex-smokers often revert to smoking after a child is born (USDHHS, 1980), it is critical to incorporate special relapse prevention counseling to deter a setback after delivery, such as providing information concerning the risks of smoking during the period the mother breastfeeds and during early infancy and childhood; suggestions for coping with the multiple stresses of early mothering; and assistance for efforts to maximize unique social supports, such as spousal support, for cessation (Orleans, 1985; Coppotelli & Orleans, 1985). Cessation manuals (e.g., those published by the National Cancer Society [see the Helpful Resources section at the end of this chapter] and Windsor [1986]) have supported quitting among pregnant women. The most successful treatments are multicomponent and often include some form of smoke holding or nicotine fading and training in nonsmoking skills and self-control techniques, with continual evaluation of their impacts on the smoker and the fetus. Materials that help the mother to understand the importance of social support during the stress of adopting her new role are particularly influential. Prenatal programs can promote continued abstinence among those who stopped smoking during pregnancy (Windsor & Morris, 1985).

Substance Abuse Treatment Facilities

Substance abusers are generally smokers as well. Alcohol- or drug-dependent clients have smoking rates 3 times higher than the general population (Joseph, Nichol, Willenbring, Korn, & Lysaght, 1990; Kozlowski, Skinner, Kent, & Pope, 1989). In fact, some evidence suggests that addictive behaviors may serve as powerful eliciting cues for one another (Battjes, 1988). Drug and alcohol abusers are at particular risk for cardiovascular diseases, respiratory diseases, and some forms of cancer. The interaction of alcohol and tobacco increases the risks for cancers of the mouth, pharynx, and larynx. (Battjes, 1988; USDHHS, 1990b).

In general, little attention is paid to the effects of smoking in substance abuse treatment settings. Some health care professionals who work in these settings feel that smoking behavior is irrelevant; others conclude that overcoming one addiction at a time is enough. Generally, however, nicotine addiction among treatment staff plays a defining role in whether programs address cigarette smoking (Jessup, 1996).

Yet, many substance abusers want to quit smoking. Bobo, Gilchrest, Schilling, Noach, and Schinke (1987) found a high level of concern about smoking in a sample of recovering alcoholics. Additionally, while many substance abusers who smoke quit on their own, many are hindered by their fear of quitting, lack of confidence in their ability to succeed, and procrastination (Tunstall, Ginsberg, & Hall, 1985). Further, smoking cessation counseling may be more effective 1 year after the alcoholic has become sober (Bobo, 1992).

Cancer Treatment Facilities

Smoking remains the leading cause of cancer in the United States, with smoking-related cancers of the lung, upper digestive tract, pancreas, bladder, kidney, uterine, cervix, and stomach accounting for 30% of all cancer mortality (USDHHS, 1989b, 1990b). Stopping smoking can reduce the risks of recurrence once a cancer has been diagnosed, particularly with early stage malignancies; it can also reduce complications associated with anesthesia, surgery, radiation, and chemotherapy (Orleans et al., 1993; Moore, 1971; Stevens, Gardner, Parkin, & Johnson, 1983; USDHHS, 1990b).

Worksites

Smoking cessation programs in worksites and communities are based on the assumption of the importance of the total social environment. Influencing social norms and other social processes at the organizational, community, or even societal level may be a more effective approach than those directed at individuals and will certainly reach more smokers (Lichtenstein & Glasgow, 1992; Biglan & Glasgow, 1991).

One unique advantage of the worksite setting is the ongoing interaction among coworkers and the potential for various environmental and incentive approaches to behavior change. The worksite, like the medical setting, has the potential to provide motivation, support, and assistance to smokers (Lichtenstein & Glasgow, 1992). The evidence is paradoxical, however. Five studies from three research groups found correlational evidence of relationships between aspects of partner, or co-worker buddy, behavior and smoking cessation but failed to find enhanced quit rates from conditions wherein coworkers or significant others were explicitly trained to be more facilitative (Lichtenstein, Glasgow, & Abrams, 1986).

For optimal effectiveness and to increase participation among employees, worksite cessation programs must be designed to fit the organization (Terborg, 1988); offer a variety of intervention options (Glasgow et al., 1991); and use organizational support, such as time off work for participation. Interventions tend to use employee steering committees to guide the program (Glasgow et al., 1991). A meta-analysis of worksite interventions revealed a modest but significant overall effect, with cessation rates at 6-month to 1-year follow-up averaging 13% (Fisher, Glasgow, & Terborg, 1990).

Important findings concerning the effects of worksite interventions on all employees who smoke, not simply on participants, are emerging. For example, a worksite-based discussion group that took place at the same time a televised cessation program on the evening news increased cessation rates (Jason et al., 1987). Worksites may also offer a context to examine the relationship between smoking policies and cessation programs. The data on the whether restrictive smoking policies increase cessation among employees at this time are inconclusive (Borland, Chapman, Owen, & Hill, 1990).

Schools

School-based programs offer an opportunity to prevent the initiation of smoking and therefore assist individuals in avoiding the difficulties of trying to stop after they become addicted to nicotine (CDC, 1994b). More effective programs target young persons before they initiate tobacco use or drop out of school, generally those in elementary school or grades 7 to 9. Since considerable numbers of students begin tobacco use at or after age 15, these programs should continue through high school.

In general, a multilevel approach—from a smoke-free school policy to prevention education to individual smoking cessation programs—tends to be most effective in reducing smoking among students (Pentz et al., 1989). Because of the multiple levels of influence found in successful programs, the involvement of teachers and parents is critical. The implementation of these approaches and their overall effectiveness are enhanced when teachers are involved in cessation curriculum development and review and are trained to deliver programs as planned (Connell, Turner, & Mason, 1985; Gold et al., 1991). This training may be supplemented with peer leaders to model social skills and to lead role rehearsals (Perry, Telch, Killen, Burke, & Maccoby, 1983; Clarke, MacPherson, Holmes, & Jones, 1986). Parents further enhance the influence of school efforts by getting involved in program development, reinforcing smoking cessation messages at home, and assessing program effectiveness (Perry, Pirie, Holder, Halper, & Dudovitz, 1990).

Successful prevention programs generally educate students about the short- and long-term negative consequences of tobacco use, the social influences on smoking, peer norms regarding smoking, and communication and refusal skills (CDC, 1994b). They tend to emphasize age-appropriate topics, with the goal of changing students' attitudes, knowledge, and skills as they develop in elementary, middle, and high schools. In elementary schools, basic knowledge about the characteristics of nicotine, the many influences on smoking, and the difficulty of stopping are emphasized. Legislative prohibitions are also emphasized to elementary school age children.

Given adolescents' orientation to the present, the short-term, rather than the long-term, effects (e.g., the immediate physiologic effects of smoking [increased heart rate, blood pressure, blood carbon monoxide levels, and vasoconstriction in hands and feet]) have been emphasized. Programs have focused on the impact of cardiac strain on athletic performance and the impact of smoking on taste, sense of smell, and one's physical appearance (e.g., smoke in the hair, stained teeth, and yellow fingers). The cost of smoking also has been emphasized. Programs have challenged teenagers to stop smoking for a specific time period to stress individual control over smoking and have taught skills necessary to negotiate with peers. Programs have used direct instruction, modeling, rehearsal, and reinforcement, as well as coaching, to assist in skill development. To counter the pressure of advertising, health education programs have encouraged young clients to analyze the advertisements.

Because of the cultural diversity found in many schools, programs to prevent smoking are most effective when they span racial/ethnic groups and genders. Since the daily smoking habits of 12th-grade girls have exceeded those of adolescent boys, school-based programs targeting this group are particularly important. Additionally, as boys and young men are increasingly attracted to smokeless tobacco, believing it to be safer than cigarettes, programs targeting the prevention and cessation of its use are necessary.

Successful programs include providing students access to cessation clinics for more intensive interventions. Effective programs for adolescents focus on immediate consequences of tobacco use, have specific attainable goals, and use contracts that include rewards.

Although most young persons who use tobacco products do not use drugs, when further involvement does occur, it is typically sequential from the use of tobacco products or alcohol to marijuana and from marijuana to other illicit drugs or prescription psychoactive drugs. School-based programs, therefore, by emphasizing cessation, may have an effect on the prevention of other drug and alcohol use.

Communities-at-Large

In general, clinical interventions—behavioral technologies implemented in formal smoking cessation treatment—have been replaced by public health approaches (i.e., promoting cessation through multicomponent interventions to a broader segment of the smoking population in health care settings, workplaces, and entire communities) (Lichtenstein & Glasgow, 1992; Shiffman, 1993). Using television, newspapers, and other media to convey stop-smoking messages may induce significant numbers of smokers to make serious quitting attempts (Jason et al., 1987; Ossip-Klein et al., 1991). Another approach is combining stop-smoking contests and competitions, which provide incentives to increase motivation and social support, with self-help programs; giving away a large grand prize, as well as humorous prizes, may increase motivation among participants (Lichtenstein & Glasgow, 1992). Efforts to encourage cessation among African-Americans have included community-based programs, which are often administered through churches and neighborhood centers (Levine, Becker, & Bone et al., 1992; Fisher, Auslander, Sussman, Owens, & Jackson-Thompson, 1992).

A recent large-scale tobacco control trial, COMMIT (Community Intervention Trial for Smoking Cessation), matched 11 community pairs in North America, assigning one at random to a comprehensive community-wide strategy designed to control tobacco, particularly among heavy smokers, and the other to a comparison site (COMMIT Research Group, 1995a, 1995b). The community interventions included public education, work with health care professionals, worksite presentations, and the provision of other cessation resources (COMMIT Research Group, 1995a, 1995b). COMMIT had a significant effect on quitting among light-to-moderate smokers; more addicted heavy smokers were not, however, affected and require more targeted clinical programs (COMMIT Research Group, 1995a, 1995b). COMMIT has formed the basis for ASSIST (American Stop-Smoking Intervention Study), another NCI-funded program, which is designed to assist in reducing cancer mortality rates 50% by the year 2000.

SMOKING CESSATION & THE HEALTH PROMOTION MATRIX

The smoking cessation script on pp. 145-147 provides a set of questions to ask a client who smokes. The script was developed by Sheinfeld Gorin (1989) and was adapted from work by Judith Ockene and others (1988). It incorporates the findings of the four-step physician (NCI) model and similar approaches for nurses (USDHHS, 1990a) and respiratory care therapists (USDHHS, 1989a). The smoking cessation script uses the dimensions of the Health Promotion Matrix, which are found in the margin, to address the special circumstances of each individual's smoking behavior.

Image Creation

The health care professional should examine the client's image of health, as well as if the client can visualize himself/herself as a nonsmoker. The health care professional also should explore how the client might feel as a nonsmoker to determine the client's readiness to quit. By asking a series of questions focused directly on smoking, the health care professional conveys her/his belief that smoking is a significant problem and that she/he would like to help the client to stop.

The health care professional's style and questions should be direct, simple, and supportive; value judgments should not be conveyed. The first priority is to understand the client's feelings about smoking, reasons for stopping, and history of cessation attempts. The health care professional should note whether feelings are positive or negative and how deeply they are expressed. These emotions may be used later, in planning ways to help clients feel good about stopping.

In asking clients' thoughts about quitting and by addressing both "the heart and the head," the health care professional helps them to discover reasons to stop and motivation (or feelings necessary) to begin the behavioral change.

Image Appraisal

The health care professional should explore past attempt(s) of and present motives for quitting. The client's responses will provide opportunities to examine past attempts to quit, to encourage present or future attempts, and to individualize the "quit smoking" message. If the client has not tried to quit smoking, the health care professional, using the HPM, should explore other attempts to change long-standing behaviors (e.g., overeating or drinking alcohol). The client's responses should be used to encourage changes in the smoking habit. The client should be encouraged to express both feelings and thoughts about quitting smoking or for modifying other unhealthy habits.

The health care professional should establish that the client is willing to develop a plan to stop smoking or decrease the number of cigarettes smoked. Many individuals are defensive about their smoking habits. If the client immediately resists any discussion, the health care professional should simply say that she/he will be available to help if the client wants to talk about stopping in the future. The health care professional should also increase the client's likelihood of quitting by developing a plan to stop. The health care professional should try not to alienate the client during the initial meeting while also not minimizing the risks of smoking or the goal of assisting the quitting process.

The health care professional should analyze the data that has been collected, and identify the resources for quitting. Most clients can be expected to say that they would quit smoking if they had an easy way to do it. When the client indicates a readiness to quit, the health care professional needs to collect more data about the client's smoking habits to formulate a realistic plan of action.

Responses to the image appraisal questions in the Smoking Cessation Script will allow the health care professional to assess three dimensions important for the individualization of treatment: (1) whether the person learned anything during prior attempts that will be helpful during the present quit effort; (2) the relapse-to-smoking event that occurred during the initial effort and how that risk can be minimized during the present effort; and (3) the role of significant others in the quit effort—whether they will aid or undermine it and whether the health care professional needs to speak with them about the program.

At the end of this step, the health care professional analyzes the data she/he has collected and identifies the individual's specific problems related to smoking cessation. This step may incorporate a diagnosis, if appropriate to the health care professional's practice or to satisfy reimbursement purposes.

Optimally, this dimension will end with an agreed upon quit date. The quit date might be the start of a particular time period, such as the beginning of a month or a special event. The health care professional must be sure to write that date on the client's index card or chart, if appropriate (see Figure 6-2 for a sample card), to make other health care professionals and staff aware of the timing of the plan and to enlist their support.

Minimize Health Depleting Patterns

With an agreed upon quit date, the health care professional may individualize a treatment plan. The health care professional should begin with the simplest, least intrusive intervention, and provide brochures and methods to overcome barriers to change. The information the health care professional collected from previous stages should give her/him a good idea of the client's strengths and weaknesses related to smoking and how each weakness should be addressed during the quit attempt.

Most clients do not realize that stopping smoking can benefit their immediate recovery. The health care professional may want to convey the message that even while the client is in the hospital, for example, cessation is worthwhile.

One message the health care professional needs to convey is that the more a person thinks about smoking, the harder quitting becomes; thus anything that distracts the smoker from cigarettes will assist the quit attempt. Two ways to handle the urge to smoke a cigarette are to do something else and to think about something else, such as taking a walk or sucking on low-calorie mints (see Table 6-2 for other

Smoker's name: _____ Date: _____
How willing is person to quit?
    Very willing _____ Somewhat willing _____ Not willing _____
Information given: _____
Quit date: _____
Follow-up: Personal visit _____ Date: _____
            Telephone call _____ Date: _____
            Postcard _____ Date: _____
Follow-up results:
    New quit date: _____ Referral: _____ More counseling _____
    Other: _____

Additional comments on reverse side of card.

Figure **6-2 Smoking status card.** (*From Stopping Smoking: A Nurse's Guide, p. 77, by S. Sheinfeld Gorin, 1989, New York: The American Health Foundation.*)

Table **6-2**

Help stop the urge to smoke	
PROBLEM	**SOLUTION**
1. Instead of puffing smoke . . .	Do breathing exercises.
2. Instead of lighting up . . .	Keep your hands busy: draw, knit, use worry beads.
3. Instead of eating . . .	Find other things to put in you mouth: chew gum, drink water.
4. Instead of being grumpy . . .	Relax and control your emotions: exercise, meditate, take a walk.
5. Instead of being bored . . .	Keep your mind busy: read, play cards, telephone a friend.
6. Instead of excuses to smoke . . .	Make excuses not to smoke.
Smoking helps me concentrate.	Smoking makes me stink.
I'm concerned about gaining weight.	Smoking costs too much.
It's too hard to quit. I don't have the willpower.	I want a cigarette because I am an addict.
I'm in agony without cigarettes.	I want to be a healthy model for my children.
Smoking helps me relax.	I want to control my life.

From *Stopping Smoking: A Nurse's Guide*, p. 75, by S. Sheinfeld Gorin, 1989, New York: The American Health Foundation.

methods). These strategies also help with weight control, an important consideration of women who smoke.

The health care professional should give the client a manual to assist with his/her quitting, such as those available through the American Lung Association, the American Cancer Society, the National Cancer Institute, and the National Heart, Lung and Blood Institute (see the Helpful Resources section at the end of this chapter). The health care professional also should review the pamphlet with the client and determine whether any changes are needed. The brochure should provide customized information according to the smoker's medical condition. For example, clients receiving a fluid-restricted diet cannot drink large quantities of water, which is suggested by some cessation programs. The client should be allowed to help modify the individual plan.

Withdrawal symptoms. The health care professional should assist with the common problems most smokers have when quitting. The health care professional also must monitor physical difficulties the client experiences during the quitting process. Most persons, though not all, experience disruptive nicotine-withdrawal symptoms when they quit smoking. The health care professional should determine how the client is handling withdrawal and decide whether additional teaching or instruction is needed to keep the client from relapsing. The person who quits using tobacco withdraws from a chemical dependence on nicotine, as well as a psychologic habit, and should be expected to have some symptoms that are both physiologic and psychologic. Anxiety, altered sleep patterns, impaired concentration, weight gain, and change in bowel habits are some of the most common complaints. Like other stress reactions, these symptoms can be reduced or eliminated. Exercise, such as brisk walking, can calm frazzled nerves while combating weight gain related to metabolic changes or overeating.

Optimize Health Supportive Patterns

In general, the health care professional can advise clients to drink plenty of water to flush the nicotine out of their bodies, to eat healthy foods, and to increase their amount of exercise. Each person's withdrawal symptoms—which might better termed recovery symptoms—will be different.

Clients are likely to have trouble either with stopping initially or maintaining abstinence. When clients describe their problems, the health care professional should combine statements of support and encouragement with suggestions for dealing with the problems.

The health care professional, as well as that of the rest of the staff, should remember that praise and encouragement reinforces the cessation message and helps to optimize health supportive patterns. This support may be the deciding factor in the client's continued willingness and efforts to stop smoking. The health care professional should identify the client's smoking status on an index card for ease of follow-up and update the Smoking Status card regularly to indicate the client's progress, with specific ways to support continued abstinence. For example, the health care professional might suggest that the water pitcher be filled frequently or that the family be asked to provide encouragement. Giving up smoking is probably one of the most difficult things the client will ever do; it requires help and encouragement from the client's significant others.

Internalize Idealized Image

The health care professional should determine the client's success at quitting and evaluate the prognosis regarding future smoking status with the client. She/he also should continue to assess the client's smoking status at the end of treatment and on every future contact, and check on the client's progress and modify the plan accordingly. If the client has not stopped smoking, the health care professional should probe for obstacles and problem-solving solutions. The health care professional should also send a follow-up postcard or telephone the client (see Figure 6-3 for sample postcards). The health care professional should tell clients that she/he will continue to check on their smoking status, and emphasize that she/he will continue to provide support for the clients' efforts to quit.

If clients cannot adhere to the plan, the health care professional should identify the specific problems and encourage them to set other quit dates. Even a handwritten note can remind clients of the health care professional's support for their cessation efforts.

If the client is succeeding, the health care professional should discuss possible temptations to return to smoking, explaining that most persons experience temptations even long after their quit date. Sometimes, even months later, the urge to light

A

POSTCARD A

Dear _____

You may remember that we spoke about your smoking _____ week(s) ago.
I hope that you are continuing not to smoke. Could you please take
3 minutes to answer the following questions? Thank you.

1. Is the plan that we negotiated helpful?
       Yes ( )   No ( )
2. What problems have you noted? _____
3. What was helpful to you? _____
4. Is there anything else I can do to help you at this time? _____
    _____

5. Do you think you will remain off cigarettes for the next six months?
       Yes ( )   No ( )

Congratulations on your healthy decision!
I am happy to help you remain smoke-free.   Call me at _____

Sincerely _____

B

POSTCARD B

Dear _____

You may remember that we spoke about your smoking _____ week(s) ago.
I'd like to follow up our discussion. Could you please answer the
following questions? Thank you.

1. Are you tapering your smoking?   Yes ( )   No ( )
2. How many cigarettes a day are you now smoking? _____
3. Is the plan we negotiated helpful?
       Yes ( )   No ( )
4. What problems have you noted? _____
5. What was helpful to you? _____
6. Is there anything else I can do to help you at this time? _____
    _____

7. Do you plan to stop smoking within the next six months?
       Yes ( )   No ( )
       7a. If yes, how will you do it? _____

I am happy to help you to become smoke-free.   Call me at _____

Sincerely _____

Figure 6-3 Sample follow-up postcards. The health care professional
should review last discussion with the client and see whether the client
wanted to stop smoking. If yes, send postcard **A**. If no, send postcard **B**
about 1 to 2 weeks after the latest client discussion. (*From* Stopping
Smoking: A Nurse's Guide, p. 78, by S. Sheinfeld Gorin, 1989, New York: The
American Health Foundation.)

up a cigarette will seem as strong as ever. The trick is not to be discouraged and to again use the same distractions—such as deep breathing or chewing gum—that helped the client deal with smoking urges in the first part of the program.

The health care professional should let clients know that she/he will make arrangements for continued monitoring of their progress. The client's knowledge that someone will be making constant inquiries is critical to long-term success.

If counseling inpatients, the health care professional should forewarn them that both leaving the hospital and returning to places associated with past smoking can be powerful inducements to resume smoking. The health care professional should help these clients to identify environmental signals (cues) to smoke (e.g., a relaxing chair in front of the television, parties, restaurants), and then prepare for discharge by helping them to plan specific steps for making a smoke-free home.

SMOKING CESSATION: *A Script*

The following script contains a series of questions that the health care professional would ask the client. When the client says, "yes" or "no," questions listed under that response are asked. By following the script and listening carefully, health care professionals can work with clients to successfully stop smoking.

"I notice that you are a cigarette smoker, Mr./Ms. _____. As you probably already know, there is no question that smoking is harmful to your health. Did you also know that it is never too late to reverse the harmful effects of smoking?"

Image Creation   How do you feel about being a cigarette smoker?

Have you ever visualized yourself as a nonsmoker?

What reasons would you have for stopping?

Image Appraisal   Have you ever stopped smoking?

YES	**NO**
When was the last time?	Have you ever made any changes in yourself or your behavior?
How did you stop?	
Did you have any problems with stopping?	When did you make those changes?
How long did the problems last?	Did you have any problems making those changes?
What helped you to stop?	
How did you feel when you stopped?	

continued

SMOKING CESSATION: *A Script—cont'd*

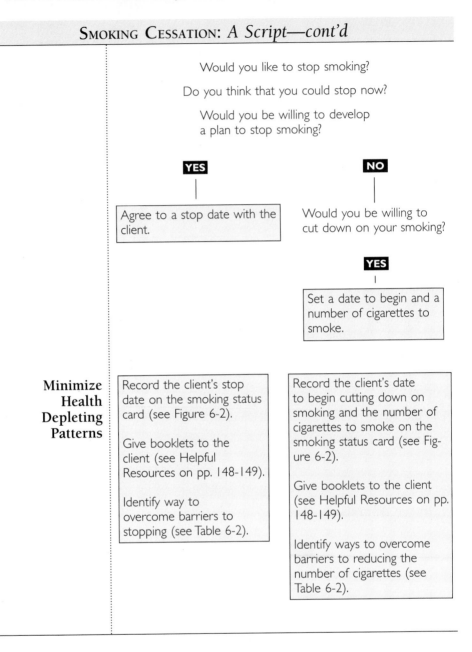

Would you like to stop smoking?

Do you think that you could stop now?

Would you be willing to develop
a plan to stop smoking?

YES

Agree to a stop date with the
client.

NO

Would you be willing to
cut down on your smoking?

YES

Set a date to begin and a
number of cigarettes to
smoke.

**Minimize
Health
Depleting
Patterns**

Record the client's stop
date on the smoking status
card (see Figure 6-2).

Give booklets to the
client (see Helpful
Resources on pp. 148-149).

Identify way to
overcome barriers to
stopping (see Table 6-2).

Record the client's date
to begin cutting down on
smoking and the number of
cigarettes to smoke on the
smoking status card (see Figure 6-2).

Give booklets to the client
(see Helpful Resources on pp.
148-149).

Identify ways to overcome
barriers to reducing the
number of cigarettes (see
Table 6-2).

SMOKING CESSATION: *A Script—cont'd*

Optimize Health Supportive Patterns

> Review the factors that may support the plan (see Table 6-1).
>
> Tell the client when you will see him/her again or follow-up with a telephone call or postcard to check his/her progress (within 1 or 2 weeks) (see Figure 6-3).

Internalize Idealized Image

Review the last discussion.

"Did you stop smoking?"

YES

Congratulations! Keep up the good work!

What problems have you noted?

What was helpful to you?

Is there anything else I can do to help you at this time?

Do you think you will remain a nonsmoker for the next 6 months?

NO

Are you tapering?

How many cigarettes a day are you smoking?

Is the plan we negotiated helpful?

What problems have you noted?

Is there anything else I can do to help you at this time?

Do you plan to stop smoking within the next 6 months?

YES

How will you do it?

Summary

The central interventions, from those designed to be used for brief exchanges to those oriented toward more intensive clinical work, rely on several features of the dynamics of smoking. The decision to smoke is multidetermined, from the economics of cigarette marketing to the physiology of nicotine addiction. Addiction and conditioning enrich each other; smoking thus becomes connected with numerous cues of daily life. This sets the stage for equally numerous cues to relapse.

Clinically, the health care professional may offer brief counseling, in some cases, a prescription and a referral. Counseling, ongoing support, and encouragement of quitting with the client and others in his/her support network will enhance the client's likelihood of stopping.

As advocates for smoke-free environments, health care professionals can have an impact not only on an individual's successful cessation, but on the creation of a healthier society. Health care professionals have the power to help clients live longer and healthier lives through smoking cessation.

HELPFUL **RESOURCES**

ON-LINE RESOURCES

The Master Anti-Smoking Page
http://www.autonomy.com/smoke.htm
This page is designed to help individuals quit smoking, with a particular emphasis toward youths. It provides many links to other tobacco control resources.

Action on Smoking and Health
http://ash.org
This is an antismoking Web site that offers resources for activists.

Doctors Ought to Care
http://www.bcm
Founded in 1977, this organization has a history in developing counteradvertising and other strategies for tobacco control. The site offers "Positive Health Strategies for the Clinic, Classroom and Community" for health care professionals and others acting for tobacco control.

CDC's Tobacco Information and Prevention Sourcepage
http://www.cdc.gov

This CDC site offers the opportunity to download guidelines for tobacco control published by the CDC and other government agencies. It also offers a multitude of "fact sheets" on tobacco control.

The National Cancer Institute
http://www.nci.nih.gov
The NCI homepage provides directories of a variety of resources for smoking cessation, as well as other cancer prevention and control approaches. The NCI has programs called "Quit for Good" to help smokers stop. (See the Additional Resources section for more information on the NCI.)

The U.S. Food and Drug Administration
http://www.fda.gov
This is a particularly useful site for recent legislation regarding children and tobacco.

The U.S. Environmental Protection Agency
http://www.epa.gov
This homepage offers directories on tobacco control legislation and initiatives.

H E L P F U L **RESOURCES—cont'd**

The American Heart Association
http://www.amhrt.org
The AHA homepage contributes a directory of materials and programs for smoking cessation. The association has developed a packet and runs programs for cessation entitled, "Calling it Quits."

American Cancer Society
http://www.cancer.org
The ACS, a voluntary organization, offers programs and other resources to help individuals quit smoking, including the "Freedom from Smoking" and "Fresh Start" programs. (See the Additional Resources section for more information about the ACS.)

The American Lung Association
http://www.lungusa.org/globa/news/report/smking
This site contains several "fact sheets," particularly about women and smoking. (See the Additional Resources section for more information about the American Lung Association.)

ADDITIONAL RESOURCES

National Cancer Institute
Office of Cancer Communications
Building 31
Room 10A16
9000 Rockville Pike
Rockville, MD 20892
Phone: (800) 4-CANCER.
The NCI offers client educational brochures and videotapes, such as *Clearing the air: How to quit smoking . . . and quit for keeps* (booklet 94-1647); *Smoking: Facts and tips for quitting* (booklet 93-3405); *Why do you smoke?* (booklet 93-1822) (quiz for selecting cessation techniques); *Smoking: Facts and quitting tips for Hispanics* (booklet 92-3405) (Spanish brochure); *Smoking: Facts and quitting tips for Black Americans*

(booklet 92-3405S) (brochure); *Beat the smokeless habit* (booklet 92-3270); and *How to help your patients stop smoking: A National Cancer Institute manual for physicians.*

National Institute on Aging
NIA Information Center
PO Box 8057
Gaithersburg, MD 20898-8057
Phone: (800) 222-2225
The NIA publishes a brochure entitled, *Smoking—It's never too late to stop.*

American Heart Association
Division of Communications
7320 Greenville Ave.
Dallas, TX 75231
Phone: (214) 373-6300.

American Cancer Society
1599 Clifton Road NE
Atlanta, GA 30329
Phone: (800) 227-2345 or (404) 320-3333.
The ACS provides client education materials such as *The most often asked questions about smoking, tobacco, and health, and . . . the answers* (brochure 2023.00); *Smokeless tobacco: A medical perspective* (brochure 2090.00); and *Tobacco-free young America: A kit for busy practitioners.*

The American Lung Association
1740 Broadway
New York, NY 10019
Phone: (212) 315-8700 or (800) 586-4872.
ALA client educational materials include *Freedom from Smoking* (a self-help smoking cessation program); *Stop smoking, stay trim: Gain your freedom, control your weight* (brochure 2102); and a *Healthy beginning counseling kit* (1989).

References

Abrams, D., Monti, P., Carey, K., Pinto, R., & Jacobus, S. (1988). Reactivity to smoking cues and relapse: Two studies of discriminant validity. *Behavioral Research and Therapy, 26* (3), 225-233.

Altman, D.G., Flora, J.A., Fortmann, S.P., & Farquhar, J.W. (1987). The cost-effectiveness of three smoking cessation programs. *American Journal of Public Health, 77,* 162-165.

Ambrosone, C.B., Freudenheim, J.L., Graham, S., Marshall, J.R., Vena, J.E., Brasure, J.R., Michalek, A.M., Laughlin, R., Nemoto, T., Gillenwater, K.A., Harrington, A.M., & Shields, P.G. (1996). Cigarette smoking, N-Acetyltransferase 2, genetic polymorphisms, and breast cancer risk. *Journal of the American Medical Association, 276*(18), 1494-1501.

Anonymous. (1996, April 24). Answer sought for "tobacco giant": China's problem. *Journal of the American Medical Association, 275,* 16, 1220-1221.

Apter, M.J. (1982). *The experience of motivation: The theory of psychological reversals.* London: Academic Press.

Asian and Pacific Islander American Health Forum. (1989, April). *Year 2000 strategic health development program for Asian and Pacific Islander Americans.* San Francisco: Author.

Axelrad, C.M., Sepkovic, D.W., Colosimo, S.G., & Haley, N.J. (1987). Biochemical validation of cigarette smoke exposure and tobacco use. In S. Sandhu, D.M. Demanni, M.J. Mass, M. Moore, & J.L. Mumford (Eds.), *Short-term bioassays in the analysis of complex environmental mixtures.* (Vol. V). New York: Plenum Publishing.

Baer, J.S., & Lichtenstein, E. (1988). Cognitive assessment. In D.M. Donovan & G.A. Marlatt (Eds.), *Assessment of addictive behaviors* (pp. 189-213). New York: Guilford Press.

Baille, A., Mattick, R.P., & Webster, P. (1990). *Review of published treatment outcome literature on smoking cessation: Preparatory readings for Quality Assurance Project Smoking Cessation Expert Committee.* (National Campaign Against Drug Abuse, National Drug and Alcohol Research Center, Working Paper No. 1). Sydney, Australia: University of New South Wales.

Bandura, A. (1986). *Social foundations of thought and action.* Englewood Cliffs, New Jersey: Prentice-Hall.

Baron, J.A., Bulbrook, R.D., & Wang, D.Y. (1986). Cigarette smoking and prolactin in women. *British Medical Journal, 293*(6545), 482-483.

Battjes, R.J. (1988). Smoking as an issue in alcohol and drug abuse treatment. *Addictive Behaviors, 13,* 225-230.

Becker, D., Hill, D., Jackson, J., Levine, D., Stillman, F., & Weiss, S. (Eds.). (1992). *Health behavior research in minority populations: Access, design, and implementation.* Washington, DC: National Heart, Lung, and Blood Institute.

Benowitz, N.L. (1992). Cigarette smoking and nicotine addiction. *Medical Clinics of North America, 76*(2), 415-437.

Bierer, M.F., & Rigotti, N.A. (1992). Public policy for the control of tobacco-related disease. *Medical Clinics of North America, 76* (2), 515-539.

Biglan, A., & Glasgow, R.E. (1991). The social unit: An important facet in the design of cancer control research. *Preventive Medicine, 20,* 292-305.

Bobo, J.K. (1992). Nicotine dependence and alcoholism epidemiology and treatment. *Journal of Psychoactive Drugs, 24,* 123-129.

Bobo, J.K., Gilchrest, L.D., Schilling, R.F. II, Noach, B., & Schinke, S.P. (1987). Cigarette smoking cessation attempts by recovering alcoholics. *Addictive Behaviors, 12,* 209-215.

Borland, R., Chapman, S., Owen, N., & Hill, D. (1990). Effects of work place smoking bans on cigarette consumption. *American Journal of Public Health, 80,* 178-181.

Boswell, T. (1990, June 10). Fastball, curve, yer out! The unhittable Gregg Olson: Orioles' ace in the pen is 'otter' this world. *Washington Post,* pp. B1, B10.

Brehm, J. (1966). *A theory of psychological reactance.* San Diego: Academic Press.

Brownson, R.C., Jackson-Thompson, J., Wilkerson, J.C., Davis, J.R., Owens, N.W., & Fisher, E.B. (1992). Demographic and socioeconomic differences in beliefs about the health effects of smoking. *American Journal of Public Health, 82,* 99-103.

Byrd, J.C. (1992). Environmental tobacco smoke: Medical and legal issues. *Medical Clinics of North America, 2,* 377-398.

Centers for Disease Control and Prevention. (1987). Cigarette smoking in the United States, 1986. *Morbidity and Mortality Weekly Report, 36*(35), 581-585.

Centers for Disease Control and Prevention. (1988). Smokeless tobacco use in rural Alaska. *Morbidity and Mortality Weekly Report, 36*(10), 140-43.

Centers for Disease Control and Prevention. (1994a). *Preventing tobacco use among young people—A report of the Surgeon General*. Atlanta: Author.

Centers for Disease Control and Prevention. (1994b). Guidelines for school health programs to prevent tobacco use and addiction. *Morbidity and Mortality Weekly Report, 43* (RR-2), 1-18.

Centers for Disease Control and Prevention. (1994c, December 23). Cigarette smoking among adults—United States, 1993. *Morbidity and Mortality Weekly, 43*(50), 925-930.

Centers for Disease Control and Prevention. (1995, November 10). Health care provider advice on tobacco use to persons aged 10-22 years—United States, 1993. *Morbidity and Mortality Weekly Report, 44*(44), 826-830.

Centers for Disease Control and Prevention. (1996, November 8). State-specific prevalence of cigarette smoking—United States, 1995. *Morbidity and Mortality Weekly Report, 45*(44), 962-966.

Centers for Disease Control and Prevention. (1997a, May 23). Cigar smoking among teenagers—United States, Massachusetts, and New York, 1996. *Morbidity and Mortality Weekly Report, 46*(20), 433-440.

Centers for Disease Control and Prevention. (1997b). *Women and smoking* [On-line]. Available: http://www.cdc.gov

Cepeda-Benito, A. (1993). Meta-analytic review of the efficacy of nicotine chewing gum in smoking treatment programs. *Journal of Consulting and Clinical Psychology, 61*(5), 822-830.

Chapman, S. (1996, April 27). Smoking in public places. *BMJ, 312,* 1051-1052.

Chassin, L., Presson, C., & Sherman, S.J. (1985). Psychosocial correlates of adolescent smokeless tobacco use. *Addictive Behaviors, 10,* 431-435.

Chollat-Traquet, C. (1992). Tobacco or health: A WHO program. *European Journal of Cancer, 28*(2-3), 311-315.

Clarke, J., MacPherson, B., Holmes, D., & Jones, R. (1986). Reducing adolescent smoking: A comparison of peer-led, teacher-led and expert interventions. *Journal of School Health, 56,* 102-106.

Clayton, S. (1991). Gender differences in psychosocial determinants of adolescent smoking. *Journal of School Health, 61,* 115-120.

Cohen, S., Lichtenstein, E., Mermelstein, R., McIntyre-Kingsolver, K., Baer, J.S., & Kamarck, T.W. (1988). Social support interventions for smoking cessation. In B.H. Gottlieb (Ed.), *Marshaling social support: Formats, processes, and effects* (pp. 211-240). Newbury Park, CA: Sage.

Cohen, S., Lichtenstein, E., Prochaska, J.O., Rossi, J.S., Gritz, E.R., Carr, C.R., Orleans, C.T., Schoenbach, V.J., Biener, L., Abrams, D., DiClemente, C., Curry, S., Marlatt, G.A., Cummings, K.M., Emont, S.L., Giovino, G., & Ossip-Klein, D. (1989). Debunking myths about self-quitting: Evidence from 10 prospective studies of persons quitting smoking by themselves. *American Psychologist, 44,* 1355-1365.

COMMIT Research Group. (1995a). Community Intervention Trial for Smoking Cessation (COMMIT). I. Cohort results from a four-year community intervention. *American Journal of Public Health, 85*(2), 183-192.

COMMIT Research Group. (1995b). Community Intervention Trial for Smoking Cessation (COMMIT). II. Changes in adult cigarette smoking prevalence. *American Journal of Public Health, 85*(2), 193-199.

Committee on Passive Smoking of the National Research Council. (Eds.). (1986). Exposure to environmental tobacco smoke and lung cancer. In *Environmental tobacco smoke: Measuring exposures and assessing health effects* (p. 223). Washington, DC: National Academy Press.

Connell, D.B., Turner, R.R., & Mason, E.F. (1985). Summary of findings of the school health education evaluation: Health promotion effectiveness, implementation, and costs. *Journal of School Health, 55,* 316-321.

Connolly, G.N., Winn, D.M., & Hecht, S. (1986). The reemergence of smokeless tobacco. *New England Journal of Medicine, 314*(16), 1020-1027.

Coppotellli, H.C., & Orleans, C.T. (1985). Partner support and other determinants of smoking cessation maintenance among women. *Journal of Consulting and Clinical Psychology, 53,* 455-460.

Covey, L., & Glassman, A. (1991). A meta-analysis of double-blind placebo-controlled trials of clonidine for smoking cessation. *British Journal of Addiction, 86,* 991-998.

Crawford, F.G., Mayer, J., Santella, R.M., Cooper, T.B., Ottman, R., Tsai, W.Y., Simon-Cereijido, G., Wang, M., Tang, D., & Perera, F.P. (1994). Biomarkers of environmental tobacco smoke in preschool children and their mothers. *Journal of the National Cancer Institute, 86*(18), 1398-1402.

Cummings, K.M., Emont, S.L., Jaen, C., & Sciandra, R. (1988). Format and quitting instructions as factors influencing the impact of a self-administered quit smoking program. *Health Education Quarterly, 15,* 199-216.

Cummings, K.M., Giovino, G., Emont, S.I., Sciandra, R., Koenigsberg, M. (1986). Factors influencing success in counseling patients to stop smoking. *Patient Education and Counseling, 8,* 189-200.

Cummings, S.R., Stein, M.J., Hansen, B., Richard, R.J., Gebert, B., & Coates, T.J. (1989). Smoking counseling and preventive medicine: A survey of internists in private practices and a health maintenance organization. *Archives of Internal Medicine, 149,* 345-349.

Curry, S. (1993). Self help interventions for smoking cessation. *Journal of Consulting and Clinical Psychology, 61,* 790-803.

Curry, S., Marlatt, A., & Gordon, J. (1987). Abstinence violation effect: Validation of an attributional construct with smoking cessation. *Journal of Consulting and Clinical Psychology, 55*(2), 145-149.

Danaher, B.G., Jeffery, R.W., Zimmerman, R., & Nelson, E. (1980). Aversive smoking using printed instructions and audiotape adjuncts. *Addictive Behaviors, 5*(4), 353-358.

Denissenko, M.F., Pao, A., Tang, M.S., & Pfeifer, G. (1996). Preferential formation of benzo[a]pyrene adducts at lung cancer mutational hotspots in P53. *Science, 274,* 430-432.

Devins, G.M. (1992). Social cognitive analysis of recovery from a lapse after smoking cessation: Comment on Haaga and Stewart (1992). *Journal of Consulting and Clinical Psychology, 60*(1), 29-31.

DiClemente, C.C. (1991). Motivational interviewing and the stages of change. In W. Miller & S. Rollnick (Eds.), *Motivational interviewing* (pp. 191-203). New York: Guilford Press.

Duryea, E.J., & Martin, G.L. (1981, February). The distortion effect in student perceptions of smoking prevalence. *Journal of School Health,* 115-118.

Eisinger, R.A. (1971). Psychosocial predictors of smoking recidivism. *Journal of Health and Social Behavior, 12,* 355-362.

Emmons, K.A., & Goldstein, M.G. (1992). Smokers who are hospitalized: A window of opportunity for cessation interventions. *Preventive Medicine, 21,* 262-269.

Ericson, E. (1950). *Childhood and society.* New York: Norton.

Expert Committee on Passive Smoking, National Academy of Sciences' National Research Council (NAS/NRC). (1986). *Environmental tobacco smoke: Measuring exposures and assessing health effects.* Washington, DC: National Academy Press.

Fagerstrom, K.O. (1988). Efficacy of nicotine chewing gum: A review. In O.F. Pomerleau, C.S. Pomerleau, K.O. Fagerstrom, J.E. Henningfield, & J.R. Hughes (Eds.), *Nicotine replacement: A critical evaluation* (pp. 109-128). New York: Alan R. Liss.

Fant, R.V., Everson, D., Dayton, G., Pickworth, W.B., & Henningfield, J.E. (1996). Nicotine dependence in women. *Journal of American Women in Medicine, 51*(1-2), 19-28.

Feyerabend, C., Higginbottam, T., & Russell, M.A.H. (1982). Nicotine concentrations in urine and saliva of smokers and nonsmokers. *British Journal of Medicine, 284,* 1002-1004.

Fiore, M.C., Novotny, T.E., Pierce, J.P., Giovino, G.A., Hatziandreu, E.J., Newcomb, P.A., Surawicz, T.S., & Davis, R.M. (1990). Methods used to quit smoking in the United States. *Journal of the American Medical Association, 263,* 2760-2765.

Fiscella, K., & Franks, P. (1996). Cost-effectiveness of the Transdermal Nicotine Patch as an adjunct to physicians' smoking cessation counseling. *Journal of the American Medical Association, 275* (16), 1247-1251.

Fisher, E., Auslander, W., Sussman, L., Owens, N., & Jackson-Thompson, J. (1992, Summer). Community organization and health promotion in minority neighborhoods. *Ethnicity and Disease, 2*(3), 252-272.

Fisher, E.B., Jr., Bishop, D.B., Goldmunz, J., & Jacobs, A. (1988). Implications for the practicing physician of the psychosocial dimensions of smoking. *Chest, 93*(2), 69S-78S.

Fisher, E., Haire-Joshu, D., Morgan, G., Rehberg, H., & Rost, K. (1990). State-of-the-art review: Smoking and smoking cessation. *American Review of Respiratory Diseases, 142,* 702-720.

Fisher, E.B., Lichtenstein, E., & Haire-Joshu, D. (1993). Multiple determinants of tobacco use and cessation. In C. Orleans & D. Slade (Eds.), *Nicotine addiction: Principles and management.* New York: Oxford University Press.

Fisher, E.B., Lichtenstein, E., Haire-Joshu, D., Morgan, G., & Rehberg, H.R. (1993). Methods, successes, and failures of smoking cessation programs. *Annual Review of Medicine, 44,* 481-513.

Fisher, E.B., & Rost, K. (1986). Smoking cessation: A practical guide for the physicians. *Clinical Chest Medicine, 7*(4), 551-565.

Fisher, K.J., Glasgow, R.E., & Terborg, J.R. (1990). Worksite smoking cessation: A meta-analysis of controlled studies. *Journal of Occupational Medicine, 32,* 429-439.

Flaxman, J. (1978). Quitting smoking now or later: Gradual, abrupt, immediate and delayed quitting. *Behavioral Therapy, 9,* 260-270.

Flay, B.R. (1993). Youth tobacco use: Risks, patterns and control. In C.T. Orleans & J. Slade (Eds.), *Nicotine addiction: Principles and management.* New York: Oxford University Press.

Fontham, E.T., Correa, P., Reynolds, P., Wu-Williams, A., Buffler, P.A., Greenberg, R.S., Chen, V.W., Alterman, T., Boyd, P., Austin, D.F. et al. (1994). Environmental tobacco smoke and lung cancer in nonsmoking women. A multicenter study. *Journal of the American Medical Association, 271*(22), 1752-1759.

Food and Drug Administration. (1996). Regulations restricting the sale and distribution of cigarettes and smokeless tobacco products to protect children and adolescents: Final rule. *Federal Register, 61,* 314-375.

Foxman, B., Sloss, E.M., Lohr, K.N., & Brook, R.H. (1986). Chronic bronchitis: Prevalence, smoking habits, impact, and antismoking advice. *Preventive Medicine, 15*(6), 624-631.

French, S.A., & Perry, C.L. (1996). Smoking among adolescent girls: Prevalence and etiology. *Journal of the American Medical Women's Association, 51*(1-2), 25-28.

Friesen, C., & Fox, H.A. (1986). Effects of smoking during pregnancy. *Kansas Medicine, 87*(1), 7-9, 21-22.

Freeman, H.P. (1989). Cancer of the breast in poor black women. *Cancer, 63,* 2562-2569.

Gerace, T., Hollis, J., Ockene, J., & Svendsen, K. (1991). Smoking cessation and change in diastolic blood pressure, body weight, and plasma lipids. *Preventive Medicine, 20,* 602-620.

Glasgow, R.E., Hollis, J.F., Pettigrew, L., Foster, L., Givi, M.J., & Morrisette, G. (1991). Implementing a year long worksite-based incentive program for smoking cessation. *American Journal of Health Promotion, 5,* 192-199.

Glascow, R.E., Lichtenstein, E., Beaver, C., & O'Neill, K. (1981). Subjective reactions to rapid and normal paced aversive smoking. *Addictive Behaviors, 6*(1), 53-59.

Glassman, A.H., Helzer, J.E., Covey, L.S., Cottler, L.B., Stetner, F., Tipp, J.E., & Hohnson, J. (1990). Smoking, smoking cessation, and major depression. *Journal of the American Medical Association, 264,* 1546-1549.

Glynn, T.J., Boyd, G.M., & Gruman, J.C. (1990). Essential elements of self-help/minimal intervention strategies for smoking cessation. *Health Education Quarterly, 17,* 329-345.

Glynn, T.J., & Manley, M. (1989). Physicians, cancer control and the treatment of nicotine dependence: Defining success. *Health Education Research, 4,* 479-487.

Glynn, T.J., & Manley, M. (1991). *How to help your patients stop smoking: A National Cancer Institute manual for physicians* (DHHS Publication No. 92-3064). Washington, DC: The National Cancer Institute.

Gold, R.S., Parcel, G.S., Walberg, H.J., Luepker, R.V., Portnoy, B., & Stone, E.J. (1991). Summary and conclusions of the THTM evaluation: The expert work group perspective. *Journal of School Health, 61,* 39-42.

Gopalaswamy, A.K., & Morgan, R. (1986). Smoking in chronic schizophrenia (letter). *British Journal of Psychiatry, 149,* 523.

Gottlieb, A.M., & Baker, J.A. (1986). The relative influence of health beliefs, parental and peer behaviors and exercise program participation on smoking, alcohol use and physical activity. *Social Science and Medicine, 22*(9), 915-927.

Graham, S., & Gibson, R.W. (1971). Cessation of patterned behavior: Withdrawal from smoking. *Social Science and Medicine, 5*(4), 319-337.

Gralnick, A.A. (1988). Nicotine addiction in the psychiatric hospitals: A preliminary report. *Psychiatric Journal of the University of Ottowa, 13*(1), 25-27.

Green, D.E. (1979). Patterns of tobacco use in the United States. In National Institute on Drug Abuse (Ed.), *Cigarette smoking as a dependence process* (Research Monograph No. 23) (DHEW [ADM] Publication No. 79-800, pp. 44-55). Washington, DC: U.S. Government Printing Office.

Gritz, E.R., & Jeor, S.T. (1992). National Working Conference on Smoking and Body Weight. Task force 3: Implications with respect to intervention and prevention. *Health Psychology, 11* (suppl.), 17-25.

Gritz, E., Klesges, R., & Meyers, A. (1989). The smoking and body weight relationship: Implications for intervention and postcessation weight control. *Annals of Behavioral Medicine, 11*(4), 144-153.

Hajek, P., Jarvis, M.J., Belcher, M., Sutherland, G., & Feyerabend, C. (1989). Effect of smoke-free cigarettes on 24h cigarette withdrawal: A double-blind placebo-controlled study. *Psychopharmacology, 97,* 99-102.

Hall, R.L., & Dexter, D. (1988). Smokeless tobacco use and attitudes towards smokeless tobacco among Native Americans and other adolescents. *American Journal of Public Health, 78*(12), 1586-1588.

Hall, S.M., Rugg, D., Tunstall, C., & Jones, R.T. (1984). Preventing relapse to cigarette smoking by behavioral skill training. *Journal of Consulting and Clinical Psychology, 52,* 372-382.

Hodgson, T.A. (1992). Cigarette smoking and lifetime medical expenditures. *The Milbank Quarterly, 70,* 81-125.

Hollis, J.F., Lichtenstein, E., Mount, K., Vogt, T.M., & Stevens, V.J. (1991). Nurse-assisted smoking counseling in medical settings: Minimizing demands on physicians. *Preventive Medicine, 20,* 497-507.

Hughes, J.R. (1993). Pharmacotherapy for smoking cessation: Unvalidated assumptions, anomalies, and suggestions for future research. *Journal of Consulting and Clinical Psychology, 61*(5), 751-760.

Hughes, J.R., Gust, S., & Pechacek, T. (1988). Prevalence of tobacco dependence and withdrawal. *American Journal of Psychiatry, 144,* 205-208.

Husten, C.G., Chrismon, J.H., & Reddy, M.N. (1996). Trends and effects of cigarette smoking among girls and women in the United States, 1965-1993. *Journal of the American Medical Women's Association, 51*(1-2), 11-18.

Jarvis, M.J., Hajek, P., Russell, M.A.H., & West, R.J. (1987). Nasal nicotine solution as an aid to cigarette withdrawal: A pilot clinical trial. *British Journal of Addiction, 82,* 983-988.

Jarvik, M., & Henninfield, J. (1988). Pharmacological treatment of tobacco dependence. *Pharmacological Biochemistry and Behavior, 30,* 279-294.

Jason, L.A., Gruder, C.L., Martino, S., Flay, B., Warnicke, R., & Thomas, N. (1987). Worksite group meetings and the effectiveness of a televised smoking cessation intervention. *American Journal of Community Psychology, 15*(1), 57-72.

Jelley, M.I., & Prochaska, A.V. (1991). A survey of physicians' smoking counseling practices. *The American Journal of the Medical Sciences, 301*(4), 250-255.

Jessup, M. (1996). Nicotine: A gateway drug? *Journal of the Medical Womens Association, 51*(1-2), 21.

Joseph, A.M., Nichol, K.L., Willenbring, M.L., Korn, J.E., & Lysaght, L.S. (1990). Beneficial effects of treatment for nicotine dependence during an inpatient substance abuse treatment program. *Journal of the American Medical Association, 263,* 1581-1583.

Joint Commission on the Accreditation of Healthcare Organizations. (1997). Comprehensive accreditation manual for hospitals: The official handbook. Chicago: Author.

Kandel, D., & Yamaguchi, K. (1985). Developmental patterns of use of legal, illegal, and medically prescribed psychotropic drugs from adolescence to young adulthood. In C. Jones & R. Battjes (Eds.), *Etiology of abuse: Implications for prevention.* (Research Monograph No. 56) (pp. 193-235). Washington, DC: U.S. Department of Health and Human Services, U.S. Public Health Service, National Institute on Drug Abuse.

Kenney, R.D., Lyles, M.F., Turner, R.C., White, S.T., Gonzalex, J.J., Irons, T.G., Sanchez, C.J., Rogers, C.S., Campbell, E.E., Villagra, V.G., Streher, V.J., O'Malley, M.S., Stritter, F.T., Fletcher, S.W. (1988). Smoking cessation counseling by resident physicians in internal medicine, family practice, and pediatrics. *Archives of Internal Medicine, 148,* 2469-2473.

Killen, J.D. (1985). Prevention of adolescent tobacco smoking: The social pressure resistance training approach. *Journal of Child Psychology and Psychiatry, 26*(1), 7-15.

Killen, J.D., Fortmann, S.P., Telch, M.J., & Newman, B. (1988). Are heavy smokers different from light smokers? *Journal of the American Medical Association, 260,* 1581-1585.

Kirn, T. (1987). Laws ban minors' tobacco purchases, but enforcement is another matter. *Journal of the American Medical Association, 257*(24), 3323-3324.

Klesges, R.C., & Klesges, L.M. (1988). Cigarette smoking as a dieting strategy in a university population. *International Journal of Eating Disorders, 7,* 413-419.

Kluger, R. (1996). *Ashes to ashes: America's hundred-year cigarette war, the public health, and the unabashed triumph of Philip Morris.* New York: Alfred A. Knopf.

Koop, C.E. (1986). The campaign against smokeless tobacco. *New England Journal of Medicine, 314*(16), 1042-1044.

Kottke, T.E., Battista, R.N., DeFriese, G.H., & Brekke, M.L. (1988). Attributes of successful smoking cessation interventions in medical practice: A meta-analysis of 39 controlled trials. *Journal of the American Medical Association, 259,* 2883-3895.

Kozlowski, L.T., Skinner, W., Kent, C., & Pope, M.A. (1989). Prospects for smoking treatment in individuals seeking treatment for alcohol and other drug problems. *Addictive Behavior, 14,* 273-278.

Leventhal, H., & Cleary, P. (1980). The smoking problem: A review of the research and theory in behavioral risk modification. *Psychological Bulletin, 88,* 370-405.

Levine, D., Becker, D., Bone, L. et al. (1992, Summer). A partnership with minority populations—A community model of effectiveness research. *Ethnicity and Disease, 2*(3), 296-305.

Lichtenstein, E. (1982). The smoking problem: A behavioral perspective. *Journal of Consulting and Clinical Psychology, 50,* 804-819.

Lichtenstein, E., & Cohen, S. (1990). Prospective analysis of two modes of unaided smoking cessation. *Health Education Research, 5,* 63-72.

Lichtenstein, E., & Glasgow, R.E. (1992). Smoking cessation: What have we learned over the past decade? *Journal of Consulting and Clinical Psychology, 60*(4), 518-527.

Lichtenstein, E., Harris, D.E., Birchler, G.R., Wahl, J.M., & Schmahl, D.P. (1973). Comparison of rapid smoking, warm smokey air, and attention placebo in the modification of smoking behavior. *Journal of Consulting and Clinical Psychology, 40,* 92-98.

Lichtenstein, E., Glasgow, R.E., & Abrams, D.B. (1986). Social support in smoking cessation: In search of effective interventions. *Behavior Therapy, 17,* 607-609.

Lichtenstein, E., & Hollis, J. (1992). Patient referral to a smoking cessation program: Who follows through? *Journal of Family Practice, 34*(6), 739-744.

Longo, D.R., Brownson, R.C., Johnson, J.C., Hewett, J.E., Kruse, R.L., Novotny, T.E., & Logan, R.A. (1996). Hospital smoking bans and employee smoking behavior: Results of a national survey. *Journal of the American Medical Association, 275*(16), 1252-1257.

Lowe, M., Green, L., Kurtz, S., Ashenberg, Z., & Fisher, E.B. (1980). Alternatives to rapid smoking: Self-initiated, cue-extinction, and covert sensitization procedures in smoking cessation. *Journal of Behavioral Medicine, 3,* 357-372.

Lynch, B.S., & Bonnie, R.J. (1994). Growing up tobacco free: Preventing nicotine addiction in children and youths. Washington, DC: National Academy Press.

Marlatt, G.A., & Gordon, J.R. (Eds.). (1985). *Relapse prevention: Maintenance strategies in the treatment of addictive behaviors.* New York: Guilford Press.

McBride, C.M., & Pirie, M.A. (1989). Postpartum smoking relapse. *Addictive Behaviors, 15,* 165-168.

McDade, E., & Keil, J. (1988). Characterization of a soup kitchen population. In American Heart Association (Ed.), *Proceedings of the American Heart Association Conference on Epidemiology.* Santa Fe, NM: American Heart Association.

McReynolds, W.T., Green, L., & Fisher, E.B. (1983). Self-control as choice management with reference to the behavioral treatment of obesity. *Health Psychology, 2,* 261-276.

Mermelstein, R., Cohen, S., Lichtenstein, E., Baer, J.S., & Kamarck, T. (1986). Social support and smoking cessation and maintenance. *Journal of Consulting and Clinical Psychology, 54,* 447-453.

Miller, W.R., & Rollnick, S. (1991). *Motivational interviewing: Preparing people to change addictive behaviors.* New York: Guilford Press.

Mittelmark, M.B., Murray, D.M., & Luepker, R.V. (1987). Predicting experimentation with cigarettes: The Childhood Antecedents of Smoking Study (CASS). *American Journal of Public Health, 77*(2), 206-208.

Mochizuki, Y. (1996, July 6). Medical students do not think they have authority to advise patients to stop smoking. *BMJ, 313,* 48-49.

Moore, C. (1971). Cigarette smoking and cancer of the mouth, pharynx and larynx. *Journal of the American Medical Association, 218,* 553-558.

Morgan, G.D., Ashenberg, Z.S., & Fisher, E.B. (1988). Abstinence from smoking and the social environment. *Journal of Consulting and Clinical Psychology, 56*(2), 298-301.

Mosbach, P., & Leventhal, H. (1988). Peer group identification and smoking: Implications for prevention. *Journal of Abnormal Psychology, 97*(2), 238-245.

Nelson, D.E., Giovino, G.A., Shopland, D.R., Mowery, P.D., Mills, S.L., & Eriksen, M.P. (1995). Trends in cigarette smoking among U.S. adolescents, 1974 through 1991. *American Journal of Public Health, 85*(1), 34-40.

Nelson, D.E., Tomar, S.L., Mowery, P., & Siegel, P.Z. (1996). Trends in smokeless tobacco use among men in four states, 1988 to 1993. *American Journal of Public Health, 86*(9), 1300-1303.

Newcomb, P.A., & Carbone, P.P. (1992). The health consequences of smoking. Cancer. *Medical Clinics of North America, 76*(2), 305-331.

Niaura, R., Rohsenow, D., Binhoff, J., Monti, P., Pedraza, M., & Abrams, D. (1988). Relevance of cue reactivity to understanding alcohol and smoking relapse. *Journal of Abnormal Psychology, 91*, 133-152.

O'Connell, K.A., Gerkovich, M.M., & Cook, M. (1995). Reversal theory's mastery and sympathy states in smoking cessation. *Image: Journal of Nursing Scholarship, 27*(4), 311-316.

O'Farrell, T.J., Connors, G.J., & Upper, D. (1983). Addictive behaviors among hospitalized psychiatric patients. *Addictive Behaviors, 8*, 329-333.

O'Malley, P.M., Johnston, L.D., & Bachman, J.G. (1995). Adolescent substance use. Epidemiology and implications for public policy. *Pediatric Clinics of North America, 42* (2), 241-260.

Ockene, J.K. (1987). Physician delivered interventions for smoking cessation: Strategies for increasing effectiveness. *Preventive Medicine, 7*, 723-737.

Ockene, J.K., Aney, J., Goldberg, R.J., Klar, J.M., & Williams, J.W. (1988). A survey of Massachusetts physicians' smoking intervention practices. *American Journal of Preventive Medicine, 4*, 14-20.

Ockene, J.K., Quirk, M.E., Goldberg, R.J., Kristellerm, J.L., Donnelly, G., Kalan, K.L., Gould, B., Greene, H.L., Harrison-Atlas, R., Pease, J., Pickens, S., & Williams, J.W. (1988). A resident's training program for the development of smoking intervention skills. *Archives of Internal Medicine, 148*, 723-737.

Onis, M., & Villar, J. (1991). La consommation de tabac chez la femme espagnole [Smoking among Spanish females]. *Rapport Trimest Statistical Sanit Mond Geneve, OMS, 44*, 80-88.

Orleans, C.T. (1985). Understanding and promoting smoking cessation: Overview and guidelines for physician intervention. *Annual Review of Medicine, 36*, 51-61.

Orleans, C.T., Kristeller, J.L., & Gritz, E. (1993). Helping hospitalized smokers quit: New directions for treatment and research. *Journal of Consulting and Clinical Psychology, 61*(5), 778-789.

Orleans, C.T., Schoenbach, V.J., Quade, D., Salmon, M.A., Pearson, D.C., & Fiedler, J. (1991). Self-help quit smoking interventions: Effects of self-help materials, social support instructions, and telephone counseling. *Journal of Consulting and Clinical Psychology, 59*, 439-448.

Ossip-Klein, D.J., Giovino, G.A., Megahed, N., Black, P.M., Emont, S.L., & Stiggins, J. (1991). Effects of a smokers' hotline: Results of a 10-county self-help trial. *Journal of Consulting and Clinical Psychology, 59*, 325-332.

Patton, G.C., Hibbert, M., Rosier, M.J., Carlin, J.B., Caust, J., & Bowes, G. (1996). Is smoking associated with depression and anxiety in teenagers? *American Journal of Public Health, 86*(2), 225-230.

Pederson, L.L. (1982). Compliance with physician advice to quit smoking: A review of the literature. *Preventive Medicine, 11*, 71-84.

Pederson, L.L., & Baskerville, J.C. (1983). Multivariate prediction of smoking cessation following physician advice to quit smoking: A validation study. *Preventive Medicine, 12*, 430-436.

Pederson, L.L., Williams, J.T., & Lefcoe, N.M. (1980). Smoking cessation among pulmonary patients as related to type of respiratory disease and demographic variables. *Canadian Journal of Public Health, 71*, 191-194.

Pentz, M., Brannon, B., Charlin, V., Barrett, E., MacKinnon, D., & Flay, B. (1989). The power of policy: The relationship of smoking policy to adolescent smoking. *American Journal of Public Health, 79*(7), 857-862.

Perkins, K.A. (1993). Weight gain following cessation. *Journal of Consulting and Clinical Psychology, 61*(5), 768-777.

Perkins, K.A., Grobe, J.E., Stiller, R.L., Fonte, C., & Goettler, J.E. (1992). Nasal spray nicotine replacement suppresses cigarette smoking desire and behavior. *Clinical Pharmacology and Therapeutics, 52*, 627-634.

Perry, C.L., Pirie, P., Holder, W., Halper, A., & Dudovitz, B. (1990). Parental involvement in cigarette smoking prevention: Two pilot evaluations of the "unpuffables program." *Journal of School Health, 60*, 443-447.

Perry, C., Telch, M., Killen, J., Burke, A., & Maccoby, N. (1983). High school smoking prevention: The relative efficacy of varied treatments and instructors. *Adolescence, 17*, 561-566.

Pierce, J.P., Gilpin, E., Burns, D.M., Whalen, E., Rosbrook, B., Shopland, D., & Johnson, M. (1991). Does tobacco advertising target young people to start smoking? Evidence from California. *Journal of the American Medical Association, 266* (22), 3154-3158.

Pirie, P.L., Murray, D.M., & Luepker, R.V. (1988). Smoking prevalence in a cohort of adolescents, including absentees, drop-outs, and transfers. *American Journal of Public Health, 78,* 176-178.

Pirie, P.L., Murray, D.M., & Luepker, R.V. (1991). Gender differences in cigarette smoking and quitting in a cohort of young adults. *American Journal of Public Health, 81,* 324-327.

Pormerleau, O.F., Collins, A.C., Shiffman, S. & Pormerleau, C.S. (1993). Why some people smoke and others do not: New perspectives. *Journal of Consulting and Clinical Psychology, 61*(5), 723-731.

Pomerleau, O.F., Fertig, J.B., & Shanahan, S.O. (1983). Nicotine dependence in cigarette smoking: An empirically-based, multivariate model. *Pharmacology, Biochemistry & Behavior, 19,* 291-299.

Pomerleau, O., & Pomerleau, C. (1987). A biobehavioral view of substance abuse and addiction. *Journal of Drug Issues, 17,* 111-131.

Prochaska, J.O., & DiClemente, C.C. (1983). Stages and processes of self-change of smoking: Toward an integrative model. *Journal of Consulting and Clinical Psychology, 51,* 390-395.

Prochaska, J.O., Velicer, W.F., Guadagnoli, E., Rossi, J.S., & DiClemente, C.C. (1991). Patterns of change: Dynamic typology applied to smoking cessation. *Multivariate Behavioral Research, 26,* 83-107.

Rachlin, H. (1991). *Introduction to modern behaviorism* (3rd ed.). San Francisco: Freeman Press.

Ramirez, A., & Gallion, K. (1993). Nicotine dependence among blacks and hispanics. In C.T. Orleans & J. Slade (Eds.), *Nicotine addiction: Principles and management* (p. 350-364). New York: Oxford University Press.

Rimer, B., Orleans, C., Keintz, M., Cristinizio, S., & Fleisher, L. (1990). The older smoker: Status, challenges and opportunities for intervention. *Chest, 97* (3), 547-553.

Robb, J.H. (1986). Smoking as an anticipatory rite of passage: Some sociological hypotheses on health-related behavior. *Social Science and Medicine, 23*(6), 621-627.

Romans, S.E., McNoe, B.M., Herbison, G.P., Walton, V.A., & Mullen, P.E. (1993). Cigarette smoking and psychiatric morbidity in women. *Australian and New Zealand Journal of Psychiatry, 27*(3), 399-404.

Rosenbaum, P., & O'Shea, R. (1992). Large-scale study of Freedom from Smoking clinics—Factors in quitting. *Public Health Reports, 107*(2), 150-155.

Rosenstock, I.M. (1991). The health belief model: Explaining health behavior through expectancies. In K. Glanz, F. Lewis, & B. Rimer (Eds.), *Health behavior and health education* (pp. 39-62). San Francisco: Jossey-Bass.

Russell, M.A.H. (1978). Self-regulation of nicotine intake by smokers. In K. Battig (Ed.), *Behavioral effects of nicotine* (pp. 108-122). Basel, Switzerland: S. Karger.

Sachs, D.P. (1986). Cigarette smoking: Health effects and cessation strategies. *Clinics in Geriatic Medicine, 2*(2), 337-362.

Schinke, S.P., Schilling, R.F., & Gilchrest, L.D. (1987). Health Effects of Smokeless Tobacco (letter). *Journal of the American Medical Association, 257*(6), 781.

Schwartz, J.L. (1987). *Smoking cessation methods* (PHS NIH Publication No. 87-2940). Washington, DC: U.S. Government Printing Office.

Schwartz, J.L. (1988). Evaluation of acupuncture as a treatment for smoking. *American Journal of Acupuncture, 16,* 135.

Schwartz, J.L. (1992). Methods of smoking cessation. *Medical Clinics of North America, 76* (2), 451-476.

Severson, H.H., & Lichtenstein, E. (1986). Smoking prevention programs for adolescents: Rationale and review. In N.A. Krannegor, J.D. Arasteh, & M.F. Cataldo (Eds.), *Child health behavior: A behavioral pediatrics perspective* (pp. 281-309). New York: John Wiley.

Sheinfeld Gorin, S. (1989). *Stopping smoking: A nurse's guide.* New York: The American Health Foundation.

Shelton, D.M., Alciati, M.H., Chang, M.M., Fishman, J.A. Fues, L.A. et al. (1995). State laws on tobacco control—United States. *CDC Surveillance Summaries, 44*(6), 1-28.

Sherman, C.B. (1992). The health consequences of cigarette smoking. Pulmonary diseases. *Medical Clincs of North America, 76* (2), 355-375.

Shiffman, S. (1986). A cluster analytic classification of smoking relapse episodes. *Addictive Behaviors, 11,* 295-307.

Shiffman, S. (1993). Smoking cessation treatment: Any progress? *Journal of Consulting and Clinical Psychology, 61*(5), 718-722.

Shimokata, H., Muller, D.C., & Andres, R. (1989). Studies in the distribution of body fat: Effects of cigarette smoking. *Journal of the American Medical Association, 261*(8), 1169-1173.

Speer, F. (1986). Tobacco and the nonsmoker: A study of subjective symptoms. *Archives of Environmental Health, 16,* 443.

Stevens, M.H., Gardner, J.W., Parkin, J.L., & Johnson, L.P. (1983). Head and neck cancer survival and lifestyle change. *Archives of Otolaryngology, 109,* 746-749.

Sutherland, G., Russell, M.A.H., Stapleton, J., Feyerabend, C., & Ferno, O. (1992). Nasal nicotine spray: A rapid nicotine delivery system. *Psychopharmacology, 108,* 512-518.

Swan, A.V., Creeser, R., & Murray, M. (1990). When and why children first start to smoke. *International Journal of Epidemiology, 19,* 323-330.

Tashkin, D.P., Clark, V.A., Coulson, A.H., Simmons, M., Bourque, L.B., Reeins, C., Detels, R., Sayre, J.W., & Rokaw, S.N. (1984). The UCLA population studies of chronic obstructive respiratory disease. VIII. Effects of smoking cessation in lung function. *American Review of Respiratory Disease, 130,* 707-715.

Terborg, J.R. (1988). The organization as a context for health promotion. In S. Oskamp & S. Spacapan (Eds.), *Social psychology and health: The Claremont Symposium on Applied Social Psychology* (pp. 129-174). Newbury Park, CA: Sage.

The Tobacco Institute. (1988). *Tobacco industry profile 1988.* Washington, DC: Author.

Thomford, P.J., & Mattison, D.R. (1986). The effect of cigarette smoking on female reproduction. *Journal of the Arkansas Medical Society, 82*(12), 597-604.

Tinn, A. (1995, July 22). Growing tobacco. *Congressional Quarterly,* 2137.

Tunstall, C.D., Ginsberg, D., & Hall, S.M. (1985). Quitting smoking. *International Journal of the Addictions, 20,* 1089-1112.

Urberg, K., & Robbins, R. (1984). Perceived vulnerability in adolescents to the health consequences of cigarette smoking. *Preventive Medicine, 13,* 367-376.

U.S. Department of Health and Human Services, U.S. Public Health Service. (1979). *Smoking and health: A report of the Surgeon General* (DHEW Publication No. 79-50066). Washington, DC: U.S. Government Printing Office.

U.S. Department of Health and Human Services, U.S. Public Health Service. (1980). *The health consequences of smoking for women: A report of the Surgeon General.* Washington, DC: Office of the Assistant Secretary for Health, Office on Smoking and Health.

U.S. Department of Health and Human Services, U.S. Public Health Service. (1984). *The health consequences of smoking: Chronic obstructive lung disease. A report of the Surgeon General* (USDHHS [PHS] Publication No. 84-50205). Washington, DC: U.S. Government Printing Office.

U.S. Department of Health and Human Services, U.S. Public Health Service. (1985). *The health consequences of smoking: Cancer and chronic lung disease in the workplace. A report of the Surgeon General* (USDHHS [PHS] Publication No. 85-50207). Washington, DC: U.S. Government Printing Office.

U.S. Department of Health and Human Services, U.S. Public Health Service. (1986a). *The health consequences of involuntary smoking: A report of the Surgeon General.* (USDHHS [CDC] Publication No. 87-8398). Washington, DC: U.S. Government Printing Office.

U.S. Department of Health and Human Services, U.S. Public Health Service. (1986b). *The health consequences of using smokeless tobacco: A report of the advisory committee to the Surgeon General* (USDHHS [NIH] Publication No. 86-2874). Washington, DC: U.S. Government Printing Office.

U.S. Department of Health and Human Services, U.S. Public Health Service. (1988). *The health consequences of smoking. Nicotine addiction. A Report of the Surgeon General* (DHHS Publication No. 88-8406). Washington, DC: U.S. Government Printing Office.

U.S. Department of Health and Human Services, U.S. Public Health Service. (1989a). *How you can help patients stop smoking: Opportunities for respiratory care practitioners* (NIH Publication No. 89-2961). Washington, DC: National Heart, Lung, and Blood Institute.

U.S. Department of Health and Human Services, U.S. Public Health Service. (1989b). *Reducing the health consequences of smoking: 25 years of progress. A Report of the Surgeon General* (DHHS Publication No. CDC 89-8411). Washington, DC: U.S. Government Printing Office.

U.S. Department of Health and Human Services, U.S. Public Health Service. (1990a). *Nurses: Help your patients stop smoking* (NIH Publication No. 90-2962). Washington, DC: National Heart, Lung, and Blood Institute.

U.S. Department of Health and Human Services, U.S. Public Health Service. (1990b). *The health benefits of smoking cessation: A Report of the Surgeon General* (DHHS Publication No. CDC 90-8416). Washington, DC: Center for Chronic Disease Prevention and Health Promotion, Office of Smoking and Health, Centers for Disease Control and Prevention, Author.

U.S. Department of Health and Human Services, U.S. Public Health Service. (1994). *Preventing tobacco use among young people: A report of the Surgeon General.* Atlanta: U.S. Department of Health and Human Services, U.S. Public Health Service, CDC, National Center for Chronic Disease Prevention and Health Promotion, Office of Smoking and Health.

U.S. Department of Health and Human Services, U.S. Public Health Service. (1995). *Healthy people 2000: Midcourse review and 1995 revisions.* Washington, DC: Superintendent of Documents.

U.S. Environmental Protection Agency. (1994). *The costs and benefits of smoking restrictions: An assessment of the smoke-free environment act of 1993 (HR 3434).* Washington, DC: Author.

Waal-Manning, H.J., & de Hamel, F.A. (1980, August 16). Psychoneurotic profiles of smokers and non-smokers (letter). *British Medical Journal, 281*(6238), 517.

Wagner, E.H., Schoenbach, V.J., Orleans, C.T., Grothaus, L.C., Saunders, K.W., Curry, S.J., & Pearson, D.C. (1990). Participation in a smoking cessation program: A population-based perspective. *American Journal of Preventive Medicine, 6,* 258-266.

Ware, J.H., Dockery, D.W., Spiro, A., Speizer, F.E., & Ferris, B.G. (1984). Passive smoking, gas cooking, and respiratory health of children living in six cities. *American Review of Respiratory Disease, 129,* 336-374.

Warner, K.E. (1981, November 18-20). *The federal cigarette excise tax: Proceedings of the National Conference on Smoking or Health.* New York: American Cancer Society.

Whyatt, R.M., & Perera, F.P. (1995). Application of biologic markers to studies of environmental risks in children and the developing fetus. *Environmental Health Perspectives, 103* (Suppl. 6), 105-110.

Willett, W.C., Green, A., Stampfer, M.J., Speizer, F.E., Coldita, G.A., Rosner, B., Monson, R., Stason, W., & Hennekens, C. (1987). Relative and absolute excess risks of coronary heart disease among women who smoke cigarettes. *New England Journal of Medicine, 317,* 1303-1309.

Wilson, D.M., Taylor, M.A., Gilbert, J.R., Best, J.A., Lindsay, E.A., Williams, D.G., & Singer, J. (1988). A randomized trial of a family physician intervention for smoking cessation. *Journal of the American Medical Association, 260,* 1570-1574.

Windsor, R. (1986). *A handbook to plan, implement, and evaluate smoking cessation programs for pregnant women.* Birmingham, AL: Department of Health Behavior, School of Public Health, University of Alabama at Birmingham.

Windsor, R.A., Lowe, J.B., Perkins, L.L., Smith-Yoder, D., Artz, L., Crawford, M., Amburgy, K., & Boyd, N.R. (1993). Behavioral impact and cost benefit of health education methods for pregnant smokers in public health maternity clinics: The Birmingham Trial II. *American Journal of Public Health, 83,* 201-206.

Windsor, R.G.C., & Morris, J. et al. (1985). The effectiveness of smoking cessation methods for smokers in public health maternity clinics: A randomized trial. *American Journal of Public Health, 75,* 1389-1392.

Winefield, H.R., Winefield, A.H., Tiggeman, M., & Goldney, R.D. (1989). Psychological concommitants of tobacco and alcohol use in young Australian adults. *British Journal of Addiction, 84*(9), 1067-1073.

Wong-McCarthy, W.J., & Gritz, E.R. (1982). Preventing regular teenage cigarette smoking. *Pediatric Annals, 11,* 683-689.

World Health Organization. (1997). *Tobacco or health: A global status report.* Geneva, Switzerland: Author.

World Health Organization Expert Committee on Smoking Control. (1979). *Controlling the smoking epidemic* (WHO Technical Report, Series 636). Geneva: Author.

CHAPTER

7

Eating Well

Lorraine E. Matthews

....
EDITORS' NOTE

Eating Well and the Family Client System.   Americans' eating patterns have changed little despite the considerable attention paid to the link between nutrition and health at the national level and in the media. Some healthy reductions in total and saturated fat intake have occurred; the diets of many ethnic minorities have not, however, changed as much. Further, individuals, particularly those of lower income, are consuming less calcium and other minerals and are eating fewer fruits and vegetables, sources of beneficial fiber and micronutrients (Norris et al, 1997).

Unhealthy eating patterns have been associated with coronary heart disease, some types of cancer, stroke, diabetes mellitus, atherosclerosis, and many other causes of morbidity and mortality. Dietary imbalances and excesses have contributed to problems such as high blood pressure, obesity, dental diseases, osteoporosis, and gastrointestinal diseases. Subgroups of the population, such as ethnic minorities, children, the poor, and the house-bound elderly, are at particular risk for these diseases due in part to their nutritional status. Environmental approaches to dietary behavior change can reach large segments of these populations through increased availability of nutritious foods, provision of quality nutrition services in workplace and health care settings, and accessible information about healthful food choices.

The family has great influence over patterns of nutrition. Throughout the life span, families teach and shape the patterns and habits that become individual decisions about nutrition. Foods may be prepared in a multitude of ways, reflecting each family's culture, preferences, and traditions. Not only are foods selected and prepared differently in the context of the family, but families also differ in the time of day meals are served, whether meals are a time for socializing, and the meaning attributed to the food. The family is the source of nurturance; nutrition is a basic means for doing this.

Eating Well and Image Appraisal.   In this chapter, author Lorraine Matthews, MS, RD, wisely discusses working with individuals—who reflect their family's patterns of eating—to analyze nutrition choices. She emphasizes the changing national nutritional recommendations and the differing perspectives among nutritionists and other health care professionals regarding an optimal diet. She recognizes the difficulties these changes and differences present to the individual, as well as the family, trying to make changes in nutrition. The health care professional's role in detailing dietary patterns and practices through a thorough nutritional assessment is instrumental in assisting client systems to examine their relationship to food and to clarify the changes they wish to make. Matthews highlights both the necessity of eating and the difficulty of making healthy choices regarding food.

Sample Case and the Health Promotion Matrix Script. Matthews' case study discusses a middle-age woman with significant health problems and family responsibilities. In the case study, a health care professional assists the woman to make small, liveable changes in her life; to reduce her overall morbidity; and to promote her health. An important aspect of Matthews' approach is how to effect positive change within the context of the client's life.

The 1988 *Surgeon General's Report on Nutrition and Health* stated that for the two out of three Americans who do not smoke or drink, eating patterns may shape their long-term health prospects more than any other personal choice (U.S. Public Health Service, 1988). The implications of this statement are staggering in terms of any health promotion program that involves modification of eating habits.

THE AMERICAN DIET

Almost every American adult and most school children will affirm that a well-balanced diet is essential for good health; however, according to a recent survey by the Food Marketing Institute (FMI), 73% of American adults believe their diet could be somewhat healthier. The same study found that consumers' greatest nutritional concern continues to be the amount of fat in foods, followed in descending order by salt, cholesterol, sugar, calories, vitamins and minerals, preservatives, and chemical additives. And although they are not completely satisfied with their diet, 77% reported that they are eating more fruits and vegetables, and 42% said they are eating fewer fats and oils (Food Marketing Institute [FMI], 1996). Ironically, despite the fact that Americans spend billions of dollars annually on the latest diet plans, books, and a variety of pills and supplements in hope of finding that "magic bullet" that will allow them to eat what they want, exercise minimally, and remain forever young, national surveys indicate that more than 33% of adults age 20 and older are overweight (U.S. Department of Health and Human Services [USDHHS], 1991). Further, approximately 11% of children ages 6 to 17 years are seriously overweight (Centers for Disease Control and Prevention, 1996).

Healthy People 2000 is a national initiative to improve the health of all Americans through a coordinated and comprehensive emphasis on prevention. In 1990 the U.S. Secretary of Health and Human Services released the first 300 objectives of the initiative. The objectives addressed three overall goals: to increase the span of healthy life for Americans, to reduce health disparities among Americans, and to achieve access to preventive services for all Americans. Twenty-one of those objectives were related to nutrition (USDHHS, 1991). Nutrition objectives fall under the larger heading of "Health Promotion," which includes those areas relating to individual life-style. A mid-point review of the *Healthy People 2000* nutrition objectives was recently completed using data from a variety of sources, including the National Health and Nutrition Examination Survey (HANES) and the U.S. Department of Agriculture food consumption surveys. The results were mixed but confirm some of what has already been discussed in the literature. Two of the Health Status objectives have had little success—the prevalence of overweight Americans is increasing and fewer overweight individuals are using appropriate methods for weight reduction. On the other hand, progress has been made in six areas—reduction of coronary heart disease deaths, reduction in cancer deaths, reduction in fat intake, availability of more informative nutrition labeling on food items, more low-fat restaurant menu choices, and a modest increase in worksite nutrition education. Two other objectives, increased calcium intake and increased breastfeeding, have had mixed results (Goldstein, 1996). Obviously, the nation still has a long way to go.

The Dilemma of Food, Nutrition, and Health

The role of food and nutrition in the promotion of health and well-being is unique. Unlike persons who must stop and avoid behaviors completely when they become problems, the person with eating problems must still continue to eat. For example, the person who abuses alcohol must come to grips with the fact that this product can no longer be used; however, the person who abuses food must somehow learn to make changes in the use of a substance that, even though it creates problems, is essential for continued life.

Another important factor regarding food is the sheer number of products available in the market today. Consumers are faced with choosing among thousands of food items in the average supermarket, and this does not include the wide variety of food that can be purchased in other commercial establishments. One could conscientiously avoid grocery stores and restaurants and still encounter food items for sale at gas stations, car washes, transportation centers, stationery stores, hardware stores, pharmacies, worksites, and the list goes on and on. This trend is not necessarily bad or good—it is simply a fact of American business. The fact that sales of food items flourish in nontraditional food stores indicates there is a market for them. The FMI study previously mentioned also notes that the patronage of alternative formats for purchasing food (e.g., buying clubs, discount stores), which accounts for less than 10% of the market, has increased by 5% since 1991 (FMI, 1996). Today, there are a lot of food products that can be produced and marketed with relatively low overhead, which means that extra shelves can turn a profit. The problem is that many of the foods sold this way are high in fat, salt, and calories and are low in nutrients. (Try to think of a place where a person can purchase a low-fat, high-fiber meal without getting out of the car. There are a few more choices now than there were 5 years ago, but not many.)

Despite all of this, Americans are concerned about their health. A recent survey of 1000 adult shoppers around the country indicated that one half had changed some factor in their diets because of health concerns. The underlying belief for making these changes was that diet is closely linked to the likelihood of having a heart attack, stroke, or high cholesterol, followed by diabetes, colon cancer, and osteoporosis (Princeton Survey Research Associates, 1996). However, the No. 1 issue remains weight control, and although there are a number of different factors surrounding eating habits, in American society today the biggest controversies in nutrition involve dieting, weight loss (or the lack of it), and body image (Ross Timesaver, 1993).

The phrase "good nutrition" instantly brings up many images in the minds of the American public—many of them negative. Consumers are bombarded on all sides of the issue by the slick, aggressive marketing of restaurant chains, grocery stores, and food companies. They hear the media sounding the alarm on even the most obscure bits of scientific information regarding nutrition—even if, in fact, the data are much more complicated than is reflected in the sound bite. They fall victim to health hucksters looking to use their confusion to make a quick buck. Additionally, unfortunately, they are often "turned off" by well-meaning health care professionals who spend too much time telling them things they don't need to know, listing what they are doing wrong, and telling them what they can't have. Consumers frequently feel that they cannot enjoy foods that they like and still maintain a healthy diet. Also, recent surveys have shown that while food shoppers generally do have positive attitudes about nutrition, they remain concerned about cost and taste. In a recent study, three out of five shoppers felt that it costs more to eat healthy foods. The same study also found that an increasing number of consumers are growing tired of "expert advice" about nutrition. About 46% of shoppers said there is too much conflicting information about which foods are good for them and that they are not sure what to eat anymore. Finally, the shoppers surveyed perceived healthy foods as being less convenient to prepare and not tasting as good (Princeton Survey Research Associates, 1996).

THE PHYSIOLOGY OF EATING

Nutrition is a relatively young science, with most of what is currently known coming after 1900, and there are still many areas in which information is incomplete (Guthrie, 1989). A lot is known about the ability of the body to extract the energy and nutrients it needs from the wide variety of available foods. For purposes of this chapter, a brief overview of this is provided.

Simply put, a person's diet must include foods that provide the nutrients required to sustain life and for the body to grow. The body requires six types of essential nutrients, which can be defined as families of molecules that are indispensible to the body's functioning and that the body cannot make for itself. Without any one of the six, the body's overall health will be impaired.

Although water provides no energy and essentially no other nutrients, it is the most abundant nutrient. It is constantly lost from the body and must constantly be replaced.

The only energy-producing nutrients are proteins, carbohydrates, and fats. Proteins also provide essential building materials that form body structures and provide the basis for many essential compounds. Some protein is found in almost all foods, but the primary food sources are meats, eggs, dairy products, and legumes. Carbohydrates and fats also provide basic components for a number of essential compounds and structures required by the body, although to a lesser degree than proteins. With the exception of milk and honey, carbohydrates are found only in plant products. Carbohydrate is generally categorized into two groups—simple sugars, which usually are found naturally in fruits and some vegetables, and complex carbohydrates, or starches, which are abundant in grain products and starchy vegetables. Fat also is present in varying amounts in almost all foods. Its primary animal sources are meat, meat products, and dairy products made from whole milk, and its primary vegetable source is the germ of most seeds and grains and of many nuts. As a rule, animal fats tend to be more highly saturated and vegetable fats tend to be more unsaturated.

Included in the general category of fats are a number of complex organic compounds that are not used for energy production but rather as building blocks of various compounds in the body. Only one of these complex organic compounds—cholesterol—is discussed in this text. Found only in animal tissues, cholesterol is an essential sterol that is part of a number of structures and compounds in the body. The human body makes cholesterol even when it is completely absent from the diet. While some is necessary, too much cholesterol in the body can cause clogged arteries and is a major risk factor for cardiovascular disease.

The last two groups of essential nutrients are vitamins and minerals, which are found in a wide variety of foods. They do not provide any energy, and all but a few are needed in very minute amounts in the body. A few minerals serve as parts of body structures (e.g., calcium and phosphorus in bones and teeth), but the primary role of vitamins and minerals is to regulate body processes. These processes include digesting food; moving muscles; disposing of wastes; growing new tissue; healing wounds; and obtaining energy from carbohydrate, fat, and protein (Sizer & Whitney, 1994).

A few other key concepts regarding nutrition that health care professionals need to understand and convey to clients include the following:

- The body is like a large chemistry laboratory that functions effectively and with much regularity. Although how it works can be considered miraculous, the body does not function through magic; there is an ordered purpose for reactions, even if health care professionals do not completely understand them.

- The foods that humans eat are also chemicals that interact with the chemicals in the body—also in an ordered manner. There are no magic foods; however, some have higher concentrations of nutrients that humans need.

- The nutrient fat is unique in that it can not be excreted or eliminated from the body. The only way to remove it is through oxidation, or burning. The loss (burning) of 1 pound of fat requires oxidizing approximately 3500 calories more than what was taken in from food (Sizer & Whitney, 1994). Most people can lose a maximum of 2 to 3 pounds of body fat in 1 week. Although weight loss may be more rapid initially when someone significantly reduces calorie intake, most of that loss is in the form of water and some muscle tissue but very little fat. Therefore diet plans that promise meaningful weight loss of several pounds a week are deceptive.

- Human bodies require regular exercise. If it is not a part of a person's regular activities (e.g., work), then it should be planned into the day. Attempts at weight reduction through eating habits are marginally effective if there is not a physical activity component (Skender et al, 1996). However, as discussed in the next chapter, the need for exercise goes well beyond just weight control. For individuals to make lasting changes in their eating behaviors, they must understand that diet and physical activity have complementary beneficial effects regarding the major chronic diseases (Blair, 1995).

For optimal health, the processes just described must occur with efficiency and regularity. This requires an adequate, consistent supply of nutrients. Some nutrients, such as vitamin C, are almost completely used up on a daily basis, with little being stored in the body. Thus symptoms of deficiency can be seen in a matter of weeks in a susceptible person who does not ingest the vitamin. Other nutrients, such as calcium, phosphorus, protein, and fat, are normally stored in the body, so an overt deficiency takes much longer to manifest itself. In reality, however, the classic deficiency diseases of scurvy (inadequate vitamin C), beriberi (inadequate thiamine), pellagra (inadequate niacin), and similar conditions are only occasionally seen today in the general population, thanks to the refinement and application of nutritional knowledge in the early part of this century. Today, in the United States, these conditions are primarily seen in at-risk groups, such as alcoholics; persons with specific diseases such as cancer, human immunodeficiency virus (HIV) infection and acquired immunodeficiency syndrome (AIDS); and persons who chronically ingest highly restrictive diets. These same high-risk clients often are on a regimen of a variety of medications that also can interfere with the efficacy of certain nutrients (Guthrie, 1989).

THE CHANGING FOCUS OF NUTRITION AND HEALTH

In the second half of the twentieth century there has been a decreased emphasis on the nutritional deficiency diseases. As the major causes of death have shifted from infectious to chronic diseases, emphasis is now focused on the maintenance of health and the reduction of the risks for chronic diseases such as heart disease, hypertension, stroke, diabetes mellitus, and some types of cancer. Improved nutritional behaviors will lower the at-risk person's potential of developing these diseases (National Research Council, 1989).

This new emphasis poses novel challenges to the health care professional, such as convincing asymptomatic clients to modify their diets to *prevent* disease. For example, if a 45-year-old man is hospitalized with severe bruising and bleeding that turns out to be scurvy or a more common occurrence, uncontrolled diabetes mellitus, in both instances immediate dietary intervention will be a key part to his recovery. The results of this treatment are fairly swift and quite dramatic. Further, when faced with the recurrence of either condition and subsequent hospitalization and treatment, he likely will be willing to make dietary modifications that will prevent recurrence of illness—at least for awhile. However, to convince a healthy 45-year-old man with no current disease symptoms that modifying his eating habits now will reduce his chances of developing a chronic disease perhaps a decade later is a lot more difficult. Unless this client has further evidence to change, such as family history of a disease, he is unlikely to be terribly concerned about making modifications.

Medical nutrition therapy plays a key role in the treatment of a variety of acute clinical outcomes (Gallagher-Allred, Voss, Finn, & McCamish, 1996). However, one of the problems that health care professionals find so frustrating is that even in persons who have long-standing chronic diseases, empowering them to change negative behaviors, including eating patterns, is extremely difficult. A 60-year-old woman with adult-onset diabetes who is unable to keep her blood glucose levels in the normal range will likely face complications such as renal failure, peripheral neuropathies, and even blindness and amputation of limbs. However, even with this information, she may be unwilling or unable to change her daily diet and activity routines to improve her chances of avoiding such complications. This is not always simply a result of obstinance. Instead, overwhelming environmental and social situations may preclude her from making major dietary changes without substantial assistance from family or the community, or both. Many clients are frequently without such a support system. For instance, a trip to the supermarket without assistance may be an insurmountable task for an older person who lives alone, and cooking for one person may become very tedious. A limited income may restrict another person from buying the foods needed to improve health. The role of the health care professional must go beyond just the basic education component; it also requires tasks such as referring clients outside the medical setting to community agencies such as congregate meal programs, senior shopping services, or emergency food cupboards.

DEFINING A HEALTHY DIET

Thus far there have been several references to "improving one's diet," but the term *healthy diet* has not really been defined. When trying to effect improvements in eating habits, it is essential that all parties involved understand the terms being used. For example, the portion sizes that most health care professionals use are commonly not the same ones clients envision. To a pregnant teenager who is being counseled about excessive weight gain, a cup of soda probably means 12 or 16 oz—not the 8 oz recommended by health care professionals. Among some health care professionals, the term "low fat" may mean a maximum of 30% of energy coming from fat, but to others it might mean 20% of energy coming from fat (Sigman-Grant, 1996). Since not all health care professionals agree on every single point of what constitutes a healthy diet, this chapter takes the middle road and uses the *Dietary Guidelines for Americans* (U.S. Department of Agriculture [USDA], USDHHS, 1995), to define a healthy diet. Briefly, the guidelines include the following:

- Eat a variety of foods.
- Balance food you eat with physical activity—maintain or improve weight.
- Choose a diet with plenty of grain products, vegetables, and fruit.
- Choose a diet low in fat, saturated fat, and cholesterol.
- Choose a diet moderate in sugars.
- Choose a diet moderate in salt and sodium.
- If you drink alcoholic beverages, do so in moderation.

These are very general guidelines, and they are useful because they can be adapted to the food preferences of a variety of ethnic groups and cultures. They are a good starting point for many health education programs; however, most persons usually need more specific information and some type of guide to put these principles into practice. So after years of promoting dietary guides such as the *Four Food Group Plan* for healthy eating, in 1995 the U.S. government introduced the *Food Guide Pyramid* (USDA, USDHHS, 1995). Now widely used in health education and in retail food advertisements, the pyramid promotes choosing a recommended number of daily servings from each of five major food groups, with the number of servings generally based on age and gender (Figure 7-1). Breads, cereals, and pastas form the base of the pyramid, and consumers are advised to select between 6 and 11 servings daily. Vegetables and fruits form the second tier of the pyramid, with recommendations of 3 to 5 daily servings and 2 to 4 daily servings, respectively; this is consistent with the message from various health organizations that recommend consumption of at least 5 servings of fruits and vegetables daily. The third tier of the pyramid is shared by the milk, yogurt, and cheese group and the meat, poultry, fish, dry beans, eggs and nuts group; consumers are recommended to eat 2 to 3 daily servings from each of these two groups. The top, or last tier, of the pyramid consists of fats, oils and sweets, with an admonition to use these food items sparingly. It is interesting to note that the last group of food items was not included in the previous food guide, because it was assumed that Americans ate adequate amounts of these items and that there was no need to provide specific amounts. The focus of the Food Guide Pyramid has shifted to emphasize that although fats, oils, and sweets can be part of a normal diet, they should be limited. One of the benefits of the pyramid is that it can be used with a variety of eating plans. Even a strict vegetarian who eats no animal products (or vegan) can effectively draw from the various categories, except for the milk group. To obtain calcium, the vegetarian could substitute

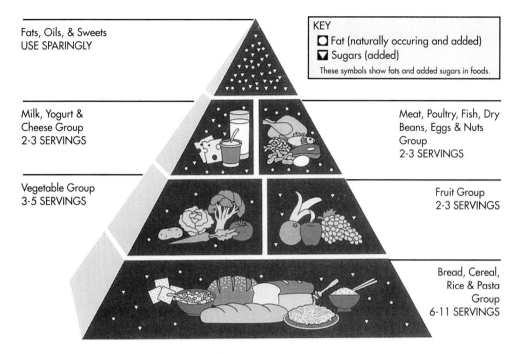

Fats, Oils, & Sweets
USE SPARINGLY

KEY
◻ Fat (naturally occuring and added)
▼ Sugars (added)
These symbols show fats and added sugars in foods.

Milk, Yogurt &
Cheese Group
2-3 SERVINGS

Meat, Poultry, Fish, Dry
Beans, Eggs & Nuts
Group
2-3 SERVINGS

Vegetable Group
3-5 SERVINGS

Fruit Group
2-3 SERVINGS

Bread, Cereal,
Rice & Pasta
Group
6-11 SERVINGS

Figure **7-1 The Food Guide Pyramid.** (*From* Nutrition and your health: Dietary guidelines for Americans *[Home and Garden Bulletin No. 232] [4th ed.], by U.S. Department of Agriculture, U.S. Department of Health and Human Services, 1995, Washington, DC: U.S. Government Printing Office.*)

products from the milk group with ample amounts of dark green leafy vegetables and soy products that have been processed with calcium sulfate.

There are at least two factors that health care professionals should keep in mind when presenting the Food Guide Pyramid to clients:

■ Many persons are confused about the number of servings and the serving sizes. The majority of serving sizes listed on the pyramid are from one half to three fourths of 1 cup, which is a lot less than many Americans eat. For example, most persons who eat rice or pasta within a meal eat at least 1 cup, which translates into 2 servings. Health care professionals must not only be able to explain the number of servings that are appropriate for a particular individual but also what constitutes a serving size.

■ There are some cultures—persons from West Africa for example—who do not use many grain products in their diets. Instead, the bulk of their high-carbohydrate foods comes from starchy vegetables such as squash, yams, and similar root vegetables. Although these foods don't show up on the base of the pyramid, they can be a healthy substitute for grain products.

EFFECTING POSITIVE CHANGE IN EATING BEHAVIOR

If health care professionals in general and nutrition professionals in particular are going to effect positive changes in eating behavior, they must realize the following:

■ The overwhelming majority of persons eat food—not just nutrients. The average person has only a passing interest in the roles of individual nutrients. If individuals are interested in improving their health status, they usually want to know which foods they need to eat—not a specific level of nutrients. This is why many persons do not do well with calorie counting to control intake. If they feel they have to emphasize particular nutrients in their diet, they often would rather take a pill than try to figure out what foods provide those nutrients.

■ Humans eat for a number of reasons that have little to do with satisfying hunger. Personal preferences, habits, ethnic heritage or traditions, social pressures, positive associations, emotional needs, values, and beliefs are all factors that have little to do with hunger but a lot to do with what a person selects to eat. For instance, food is a central focus during most religious holidays—no matter what the religion—and an individual's cultural background has a strong impact on decisions about what is appropriate to eat. Wherever possible, factors such as these must be respected and incorporated into an eating plan.

■ Health care professionals sometimes forget that while it is their chosen work to spend all day thinking about health issues, it is usually not their clients' primary focus. Other persons have different careers and issues to occupy their minds. A busy executive with diverticulosis, for example, does not need to know all the chemical properties of every type of dietary fiber, but this person does need to know how to select high-fiber foods from a restaurant menu.

■ Most adults must have a role in the planning process to make changes in the way they eat. A person's own and cultural preferences must be considered and valued. Telling a pregnant woman who does not drink milk to follow a standardized diet sheet that recommends obtaining calcium from milk as a beverage 2 or 3 times daily will not be met with much success. A more successful approach would be to determine the foods she does eat, note which ones contain the most calcium, and help her to emphasize those foods in her diet. Some persons do not make the connection between milk and foods such as yogurt and cheese. Additionally, some do not understand that the milk that they dislike as a beverage tastes OK as a part of foods such as puddings and cream soups. The health care professional must remember that persons may be willing to try some new foods, but they also want to see familiar ones.

■ Persons make changes to improve their diets and thus health from a variety of starting points that directly influence how much improvement will be achieved. A client may begin making these changes while suffering from disease or when illness is absent. For example, the middle-age person who contracts one or two chronic conditions such as diabetes or hypertension will greatly improve outcome in most cases through an improved eating plan. On the other hand, the young healthy adult who exercises on a regular basis and eats a reasonable healthy diet probably will not see significant improvement in current health status; benefits for this person are much more long range.

■ For successful, long-term change, the consumer must be satisfied that the proposed modifications can be incorporated into an existing life-style without major sacrifices. The first step in improving anyone's diet, no matter what a person's health status is, may be as simple as suggesting that an effort be made to eat at least 5 fruits and vegetables a day. If this is not a normal part of the person's current routine—and lots of studies indicate that it isn't—this small change will make a significant improvement in a person's diet (Princeton Survey Research Associates, 1996). Eating more vegetables and fruits also may make some small differences in the way a person feels. If nothing else, a diet that includes more fruits and vegetables often improves regularity. Since long-term positive changes are best accomplished in small increments that can be internalized, more changes can be added when a step such as this becomes a routine part of daily activity.

Health care professionals must be able to recognize severe nutrition problems and make a referral to an appropriate specialist. Dysfunctional eating is a relatively recent concept that incorporates abnormal and inappropriate eating behaviors. Berg (1996) calls it a disruption of normal eating, but it can also include restrained eating, disordered eating, and chronic dieting syndrome. It is most prevalent among girls and women and appears to be increasing and occurring at younger ages, as cultural pressures to be thin continue (Berg, 1995). However, the person who develops a problem with a particular food or group of foods does not always have an eating disorder.

Sometimes, dietary interventions are contradictory to traditional nutrition teachings. A chronic disease that has occurred because of lifelong habits other than eating patterns may necessitate a significant dietary intervention that can be challenging for a client. For example, the regular smoker who develops chronic obstructive pulmonary disease (COPD) often needs dietary manipulation that is almost the direct opposite of what is normally considered a healthy diet for the average adult. The person with COPD needs a diet that eases breathing by lowering the production of carbon dioxide (i.e., a diet high in fat and low in carbohydrate) (Williams, 1997). Since this is the opposite of what persons have been taught, it often takes some convincing to get clients and families to accept such an eating plan. In one case, a 63-year-old female home care client with COPD who weighed less than 60 pounds and was so weak that she had difficulty expelling bowel movements resisted ingesting a high-fat diet because she feared it might "make her cholesterol go up." Persons with HIV must sometimes be persuaded to ingest a very high-calorie diet even though a high-calorie, high-protein diet may delay conversion to AIDS (American Dietetic Association, 1992).

THE PROBLEM OF FUNDING NUTRITIONAL INTERVENTIONS

Another major issue that must be considered in today's health care environment is funding. There is rarely third-party reimbursement for individualized counseling for preventive behavior change; however, when counseling becomes therapy for a specific condition, coverage is more likely. For example, an insurance company or health maintenance organization is unlikely to pay for generalized weight loss counseling for an obese individual, although it may give reduced rates or rebates to local health clubs or similar facilities. When that same individual develops a condition such as hyperlipidemia or hyperglycemia, however, then reimbursement for weight loss counseling is more likely (Philadelphia Dietetic Association, 1994). Reimbursement for nutritional counseling may become more prevalent because of changing government regulations.

The health professional must be very pragmatic in planning education regarding behavior change. A key factor to consider is the foci of intervention found in the Health Promotion Matrix (HPM). Although ongoing personalized counseling may be the ideal, it is certainly not the norm. Often, general preventive information such as the *Food Guide Pyramid* (USDA, USDHHS, 1995) must be presented in a group setting because individualized teaching would not be cost-effective. This requires innovative teaching techniques that involve group members and give them a stake in the outcome. A straight classroom lecture format is rarely effective, but if clients can be involved in the activity—preparation of healthy menu items, for example—then learning and behavior change is more likely.

While individual counseling for a client with specific problems may be covered by an insurance program, the health professional may only be allowed one reimbursed session. This is often less than satisfactory, but it is an economic reality. The need to cover as much as possible in one session must be carefully balanced with the reality of how much the client can absorb in that time.

WORKING FOR POSITIVE DIETARY CHANGE

On the surface, bringing about long-term positive dietary change seems difficult, if not hopeless. Particularly in the area of obesity treatment, some health care professionals and consumer advocates have gone so far as to say that the whole concept of dieting per se is dangerous and usually destined to failure. Some advocates have urged that all dieting be discouraged and, instead, clients be taught to accept and love their bodies as they are. They advocate efforts to help clients be comfortable with their current size, to try to live a healthy life-style, and to stop worrying about their weight and get on with their lives (Erdman, 1995). Although not totally acceptable, this argument has some validity. It is true that persons who suffer from obesity often do not fare well in American society, which places tremendous emphasis on thinness; this is especially true for women and girls (Fallon, 1994). Obese persons are apt to spend inordinate amounts of money and time on diet plans that have only a marginal chance of working, thus increasing these persons' frustration and self-doubt (Berg, 1995). However, the health risks of obesity and its chronic complications are well-documented (National Heart, Lung, and Blood Institute, 1992; Berg, 1995), so it is not enough to simply say, "I'm comfortable with myself, and I don't have to bother any more." Health care professionals must continue to search for rational methods to enable overweight persons to be physically and mentally healthy while gradually managing some weight loss and to refer to specialized weight loss clinics, where appropriate.

Dietary change is commonly a major issue for persons with conditions other than obesity. Learning to eat foods with less salt and conscientiously reducing the amount of saturated fat in one's diet can be very difficult for adults who have spent a lifetime eating high-salt and high-fat foods. The issues of proper nutrition take on major importance for a child who develops diabetes mellitus. The pregnant woman who may be dealing with a variety of positive and negative emotions and physical changes often finds the increased emphasis on healthy eating a difficult issue to handle.

Health care professionals have a responsibility to help their clients search for practical and realistic ways to improve their health (Parham, 1996). In her review of research on intervention models, Sigman-Grant (1996) considers a number of intervention approaches and relates them to the stages of change model (Prochaska, Velicer, Rossi, Abrams, & Follick, 1994). As discussed in Chapter 2, this is a model that explains how individuals make and internalize behavior changes. Briefly, the stages include precontemplation (no changes are considered); contemplation (awareness of problem and consideration of action); preparation (plans are made to take action in the next 30 days and small changes may have been made); action (noticeable efforts to change targeted behavior); and maintenance (period for trying to stabilize the behavior change and prevent relapses). Sigman-Grant points out that many individuals get stuck in the early stages, particularly in contemplation. Also, recycling between stages is common, especially in individuals struggling with weight loss or trying to adopt an exercise program (Sigman-Grant, 1996).

So, with all the potential roadblocks listed previously, how does the intrepid health care professional proceed? How does one make the most effective use of one's limited time and access without totally overwhelming the client? At this point it should be clear that no two clients will have exactly the same problems or issues when it comes to intervention in the way they eat. Using the Health Promotion Matrix (see Figure 5-1, p. 92) as the overall guide, the health care professional can develop and cultivate procedures to make a counseling session as beneficial as possible, as illustrated in the following example.

EATING WELL & THE HEALTH PROMOTION MATRIX*

Mrs. R. is a 54 year-old woman who has a primary diagnosis of hypercholesterolemia, degenerative joint disease, and moderate obesity (approximately 50 to 55 pounds more than ideal body weight range). She has become frustrated with her physician because he chastised her for gaining 2 pounds since her last visit; however, she maintains it was just because she had attended a family graduation ceremony and party. He has also insisted that she be placed on a low-calorie diet. She is visiting another health care professional (in this case, a registered dietitian) in a community health center for the first time.

Image Creation

The health care professional greets the client and initiates communication to establish a constructive rapport between them. It is usually helpful to determine the client's perception about why he/she has come to see the health care professional. This initial contact is described as understanding the client's agenda. The following questions can also lead to a clarification of the client's own image of health.

UNDERSTANDING THE CLIENT'S AGENDA

Q. *Why are you here?*

Sample Responses

1. *"I am concerned about the increase in my weight and cholesterol."*
2. *"I am worried that I am going to have a heart attack."*
3. *"I don't know why! My doctor said I had to see you before I go home."*

Health Care Professional's Response:

"I understand your frustration Mrs. R; I'm really sorry you had to wait so long. Let's see what we can do to help you get on track and be as healthy as possible. First, I have to ask you some questions such as the purpose for your visit so that between us we can develop an eating guide that is comfortable for you to follow. First, how do you feel today?"

*Adapted from L.E. Matthews by J. Arnold and S. Sheinfeld Gorin.

Mrs. R. could respond to why she made the appointment to see the health care professional in a variety of ways. She may express concern about her increase in weight and cholesterol or express worry that she is going to have a heart attack. She may say: "I don't know why! My doctor said I had to see you before I go home." The health care professional could then express acceptance and understanding for Mrs. R's frustration and a desire to help Mrs. R be as healthy as possible. To put the client at ease and to demonstrate that their mutual goal is improved health, the health care professional may ask about the client's family or job.

DETERMINING CLIENT'S SELF-IMAGE

Q. What changes would you like to make in yourself?

Sample Responses
1. "I would like to lose 100 pounds and look like I did before I was married."
2. "I would really like to be able to go up and down the steps without my legs hurting so much and not being so tired."
3. "I am an old woman, and I really don't care too much about how I look."

Image creation requires that the client determine a desired self-image and how that relates to improved health. To determine the client's self-image, the health care professional would ask: "What changes would you like to make in yourself?" Mrs. R. responds: "I would really like to be able to go up and down the steps without my legs hurting so much and not be so tired." Mrs. R. expresses that feeling better is her priority. Frequently, clients have totally unrealistic images (i.e., "I would like to lose 100 pounds and look like I did before I was married") or feel incapable of imagining themselves differently (i.e., "I am an old woman and I really don't care too much about how I look"). The health care professional must guide clients in establishing a realistic image of where they are and what they desire to become.

Image Appraisal

The client must move from image creation to image appraisal. This is where the client must be grounded in reality. Most women are never going to have the body and face of a supermodel no matter how much weight they lose; yet a healthy diet coupled with an exercise program can improve their looks and energize them in a way that extreme dieting will not. Thus an effective image appraisal helps clients to see where they really are in comparison to where they want to be and what changes they can make. In this situation, the client has made realistic choices about her status and what she can improve. Mrs. R wants to increase her mobility without experiencing leg pains and have more energy.

The health care professional explains that it will be necessary to ask a number of questions to more fully understand the client's current situation. The client must understand that the questions are not meant to criticize and judge but simply to set up a pattern that the two of them can use to effect changes that will improve outcome. This information-gathering process can be separated into subjective data (a description of how the client feels about his/her status) and objective data (actual test results and observations regarding the client). Although in real situations all of the questions are asked at the same time, it is often useful to separate the information for documentation purposes, as done here.

GATHERING A DATABASE (SUBJECTIVE)

Q. How would you say you feel most of the time?

Sample Responses
1. *"I get very tired and my knees hurt so bad."*
2. *"All right, but I do worry about getting sick again."*
3. *"I feel all right most of the time."*

Health Care Professional's Responses
Q. Who does most of the shopping and cooking in your house? (Client, significant other, or other family member).

Q. Do you have other persons dependent on you? (Is client independent or responsible for the care of dependents—parents, children, grandchildren?)

Q. Do you work outside the home and if so, what hours? (Yes or no, does not have a job.)

The subjective data-gathering phase may reveal that Mrs. R feels all right but that she worries about getting sick again. Mrs. R admits that she has been sick in the past, and she is scared of being hospitalized again. She is a widow, but her adult daughter and three small children live with her in the family home. She and her daughter share the responsibilities of shopping and cooking, and she helps with the children when her daughter works. She worked as a housekeeper for many years, but now because of her leg pains, she only occasionally takes on a day's work. They get by on her daughter's salary and her survivor's pension. Mrs. R admits she doubts she will be able to do anything about her weight since she has had little success in changing her health status so far. She also notes that her family doesn't need to go on a diet and they might object to "diet foods." She adds that her daughter frequently brings home "fast foods" at night for dinner when she doesn't feel like cooking. Mrs. R also confides that she has gotten into the habit of consuming a bag of microwave buttered popcorn and iced tea at night while she watches television.

To plan meaningfully for an eating well guide, the health care professional must be able to determine from the client which life-style factors affect her eating behaviors. The health care professional responds with an understanding of the stresses facing Mrs. R. They chat briefly about what children eat today and how "no one cooks anymore." The health care professional also explains that any changes that the client might make should be done very gradually and that their next step would be to set up goals that she can live with successfully. The health care professional stresses that the eating plan will include foods that the entire family can benefit from and enjoy.

GATHERING A DATABASE (OBJECTIVE)

Q. Can you give me some basic physical information about yourself (e.g., age, height, weight, recent weight changes, any medical problems, medication use)?
NOTE: *Some of this information may come from a medical record or from measurement at the time of the session.*

Objective data are gathered through physical examination and testing. Some of this information may come from a health care or medical record or from measurement at the time of the session. As noted, Mrs. R has been diagnosed with hypercholesterolemia, degenerative joint disease, and moderate obesity. The health care professional asks the client to share basic physical information, such as age, height, weight, recent weight changes, medical problems, and medication use. Other data may be collected from a food diary or laboratory tests. Mrs. R is 64 inches tall, and she weighs 201 pounds. Her serum cholesterol level is 320 mg/dl. She is postmenopausal, with a history of high blood pressure and a strong family history of noninsulin dependent diabetes. She is currently taking an over-the-counter analgesic for her knee pain and a cholesterol lowering medication.

Minimize Health Depleting Patterns

A key part of the health care professional's goal is to help the client identify patterns that are detrimental, or health depleting patterns, and to minimize their occurrence. However, the health care professional must be reasonable—trying to resolve too many problems at once can be overwhelming. Solving one or two problems at a time is often better. In Mrs. R's case, this means speaking to the physician who ordered a very low calorie diet and explaining that they are going to approach this gradually, since a very restricted diet has not worked in the past.

DETERMINING A PROBLEM LIST

Q. What are your priority problems?

Sample Responses
1. *"My cholesterol is too high, I have to lose weight, and I have high blood pressure. I don't get enough exercise, and I think I use too much sugar."*
2. *"I think the major problems I have right now are high cholesterol and high blood pressure."*
3. *"I don't know; you decide."*

Setting up a problem list is one way of establishing priorities. The health care professional can ask what are the priority problems as determined by the client. Mrs. R responds that right now her problems are high cholesterol and high blood pressure. Mrs. R recognizes that addressing these two problems will be a major accomplishment for her overall health at this time. Although she may be anxious to lose weight, focusing on priority problems seems satisfying.

The health care professional and the client begin to establish mutually agreeable simple goals. In the situation of Mrs. R, the goals may be to reduce her cholesterol level 5 points by the next visit, limit salt intake every day, and do 15 minutes of physical activity daily. Reducing cholesterol may be accomplished by Mrs. R's increasing fruits and vegetables to at least 5 servings a day and finding at least two recipes for cooking chicken and fish without frying it. Salt (sodium) intake can be limited when Mrs. R agrees to not use any kind of salt in cooking or at the table and to try cooking with some new herbs. Once the physician approves a physical activity plan, Mrs. R could agree to try arm chair exercises every day and look into arthritis water classes at the local community center.

The health care professional and the client come to agree on simple changes in eating patterns and life-style that the client believes are realistic and that do not present inherent obstacles. The key to success is in the client's determination of priorities and in selecting strategies that do not present obstacles that would limit the success for change.

Optimize Health Supportive Patterns

ESTABLISHING MUTUALLY AGREEABLE SIMPLE GOALS

A. Reduce Cholesterol Level 5 Points by Next Visit

Sample strategies

1. *"I will increase the fruits and vegetables that I eat to at least 5 servings a day."*
2. *"I will find at least two recipes for cooking chicken and fish without frying."*

B. Limit Salt (Sodium) Intake Every Day

Sample strategies

1. *"I won't use any kind of salt in cooking or at the table."*
2. *"I will try cooking with some new herbs."*

C. Include 15 Minutes of Physical Activity Daily (after checking with the physician)

Sample strategies

1. *"I will try arm chair exercises every day."*
2. *"I will look into arthritis water classes at the community center."*

It is essential for the health care professional to work with the client in establishing goals that they both feel are meaningful and workable. Positive patterns that are supportive of health should be emphasized, but they should come in small, measurable steps. In this case, Mrs. R is agreeable to trying to eat more fruits and vegetables since both she and her family like them. To her, this seems like a relatively painless change to make, and she is willing to substitute fruit for popcorn in the evenings. Since she likes to cook, she is willing to start looking at other ways to prepare meats and poultry besides frying them. Also, she is interested in trying some new spices and herbs in cooking. She will tell her daughter that cutting down on "fast foods" would be better for the whole family and will save money. In this client's case, walking is rather painful; however, Mrs. R is willing to try upper body–

strengthening exercises. Since she realizes that she has a role in planning what changes she will make to improve her health and has identified her strengths and capabilities, Mrs. R is more receptive to the dietary intervention process.

Internalize Idealized Image

....

BUILDING IN SAFEGUARDS

How to manage little problems before they become failures.
The client needs to know that anyone can have a bad day—it does not negate the process, and it does not make him/her a bad person.

....

Building in safeguards is also an important strategy. The client needs to know that anyone can have a bad day—which does not negate the process and does not make her a bad person or a failure. Most reasonable persons would agree that no one is perfect, and people do make mistakes. Usually, they stop what they are doing, take a quick look, make some course adjustments, and proceed toward their goal. Unfortunately, lots of persons, including many health care professionals, are not so forgiving when someone who is trying to make changes in the way he/she eats has a few bad days. Obviously, the seriousness of this depends on the severity of the person's condition, but in most cases, the best advice is to say, "Let's see if you can do better tomorrow." While everyone, especially the client, is anxious for success, directing blame toward the client is not productive. In fact, it can make the client react negatively as it appears that he/she can't do anything right.

The health care professional must instill in the client, that if things go wrong, just start over. Failure to provide this kind of support will damage the client's ability to internalize the idealized image of health. For example, when Mrs. R returns to the health care professional, her blood pressure is within normal range and she has lost 2 pounds; however, her cholesterol has remained at the same level. She is somewhat disappointed because she thought she had been doing everything that they had agreed upon.

The health care professional praises Mrs. R because she obviously has been making an effort to change the way she and her family eat (i.e., to internalize behaviors she believed to be ideal). Further, Mrs. R is told that sometimes cholesterol levels can take awhile to decrease and the fact that she has lost weight indicates that she is moving in the right direction. It is important to reaffirm the new changes so that the client does not backslide and so that these life-style changes can become internalized.

Eating Well: *A Script**

A good diet is important for a person's health. It can help a person maintain a healthy weight and prevent diseases such as cancer and heart disease.

Image Creation : What changes would you like to make in yourself?

Do these desired changes require that you alter your eating patterns?

YES   **NO** ────────────────────────────┐

When you imagine yourself eating well, what does it look like?

Image Appraisal : How do you feel about eating? ──────────────────┘

Could you choose a typical day from this or last week and tell me what you ate?

YES   **NO** ──────────────────┐

Record foods eaten, by size on the "food diary" (Figure 7-2).	What is the first food you usually eat in the day?
	Where do you eat during the day?
	What do you usually have when you eat there?

Who prepared(s) most of the foods you ate on this day or that you generally eat?

Record on "food diary," next to each food.

Did/Do you (generally) eat alone or with others?

Record on "food diary," next to each food.

Are there foods you ate (eat) that you really enjoy(ed)?

Record on "food diary," with a **+** next to each food.

*Script adapted from L.E. Matthews by S. Sheinfeld Gorin and J. Arnold. Parts were also adapted from *Second Report of the Expert Panel on Detection, Evaluation, and Treatment of High Blood Cholesterol of Adults* (Adult Treatment Panel II) (NIH Publication No. 93-3095), 1993, by National Cholesterol Education Program, Bethesda, MD: National Heart, Lung and Blood Institute.   *continued*

Date: _____

	Food(s) eaten	Time	Amount	Intake*	Prepared by	Ate alone/ with other(s)	Feelings at time	Like/ dislike	Adequacy†
Example	Oatmeal	8 AM	8 oz	Cereal	Self	Alone	Calm	+	kcal; mg/dl; g/dl
Meal 1									
Meal 2									
Meal 3									
Meal 4									
Meal 5									
Meal 6									

* Intake includes the following categories: grains, cereals, and breads; fruits; vegetables; meat and meat substitutes; dairy products; sugars, fats, and snack foods; soft drinks; alcoholic beverages.

† Adequacy concerns the following characteristics: energy (kcal); fat (% cal); saturated fat (% kcal); cholesterol (milligrams [mg]/deciliter [dl]); sodium (grams [g]/dl); and fiber (g/dl). The health care professional completes this column.

Figure 7-2 Food Diary.

EATING WELL: *A Script—cont'd*

Are there foods that you dislike(d)?

Record on "food diary," with a − next to each food.

Measure height and weight, alcohol use (Chapter 11), physical activity level (Chapter 8), blood pressure, blood cholesterol profile, and blood glucose level, if necessary; ask about age, work schedule, use of prescribed and over-the-counter medications, medical problems (if not already known), and any weight changes.

Would you be willing to fill out a "food diary" similar to ours over the next week to record what you eat?

YES   **NO**

Please take a few minutes to review the "food diary" with me now.

Health care professional can conduct a "rapid screen for dietary intake" and/or a "rapid screen for dietary adequacy" (National Cholesterol Education Program [NCEP], 1993 [see Helpful Resources on pp. 182-183.]) with the food diary. She/he compares client age, sex, weight, and height to recommendations, (e.g., USDHHS [1994] [see Helpful Resources section], and she/he evaluates for obesity, using current weight/desireable weight for height × 100.

I'm glad to see that your diet contains a good balance of (specify).

I'm also a bit concerned that your diet may be making it hard for you to (lose weight, lower your cholesterol, etc).

Would you be willing to change your diet at this time? What changes do you think you might be able to make right now?

Minimize Health Depleting Patterns

What do you see as obstacles to making this change now?

Review each, return to Optimize Health Supportive Patterns.

Is there someone in your household who can help you make this change?

continued

EATING WELL: *A Script—cont'd*

YES   **NO** – Could we list the persons with whom you spent the most time this week to identify someone to help?

Explore *one or two* key substitute behaviors that will be acceptable to the client (e.g., "I see that you like to drink milk. Have you ever tried low-fat or skim milk at least part of the time? Could you try skim milk with your cereal?" "I see that you fry foods a lot. Have you ever tried baking or broiling these foods? Do you think you could sometimes try to bake or broil instead of frying?")

Optimize Health Supportive Patterns

Enrich physical activity (see Chapter 8).

Identify supportive person(s) for changes.

Suggest eating more of something a client likes (i.e., "Your diet could be improved easily if you ate more fruits and vegetables every day. What are your favorite fruits, vegetables? Do you think you could eat more [specify]?")

Discuss sample menus for client to prepare for 1 week, with preparation suggestions to maximize nutrition.

Explore existing supportive eating patterns to extend and improve them (e.g., eating alone or with some else, eating at a usual time and place, shopping for food at regular intervals.)

Detail specific approaches to enhance eating behavior (e.g., touching stomach to perceive hunger, sitting at a table to eat, using small dishes, monitoring all portion sizes, varying diet).

Internalize Idealized Image

Can you share with me the dietary changes you have made in your life-style?

Review 1 week of the client's "food diary," and congratulate client on positive changes. Support client on any movement toward positive change.

EATING WELL: *A Script—cont'd*

> Out of the goals you initially set for yourself, which do you continue to value most?
>
> | Review client's list of priorities for change. |
>
> Even though this is now your new way of eating, are there times when you resumed some of your old habits? When? How?
>
> | If the client's changes have been negligible after 3 months, refer him/her to a nutrition specialist or a specialized program. Continue to follow-up with the client. |

EFFICACY OF NUTRITION INTERVENTIONS

It is obvious that effecting change in eating patterns is a difficult process, particularly when the change requires restricting a food or foods previously eaten as desired. The numerous approaches referenced in this chapter show the difficulties faced by clients and health care professionals alike. Nowhere is this more apparent than in the area of weight loss and control. A recent review demonstrated that long-term weight loss after any type of intervention was limited to a small minority of obese persons studied (Miller, 1997). Based on working with clients of all ages during a span of 2 decades, it is this author's opinion that the best focus for changing most persons' eating habits is to emphasize improved overall health. Demonstrating practical ways to eat a healthy diet that meets a person's lifestyle requirements and encouraging increased physical activity, however small the increase may be, is usually more frequently embraced by most clients. In some cases, it is more effective in the long run to downplay the emphasis on weight loss until the client is able to master the basics of dietary and life changes. Embracing a model such as the HPM and mastering its basic educational principles can be beneficial for the client and the health care professional (review in Simons-Morton, Mullen, Mains, Tabak, and Green, 1992).

However, the administrative and financial sides of health promotion and health care require more concrete measures of outcome. In considering the previously mentioned processes, how does a health care professional measure success or failure? A study of the outcome and cost-effectiveness of a diabetes education program looked at this issue. A community hospital with a multidisciplinary team approach to teaching diabetic clients self-management techniques in its outpatient center randomly compared charts of 30 participants in the diabetes self-management program with 30 charts of clients with diabetes who had received instruction (e.g., self-help brochures) only in physicians' offices. In 1 year, the average fasting blood sugar (FBS) for the clients who participated in the self-management program was 95 mg/dl less than the level before the program. This same group also lost an average of 16 pounds. For clients who were educated in the physicians' offices only, there was an average drop in FBS of only 5.4 mg/dl and a mean weight gain of 0.6 pounds (Crossan, personal communication, April 11, 1997). This study clearly demonstrated that the ongoing multidisciplinary teaching helped the clients in the program to manage and improve their overall health.

To evaluate outcome, there must be clearly measurable goals in place; otherwise both the client and the health care professional are setting themselves up for failure. As previously stated, it is usually better to have several small goals than one or two large ones. Consider the goals that were established with Mrs. R in the HPM section. When the client returned to the clinic, these goals either were achieved or they weren't. On the other hand, if the only stated goals were, "Client will improve overall health" or "Client will lose 50 pounds," it would be difficult to have any success to measure. The first one is too vague, and the second is probably unrealistic. Also, a definite time frame usually needs to be included. Once goals are achieved, they can be modified or expanded to take the client to the next level.

One could argue that proceeding in this manner is not addressing the major problem, which in the case of Mrs. R is the need for significant weight loss. However, Mrs. R's history has demonstrated that this single goal is not achievable at this time, so it is better to set up a number of small successes rather than doom her to failure for being unable to lose a lot of weight quickly. Also, these small successes may reduce her need for at least one of her medications, which would save money and might improve the way she feels.

Summary

Effecting change in human behavior of any kind is difficult. Helping someone to change lifelong eating habits is sometimes one of the most challenging tasks faced by health care professionals. Yet clients do willingly make changes if they perceive a need and if there is a practical, relatively simple way to do it. Health care professionals will be more successful in bringing about positive changes in behavior if they can adapt a model such as the Health Promotion Matrix to their client populations. In addition, for positive change to occur, the client must be an equal partner in the process. The health care professional must alternately function as a teacher, cheerleader, and partner in the process; however, the primary goal should be to give the client the tools he/she needs to succeed.

HELPFUL **RESOURCES**

CLIENT EDUCATION MATERIALS
American Heart Association
7272 Greenville Ave.
Dallas, TX 75231-4596
Phone: (800) 242-8721
American Heart Association Diet: An eating plan for healthy americans and *how to read the new food label* (Brochure No. 51-1075); *A guide to losing weight* (Brochure No. 50-1035 in English and Spanish); *Taking it off* (Brochure No. 50-079A).

Eat more fruits and vegetables: 5 a day for better health (Brochure No. 92-3248). *Diet, nutrition and cancer prevention* (NIH Publication No. 87-2878). Washington, DC: U.S. Government Printing Office.

National Diabetes Information Clearinghouse
1 Information Way
Bethesda, MD 20892-3560
Phone: (301) 468-2162
Insulin-dependent diabetes (Booklet No. 94-2098); *Non-insulin dependent diabetes* (Booklet NIH No. 92-241).

American Academy of Family Physicians
8880 Ward Parkway
Kansas City, MO 64114-2796
Weight control: Losing weight and keeping it off. Diabetes: Taking charge of your diabetes (Brochure No. 1530); *Diabetes and your body: How to take care of your eyes and feet* (Brochure No. 1553).

National Center for Nutrition and Dietetics
216 W. Jackson Blvd.
Chicago, IL 60606
(800) 366-1655
On-line: www.eatright.org

HEALTH CARE PROFESSIONAL'S RESOURCES

American Academy of Pediatrics. (1993). *Pediatric nutrition handbook.* Elk Grove, IL: Author.

American Diabetes Association. (1993). Office guide to diagnosis and classification of diabetes mellitus and other categories of glucose intolerance. *Diabetes Care, 16* (Suppl. 2), 4.

Clinician's Handbook of Preventive Services. (1994). *Height and weight tables for adults age 25 and over.* Washington, DC: U.S. Department of Health and Human Services.

Hamill, P.V.V., Drizd, T.A., Johnson, C.L., Reed, R.B., Roche, A.F., & Moore, W.M. (1979). Physical growth: National Center for Health Statistics percentiles. *American Journal of Clinical Nutrition, 32,* 607-629. (Available as weight and length charts for boys and girls, ages 0-36 months from Abbott Laboratories, Ross Products Division, Columbus, Ohio.)

Joint National Committee on Detection, Evaluation, and Treatment of High Blood Pressure. (1993). The fifth report of the Joint National Committee on Detection, Evaluation, and Treatment of High Blood Pressure (JNCV). *Archives of Internal Medicine, 153,* 154-183.

National Cholesterol Education Program. (1993). *Second report of the expert panel on detection, evaluation, and treatment of high blood cholesterol of adults (Adult Treatment Panel II).* (NIH Publication No. 93-3095). Bethesda, MD: National Heart, Lung and Blood Institute.

National Research Council, Food and Nutrition Board. (1989). *Recommended dietary allowances* (10th ed.). Washington, DC: National Academy Press.

Shils, M., Olson, J.A., & Shike, M. (1993). *Modern nutrition in health and disease* (8th ed.). Baltimore, MD: Williams & Wilkins.

U.S. Department of Agriculture and U.S. Department of Health and Human Services. (1990). *Nutrition and your health: Dietary guidelines for Americans.* (Home and Garden Bulletin No. 232, GPO 1990-273-930). Washington, DC: U.S. Government Printing Office.

U.S. Department of Agriculture. (1992). *The food guide pyramid.* (Home and Garden Bulletin No. 252). Hyattsville, MD: Human Nutrition Information Service (Order from U.S. Food and Drug Administration [product FDA 93-2259]. Information and Outreach Staff, HFE-88, Room 16-63, 5600 Fishers Lane, Rockville, MD 29857; (301) 443-3170; or [on line] http://www.nal.usda.gov/fnic/Fpyr/pyramid.html

Woolf, S.H., Jonas, S.J., & Lawrence, R.S. (1996). *Health promotion and disease prevention in clinical practice.* Baltimore, MD: Williams & Wilkins.

References

American Dietetic Association. (1992). Position of the American Dietetic Association: Nutrition intervention in the treatment of human immunodeficiency virus infection. In *Handbook of clinical dietetics* (2nd ed.). Chicago: Author.

Berg, F.M. (1996). Dysfunctional eating: a new concept. *Healthy Weight Journal, 10*(5), 88-92, 99.

Berg, F.M. (1995). Thinness: a cultural obsession. In *Health risks of weight loss* (pp. 89-98). Hettinger: ND: Healthy Weight Journal.

Blair, S.N. (1995). Diet and activity: The synergistic merger. *Nutrition Today, 30*(3), 108.

Centers for Disease Control and Prevention. (1996). Prevalence of overweight among adolescents—United States, 1988-91, *CDC Morbidity and Mortality Weekly Report, 45*, RR-9, 3.

Erdman, C.K. (1995). *Nothing to lose. A guide to sane living in a larger body.* New York: Harper Collins.

Fallon, P., Katzman, M., & Wooley, S. (Eds.). (1994). *Feminist perspectives on eating disorders.* New York: Guilford Press.

Food Marketing Institute. (1996). *Food Marketing Institute. Trends in the United States: Consumer attitudes and the supermarket, 1996.* Washington, DC: Author.

Gallagher-Allred, C., Voss, A.C., Finn, S., & McCamish, M. (1996). Malnutrition and clinical outcomes: The case for medical nutrition therapy. *Journal of the American Dietetic Association, 96*, 361-366, 369.

Goldstein, S.M. (1996). *Healthy people 2000: Are we anywhere near meeting the objectives? Nutrition Education for the Public Networking News, 18*, 1,6.

Guthrie, H.A. (1989). *Introductory nutrition* (7th ed.). St. Louis: Mosby.

Miller, W. (1997). The history of dieting and its effectiveness. *Healthy Weight Journal, 11*(2), 28-29.

National Center for Health Statistics. (1995). *Health, United States, 1994.* Hyattsville, MD: U.S. Public Health Service.

National Cholesterol Education Program. (1993). *Second report of the expert panel on detection, evaluation, and treatment of high blood cholesterol of adults (Adult Treatment Panel II).* (NIH Publication No. 93-3095). Bethesda, MD: National Heart, Lung and Blood Institute.

National Heart, Lung, and Blood Institute. (1992). *NIH strategy development workshop for public education on weight and obesity* (p. 51). Hyattsville, MD: U.S. Public Health Service.

National Research Council. (1989). *Diet and health. Implications for reducing chronic disease risk.* Washington, DC: National Academy Press.

Norris, J., Harnack, L., Charmichaekm, S., Pouane, T., Wakimoto, P., & Block, G. (1997). U.S. trends in nutrient intake: The 1987 and 1992 National Health Interview Surveys. *American Journal of Public Health, 87*(5), 740-746.

Parham, E.S. (1996). Is there a new weight paradigm? *Nutrition Today, 31*(3), 155-161.

Philadelphia Dietetic Association. (1994). *Medical nutrition therapy improves health and reduces cost: Evidence from the Philadelphia region.* Philadelphia: Author.

Princeton Survey Research Associates. (1996). *Shopping for health, 1996.* Washington, DC: Food Marketing Institute.

Prochaska, J.O., Velicer, W.F., Rossi, J.S., Abrams, D.B., & Follick, M.J. (1994). Stages of change and decisional balance for 12 problem behaviors. *Health Psychology, 13*, 39-46.

Ross Timesaver. (1993). Body image and weight control. *Dietetic Currents, 20*, 1.

Sigman-Grant, M. (1996). Stages of change: A framework for nutrition interventions. *Nutrition Today, 31*, 162-170.

Simons-Morton, D.G., Mullen, P.D., Mains, D.A., Tabak, E.R., & Green, L.W. (1992). Characteristics of controlled studies of patient education and counseling for preventive health behaviors. *Patient Education and Counseling, 19*(2), 175-204.

Sizer, F.S., & Whitney, E.N. (1994). *Hamilton and Whitney's nutrition concepts and controversies* (6th ed.). St. Paul, MN: West.

Skender, M.L., Goodrick, G.K., Del Junco, D.J., Reeves, R.S., Darrell, L., Gotto, A.M., & Foreyt, J.P. (1996). Comparison of 2-year weight loss trends in behavioral treatments obesity: Diet, exercise, and combination interventions. *Journal of the American Dietetic Association, 96*, 342-346.

U.S. Department of Agriculture, U.S. Department of Health and Human Services. (1995). *Nutrition and your health: Dietary guidelines for Americans* (Home and Garden Bulletin No. 232) (4th ed.). Washington, DC: U.S. Government Printing Office.

U.S. Department of Health and Human Services. (1988). *The Surgeon General's report on nutrition and health.* (Publication No. (PHS) 88-50210). Washington, DC: U.S. Government Printing Office.

U.S. Department of Health and Human Services. (1991). *Healthy people 2000: National health promotion and disease prevention objectives* (DHHS Publication No. PHS 91-50213). Washington, DC: U.S. Government Printing Office.

Williams, S.R. (1997). *Nutrition and diet therapy.* (8th ed.) St. Louis: Mosby.

Physical Activity

Karen J. Calfas

EDITORS' NOTE

Physical Activity and the Individual Client System. Clients and health care professionals share a widespread belief in the importance of physical activity to promoting health. Yet, few health care professionals have confidence in their ability to counsel clients in steps toward more effective physical activity. Moreover, clients who do elect to engage in physical activity programs often turn to health clubs, trainers, videos, and television for direction. Some individuals devise their own physical activity routine. Many others lead more sedentary lives or exercise sporadically. Physical activity is often linked to recreational interests and events. Rarely do individuals consult their health care professional to plan a systematic physical activity regimen. The individual more often self-prescribes physical activity in isolation from health care professionals. Additionally, health care professionals tend to offer limited advice, if any at all, about maximizing the effectiveness of physical activity for each individual.

Physical Activity and Minimizing Health Depleting Patterns/Optimizing Supportive Patterns. Author Karen Calfas, PhD, reminds us that when health care professionals work with clients, an individualized approach to using the dimensions of the HPM is essential. Client movement through the dimensions is variable for each of the nine behaviors. Through the PACE (Physician-based Assessment and Counseling for Exercise) approach, Calfas details a plan for minimizing health depleting patterns and optimizing health supportive patterns for individual clients with different needs. The PACE approach explores the staging of physical activity from precontemplation to contemplation to active. In the contemplation stage, individuals are encouraged to set a goal for physical activity, reinforce its benefits, and find solutions for roadblocks. As in the HPM, clients work with health care professionals to identify supports for physical activity in their lives and barriers to adopting these new behaviors.

Protocol for Adults in Primary Care Settings and the Health Promotion Matrix Script. In keeping with the PACE approach, Calfas has presented an empirically tested protocol for health care professionals to instruct their clients who differ in their acceptance of physical activity so that they move from one stage of activity to the next. The script in this chapter integrates the PACE protocol with the Health Promotion Matrix (HPM).

Being "healthy and vital" requires being able to perform physical activities, which bring enjoyment and satisfaction to life. In fact, restrictions in physical activity (or the ability to perform basic physical activities of daily living) are associated with substantial decreases in quality of life. Despite the high value Americans place on maintaining vigor, they do little to protect it. Americans are less physically active than in previous years, and an aging population will become more dependent on others for basic needs if they don't become more active now.

Health care professionals can have a big impact on the amount of physical activity their clients perform and in turn improve their clients' quality of life. Whereas some health care professionals do not see counseling on this topic as their responsibility, many find it quite important. In fact, some would argue that it is not only the responsibility of primary health care professionals but that it is bad medicine if they don't counsel about physical activity.

Counseling about healthful life-styles is essential for the prevention of chronic disease, and all members of the primary care team can be involved. This chapter focuses on contributions that can be made by nurses, physicians, physician assistants, and health educators, to name a few. Any health care professional interested in helping her/his clients adopt and maintain a physically active life-style will be able to use the principles described in this chapter.

These principles are meant to be used in conjunction with topics presented in other chapters of this text. Obviously, every health behavior topic cannot be addressed in the context of one client encounter. Rather, the health care professional should prioritize the behavioral health issues based on the client's needs and interests.

This chapter specifically addresses physical activity counseling in the primary care setting—broadly defined as any clinical setting where clients seek preventive health care. The chapter is organized into six sections. The first deals with specific health benefits and the epidemiology of physical activity in the United States. The second section describes theoretical models used to understand physical activity behavior. The third section describes provider barriers to counseling and reviews studies of different counseling approaches used in primary care and their efficacy. The fourth section discusses how to use Project PACE protocols to counsel apparently healthy adults in an outpatient setting and includes example scripts. The fifth section includes an overview of physical activity counseling for children and older adults. The final section focuses on future directions for physical activity in health promotion.

HEALTH BENEFITS AND EPIDEMIOLOGY OF PHYSICAL ACTIVITY
Cardiovascular Benefits

In 1992 the American Heart Association named physical inactivity an independent risk factor for cardiovascular disease (Fletcher et al., 1992). This means that regardless of smoking status, family history, and the presence of other related diseases, if someone is inactive, his/her risk of developing cardiovascular disease is higher than that of an active person with similar characteristics. The relative risk of developing coronary heart disease associated with physical inactivity is approximately 1.8 (Berlin & Colditz, 1990), so those who are inactive are almost twice as likely to develop cardiovascular disease.

Also, there appears to be a dose response relationship between physical activity and the incidence of cardiovascular disease (U.S. Department of Health and Human Services [USDHHS], 1996) (i.e., more physical activity leads to greater benefits). In one study (Paffenbarger, Hyde, Wing, & Hsieh, 1986) participants who expended 71 to 143 kilocalories of energy per day had a 22% reduction in overall mortality, whereas those who expended 143 to 214 kilocalories per day had a 27% reduction.

Other Benefits

While the most compelling evidence suggests that physical activity reduces the risk of cardiovascular disease, especially coronary heart disease, there are many other benefits associated with an active life-style (USDHHS, 1996). There is clear evidence that physical activity is associated with decreased risk of colon cancer and decreased risk of developing non–insulin-dependent diabetes mellitus. Physical activity is associated with improved joint function, and weight bearing exercise is associated with achieving and maintaining peak bone mass. Physical activity also is an important factor in achieving and maintaining a healthy weight. In fact, studies of weight loss suggest that regular physical activity is essential for weight loss maintenance (Brownell, 1995). Finally, physical activity is associated with reduced symptoms of depression and anxiety, and it appears to improve health-related quality of life and psychological well-being (USDHHS, 1996).

How Much Physical Activity is Enough?

Although research on this issue is not entirely clear, experts agree that some activity is better than no activity (USDHHS, 1996). There is recent evidence to suggest that many health benefits can be derived from moderate-intensity activity (Blair et al., 1995) and that this type of activity can be broken up into two or three short bouts during the course of a day (Debusk, Stenestrand, Sheehan, & Haskell, 1990; Ebisu, 1985).

The Centers for Disease Control and Prevention and the American College of Sports Medicine recently revised physical activity recommendations for adults (Pate et al., 1995), emphasizing the importance of moderate activity. These organizations state, "Every U.S. adult should accumulate 30 minutes or more of moderate-intensity physical activity on most, preferably all, days of the week" (Pate et al., 1995). This new guideline is not intended to replace the more familiar guideline of 20 minutes of vigorous physical activity 3 or more times per week (Pate et al., 1995). However, those who already meet the moderate guidelines will benefit even more by increasing their activity level.

Experts agree that expending between 150 and 200 kilocalories per day can provide many health benefits. Examples of activities that burn 150 kilocalories include walking 2 miles in 30 minutes, gardening for 30 to 45 minutes, washing windows or floors for 45 to 60 minutes, pushing a stroller 1.5 miles in 30 minutes, or bicycling 5 miles in 30 minutes (USDHHS, 1996). These activities can be broken down into 2 or 3 shorter bouts but must accumulate to at least 30 minutes per day, or nearly every day, to meet the minimum guidelines for improved health.

From a behavioral point of view, research identifying the benefits of moderate-intensity physical activity is good news. Many Americans engage in little or no leisure-time physical activity (USDHHS, 1996); however, for these persons, participation in moderate physical activity may be more acceptable and achievable. Moderate activity, such as gardening or walking, is often very acceptable to those not interested in "exercise." For this reason, recommending moderate activity to clients is a good place for the health care professional to begin, and if clients are interested in and able to perform vigorous activity, such as jogging or swimming, that also can be recommended.

How Active are Americans?

Despite the known benefits of a physically active life-style and guidelines established by experts, more than 60% of adults do not perform the recommended amount of regular physical activity. In fact, 25% of all adults are completely sedentary in their leisure time (USDHHS, 1996). Physical activity decreases with age, and women and those with lower income and less education are less active than men and those with higher income and education. According to the U.S. Surgeon General's Report on physical activity (1996), approximately 22% of U.S. adults meet the moderate physical activity guideline (i.e., 30 minutes of moderate activity most days of the week), and only 15% of adults engage in vigorous activity on a regular basis (i.e., 20 minutes, 3 times a week) during their leisure time.

Healthy People 2000

Physical activity is one of the targeted areas in the Year 2000 objectives for the nation (USDHHS, 1990). In addition to increasing the proportion of physically active Americans, one of the goals is to "increase to at least 50 percent the proportion of primary care providers who routinely assess and counsel their patients regarding the frequency, duration, type and intensity of each patient's physical activity practices" (USDHHS, 1990, p. 92). Estimates about the number of primary health care professionals who currently counsel their clients vary greatly (Lewis, Wells, & Ware, 1986; Marcus et al., 1995; Orleans, George, Haupt, & Brodie, 1985; Rosen, Logsdon, & Demak, 1984). According to *Healthy People 2000*, in 1988 approximately 30% of physicians counseled their sedentary clients about physical activity (USDHHS, 1991). Estimates of those who routinely counsel all of their clients are likely lower. Physicians' beliefs about health habits influence their counseling practices. For example, physicians who currently practice a healthy life-style or are in the process of improving their life-style are more likely to counsel their clients about health habits (Wells, Lewis, Leake, & Ware, 1984; Lewis et al., 1986). Unfortunately, many health care professionals may use counseling techniques that are ineffective because they do not incorporate methods already known to promote health behavior acquisition (Orleans et al., 1985).

THEORETICAL MODELS FOR UNDERSTANDING PHYSICAL ACTIVITY

There are many theories about how persons change health behaviors. Increasing knowledge about the risks or benefits of a health behavior is generally considered to be necessary but insufficient to change that behavior. This section focuses on three theoretical models of health behavior change that are known to influence health behaviors and applies them to physical activity counseling.

Determinants of Physical Activity

If health care professionals ask sedentary clients why they don't exercise, they will probably give a list of barriers, including lack of time, poor motivation, lack of support from family and friends, bad weather, and their displeasure for physical activity. In fact, competing demands are among the most common reasons persons are not physically active (USDHHS, 1996; Calfas, Sallis, Lovato, & Campbell, 1994). Additionally, there are few things about modern society that promote physical activity. Electric garage door openers, escalators, and televisions—including their remote controls—all encourage persons to be sedentary, therefore one's environment also can be a barrier to an active life-style. Because so many factors influence participation in physical activity, it is a difficult behavior to change. Successful attempts to change activity patterns require modification of personal, social, and environmental factors. To maximize its effect, an intervention must have a theoretical foundation, target known mediators of the behavior, and apply the most effective intervention approaches.

Behavioral theories have been applied to the study of physical activity determinants (or correlates). These theories, or models, have been used to generate hypotheses about how to best help someone adopt (or maintain) physical activity. Three theories are discussed here: social cognitive theory, the transtheoretical model, and the health belief model.

Social Cognitive Theory

Social cognitive theory states that personal factors and the environment interact to determine behavior and that all three can influence each other (Bandura, 1986). This theory takes into account the complexity of behaviors such as participation in physical activity. A key component of social cognitive theory is self-efficacy. Self-efficacy is the belief in one's ability to competently perform a behavior. To determine a client's self-efficacy, the health care professional could ask, "How confident do you feel about meeting this exercise goal over the next 2 weeks?" If the client is highly confident, then he/she is experiencing high self-efficacy, and research suggests that those who experience high self-efficacy are more likely to be physically active (Sallis, Hovell, Hofstetter, Faucher et al., 1989).

Other determinants of physical activity include social support, perceived barriers and benefits, and enjoyment. Research indicates that social support (e.g., exercising with a friend, praising a friend for being active, or doing a chore for a family member so that he/she has time to be active) is consistently associated with increased physical activity (Sallis, Hovell, & Hofstetter, 1992). Perceived benefits of physical activity (e.g., endorsing statements such as, "I know if I exercise this morning, I'll feel good all day") also have been consistently positively associated with participation in physical activity (Ali & Twibel, 1995). Similarly, perceived barriers to activity are negatively associated with physical activity (Dishman & Steinhardt, 1990). Finally, enjoyment also is consistently positively associated with physical activity (Courneya & McAuley, 1994). These determinants, or predictors, of physical activity are modifiable and should be targeted during an intervention aimed at improving adherence to an activity program.

Transtheoretical Model

The second model is called the transtheoretical model, developed by Prochaska and Di-Clemente (1982). In this model, behavior change is conceptualized as progressing through five "stages of change." With respect to physical activity the five stages are described as follows: (1) precontemplation, when one is not engaging in physical activity and is not interested in doing so in the near future; (2) contemplation, when one is not engaging in activity (or is irregularly active) but is interested in becoming more active; (3) preparation, when one is making small changes in physical activity; (4) action, when one is beginning a new activity program; and (5) maintenance, when one has been regularly active for more than 6 months (Marcus, Rakowski, & Rossi, 1992). Persons may progress through these stages out of order and revert back to earlier stages. An important implication of the stages of change model is that clients need different intervention messages, depending on their current stage of change or "readiness to change." By assessing stage of change, the health care professional will be able to identify a client's current behavioral patterns, his/her interest in changing those patterns, and his/her likelihood of actually changing those behavioral patterns.

The behavioral science literature also teaches that when persons acquire new health behaviors, certain methods are more effective in motivating persons to acquire new behaviors. Some health education approaches focus on giving information to clients. This is certainly necessary and appropriate but is usually insufficient to change behavior, and changing behavior is necessary to obtain the desired outcome, or the idealized image of health. Rather, interventions that target improved behavioral skills are more likely to lead to behavior change. For example, helping a client increase his/her social support (e.g., by identifying a friend or family member who will encourage him/her) and increase his/her self-efficacy (e.g., by setting realistic and measurable goals) will do more to increase physical activity than just by telling a client to be more active. In fact, a review of the literature compared didactic, knowledge-based interventions with behavioral skill-based interventions and showed that the latter were more than twice as likely to lead to behavior change (Mazzuca, 1982).

Health Belief Model

The health belief model is a widely used model to explain health behavior. It is based on the assumption that one's beliefs influence behavior (Rosenstock, 1990). According to the Health Belief Model, behavior change is most likely to occur if one believes he/she is susceptible to a disease or condition; that the condition has serious, unwanted consequences; and that there are relatively more benefits than barriers to taking action. Research on the Health Belief Model has yielded mixed results. It is successful in predicting health behavior change in some instances (Cummings, Jette, Brock, & Haefner, 1979), but when the health behaviors are more complex (e.g., smoking cessation) it is often unsuccessful at predicting change (Flay, 1985).

The PACE program (described in detail later in this chapter) uses the stages of change model to identify where clients are on the continuum of readiness to change and also targets known determinants of physical activity specifically for each stage using concepts from social cognitive theory.

HEALTH CARE PROFESSIONAL PHYSICAL ACTIVITY COUNSELING

Clients report that they value their physician's advice and want to receive counseling about physical activity (Godin & Shephard, 1989). Currently much of the information about physical activity delivered to the American public comes from infomercials and other unreliable sources. In surveys, clients report that they welcome information about physical activity from the primary care setting because they see their health care professional as a credible source of health information (Gilmore, 1983).

Barriers to Health Care Professional Counseling

There are many reasons why primary care providers do not regularly counsel their clients about physical activity. Surveys estimate that one half to two thirds of physicians cite time as the primary barrier against counseling clients about physical activity (Orleans et al., 1985; Lewis et al., 1986). Certainly as constraints from managed care and restrictive measures of efficiency are introduced into more medical settings, spending even 5 minutes during a 15-minute client encounter may be unrealistic, especially if it is nonreimbursable time. Lack of time and reimbursement are not the only barriers. Many health care professionals are not trained to deliver behavioral counseling, there are no standard protocols to follow, health care professionals are pessimistic about clients' ability to change their life-styles, and some primary health care professionals do not see it as their job to provide this counseling (Orleans et al., 1985).

Efficacy of Current Physical Activity Counseling Approaches

Despite the formidable competing demands, some health care professionals do counsel their clients; however, only a few studies have explored the efficacy of this type of counseling. Four studies have examined physical activity counseling in primary care settings. The first was a quasi-experimental study conducted by Logsdon, Lazaro and Meier (1989) and was designed to focus on several behavioral risk factors in addition to physical inactivity. Experimental and control practices were matched and included 72 primary care physicians. Intervention providers were trained during a continuing medical education (CME) program and received written materials for themselves and their clients. Intervention clients (n = 1409) received at least 15 minutes of physician advice during a free prevention visit, whereas control clients (n = 809) did not receive any risk factor counseling. During the 12 months of the trial, 34% of the sedentary intervention clients who received counseling began exercising, compared with 24% of control clients ($p < .05$).*

In another quasi-experimental study, Lewis and Lynch (1993) compared clients who received counseling (n = 162) from 24 family practice residents with those who did not (n = 221). The residents received 15 minutes of individual training, a laminated card of the counseling protocol, and client education material placed in the chart to act as a prompt to counsel. Clients received 2 to 3 minutes of exercise advice from residents and written materials. More clients who received advice began exercising, compared with those in the control group (+10% [study group] vs. +2% [control group], $p < .04$). Additionally, clients who received advice from residents reported a greater increase in duration of exercise per session (+27 minutes versus −5 minutes, $p < .01$) and in total weekly minutes of exercise (+109 minutes versus −24 minutes, $p < .01$).

The third study compared the effects of routine care, video, and video plus written materials on exercise behaviors (Graham-Clarke & Oldenburg, 1994). Eighty general practitioners in Australia were randomly selected according to practice. Intervention physicians

---

*A p value $<.05$ means that there is less than a 1 in 20 probability that this result would have occurred by chance alone.

were trained during workshops to assess risk factors, provide feedback, tailor advice to client needs, and use the video and written materials. Clients in the two experimental groups that included videos also received a risk assessment from their physician, which included information about nutrition and smoking in addition to physical activity. Clients were assessed at 4 and 12 months. Results showed that physician advice and additional educational materials had no effect on clients' level of physical activity.

The fourth counseling approach to be evaluated was Project PACE. Two studies have been conducted to date on this intervention. The first was an acceptability trial designed to test the feasibility and utility of the PACE intervention materials among providers, office staff, and clients (Long et al., 1996). Primary health care professionals (92 physicians and 8 nurse practitioners) were recruited and trained in four parts of the United States—Rhode Island, Michigan, Tennessee, and California. Providers used the PACE materials with their apparently healthy adult clients for 5 months. Providers, clients, and office staff were assessed after the trial period.

Results indicated that the materials were highly acceptable and usable to health care professionals. Most providers reported that the suggested counseling was easy to do and that it improved their ability to perform physical activity counseling. Seventy-five percent reported that they would recommend PACE to other health care professionals and 80% said that their clients were "receptive" or "very receptive" to counseling. Client assessment of the PACE process was uniformly positive, with 80% of clients reporting that the forms were "easy" or "very easy" to understand, and 72% reporting that the counseling was helpful. However, only 35% of health care professionals reported that office staff were able to adopt PACE with minimal difficulty. Similarly, more than one third of office staff reported difficulty with paperwork or procedures related to PACE (Long et al., 1996). Although the PACE materials are acceptable and usable to providers, the process is heavily dependent on the office staff, thus a subsequent study of PACE included more specific procedures and training for office staff.

The second PACE study was designed to determine its efficacy, or effect on clients' physical activity level if the intervention was delivered as written (Calfas, Long et al., 1996). In this quasi-experimental study, 212 apparently healthy sedentary adults either received PACE counseling during a scheduled "well visit" or received standard care. Seven control health care professionals were matched to 10 intervention health care professionals according to medical specialty, geographic location in San Diego County, and client demographics. Health care professionals were trained individually during a 30 to 60 minute session. Office staff were trained separately. Clients were assessed before and 4 to 6 weeks after their scheduled appointment. Compared with control clients, those who received PACE counseling increased their use of cognitive and behavioral strategies to increase physical activity; behavioral methods and improved self-efficacy were associated with an increase in physical activity (Calfas, Sallis, Oldenburg, & Ffrench, 1997). Clients who received PACE counseling reported more minutes of walking for exercise compared with those who did not receive counseling (75.4 minutes versus 42.2 minutes/week, $p <$ .05). Whereas all patients were in the contemplation stage of change at baseline, more participants in the intervention group moved into the action stage of change compared with those in the control group (52% versus 12%, $p < .001$).

In summary, there are very few outcome studies of physical activity counseling in primary care settings. The research to date is mixed but generally supports the efficacy of this type of counseling. Currently, the PACE intervention is being studied in an HMO setting with longer-term follow-up. Other interventions are also being developed, as described later in this chapter. It is certainly appropriate for health care professionals to begin or continue advising their clients about the benefits of physical activity. The next section describes the PACE counseling approach in more detail.

PACE COUNSELING APPROACH
Overview of PACE

PACE counseling was developed in response to the health objective for the year 2000 that calls for a greater proportion of physicians to counsel their clients about physical activity. The focus of PACE is to alter known determinants of physical activity using a simplified version of the stages of change approach to categorize clients into one of three stages of readiness for change (precontemplators, contemplators, and actives). A different counseling approach was developed for clients in each of the three stages, and these corresponded to three counseling protocols. A one-page assessment tool is used to identify clients' stage of change. The back of the assessment page includes the Physical Activity Readiness Questionnaire (PAR-Q) (Chisholm, Collis, Kulak, Davenport, & Gruber, 1975), which screens for contraindications to exercise and is meant to be a risk assessment for the provider to use in addition to the medical record and the provider's knowledge of the client and his/her medical history.

PACE was developed for use by health care professionals with their apparently healthy adult clients in an outpatient setting. Although the original purpose of the PACE project was to develop tools for physicians to use, it is appropriate for nurses, health educators, and other members of the primary care team to conduct this counseling. The PACE approach has been adapted for use in many other medical settings, including diabetes management and physical therapy settings, to name a few. The goal of PACE is to promote modest increases in physical activity, therefore health care professionals often recommend that clients begin a program of moderate physical activity. For clients already doing moderate or vigorous physical activity, recommendations that include vigorous activity may be made, as appropriate.

The PACE Process

Clients are given the one-page PACE assessment tool (a measure of interest and their level of physical activity) when they arrive for their well visit (Figure 8-1). They complete it and return it to the receptionist who notes their stage of change and gives the clients the appropriate one-page counseling protocol. The first side contains stage-relevant questions about physical activity, which the client is asked to complete and return to the receptionist. The back of the protocol contains stage-relevant information for the client's use at home. The protocol is printed in duplicate, with one copy for the client and one copy for the medical record, if desired.

After the client completes the first half of the protocol in the waiting room and returns it to the receptionist, it is placed in the chart for the health care professional to review before entering the examination room. The counseling takes 2 to 5 minutes, depending on the protocol. During counseling, the health care professional discusses stage-tailored content with the client and they come to an agreement about a physical activity goal, if one is to be set.

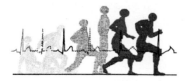

_____   _____
          Patient's Name   Date

What is Your PACE SCORE?

This form will help your doctor understand your level of physical activity. Please read the entire form and then choose the number below that best describes your *current* level of physical activity or your interest in physical activity. Do *not* include activities that you do as part of your job.

"**Vigorous**" exercise includes activities like jogging, running, fast cycling, aerobic classes, swimming laps, singles tennis, and racquetball. Any activity that makes you work *as hard as jogging* and lasts *20 minutes* at a time should be counted. These types of activities usually increase your heart rate, and make you sweat, and you get out of breath. *(Do not count weight lifting.)*

"**Moderate**" exercise includes activities like brisk walking, gardening, slow cycling, dancing, doubles tennis, or hard work around the house. Any activity that makes you work *as hard as brisk walking,* and that lasts at least *30 minutes* at a time, should be counted.

Circle One
Number Only

Current Physical Activity Status

1. I do not exercise or walk regularly now, and I do not intend to start in the near future.

2. I do not exercise or walk regularly, but I have been thinking of starting.

3. I am trying to start to exercise or walk. *(or)* During the last month I have started to exercise or walk on occasion *(or on weekends only)*.

4. I have exercised or walked infrequently *(or on weekends only)* for over one month.

5. I am doing vigorous or moderate exercise, less than 3 times per week *(or moderate exercise less than 2 hours per week)*.

6. I have been doing moderate exercise, 3 or more times per week *(or more than 2 hours per week)* for the last 1-6 months.

7. I have been doing moderate exercise, 3 or more times per week *(or more than 2 hours per week)* for 7 months or more.

8. I have been doing vigorous exercise, 3-5 times per week for 1-6 months.

9. I have been doing vigorous exercise, 3-5 times per week for 7-12 months.

10. I have been doing vigorous exercise, 3-5 times per week for over 12 months.

11. I do vigorous exercise 6 or more times per week.

Rev. 3/96

Please Complete Other Side

Figure **8-1** PACE assessment tool. *(From* Project PACE (physician-based assessment and counseling for exercise): Physician manual *by K. Patrick, J. Sallis, B. Long, K. Calfas, W. Wooten, & D. Sharpe, 1992, San Diego: San Diego State University and Centers for Disease Control, Cardiovascular Health Branch.)*

PHYSICAL ACTIVITY READINESS QUESTIONNAIRE (PAR-Q)*

A SELF-ADMINISTERED QUESTIONNAIRE FOR ADULTS

PAR-Q is designed to help you help yourself. Many health benefits are associated with regular exercise, and the completion of PAR-Q is a sensible first step to take if you are planning to increase the amount of physical activity in your life.

For most people, physical activity should not pose any problem or hazard. PAR-Q has been designed to identify the small number of adults for whom physical activity might be inappropriate or those WHO SHOULD HAVE MEDICAL ADVICE CONCERNING THE TYPE OF ACTIVITY most suitable for them.

Common sense is your best guide in answering these questions. Please read them carefully and check YES or NO opposite the question as it applies to you.

YES	NO		
☐	☐	1.	Has a doctor ever said that you have a heart condition and recommended only medically supervised activity?
☐	☐	2.	Do you experience chest pain as a result of physical activity?
☐	☐	3.	Have you experienced chest pain in the past month?
☐	☐	4.	Do you tend to lose consciousness or fall over as a result of dizziness?
☐	☐	5.	Do you have a bone or joint problem that could be aggravated by the proposed physical activity?
☐	☐	6.	Has a doctor ever recommended medication for high blood pressure or a heart condition?
☐	☐	7.	Are you aware through your own experience, or a doctor's advice, of any other physical reason against your exercising without medical supervision?

Note: If you have a temporary illness, such as a common cold, or are not feeling well at this time — Postpone.

You are participating in a national program that is designed to increase physical activity among adults. We need to know what you think of the information you receive from your healthcare providers today. If you would be willing to talk to a researcher over the telephone in the near future, please sign below and provide us with a phone number and time of day that you prefer to be contacted.
Thank you for your help.

_____
Patient's Name

Telephone # _____ (Home/Work) *please circle*

_____ (A.M./P.M.)
Time of Day

Figure 8-1. For legend, see opposite page.

General Principles for PACE Counseling

PACE was developed to address the many barriers physicians have to this type of counseling. There was little researchers could do about the reimbursement issue. However, researchers could develop standardized counseling protocols, good training, and minimize the time required to conduct the counseling.

The first general principle is *time efficiency*. The challenge with any type of health behavior counseling in primary care is that it needs to be brief enough for health care professionals to actually do it, yet it needs to have enough substance to change client behavior. Imbalance in either direction will produce little or no change in physical activity. Primary care providers want to do the best thing for their clients, and if they believe that it is important for a specific client to address the issue of physical activity and that spending a few minutes will produce change in the client, they are usually willing to try it. The PACE protocols are based on theories of behavior change known to affect physical activity, and they can be delivered in 2 to 5 minutes.

Another general principle is that it must be a *team effort*. If the office staff is not fully aware and willing to distribute and collect the assessment and counseling forms, the process will not work. Likewise, different health care professionals in the same office may deliver different parts of the message. Generally, there are two parts of the PACE message—the advice, or recommendation, to be active and the counseling about how to be or stay active. In some settings, the physician may give the recommendation and a nurse or health educator may do the rest of the counseling. In other settings the nurse or physician will deliver both the advice and counseling, and that is how the PACE process is described here. The point is that this counseling is delivered in the primary care setting and that the health care professional should use whatever resources are available to deliver the counseling in whatever manner makes the most sense for that setting. The PACE materials were designed to accommodate different settings and have been used by a variety of health care professionals, including physicians, nurse practitioners, nurses, health educators, and physical therapists.

A third principle is *to get the right message to the right person*. In almost every encounter, time is premium. Health care professionals don't have time to waste giving detailed advice to clients who are not interested, but that is what many health care professionals do. They do not take into account how "ready" the client is to deal with a particular clinical issue. Similarly, they should not spend time extolling the benefits of physical activity to someone who is already active (i.e., "preaching to the choir"). The PACE approach allows the health care professional to target her/his message to meet a client's unique needs.

The PACE materials use a modified version of the stages of change theory to divide clients into one of three groups, or stages: (1) "precontemplators," those not active and not interested in becoming active; (2) "contemplators," those not active or irregularly active but interested in beginning an activity program; and (3) "actives," those already active at some level. As previously stated, a different message has been specifically designed to be relevant to clients in each stage. The stages were collapsed into three because the intervention message was not significantly different between preparers and contemplators or for those in action or maintenance, and three protocols (messages) were more practical for use in a medical setting than five. See Table 8-1 for a summary of PACE counseling by stage.

The value of identifying clients as part of one of these groups is that health care professionals can spend the most time with the middle group, the contemplators. They are the most "ready" for change and are the most likely to adopt an activity program based on

Table **8-1**

Summary of PACE counseling by stage

	PRECONTEMPLATOR	CONTEMPLATOR	ACTIVE
Title of PACE protocol	"Getting out of your chair"	"Planning the first step"	"Keeping the PACE"
PACE assessment score (scored 1-11)	1	2-5	6-11
Goal for the client	Think about the benefits of physical activity	Plan for a moderate physical activity program and identify roadblocks and potential solutions	Maintain physical activity and avoid relapse
Primary behavioral strategies to use	Listening, identifying benefits, problem-solving	Goal-setting, self-efficacy, social support, praise	Relapse prevention, goal-setting, self-efficacy, praise
Message/ recommendation	Health care professional identifies potential benefits of physical activity; gives a personalized message for client to consider beginning a program of moderate physical activity	Health care professional praises client for intending to begin a program; recommends moderate physical activity program based on client's interests; together with client agrees on a realistic goal, identifies who will help client be active, reinforce benefits, and problem-solve around anticipated barriers	Health care professional recommends continued physical activity at client's current level (or any other suggestions); Reviews current physical activity program and recommends changes, if appropriate (encourages variety, enjoyment, and convenience); identifies potential sources of relapse and problem-solves around them; advises client about sport-related overuse injury prevention

Continued

Table 8-1

Summary of PACE counseling by stage—cont'd		
	PRECONTEMPLATOR	**CONTEMPLATOR**	**ACTIVE**
Action	No specific goal is set	Health care professional records physical activity goal for a specified period at bottom of protocol; both sign	Health care professional records physical activity goal (set for longer period)
Materials	Protocol only	Protocol plus walking handout (or others)	Protocol and other handouts, as appropriate
Time	1-2 min	5 min (or more if available)	2-4 min

their health care professional's recommendation. Also, clients moving from mostly sedentary to moderately active life-styles will derive the most benefit (Blair et al., 1995). Using this "tailoring" approach allows health care professionals to be more efficient with time because they do not waste time outlining an exercise program for a precontemplator, nor do they waste time by espousing the benefits of activity to someone in the active stage.

The final general principle is *to involve the client.* Persons are more likely to meet goals if they are able to participate in setting them. PACE counseling uses an interactive approach in which the health care professional and client agree on the physical activity goals, using recommendations from the health care professional and information from the client about what would be most enjoyable and doable given a particular life-style. Involving the client in the decision-making process makes him/her more accountable for the result and encourages him/her to take responsibility for his/her own health.

PACE PROTOCOLS & THE HEALTH PROMOTION MATRIX*

The original PACE materials were developed using social cognitive theory (Bandura, 1986) and the stages of change model (Prochaska & DiClemente, 1982). Health care professionals give stage-relevant messages designed to increase known behavioral determinants of physical activity. What follows is a description of the PACE counseling from the perspective of the Health Promotion Matrix; therefore it is conceptually and may be empirically different from the original PACE counseling protocols.

Image Creation

Image creation fosters a client's ability to identify an ideal image of himself/herself in relation to health. The PACE model enables a realistic self-assessment of physical

*Adapted from K.J. Calfas by J. Arnold and S. Sheinfeld Gorin.

activity goals. The model rests on an understanding of differing images of self in relation to physical activity and differing motivations to alter these images. The precontemplator does not imagine the self as active. The minority of clients, probably about 10%, can be considered precontemplators (i.e., their expressed interest in physical activity is minimal or absent). The health care professional is careful not to place pressure on clients who are declared precontemplators. Further, the health care professional cannot express disappointment or frustration with the precontemplator but rather realign expectations for client goal attainment and express acceptance of the personal image the client describes.

Contemplators imagine themselves becoming more physically active. Contemplators, probably about half of clients encountered, indicate a desire to change. They may desire more energy, weight loss, or reduction of risk factors for certain diseases found in their family histories.

Actives already have a positive personal image with regard to their physical activity status. They may also wish to increase or change activity. Actives, probably constituting 40% of clients, create an image consistent with their current level of physical activity, hoping to maintain their practices, and avoid physical injury.

Image Appraisal: PACE Assessment

The PACE model provides for specific assessment protocols for all clients. The protocol for precontemplators (PACE score = 1) is called "Getting out of your chair;" the underlying principle is to get precontemplators to think about beginning a program of physical activity, not to agree to a program. Clients appreciate not being pressured to begin exercise. Clients complete part of the PACE protocol in the waiting room, including listing two potential benefits of being physically active, reasons they are not currently active, and two ways they can get around their roadblocks. If they can't think of how to get around roadblocks, examples are listed on the back of the protocol.

The protocol for contemplators is called "Planning the first step" (PACE score = 2 to 5). Clients are asked to identify two benefits of physical activity and what type of program they would like to begin. They are asked to be fairly specific, identifying activities they enjoy, where they will be active, a realistic frequency of activity, duration, and who in their life can provide social support for their program. The health care professional could begin by praising them for wanting to begin: "Mr. Jones, it is great that you are thinking about starting a walking program. You indicated on your form that you would like to have more energy, and being physically active will help you do that. I'd like to help you get started. Are there other things you would like to gain by being active? (Client responds.) In addition to having more energy, being active will help you control your weight, reduce the risk of cardiovascular disease, and even help you sleep better at night."

The protocol for actives is called "Keeping the PACE" (PACE score = 6 to 11). The goal for this intervention is to review their current program; make suggestions for changes, if appropriate; and discuss ways to avoid relapse. Clients are asked to document the type, intensity, frequency, and duration of their current activity program; with what aspects of their program they are most and least satisfied; and any changes they desire to make their activity program more convenient, enjoyable, or safe.

Minimize Health Depleting Patterns

Once the precontemplator has identified roadblocks, or depleting patterns, the health care professional works with this client to clarify the reasons he/she is not currently active and reviews in greater depth the two ways he/she has identified to get around these roadblocks. Together the client and health care professional clarify the special circumstances pertinent to the client's life. Plans are created together that address each obstacle. Again, the goal of the PACE protocol is not to encourage the precontemplators to agree to a program of physical activity, but to get them to think about beginning one. The health care professional gives personalized advice for thinking about beginning a moderate program of physical activity. The health care professional may present specific information to improve client health status to strengthen this dialogue. After reviewing a client's protocol a health care professional might say, "Ms. Smith, I understand that you are not interested in starting a walking program now. However, since you are overweight and are taking medication for high blood pressure, walking regularly—even just 15 minutes per day to start—will help both of these conditions. You listed lack of time and interest as barriers to beginning a program. I'd like you to look over the potential ways to get around these barriers on the back of this sheet and think about starting a walking program. It is important to your health."

Contemplators have already been able to identify two benefits of physical activity and the type of program they would like to begin. The client and the health care professional should review the proposed plan. Some clients will write a plan that is too ambitious or not challenging enough. The health care professional should negotiate with the client: "I know you are anxious to get started, and that's great, but why don't you start out with walking 2 to 3 days per week for 15 to 20 minutes each time, instead of every day. Once you've mastered that, you can gradually increase." Next, it is also important to assess the clients' social support: "Who will help you stick to your physical activity program? What kinds of things would you specifically not like them to do?" If the client does not express confidence in his/her ability to carry out the plan (i.e., he/she is less than 90% sure he/she can do it), the health care professional adjusts the goal to something easier to accomplish.

Next, the client names barriers that might get in his/her way of meeting the goal. Planning in advance for these barriers is much more powerful than waiting for them to happen. The health care professional might say, "You indicated that being too tired when you come home from work and being bored with exercise are barriers for you. You also said that you might try exercising in the morning. I think that's a great idea. You'll feel good all day knowing you have done something good for yourself. Another way people deal with this problem is to exercise before they go home at night, so take your walking shoes with you to work and walk there before you leave or meet a friend at a park. Just avoid going home and sitting down in front of the television, because you're right, you might not leave to do your walk. The other thing you mentioned is that exercise can be boring. Try to vary what you do—walk one day, swim the next—and where you do your activity. That will take the routine out of it."

After agreeing on the frequency, intensity, type, and time (duration) of physical activity, both the health care professional and client sign the protocol, indicating the client's commitment to keep this goal for a specified period. The back of the protocol contains suggestions of moderate or vigorous activities and how to get around road-blocks and an activity log. This protocol takes approximately 5 minutes to complete.

For actives, the health care professional makes recommendations about the client's level of activity. In some cases it may be necessary to recommend decreasing current activity: "I see that you run 5 miles 6 to 7 times per week. That's a lot of exercise, and I'm concerned that you might get a sports-related injury. What is prompting you to exercise that much? Have you encountered any problems?" Assess social support and potential relapse situations by asking, "Who can help you accomplish this goal?" and "What is most likely to interfere with your activity program? What has caused you to stop exercising in the past? What did you do to get back on track the last time you stopped exercising for a while?" The health care professional can make suggestions based on the back of the protocol.

Optimize Health Supportive Patterns

For precontemplators, the door is always open regarding client interest in beginning an exercise program. The health care professional values the importance of physical activity for client health and communicates this position clearly and repeatedly to the client while accepting the client's personal image and practice of physical inactivity. This openness and acceptance is key to continuing a relationship with the client and to supporting the client in thinking about beginning a program of physical activity. The health care professional supports the client to think about the benefits of physical activity and to consider getting started. The health care professional can say, "When, or if, you decide you'd like to begin, come back and see me and I'll help you get started." If the client even thinks about it before the next visit, the health care professional will have succeeded.

When working with contemplators, health care professionals should ask about enjoyment: "You need to choose an activity that you enjoy doing. What kind of activities have you done and enjoyed in the past?" Once the contemplator has identified an enjoyable activity, the health care professional can determine the client's confidence in performing it. A good way to assess self-efficacy is to ask the client, "How confident are you that you can do this plan for the next 2 weeks?" If the client expresses definite confidence in carrying out the plan, the health care professional supports the client's confidence. Next the health care professional assesses the client's social support: "Who will help you stick to your physical activity program? What kinds of things can they do which will be helpful to you?"

When working with actives, the health care professional might recommend that they continue with the same level of activity: "I see here that you are walking 3 times a week for half an hour. That's a good level for you. Keep up the good work." The health care professional might also suggest they increase current activity: "I see that you are riding your bike 2 times per week. Have you considered adding another exercise time to your schedule? Given your medical history and current physical condition, you can safely exercise 3 times per week. Finally, the health care professional assesses their self-efficacy: "On a scale from 1 to 5, how confident are you that you can continue doing regular physical activity for the next 3 months?" Again, if clients are not highly confident, the health care professional readjusts the goal for success. The health care professional notes the agreed upon program in the box at the bottom of the protocol. Provide handouts that address patient questions the health care professional does not have time to answer fully. A list of resources is found at the end of this chapter.

Internalize Idealized Image

Reaching an idealized image of physical activity differs considerably for precontemplators, contemplators, and actives. The precontemplator's receptivity may be strengthened, resulting in greater willingness and readiness to take action. The contemplator may realize a program of greater physical activity that is doable in his/her life-style and may integrate these changes into a more physically active way of life. The active client may refine a physical activity program already valued and enjoyed and may learn ways to alter exercises to avoid injury and to prolong interest in the program. Self-satisfaction and intrinsic gains may further commit the active client in living a physically active life.

PHYSICAL ACTIVITY: *A Script**

Image Creation	On a scale measuring physical activity, are you "inactive," "moderately active," or "very active?" If you are "inactive" or "moderately active," can you imagine yourself participating in more physical activity, or are you interested in participating in more physical activity?
	If you selected *inactive* as the level that describes you best, would you consider learning about how physical activity could benefit you?
	If you selected *moderately active* as the level that describes you best, would you consider learning about a physical activity plan specifically designed for you?
	If you selected *very active* as the level that describes you best, would you consider assistance in reviewing your current program for suggested changes, if needed?
Image Appraisal	While you are waiting, would you consider filling out this protocol about your physical activity/inactivity patterns? It is important that you be honest about your answers because it will help me learn more about you and to suggest ways that I may be helpful to you.

(Clients complete the appropriate PACE protocol; the health care professional places them in the appropriate category according to their score: "Getting out of your chair" for precontemplators; "Planning the first step" for contemplators; or "Keeping the PACE" for actives.)

---

*Adapted from K.J. Calfas by S. Sheinfeld Gorin and J. Arnold.

Physical Activity: *A Script—cont'd*

For Precontemplators:

Will you identify two potential benefits of being physically active?

Can you identify reasons why you are not currently active?

YES*   **NO**

> Refer client to the back of the PACE protocol.

For Contemplators:

What physical activities do you enjoy?

Where do you engage in physical activity?

How frequently do you engage in physical activity?

In general, how long are you physically active (the duration of these activities)?

Who is supportive of your activity and encourages you?

For Actives:

> Document the type, intensity, frequency, and duration of the client's current activity program.

Who is supportive of you in maintaining this exercise program?

Have any injuries resulted from your exercise program?

What aspects of your program are most satisfying to you?

What aspects are least satisfying to you?

Are there any changes you would like to make in the activity program in which you currently engage?

Do you think your activity program is convenient? Safe? Enjoyable?

YES†   **NO**

Which aspects are not convenient? Why?

Which are not safe? Why?

Which are not enjoyable? Why?

continued

*See Precontemplators section under Minimize Health Depleting Patterns.
†See Actives section under Minimize Health Depleting Patterns.

Physical Activity: *A Script—cont'd*

Minimize Health Depleting Patterns

For Precontemplators:

> Give the recommendations to consider being more physically active.

As your health care professional, I would like to encourage you to consider beginning a physical activity program. Physical activity is likely to improve your _____ (give example of medical condition or other benefit the client will personally receive). This is why I think it is so important.

> Clarify what you mean by being "more physically active."

I'm not talking about running a marathon. Many of the health benefits can be gained by brisk walking 30 minutes most days of the week, but you could start with less than that and still get some benefits.

> Ask about barriers

Together, let's look at each roadblock you have identified and ways around it.

> For each barrier to participation, the health care professional asks the client to identify an alternative, using the PACE protocol and the Helpful Resources list at the end of this chapter.

Do you think you will consider beginning a physical activity program?

YES   **NO**

That's great. May I answer any other questions about physical activity or inactivity?

> The health care professional reviews each barrier to identify other alternatives.

For Contemplators:

How realistic is your plan? Is it too ambitious? Is it not challenging enough?

> The health care professional should assess the plan to determine whether it is medically and behaviorally appropriate and suggest and agree upon alterations, as necessary.

Physical Activity: *A Script—cont'd*

Are you more than 90% confident that you can carry out your plan for physical activity?

YES   **NO**
| |
| Do you feel you would be more successful if we
| adjusted the goal to something easier to accomplish?

What could you say to persons in your support network to help them learn about the kinds of things you would like them to do to further encourage you to successfully carry out your plan?

What barriers have you identified that might get in the way of meeting your physical activity goals?

How can you adjust your daily patterns to plan ahead so that these barriers do not limit your success?

Will you sign this plan to indicate your commitment to your goals?

YES *   **NO**
                                |

| Renegotiate the goal toward something the client will do. |

For Actives:

What aspects of your activity program are the least satisfying?

What has caused you to stop exercising in the past?

What would you change about your activity program to make it more convenient?

What would you change to make it more enjoyable?

| Suggest that client try listening to music, talking with a friend, or doing physical activity at a location with nice scenery. |
| If you are exercising hard, you can try to go a little slower or vary the intensity of your exercise to make it more enjoyable. |

What would you change to make it safer?

Do you think your activity program may be too vigorous or simply too much exercise?

| Given your activity program, you could be at risk for certain sports injuries. |
| Identify modifications of or alternatives to the program selected, using the Helpful Resources list. Refer to a physical activity specialist if necessary. |

---

*See Contemplators section under Optimize Health Supportive Patterns.   *continued*

PHYSICAL ACTIVITY: *A Script—cont'd*

If you have encountered any barriers to your activity program, what could you do to avoid them?

> Review each barrier with the client.

Optimize Health Supportive Patterns

For Precontemplators:

You identified two benefits of being physically active. In what ways are these two benefits important to you?

Your interest in listening and learning about the benefits of physical activity is impressive. May I answer any other questions about physical activity or inactivity?

For Contemplators:

Since experiencing success is so important, how confident are you that you can carry out the activity program we have planned?

Your support network is vital to success in carrying out the plan. Have you shared your interest in exercise with others you care about to enlist their support for your plan?

YES　　　　　**NO**

Good. That support will help you maintain your program.

> Let's list each person in your support network and how each could support your plan.

Could you sign the protocol, indicating your commitment to your activity program?

YES*

For Actives:

Is there anything about your physical activity program that you find especially satisfying?

Is there anything in your current physical activity program you would like to alter?

A support network is important to success. Who helps you to accomplish your physical activity goals?

What did you do to get back on track the last time you stopped exercising for a while?

How confident are you that you can continue your activity program?

---

*See Contemplators section under Internalize Idealized Image.

Physical Activity: *A Script—cont'd*

Internalize Idealized Image	**For Precontemplators:**
	When may we talk again about your physical activity?
	For Precontemplators and Actives:
	How would you evaluate your progress in maintaining your physical activity goals?
	How have you solved the problems you encountered with your physical activity program?
	When may we talk again to discuss your progress?

PACE Follow-up

PACE counseling includes a brief follow-up, which may be done in person or over the phone. If there is a reason for the client to return to the clinic, that is ideal but not necessary. In the PACE efficacy study (Calfas et al., 1997) a trained health educator conducted the follow-up during 10-minute phone interviews 2 weeks after the office visit. Follow-up can be done by any trained health care professional. It does not have to be the same health care professional who conducted the original counseling. The purpose of the follow-up is to ask how a client's activity goals are progressing, to identify problems and solutions, and to provide support. If formal follow-up is not possible, it is recommended that health care professionals send a postcard follow-up and be sure to ask about physical activity at the client's next office visit. Ideally, clients should complete a new PACE protocol at every well visit. This allows the health care professional to continue tailoring the exercise program to meet the client's changing needs. This may not be practical in some settings, but the health care professional should at least ask about physical activity at every well visit.

Making PACE Part of the Clinical System

An effective protocol will not help if health care professionals do not use it. The use of these kinds of protocols and prevention efforts in general will increase as their relative importance increases in the health care field. As medicine changes from a system in which reimbursement occurs only when persons are sick to a captitated system in which a profit is made by keeping clients well, these protocols will be in more demand. If they are effective, time will be provided for health care professionals to conduct this counseling.

Additionally, the literature on exercise adoption and maintenance is relatively scant compared with that of smoking cessation and diet intervention. Physical activity was only recently recognized as an independent risk factor for cardiovascular disease. It took many years for smoking cessation recommendations from physicians to become part of the "routine" primary care visit. It is this author's hope that physical activity will follow suit.

There are four practical factors that can significantly increase the likelihood of PACE counseling occurring as planned. First, health care professionals should use chart stickers to identify clients who are being "paced." This will alert any health care professional to ask about physical activity at every visit. Second, during counseling visits, the completed protocol should be put on (or in) the chart as a reminder to health care professionals to do the full PACE counseling. Third, the health care professional decides which clients will receive PACE counseling routinely in her/his clinic. Good candidates may be clients receiving annual pap smears, routine physical examinations, or routine blood pressure checks for controlled hypertension. Fourth, the physical activity level (PACE score) is included with vital sign measurements, similar to how smoking status is recorded as a "vital sign" in many clinic settings today. Finally, no system can be designed to accommodate all possible settings, so the system can be changed so that it works in any setting.

PHYSICAL ACTIVITY COUNSELING FOR CHILDREN, ADOLESCENTS, AND OLDER ADULTS
Children and Adolescents

Adolescents benefit from physical activity and should be physically active daily, or nearly daily, and engage in 20 minutes of moderate to vigorous physical activity at least 3 times per week (Patrick & Sallis, 1994). The *Guidelines for Adolescent Preventive Services (GAPS)* (American Medical Association, 1992) recommends that adolescents (ages 11 to 21 years) receive annual preventive services visits that address both medical and behavioral aspects of health. With respect to physical activity, GAPS recommends that "all adolescents should receive health guidance annually about the benefits of exercise and should be encouraged to engage in safe exercise on a regular basis."

Project PACE is currently developing a web-based physical activity and nutrition intervention for health care professionals to deliver to adolescents. It is currently in the early stages of development and will not be available for several years. However, the *Clinician's Handbook of Preventive Services: Put Prevention Into Practice* (USDHHS, 1994) outlines an approach to use specifically with children and adolescents. Nine of their counseling recommendations are paraphrased here. Health care professionals should do the following.

1. Inquire about physical activity at every visit (for both children/adolescents and their parents).
2. Stress that smaller children need only a safe place to be active and play, whereas older children should be encouraged to engage in 20 to 30 minutes of vigorous physical activity at least 3 times per week.
3. Emphasize participation in physical activities that are enjoyable—not just competitive; recognize that unpleasant experiences with competition can discourage physical activity in general.
4. Encourage physical activities that can be enjoyed into adulthood (e.g., walking, swimming, cycling).
5. Encourage physical activities that can be done as part of a daily routine all year.
6. Encourage parents and children to engage in a variety of physical activities.
7. Counsel on the appropriate use of safety equipment such as helmets and protective pads.
8. Should encourage children with disabilities to participate fully in appropriate physical activities.
9. Advise students engaged in "power" sports such as football of the dangers of anabolic steroids.

Older Adults

Counseling older adults about physical activity is similar to counseling younger adults with few exceptions. For one, older adults are more likely to require physician approval to begin a physical activity program. Once obtained, many seniors lead very active life-styles. For this age group, health care professionals should emphasize the benefits of moderate physical activity. Brisk walking, gardening, and some forms of housework can lead to health benefits. Living independently is very important to this age group. Strength training exercises can help older adults maintain independence by increasing muscle strength to perform activities of daily living such as maintaining personal hygiene, maintaining a household, and transportation. Health care professionals should encourage older clients to think of each physical challenge, such as lifting groceries into their car or reaching for something on the top shelf, as an opportunity to maintain their muscle strength and independence. The American Association of Retired Persons and the Arthritis Foundation have good information and physical activity programs available for senior citizens. Michael Goldstein, MD, and other researchers at Brown University are developing provider-based physical activity counseling protocols specifically for use with older adults.

FUTURE DIRECTIONS FOR HEALTH PROMOTION IN PHYSICAL ACTIVITY

One of the most important goals for the health promotion field is to develop counseling protocols that work. To date only a few studies have been conducted, with promising but very preliminary results. Before the health promotion field can ask health care professionals to spend valuable time doing these kinds of interventions, the field needs to demonstrate more fully that these interventions work. Project PACE is evolving. Two new research studies have been funded to (1) include nutrition messages along with physical activity counseling and (2) to adapt PACE counseling (both nutrition and physical activity) to an adolescent population. The new protocols are being developed and evaluated and will not be available for approximately 3 years. Although these protocols are not yet available, the general counseling principles can be used with many health promotion topics and adapted for other populations and age groups.

A very important clinical issue in preventive medicine is how to manage all of the demands for preventive medicine counseling. Physical activity is only one of many important health topics about which providers and clients should be talking and planning. Eight other health behaviors/topics are outlined in this text, and each deserves special attention. *Put Prevention into Practice* (USDHHS, 1994) was developed at the Office of Disease Prevention and Health Promotion. Its purpose was to create a system of preventive care that could be adopted by primary care settings. It uses a "prevention passport," which documents the prevention topics to be addressed for a given patient. It also gives well-researched guidelines on what types of interventions are recommended for many behavioral health topics including nutrition, physical activity, drug and alcohol use, tobacco, safety, sexually transmitted disease, and others. There are no rules about what topic to address first. Most health care professionals make that decision based on clinical relevance to their clients and their clients' level of interest.

The future of health promotion and the delivery of medical services in general will be shaped by the research presented in this text, as well as other sources. The National Committee for Quality Assurance (NCQA) is a national group devoted to reporting on the quality of managed care plans. It has developed a set of standardized performance criteria to compare the quality of care provided by different health care plans. These performance standards are called HEDIS (Health Plan Employer Data and Information Set). Currently, there are no performance standards for physical activity counseling, but there are standards for smoking cessation and other health promotion topics. These standards will provide a rationale for the provision of health promotion counseling in primary care settings and will have a large impact on the quantity and quality of such counseling. Additional information about HEDIS can be obtained on the Internet at www.ncqa.org/hedis.htm and in Chapter 2.

Whatever the future standards include, health care professionals need to tailor the message to meet the needs of their clients and remember that they can have a significant impact on the health of their clients.

Summary

Physical activity is a major factor in risk reduction for cardiovascular disease, colon cancer, and non–insulin-dependent diabetes mellitus. It is a key element of weight control and maintenance of bone mass. Physical activity is related to reduced symptoms of depression and anxiety and overall psychological well-being. Yet more than 60% of all adults do not perform the recommended moderately intense activity, such as gardening or walking 30 minutes or more every day. A common barrier to activity is competing time demands.

The transtheoretical model, which focuses on the stages of change through which a client moves in adopting physical activity, is the foundation of the PACE model described in this chapter. Several studies have demonstrated its efficacy with adults in outpatient settings. The client's stage of change, from precontemplation to contemplation to active, determines the approach each health care professional adopts. The PACE script presented here incorporates principles of the HPM and guides clients through a multifaceted behavioral change.

HELPFUL **RESOURCES**

Project PACE
San Diego State University
San Diego, CA 92182-4701
Phone: (619) 594-5949.
Fax: (619) 594-5613
PACE *physician's manual.* Outlines the PACE process in more detail.

Put prevention into practice, education and action kit. Published by the U.S. Public Health Service (stock number: 017-001-00492-8). Contains 5 health guides, one *Clinician's Handbook,* and samples of all other materials.
Fax: (202) 512-2250.

How to start a walking program (No. 1002). The physician and sportsmedicine, 1991. Copywritten handout, single-page tear-offs. McGraw-Hill.
Phone: (800) 525-4776

Parlay International. Provides non-copywritten, one-page exercise handouts. These can be copied onto letterhead and given to clients, as appropriate. Topics include dressing for exercise in warm/cold weather, buying good walking/running shoes, stretching, injury prevention.
Phone: (800) 457-2752.

HELPFUL **RESOURCES**

NATIONAL ORGANIZATIONS

American College of Sports Medicine, (327) 637-9200

American Heart Association, (800) 233-1230

YMCA Program Store, (800) 872-9622

American Alliance for Health, Physical Education, Recreation, and Dance (AAHPERD), (800) 321-0789

President's Council on Physical Fitness, (202) 273-3424

• • •

The author of this chapter wishes to acknowledge the team of PACE researchers: Kevin Patrick, MS, MD; James F. Sallis, PhD; Barbara J. Long, MD, MPH; and Wilma J. Wooten, MD, MPH.

References

Ali, N.S., & Twibell, R.K. (1995). Health promotion and osteoporosis prevention among postmenopausal women. *Preventive Medicine, 24,* 528-534.

American Medical Association, Department of Adolescent Health. (1992). *Guidelines for adolescent preventive services* (pamphlet). Chicago: Author. Order No. NL018292.

Bandura, A. (1986). *Social foundations of thought and action.* Englewood Cliffs, NJ: Prentice-Hall.

Berlin, J.A., & Colditz, G.A. (1990). A meta-analysis of physical activity in the prevention of coronary heart disease. *American Journal of Epidemiology, 132,* 612-628.

Blair, S.N., Kohl, H.W., Barlow, C.E., Paffenbarger, R.S., Gibbons, L.W., & Macera, C.A. (1995). Changes in physical fitness and all-cause mortality: A prospective study of healthy and unhealthy men. *Journal of the American Medical Association, 273,* 1093-1098.

Brownell, K.D. (1995). Exercise in the treatment of obesity. In K.D. Brownell, & C.G. Fairburn (Eds.), *Eating disorders and obesity: A comprehensive handbook* (pp. 473-478). New York: Guilford Press.

Calfas, K.J., Long, B.J., Sallis, J.F., Wooten, W.J., Pratt, M., & Patrick, K. (1996). A controlled trial of physician counseling to promote the adoption of physical activity. *Preventive Medicine, 25,* 225-233.

Calfas, K.J., Sallis, J.F., Lovato, C.Y., & Campbell, J. (1994). Physical activity and its determinants before and after college graduation. *Medicine, Exercise, Nutrition, and Health, 3,* 323-334.

Calfas, K.J., Sallis, J.F., Oldenburg, B., & Ffrench, M. (1997). Mediators of change in physical activity following an intervention in primary care: PACE. *Preventive Medicine, 26,* 297-304.

Chisholm, D.M., Collis, M.L., Kulak, L.L., Davenport, W., & Gruber, N. (1975). Physical activity readiness. *British Columbia Medical Journal, 17,* 375-378.

Courneya, K.S., & McAuley, E. (1994). Are there different determinants of the frequency, intensity, and duration of physical activity? *Behavioral Medicine, 20,* 84-90.

Cummings, K., Jette, A., Brock, B., & Haefner, D. (1979). Psychosocial determinants of immunization behavior in a swine influenza campaign. *Medical Care, 17,* 639-649.

Dishman, R.K., & Steinhardt, M. (1990). Health locus of control predicts free-living, but not supervised, physical activity: A test of exercise-specific control and outcome-expectancy hypotheses. *Research Quarterly for Exercise and Sport, 61,* 383-394.

Debusk, R.F., Stenestrand, U., Sheehan, M., & Haskell, W.L. (1990). Training effects of long versus short bouts of exercise in healthy subjects. *American Journal of Cardiology, 65,* 1010-1013.

Ebisu, T. (1985). Splitting the distance of endurance running: On cardiovascular endurance and blood lipids. *Japanese Journal of Physical Education, 30,* 37-43.

Flay, B.R. (1985). Psychosocial approaches to smoking prevention: A review of findings. *Health Psychology, 4,* 449-488.

Fletcher, G.F., Blair, S.N., Blumenthal, J., Caspersen, C., Chiatman, B., Epstein, S., Falls, H., Froelicher, S., Froelicher, V.F., & Pina, I.L. (1992). Benefits and recommendations for physical activity programs for all Americans: A statement for health professionals by the Committee on Exercise and Cardiac Rehabilitation of the Council on Clinical Cardiology, American Heart Association. *Circulation, 96,* 340-344.

Gilmore, A. (1983). Canada fitness survey finds fitness means health. *Canadian Medical Association Journal, 129,* 181-183.

Godin, G., & Shephard, R. (1989). An evaluation of the potential role of the physician in influencing community exercise behavior. *American Journal of Health Promotion, 4,* 225-229.

Graham-Clarke, P., & Oldenburg, B. (1994). The effectiveness of a general-practice-based physical activity intervention on patient physical activity status. *Behavior Change, 11,* 132-144.

Lewis, B.S., & Lynch, W.D. (1993). The effect of physician advice on exercise behavior. *Preventive Medicine, 22,* 110-121.

Lewis, C.E., Wells, K.B., & Ware, J. (1986). A model for predicting the counseling practices of physicians. *Journal of General Internal Medicine, 1,* 14-19.

Logsdon, D.N., Lazaro, C.M., & Meier, R.V. (1989). The feasibility of behavioral risk reduction in primary medical care. *American Journal of Preventive Medicine, 5,* 249-256.

Long, B.J., Calfas, K.J., Wooten, W., Sallis, J.F., Patrick, K., Goldstein, M., Marcus, B., Schwenk, T., Carter, R., Torez, T., Polinkas, L., Heath, G. (1996). A multisite field test of the acceptability of physical activity counseling in primary care: Project PACE. *American Journal of Preventive Medicine, 12,* 73-81.

Marcus, B.H., Pinto, B.M., Clark, M.M., DePue, J.D., Goldstein, M.G., & Simkin-Silverman, L. (1995). Physician-delivered physical activity and nutrition interventions. *Medicine, Exercise, Nutrition, and Health, 4,* 325-334.

Marcus, B.H., Rakowski, W., & Rossi, J.S. (1992). Assessing motivational readiness and decision making for exercise. *Health Psychology, 11,* 257-261.

Mazzuca, S.A. (1982). Does patient education in chronic disease have therapeutic value? *Journal of Chronic Diseases, 35,* 521-529.

Orleans, C.T., George, L.K., Haupt, J.L., & Brodie, K.H. (1985). Health promotion in primary care: A survey of U.S. family practitioners. *Preventive Medicine, 14,* 636-647.

Paffenbarger, R.S., Hyde, R.T., Wing, A.L., Hsieh, C.C. (1986). Physical activity, all-cause mortality, and longevity of college alumni. *New England Journal of Medicine, 314,* 605-613.

Pate, R.R., Pratt, M., Blair, S.N., Haskell, W.L., Macera, C.A., Bouchard, C., Buchner, D., Ettinger, W., Heath, G., King, A., Kriska, A., Leon, A., Marcus, B., Morris, J., Paffenbarger, R., Patrick, K., Pollock, M., Rippe, J., Sallis, J., & Wilmore, J. (1995). Physical activity and public health: A recommendation from the Centers for Disease Control and Prevention and the American College of Sports Medicine. *Journal of the American Medical Association, 273,* 402-407.

Patrick, K. & Sallis, J. (1994). Physical activity guidelines for adolescents: Consensus statement. *Pediatric Exercise Science, 6,* 302-314.

Prochaska, J.O., & DiClemente, C.C. (1982). Transtheoretical therapy: Toward a more integrative model of change. *Psychotherapy: Theory, Research and Practice, 20,* 161-173.

Rosen, M.A., Logsdon, D.N., & Demak, M.M. (1984). Prevention and health promotion in primary care: Baseline results on physicians from the INSURE Project on lifecycle preventive health services. *Preventive Medicine, 13,* 535-548.

Rosenstock, I.M. (1990). The health belief model: Explaining health behavior through expectancies. In K. Glanz, F.M. Lewis, & B.K. Rimer (Eds.), *Health behavior and health education: Theory, research and practice.* San Francisco: Jossey-Bass.

Sallis, J.F., Hovell, M.F., Hoffstetter, C.R. (1992). Predictors of adoption and maintenance of vigorous physical activity in men and women. *Preventive Medicine, 21,* 237-251.

Sallis, J.F., Hovell, M.F., Hoffstetter, C.R., Faucher, P., Elder, J.P., Blanchard, J., Casperson, E.J., Powell, K.E., & Christenson, G.M. (1989). A multivariate study of determinants of vigorous exercise in a community sample. *Preventive Medicine, 18,* 20-34.

U.S. Department of Health and Human Services, U.S. Public Health Service. (1991). *Healthy people 2000: National health promotion and disease prevention objectives* (DHHS Publication No. PHS 91-50213). Washington, DC: U.S. Government Printing Office.

U.S. Department of Health and Human Services, U.S. Public Health Service, Office of Disease Prevention and Health Promotion. (1994). *Clinician's handbook of preventive services: Put prevention into practice,* Washington, DC: U.S. Government Printing Office.

U.S. Department of Health and Human Services. (1996). *Physical activity and health: A report of the surgeon general,* Atlanta: U.S. Department of Health and Human Services, Centers for Disease Control and Prevention, National Center for Chronic Disease Prevention and Health Promotion.

Wells, K.B., Lewis, C.E., Leake, B., & Ware, J.E. (1984). Do physicians preach what they practice? A study of physicians' health habits and counseling practices. *Journal of the American Medical Association, 252,* 2846-2848.

Sexual Awareness

Jacqueline Rose Hott

EDITORS' NOTE

Sexuality and the Family Client System.   Sexual behavior originates in utero and continues until death. Sexuality is central to one's sense of self and begins with the cognizance of the genitals then progresses to the creation, and oftentimes re-creation of the gender identity, to the joining with others in the discovery of the sexual union and includes the modification in sex drive.

   The family is the social agent for education and values for the sexual self. In many families, sex is not discussed, and sexual identity is denied. Children are viewed as asexual. As a result, sexual selves are formed in the context of peers, members of the extended family, or through images in the media.

   Gender relationships, too, whether same sex or heterosexual, are created within the context of the family. Early formative experiences observing parents are the template for future sexual behaviors expressed outside the family.

Sexual Awareness and Image Creation.   Author Jacqueline Rose Hott, RN, CS, PhD, FAAN, explores human sexuality across the lifespan, highlighting each phase of development and the influence each wields on the creation of a sexual self. It is within the family that one uncovers one's sexual identity, but it is also within the family that one's sexual identity can be denied, suppressed, or abused, thus profoundly influencing one's sexual image. An important aspect of sexual growth is the challenge of shaping one's own unique image with the support one obtains through family life or in opposition to the forces of family connectedness.

Case Materials for Gay/Lesbian/Bisexual Teens and the Health Promotion Matrix Script.   Hott, through a candid application of the Health Promotion Matrix (HPM), provides questions that will stimulate discussion of sexual identity for teens struggling with their sexuality. In general, a recent review of school-based programs in sex education revealed that not all sex and AIDS education programs have significant effects on adolescent sexual risk-taking behavior, but specific programs may delay the initiation of intercourse, reduce the frequency of inter-course, reduce the number of sexual partners, or increase the use of condoms or other con-traceptives (Kirby, 1994). Given the increase in sexually transmitted diseases—especially HIV infection—and the relative vulnerability of the young, health care professionals need to discuss clients' sexual images as formidable influences on their behavior. The script applies the HPM to sexual awareness.

Sexuality in humans is more than just sex. It's a part of everything humans are, ever have been, or ever will be. It's who humans are from the top of their heads to the toes of their feet. Sexuality is a part of humans' lives from the womb until death. A major concern for the health care professional regarding sexuality is that although most practitioners acknowledge and laugh at sexual humor and can probably repeat a sexual joke, they are not able to talk seriously about sexuality and do not feel comfortable responding to their clients' sexual concerns. As *Sexual Etiquette 101* (Hatcher, Atkinson, Cates, Glasser, & Legins, 1993) points out, Americans have always been taught to be discreet about their sexuality and therefore find it hard to have an open, constructive discussion about sexual matters. The consideration of sexuality is as significant as any other aspect of total health to include in client assessment. Sexuality is an activity of daily living (ADL)—a healthy, natural part of human life.

The Sexuality Information and Education Council of the United States (SIECUS) (1996) affirms the aforementioned philosophy. SIECUS develops, collects, and disseminates information; promotes comprehensive education; and advocates the rights of individuals to make responsible sexual choices. At its September 1995 Board of Directors meeting, SIECUS updated and approved position statements on issues relating to human sexuality, sexual health, and sexuality education and information.

> Human sexuality encompasses the sexual knowledge, beliefs, attitudes, values, and behaviors of individuals. Its various dimensions include the anatomy, physiology, and biochemistry of the sexual response system; identity, orientation, roles, and personality; and thoughts, feelings and relationships. The expression of sexuality is influenced by ethical, spiritual, cultural, and moral concerns (SIECUS, 1996, p. 21).

This chapter looks at sexuality as a healthy dimension of being human and uses the HPM to focus on sexual attitudes, beliefs, and behaviors and how they are influenced throughout the lifespan physiologically, psychologically, socioculturally, and spiritually.

PSYCHOSEXUAL DEVELOPMENT

Psychosexual development is a continuous process by which humans become the sexual beings they are (see Table 9-1 for a summary of sexual issues over the lifespan). At any point in the human lifespan, sexuality can represent the cumulative effects of many forces, and it is one aspect of psychologic and maturational development that is constantly being shaped and directed by a trio of forces acting simultaneously. One force is biologic, including physiologic and hormonal influences, innate maturational timetables, and cognitive maturation. The second force is cultural, including social learning in the family and influences outside the family. The third force is intrapsychic, including normal developmental conflicts; unconscious fantasies, conflicts, and attitudes; and the influences of all earlier experiences and emotions that help individuals approach and cope with each new biologic, cultural, and intrapsychic event (Gadpaille, 1981).

Prenatal Period and Infancy

This section briefly explores the prenatal influences that determine sexual development. The presence of normal sex chromosomes (XY or XX) determines whether the undiffer-

Table 9-1

Summary of primary sexual concerns over the lifespan

	CONCERNS
Prenatal	Differential valuing; preference for males, females
	Transmission of HIV/AIDS from mother to infant
Toddlerhood (18 months to 3 years)	Genital exploration
	Purposeful masturbation
	Gender dysphoria
Preschool period (3½ to 6 years)	Sexual abuse
	Heterosexual fantasies
	Cryptorchidism
School years (6 years to puberty)	Preference for same sex
	Drug involvement
	Sexual experimentation
	Assaults on body image
	Sexual abuse
Adolescence (puberty)	HIV/AIDS, other STDs, Risky sexual practices
	Pregnancy
	Date rape
	Oedipal sexual conflicts
	Same sex, bisexual or transsexual orientation

SUGGESTED APPROACHES

Advocate for changes in practices toward women
Promote family's healthy acceptance of either gender
Counsel mother on safe sex practices
Advise avoidance of drugs, needles (see Chapter 11)
Advise few partners, safe sexual practices
Advise avoidance of sex with prostitutes, anal sex
Specialized medical assessment, treatment for baby

Teach family to:
    Use correct language to identify genitals
    Accept, rather than show disgust
    Avoid overt or covert disparagement of either gender

Good touch/bad touch programs
Encourage family to:
    Display openly warm welcoming attitude toward child's budding interests
    Let child know that parents' intimacies reserved for one another
Evaluate, discuss orchiopexy, prosthesis

Provide professional guidance in acceptance and adaptation, support for family

Teach family to:
    Support changes as positive
    Avoid blame, secure professional help
Health care professional must report

Advise adolescent to:
    Avoid drugs and needle sharing
    Avoid sex until ready, say no to pressure
    Avoid sex with prostitutes, anal sex
Advise few partners, safe sexual practices
Encourage sex education, family planning courses in school, community
Health care professionals must report
Consider "morning after" postcoital regimen
Recommend professional counseling
Encourage family members to discuss and resolve feelings
Use nonjudgemental approach
Provide realistic, educational discussions with family
Recommend psychiatric evaluation, as necessary

Continued

Table **9-1**

Summary of primary sexual concerns over the lifespan—cont'd	
	CONCERNS
Young Adulthood (20s)	Sex role not reversible Primary sexual problems Secondary problems from the relationship HIV/AIDS, STDs Infertility Sexuality and pregnancy
Middle and Later Adulthood (30-50 years of age)	Extramarital relationships Diminished sexual gratification Men: erectile dysfunction, ejaculatory retardation Women: anorgasmia, dyspareunia, Perimenopause, menopause HIV/AIDS/STDs
Aging (older than 65 years)	Men: ejaculatory response Women: lubrication slower, orgasmic phase shorter, fragile vaginal tissues, clitoral stimulation painful HIV/AIDS/STDs

entiated gonadal anlage develops into testes in the XY embryo, producing androgens at about 6 weeks, or into ovaries in the XX embryo somewhat later. External genitalia of both genders form from the same embryologic tissue, but in the presence of fetal androgens, the genital tubercle enlarges and becomes a penis with the urethra enclosed in the underside of the urogenital folds. By the end of the 14th week of fetal development, external male genital morphology is complete and irreversible. With the female, in the absence of androgens, the genital tubercle becomes a clitoris. The vaginal introitus develops from the open urogenital groove while the urogenital folds and labioscrotal swellings, instead of fusing as they do for the male's scrotum, remain unfused and enlarge to form the labia minora and labia majora. Female genital morphology, like that of the male's, is complete and irreversible by the 14th week.

At about 6 weeks, but probably extending for a longer period, fetal androgens start organizing parts of the developing brain, particularly in the hypothalamus and limbic system, which may mediate behavior and temperament more characteristic of males than of females. A comparable central nervous system is organized in the female but without fetal androgen so that at puberty gonadotropins accounting for the menstrual cycle, character-

SUGGESTED APPROACHES

Encourage acceptance in family, finding satisfying partner
Provide information, medical evaluation; condition new behaviors
Encourage client to increase communication, understanding, intimacy

Address in context of relationship, with approaches similar to those for adolescents
Focus discussion on achieving a loving relationship; discuss medical referral, adoption options
Provide anticipatory guidance, counseling with both partners
Provide family planning education

Encourage discussion and renegotiation of relationship
Provide therapy, education, permission, and reassurance
Provide medical referral, medication review, counseling

Provide medical referral, medication review, counseling
Discuss lubrications, estrogen replacement therapy decisions
Address issues with approaches similar to those in early adulthood

Discuss more direct stimulation, medical referral, medication use, losses
Address need for available and interested partner, or masturbation and same sex relationships
Discuss lubrication, medication use
Address issues with approaches similar to those in early adulthood

istically female behavior, and feminine temperament may be mediated; however, Gadpaille (1981, p. 18) cautions:

> In considering sexual development one must distinguish maleness and femaleness from masculinity and femininity. Maleness and femaleness are physical and physiological; for instance, childbearing is a female characteristic. Masculinity and femininity are sex-linked psychological and social behaviors not directly related to copulation and reproduction.

According to this statement, masculinity and femininity are not polar opposites; brain structures and functions that mediate masculinity and feminity probably exist normally in both genders. Biology is not necessarily destiny.

Sex-role identification. Sex-role identification is greatly influenced by the interactions of parents and others toward the infant. There is sufficient evidence to show that from the moment of birth, the parents' treatment of their child is based on the newborn's biologic sex. Worldwide (Ridley, 1993), the male is more valued than the female as a firstborn. Almost immediately, parents place their newborn in a male or female category by giving the infant a name that clearly indicates the newborn's gender. The infant is further classified as "he" or "she." Adults appear to need specific classifications of gender to know how to react to an infant. For example, Lois Gould (1978) wrote a thought-provoking essay in *MS Magazine* about a family who chose not to reveal their baby's gender and reared the infant as "X". "X" was loved by classmates but despised by adults because no one knew whether "X" was a boy or a girl. Colors also are used to designate gender. Although there are efforts to change the traditional colors used to differentiate boys from girls to unisex colors such as white and pastel shades of yellow and green, blue for boys and pink for girls still predominate in the United States. Gender classification conveys a sexual identity to the child and to the world, and a set of sex-related attitudes toward the child emerges. The expectations of parents—and in some families, caretaker grandparents—regarding sex-appropriate behaviors, acquired from their own upbringing, influence the manner in which they react to their infant, in both subtle and and more obvious ways.

Developmental theorists, too, have been criticized for recognizing maturation as separation and individuation (e.g., Gilligan, 1982; Berger et al 1994). To girls, however, social interaction and personal relationships are vital to normal development.

Learning core-gender identity—the sense of being male or female—is also directly sexual. There are physiologic differences in newborns, such as boys' greater muscular strength and irritability and girls' more frequent vocalizations, spontaneous smiling—even during sleep—and greater tactile sensitivity. Having a male or female body determines other sexual experiences during infancy. For example, the mostly invisible and internal female sex organs with their diffuse and vague sensations are in contrast to the more external, visible male genital organs and their more localizable sensations. This lays an early base for differences in sexual self-concept, body image; and sexual attitudes, qualities, and vulnerabilities felt by females and males (Gadpaille, 1981; Sherwen, Scolaveno, & Weingarten, 1991). Some genital focusing takes place later in infancy and is apt to continue randomly until the infant learns that certain spots produce pleasurable feelings more intensely than others. Under the guidance of adults, genital focusing may become more clearly established. For example, some infant caretakers may have fondled their infant charges to quiet them (Shope, 1975). There are few indications that infant sexual responses are dependent on maleness or femaleness, although there has been discussion that because the penis protrudes, it may produce greater sexual awareness in male babies. In either gender, once the infant experiences a satisfactory response, the stimulus is apt to be repeated and the response becomes a source of both arousal and relief.

Whaley and Wong (1997) identify components of the self-concept and body image, which appear to be involved in the development of sex roles. Children learn to apply an appropriate gender label to themselves, acquire sex-appropriate standards of behavior, develop a preference for being the sex that they are, and identify with their parent of the same sex. Children's significant others exert the most influence on their body image and sex role. Thus single parents may be challenged with finding an appropriate role model of the same sex of the parent who is absent for the young child. Both boy and girl infants first identify with the mother in their earliest months. Boys must then disidentify with the mother to achieve a male identity—an intrapsychic task unnecessary for girls. Because of this, males have more difficulty establishing a sex-appropriate identity and once established, that identity is more vulnerable to emotional stressors. Infancy is probably the optimal period to achieve trust and enjoy physical closeness with a child, as well as the best capacity to form loving, healthy bonds and for an individual to acquire a core-gender identity. Although gender development may continue into toddlerhood, it is usually irreversible by 18 months to 2 years of age. This has major significance in the care of the infant born with ambiguous genitalia and who may need surgical intervention for sexual re-assignment. Health care professionals face difficulty in providing interventions to promote a family's healthy acceptance of such an infant. A well-trained multispecialty clinical team is essential. Helping parents and family when an infant is born with this congenital sexual anomaly requires a sensitive approach and poses challenging diagnostic and therapeutic issues for the health care professional (Donahoe & Schnitzer, 1996).

Toddlerhood

Much of the experience of the toddler, from 18 months to 3½ years, is specifically sexual as his/her body autonomy emerges and he/she learns to balance self-control with the ac-ceptance of social controls. During this time, most children become aware of anatomic sex differences, and enormous curiosity is stimulated. Many toddlers may be in circum-stances where their families are experiencing pregnancy and birth and are intrigued by this. There is increased genital exploration and purposeful (no longer random) masturba-tion, and sex play with others is part of the "you show me yours, and I'll show you mine" mind-set. Toilet training and all its conflicts has sexual implications because of the prox-imity of sensations to the function of elimination. There is a greater emotional hazard for girls than for boys to associate statements such as, "It's dirty down there," to bowel func-tions and sexual sensations. Parents who respond in a way that displays disgust or dis-comfort toward the child's touching or exploring genitals, pelvic thrust movements, and sexual arousal may create shame and doubt about the child's body image, giving the child the sense that part of his/her body is untouchable, undesirable, and dirty. Using correct language to identify genitals shows acceptance of one's body. For example, whereas body parts above the umbilicus and below the knees are called by their accurate anatomic names, genitalia and the body functions associated with them are given double-syllable attributions such as "wee-wee," "pee-pee," and "ka-ka" that diminish their importance. The American Academy of Pediatrics recommends that at 18 months, children should be taught proper names for body parts and at 3 to 5 years, children should be taught about "private" parts of the body and how to say "no" to sexual advances (American Medical Association, 1992).

Toddlerhood is also a time for socialization and for sex roles to become more signifi-cant as the child processes information and instruction and becomes more mobile and ac-tive within the family, developing gender-typical behaviors. Which sex he or she belongs to is already determined; what it means to be that sex is the new horizon (Fogel & Lau-ver, 1990; La Freniere, Strayer, & Gauthier, 1984). Toddlers identify with and imitate the same-sex parent. Temporary periods of cross-sex identification are normal; persistent cross-sex identification may be an early indicator of gender dysphoria. Toddlers are af-fected by how the family treats each other on the basis of sex. Many families encourage and reward toddlers for sex-appropriate behavior and ridicule or punish them for devia-tions. Valuing or devaluing one's gender and one's self-concept as male or female is rooted in consistent overt or covert praise or disparagement of one's own or opposite sex.

Preschool Period

The period of 3½ to 6 years is known as the genital, or phallic, stage (as described by Sig-mund Freud) because some subtle but important maturational changes in sexual physiol-ogy occur. There is an increase in masturbatory activity and an associated genital eroti-cism. There is probably a slight increase in androgen production in both genders, which sensitizes the penis and clitoris to tactile stimulation and enhances the child's sexual drive (Gadpaille, 1981). Heterosexual fantasies are likely to appear at this time, and it is not unusual to hear the child say, "When I grow up I want to marry Daddy" or "When Daddy dies, I'm going to marry Mommy" as he/she tries to resolve his/her Oedipal issues. There is no reason to teach the child that these feelings about the parent of the opposite sex are bad or for the other parent to be jealous. Instead parents should display an openly welcoming attitude toward the child's budding heterosexual interests. Gadpaille (1981, p. 24) points out that "the child also should be shown gently but firmly that the parents' physical intimacies are reserved for one another and that, while the child's sexuality is accepted, it must be deferred and eventually directed toward a different partner." This is also a time when parents may want to teach their preschooler about how to respect his/her body, body integrity, and sexual health through "good touch/bad touch" programs. Becoming an "askable" parent or caregiver and responding to the child's questions openly and clearly without instilling fear or guilt is a challenge. The American Academy of Pediatrics (1988) offers helpful information about teaching children to avoid sexual abuse without making the child unduly upset or fearful.

Since this is a time when boys tend to compare their own genitals with those of peers, they may find themselves different if one of their testicles is undescended (cryptorchidism). Often, parents have maintained a conspiracy of silence and have not discussed this condition with the child after the pediatrician has diagnosed it, or they have alarmed the child with their own frequent checks to see whether the testicle has descended into the scrotum. There is disagreement about the best time to perform the surgery (orchiopexy) to correct this condition; however, if the testes are not descended after puberty, although testosterone production will not be impaired, infertility will result (Siemens & Brandzel, 1982). It is possible that if there is a congenital absence of the testes or if they were not successfully brought down surgically, the young boy or adolescent may need a testicular prosthesis (a sac filled with silicone gel in the appropriate size) so that he is not embarrassed by his body image when his genitals are exposed in the locker-room shower or at the urinal or in later years with a sexual partner.

School Years

Although Freud referred to the period of about 6 years to puberty as sexual latency, cross-cultural studies and investigations of school-age children in Western culture do not sustain that view. Pipher (1994) described her own and her daughter's experiences during these years as anything but latent.

> I think of my daughter Sara during those years—performing chemistry experiments and magic tricks, playing her violin, starring in her own plays, rescuing wild animals and biking all over town. I think of her friend Tamara, who wrote a 300 page novel the summer of her sixth-grade year. I remember myself, reading every children's book in the library of my town. One week I planned to be a great doctor like Albert Schweitzer. The next week I wanted to write like Louisa May Alcott or dance in Paris like Isadora Duncan. I have never since had as much confidence or ambition (p. 18).

Although Pipher is not specifically referring to sexual experiences, her description could be used as a framework for the changes girls experience as they view their bodies at this time; they are the same as boys, only without a penis, and they feel can do anything a boy can do. Some gender differences, however, are particularly apparent in these years. Girls tend to exhibit greater sensitivity to touch, timidity or anxiousness, and compliant or nurturant behavior. Boys tend to be more active, competitive, and concerned with dominance in their relationships (Fogel & Lauver, 1990).

This is also a period when same-sex friendships expand sex roles and initiate activities and behaviors that may indicate a sexual preference for a partner of the same sex. Sexual health promotion calls for understanding that same-sex attachment at this age is a way of feeling secure among one's peers and may serve to protect the school-age child from involvement in heterosexual activities for which he/she is not ready. Usually, experimentation in same-sex behaviors is considered within the range of normal during late childhood. If indeed there is an orientation for the same sex, the health care professional needs to provide guidance to the parents in accepting and adapting to their child's sexual preference and to help the parents and the child find the psychosocial support necessary (Fogel & Lauver, 1990).

Since school-age children are still receptive to information from their parents, the health care professional can help parents by recommending they discuss the following points with their preteen (Whipple & Ogden, 1989):

1. Stay away from street drugs and needles.
2. Abstain from sex until the child feels he/she is ready and responsible.
3. Avoid having sex with someone unless the preteen can be positive that person does not have the AIDS virus.
4. Be sure to use contraceptives, including a condom for the male and a spermicide for the female, during intercourse.
5. Do not have intercourse with a lot of different people.
6. Do not have sex with a prostitute.
7. Do not have anal sex.
8. Say "no" to anyone's pressure to have sex.

On average, at about 10 to 12 years of age, girls are approaching puberty—2 years earlier than boys. Their self-image is constantly changing and begins to crumble by the inadequacies and insecurities generated by their growth process and peer group reactions, which they fear are critical and negative. Supportive parents and health care professionals can do much to prepare the prepubertal child for this uncertain time and the experiences of assaults on his/her body image.

A recent national telephone survey of children estimated that 3.2% of girls and 0.6% of boys are sexually abused before they reach 16 (Finkelhor & Dziuba-Leatherman, 1994). Among female adolescents in a Midwestern state, 1% were experiencing sexual abuse in an ongoing situation (Luster & Small, 1997). These are probably conservative estimates since many incidents of sexual abuse are never reported. Child sexual abuse is any sexual behavior directed toward a child by a person who has power over that child and always involves betrayal of the child's trust. Some forms of sexual abuse involve physical contact such as masturbation, intercourse, fondling, oral sex, and anal or vaginal penetration with objects; other types include exhibitionism, leering, and sexual suggestiveness but not necessarily with physical contact. Abusers need not be strangers to the child. They can be anyone in a position of power or trust: a father, uncle, cousin, stepfather, mother, sibling, teacher, babysitter, neighbor, grandparent, peer, clergy, or health care professional. Many children do not get the help that they need at the time of the abuse but instead are met with disbelief, lack of concern, and even blame. Sexual abuse of a child is never a child's fault; for whatever reasons, if the abuse is not dealt with at the time it occurs, its damaging consequences will be felt many years later.

Box 9-1

Indicators of sexual abuse

PHYSICAL INDICATORS
Torn, stained, or bloody underclothing
Pain or itching in genital area
Difficulty walking or sitting
Bruises or bleeding in external genitalia
Venereal disease
Frequent urinary or yeast infections

BEHAVIORAL INDICATORS
Withdrawal, chronic depression
Excessive seductiveness
Role reversal, overly concerned for siblings
Poor self-esteem, self-devaluation, lack of confidence
Peer problems, lack of involvement
Massive weight change
Threatened by physical closeness
Suicide attempts, especially among adolescents
Hysteria, lack of emotional control
Sudden school difficulties
Inappropriate sex play or premature understanding of sex
Promiscuity

The health care professional must be aware of the need to report abuse of a child younger than 18 years in general and sexual abuse in particular (see Box 9-1 for indicators of abuse). Although specific state laws vary, the Social Services Law (1988) of New York State can be used as a guide for indicators of a child's potential need for protection. Additionally, health care professionals should give clients the telephone numbers of abuse hotlines, and/or refer clients to community resources, such as "safe houses" or emergency foster care for abused or neglected children, as well as for abused adult women or elders.

Adolescence

Adolescence is a developmental phase that spans a 10-year period, beginning with puberty. Puberty is the biologic surge of maturation resulting in being able to reproduce and have an adult physical appearance. Arbitrarily, its midpoint is defined as menarche in girls and seminal emission in boys. Adolescence is the psychologic and social response to this biologic surge—the latter somewhat similar throughout the human species but the former varying widely across individuals and cultures.

In females the body changes associated with this phase of physiologic development start with ovarian growth stimulated by estrogen. Breast budding, which may have started as early as 8 years or as late as 13 years, precedes the development of breasts, hip fat, and axillary and pubic hair. The average age of the first menstrual period is a little past the 12th birthday. Girls' rapid growth and development result in them towering over their male peers, forcing psychosexual adjustments that they are not emotionally mature enough to make. For males, the first external evidence of puberty is the enlargement and increased sensitivity of the testicles, with an associated increase in the length of the scrotum. When pubic hair begins to grow, it is straight, then after testicular enlargement and elongation of the penis, the pubic hair becomes kinky in texture, the first ejaculation occurs, and the growth spurt is obvious. Estrogen and androgen are responsible for some of the changes in both genders. Fatty body deposits and breast tissue development in both genders are stimulated by estrogen; testosterone is responsible for the masculinization of boys and promotes development of pubic hair, the clitoris, and the labia majora in girls. Sexual arousal in both genders is stimulated by androgens (Siemens & Brandzel, 1982).

Although they may see themselves as Romeo and Juliet, adolescents experience self-centered sexual discovery and self-discovery. Masturbation increases, primarily among boys, and homoerotic play becomes the most common form of sexual exploration, at least among adolescents in the U.S. middle class (Gadpaille, 1981). This is a period of considerable emotional stress for many nonsexual reasons, but sexual conflicts predominate. Oedipal feelings resurface—only now the son may be more handsome and stronger than the father and the daughter more attractive than the mother. These feelings need to be resolved before youngsters move into adolescent socialization and heterosexual pairing.

Each year in the United States, more than 1 million teenagers become pregnant, and half of those give birth (Henshaw, 1997; Forrest & Singh, 1990). More than 80% of those births result from unintended pregnancies (Henshaw, 1997; Forrest & Singh, 1990). Because intercourse among adolescents is usually unplanned, they are unlikely to seek contraceptive counseling before engaging in sexual activity. Almost half of the unplanned pregnancies among adolescents occur within the first 6 months of sexual activity, with female teens who are sexually active without contraception having a 66% chance of becoming pregnant within 2 years of their first sexual encounter (Furniss, 1996).

The World Health Organization estimates that about half of all AIDS infections to date first occurred in 15- to 24-year-olds, and infections in young persons are increasingly driving the epidemic. In developing countries the peak age of infection tends to be lower in girls than in boys. In industrialized countries, where same-sex relationship contact and needle sharing used to account for the majority of infections, there is an ominous rise in heterosexual transmission (American Academy of Nursing [AAN], 1994).

Sexually active teens are also at an increased risk for a number of other sexually transmitted diseases. The cervical squamocolumnar junction emerges in adolescence, and this may make the teenage girl more vulnerable to chlamydial and gonorrheal infection. Since the human papilloma virus is particularly prevalent during adolescence, girls may be in greater jeopardy for developing cervical cancer later in life (Moore, 1996). Teaching about the use of condoms for "safer sex" has become an issue in many schools and communities. For teens, or those in any age group, who do not choose abstinence, teaching about the proper use of the condom for prevention of an unintended pregnancy and using a condom or latex dental dam to prevent a potentially life-threatening sexually transmitted disease is essential to health promotion. *Sexual Etiquette 101* (Hatcher et al., 1993, p. 158) recommends "safer sex" practices such as massage, hugging, body rubbing, dry kissing, masturbation, hand-to-genital touching, mutual masturbation, and erotic books and movies. Unsafe practices include any intercourse without a latex condom; oral sex (fellatio) without a latex condom; oral sex on a woman during menses or a vaginal infection without a latex barrier (dam); semen in the mouth; oral-anal contact; sharing sex toys or douching equipment; blood contact of *any* kind, including menstrual blood; sharing needles; and any sex that causes tissue damage or bleeding.

In response to the query, "Won't sex education in the schools encourage early or increased sexual activity in young persons?", WHO has recently spoken strongly on this subject. A document summarizing 19 studies shows that talking seriously to young persons about sexuality leads to postponement of sexual activity or to an increase in responsible sexual behavior. In other words, it helps protect teenagers not only from unwanted pregnancy but also from a potentially fatal disease (AAN, 1994).

Eng and Butler (1996) have described risky sex practices as "The Hidden Epidemic" in the United States and state that the United States has failed to respond adequately to sexually transmitted diseases (STDs) even though it has the highest rates of infection in the developed world. According to Eng and Butler (1996), 12 million persons in the United States, one fourth of them adolescents, get STDs each year. The U.S. rate of infection is 50 to 100 times that of other developed nations. For example, in Sweden the rate for gonorrhea is 3 per 100,000; in Canada, 18.6 per 100,000; and in the United States, 150 per 100,000. Eng and Butler (1996) state that only a concerted effort to screen persons for STDs, treat them, and educate others about the risks of infection will stem the tide of disease. For example, *Chlamydia*, the nation's most common bacterial STD, is transmitted 4 million times annually, yet 80% of the women and 40% of the men infected experience no initial symptoms and may unknowingly infect someone else. Because so many cases are undetected, in 1 million women annually, the disease progresses to pelvic inflammatory disease. Eng and Butler (1996) assert that a moralistic approach to STDs— where they are seen as symbols of sinful behavior—may deter persons from seeking information and treatment and thus hinders efforts to control this "hidden epidemic."

Perhaps the most significant aspect of adolescent sexuality is emotional readiness, and many adolescents can sensibly postpone sexual experiences that could be damaging. As Gadpaille (1981, p. 28) notes, "It is an individual's family experience and ego development that determine the impact of sexual experience." Although the concerns adolescents have regarding sexuality may be "too much, too soon," as individuals move into adulthood, the sexual issues can sometimes become "too little, too late." It is important for parents to convey to their child that they will always be there to help, no matter what the crisis. And if the parents cannot deal with their teenager's sexuality, or the conflicts they may be having with their own sexuality and resulting consequences, then teens need to know where and to whom they can go for help and whom they can trust. Many times it is the health care professional in the school nurse's office, at the pediatrician's office, or at the family planning clinic, or it could be a well-informed family member, teacher, or school counselor who provides this support. If this is the case, the emphasis must be on confidentiality, trust, and the provision of accurate factual information in these relationships.

Dating violence. Because dating violence in teen relationships is such a serious and prevalent problem, all health encounters with female adolescents should include screening for dating violence. Furniss (1996) defines dating violence as physical, sexual, emotional, and/or verbal abuse between persons who are or have been in a casual or serious dating relationship. Teen dating abuse begins on average at age 15. About 50% of rape victims are between 10 and 19 years old, an indicator of adolescent girls' vulnerability to violence and sexual abuse (Furniss, 1996). Health care professionals are required to report rape or abuse of a minor. It is essential for the health care professional to maintain knowledge about current medicolegal requirements regarding the care of the victim of assault, as well as conception-prevention protocols—known as the "morning after" emergency postcoital regimen—to assist the traumatized teen or adult woman to deal with the emotional and behavioral responses that follow sexual assault. Even though large doses of mifepristone (RU-486) followed by misoprostol, or the Yuzpe method (2 doses of combined oral contraceptives 12 hours apart) are known to induce an abortion, many physicians are willing to prescribe these doses in a sexual assault crisis (guidelines for emergency contraception in American College of Obstetrics and Gynecologists, 1997).

In the past, rape was regarded merely as an act of sexuality. Later, experts refuted that argument and maintained that rape was an act of aggression in which the perpetrator was motivated by a desire to dominate, control, and degrade a victim. Today, most persons who work in the field of violent sexual crime assert that it is a combination of the two. One working definition of rape is the "sexual expression of aggression" (Congressional Caucus for Women's Issues, 1991).

Sexual orientation. Many sexologists have tried to discover causes of sexual orientation. Studies of monozygotic and dizygotic twins, some reared separately and some together, suggest that there may be an inherited component of same-sex orientation. Other studies, particularly those concerned with the evolution of human sexuality, question such a possibility. A further question arises from the fact that a large part of the human population is involved in neither an exclusively same sex relationship nor an exclusively heterosexual one (Haynes, 1995). Sexual orientation is a concern during teen years when an adolescent consciously realizes he/she may be attracted to members of one's own sex. This is a stressful recognition that can lead to identity confusion, emotional crisis, and possible disconnection and alienation from friends, family, and society. Furniss (1996) cautions health care professionals to be aware of and sensitive to same sex relationship adolescents' needs.

> In taking the health history, providers must assume a nonjudgmental role. They must also remember not to make assumptions about orientation. Heterosexuality, same sex relationships, and bisexuality are often issues and choices for the same client. It is essential therefore to cover topics such as pregnancy and STDs with all adolescents (p. 6)

According to Landau (1986), 10% of the adult male population may be in predominantly same sex relationships, with about 5% of women choosing same-sex life-styles. Many same sex relationship clients tend to conceal their sexual orientation from the health care professional because they fear disapproval and less-than-adequate and empathetic care. The same sex relationship client's sexual experience is diverse, and there are as many different kinds of personalities among same sex relationships as there are among heterosexuals. It is impossible to predict the nature of the client's personality, social adjustment, or sexual functioning from sexual orientation. "We are all more human than otherwise" (Green & Schiavi, 1995). Putting away one's stereotypes and caricatures becomes an essential aspect of health promotion in providing effective care.

Adolescent males who cross-dress are not necessarily programmed for lifelong transvestism or a life of same sex relationships. The boy's fantasies about becoming a woman (transsexualism) may blur with transvestism. The onset of pubertal changes and secondary sex characteristics can pose a life crisis for the adolescent boy because they are dissonant with his identity and tend to be associated with females. Realistic, educational discussions with the adolescent's parents plus a thorough psychiatric evaluation that provides an opportunity for the teen to reversibly test contra-sexed identity may be helpful (Green & Schiavi, 1995). A 1990 survey revealed that about 2% of sexually active adults reported being exclusively in same-sex or bisexual relationships in the year before the survey, with 5% to 6% exclusively in same-sex or bisexual relationships since age 18 years (Smith, 1991).

Young Adulthood

By the time most persons have entered their 20s, they have adopted a sexual orientation that is either same sex or heterosexual, although these choices are not irreversible in later adulthood. The classic studies of human phases of the sexual response cycle were compiled by researchers such as Kinsey, Pomeroy, and Martin (1948); Masters and Johnson (1966); and Kaplan (1974) by observing and recording volunteer male and female subjects, of both sexual orientations, married and unmarried, and across all socioeconomic groups.

Drawing on the clinical research of Masters and Johnson (1966) and Kaplan (1974), five phases of the sexual response cycle (SRC) are seen in adults: desire, excitement, plateau, orgasm, and resolution. Most of the time, the individual is sexually at rest. The desire phase, characterized by sexual thoughts about intimacy and sexual gratification, is followed by excitement and arousal, which are marked by increasing vasocongestion in the genitals in both genders and rising myotonia—or increase in muscle tension, particularly genitally, but in other areas as well. The chief signals of genital arousal are penile erection and vaginal swelling and wetness. Physical conditions such as fatigue and illness or medications can affect vasocongestion and/or myotonia and therefore sexual response. Excitement is affected by the five senses—sight, touch, hearing, smell, and taste—and by fantasies.

Rising excitement levels out over the plateau stage, which is affected by desire, social learning, continued sexual stimulation, and individual needs to either greatly extend this period to delay orgasm or to end it in striving to reach orgasm quickly. From the plateau phase, the response cycle procedes to the brief release of tension, which results in the explosive orgasmic phase in which psychologic and muscle tension climax. In men, increased stimulation of the penis can lead to orgasm, which usually includes ejaculation; in women, orgasm is most commonly triggered by clitoral stimulation and results in contractions of the muscles around the vagina and the perineum. Perry and Whipple (1981; Whipple & Ogden, 1989) have described simultaneous stimulation of the clitoris and Grafenberg spot (G spot) as a source of female ejaculation of a fluid from the urethra. The orgasmic phase lasts only 3 to 15 seconds, is involuntary, and cannot be consciously controlled. Women are capable of maintaining orgasms for longer periods than men and can experience multiple orgasms.

The resolution phase follows ejaculation and is experienced differently by men and women. For women, if they are erotically stimulated sufficiently they can reexperience effective stimulation; for men the refractory period is longer and extends with aging (Gotwald & Golden, 1981; Diamond & Karlen, 1981).

Sexuality is integral to the total relationship of two sexual partners. When partners experience problems, they are generally either primary or secondary. Primary sexual problems are those where the basic issue is specifically sexual (i.e., premature ejaculation, vaginismus) and are of sufficient significance to cause severe discord in a relationship. These sexual problems usually have existed for one or both of the partners since the beginning of their relationship or even before. Secondary sexual problems are those stemming from other difficulties in the relationship (infidelity, extended family stress) and arise from conflicts that cause resentment, anxiety, anger, and guilt. Primary sexual problems usually are associated with lack of information, misinformation, ignorance, or faulty learning or conditioning. Because they are ashamed, embarrassed, or fear rejection, many couples are inhibited about talking about sex, so their communication about it is virtually nonexistent. Often, couples have unrealistic expectations of what the other expects or what the other should be able to give. In problems that are secondary, assessment of the nature of the couple's interaction and any behavior that would engender hostility, disrespect, and anxiety when intimacy, tenderness, and understanding are needed becomes the focus of the intervention (Group for the Advancement of Psychiatry, 1973). In some cases, this hostility may become manifest in intimate-partner physical violence or emotional abuse, particularly to the younger woman (age 18 to 30 years) (CDC, 1996b). Several studies suggest that 30% of women treated in emergency departments have injuries or symptoms related to physical abuse (CDC, 1993).

Sexual decisions. Courtship; selecting a mate or a sexual partner; marrying; staying single; living with one's sexual partner; staying celibate; becoming a married parent or a single parent; or remaining as a nonparent are all sexual decisions that young adults, as well as those in later years, must face. The most common sexual issues that evolve during young adulthood relate to preventing unwanted pregnancy and sexually transmitted diseases—issues that were of concern during adolescence when individuals were emotionally immature and more likely to engage in impulsive, unsafe sexual behaviors. Each phase of the sexual response cycle is vulnerable to psycho/social/physiologic problems. Fears of unwanted or unplanned pregnancy in or out of marriage can affect the sexual desire phase for both men and women. A stable monogamous sexual relationship between partners and the use of a latex condom in a new relationship while the partners await AIDS clearance confirmation may enhance freedom from the fears inhibiting either partner's desire. Desire is also affected by depression, fatigue, anger, and conflict in the relationship. Because of the dependent nature of the male's erection on vasocongestion, fear, anxiety, fatigue, and drugs can all interfere with erectile functioning. In the female, vaginal swelling and lubrication, similarly affected by physiologic and psychologic factors, can interfere with the excitement and plateau phases of the sexual response cycle. Common problems for the male that cause premature or retarded ejaculation relate to psychologic and sociologic conditioning, or in some cases, to alcohol and drugs that affect muscular contractions. For women, dyspareunia (painful or difficult intercourse) and vaginismus (painful spasm of the vagina) appear with diminished lubrication and excessive anxiety, inhibiting intercourse and sexual pleasure. Both partners' need to express love, care, intimacy, and sex play as a significant part of adulthood and commitment in a relationship.

Although there are anticipated sexual problems associated with an unwanted pregnancy, the couple desiring to have children who are experiencing fertility problems, whether primary or secondary, may suffer unanticipated stresses in their sexual relationship. Having to make love and be "potent on demand" may strain the male partner. The fertility tests, painful injections, financial strains, and emotional losses create stress for both the woman and her partner. Decisions about reproductive technology or perhaps the ultimate decision to give up on their plans to bear their biologic child and resolve the conflict with adoption or a decision to nonparent all have ramifications on a couple's sexual relationship as they experience depression, anger, loss, and anxiety. The pregnancy that may ensue after years of trying may become so dear that it may itself be a deterrent to the couple's sexual relationship. Health care professionals need to be sensitive to these issues and help the couple achieve the loving relationship that may have been sacrificed when all their efforts became focused on getting pregnant and then having a baby.

Sexuality and pregnancy. When pregnancy does occur, the health care professional must be aware of the bio/psycho/social variables that affect sexuality. For most women who are having an uncomplicated normal pregnancy, with no history of bleeding, pain, or previous abortion, manipulation or coitus to orgasm is not contraindicated. Hogan (1980) emphasizes the need to counter myths and misconceptions about sex during pregnancy, explaining that the fetus is not harmed by coitus. The more the father, in particular, knows about pregnancy changes, the more supportive he can be to his partner and the better the couple's sexual adjustment throughout the pregnancy. "When a couple is advised to abstain 4 to 6 weeks before and after delivery, they may experience severe strain in their relationship in terms of lack of sexual outlet for both partners. It is at times like this that the man may seek outside release for the first time" (Hogan, 1980, p. 484). This viewpoint validated previous clinical observations (Hott, 1972).

Sexuality also is altered during the postpartum phase. Anticipatory guidance is necessary to make resumption of sexual activity postpartum comfortable and less anxiety provoking. If the mother is breastfeeding, she may experience erotic responses to the infant's nursing and her vaginal lubrication will be decreased, causing dryness and discomfort. The health care professional can recommend using a water-soluble gel or contraceptive cream or jelly, as well as changing coital positions to make sex most comfortable for the new mother. The health care professional also can teach the woman to perform Kegel exercises, the technique to strengthen the woman's pubococcygeal muscle, to help prevent relaxation of pelvic support as the woman ages.

Family planning choices and birth control are major concerns throughout a woman's menopausal years; for men, fertile sperm can still be produced well into the geriatric years. Reproductive technology has extended potential fertility and has become another alternative for couples seeking to have children in late adulthood. Providing accurate information about planning options objectively and sensitively is essential to health care promotion. There is no ideal method of contraceptive control for everyone. Helping the couple who use contraception infrequently or not at all and who are dealing with contraceptive failure are sensitive issues that demand the health care professional's tolerance and understanding. Sex is increasingly valued as a form of recreation and intimacy among married couples who have options to control their fertility through contraception, sterilization, and abortion. Sexuality is increasingly seen as separate from reproduction, particularly among married couples, and therefore holds significant influence over the quality of sexual relationships.

Rather than declining steadily, sexual satisfaction appears to fluctuate cyclically during a long, stable marital relationship, with a drop occurring during the early years of parenthood, reaching a low point when their children are teenagers (and at their own sexual peak), and then rising again when children leave home. Although parenting may be rewarding, the demands of a two- and three-career family and maturational conflicts can divert emotional and sexual energy away from the couple's conjugal relationship. Often the "empty nest" provides couples with an opportunity for sexual renewal and reinvestment in the relationship.

Middle and Late Adulthood

By their 30s and 40s, most persons are married or have been in one or more intimate relationships. During this time, family life and work are reassessed. A woman's career may be interrupted by her marriage and childrearing, yet she may accomplish the developmental tasks of separation and individuation—accomplished earlier in a man's life—during this period of her life cycle. This change may create tension in a relationship (Chehrazi, 1987). Extramarital relationships become more common, indicating the couple's need to deal with problems in their relationship and sexual adjustments (Laumann, Gagnon, Michael, & Michaels, 1994). Because of the physiologic changes and body image alterations that occur in the middle years, sexual desire and activity often decrease and there is a decrease in sexual gratification. Men usually have increased their capacity to control ejaculation, however, so the quality of their sexual encounters may have improved. Most men who seek therapy in the middle years are experiencing erectile dysfunction; for women in this age group the more common concerns are lack of desire, anorgasmia, dyspareunia, and infidelity, whether theirs or their partner's.

Although acute or chronic physical illness can interfere with sexual desire or ability because of organic, psychologic, or interpersonal factors at any point along the life cycle, sexual function may diminish or cease in adult years because of pain, fatigue, depression, immobility, changes in body function, disfigurement, body image changes, or the demands of coping with a temporary or permanent disability. When these factors are ameliorated by therapy, education, permission, and reassurance, total or partial sexual activity can be resumed. Levay, Sharpe, & Kagle (1981) state:

> The patient's emotional response almost always affects sexual functioning, but there are no simple correlations. Anxiety arising from physical illness often leads to concern about current or future sexual functioning. There may be loss or increase in desire, or a shift to more aggressive or passive sexual behavior. Being more demanding may be expressed in increased sexual contact as a way of becoming close, or in decreased sexual contact with the wish to be taken care of in nonsexual ways by the spouse (p. 169).

Illnesses can affect sexual functioning by direct physical sexual dysfunction (organic), such as paraplegia and postsurgical conditions (e.g., non-nerve sparing radical prostatectomy, where the nerves responsible for sexual response have been affected). Others, such as cardiovascular disease and bronchopulmonary conditions, cause psychologic reactions, such as "performance anxiety," that lead to psychogenic dysfunctions, even though there is no direct organic component related to erectile, lubricatory, or orgasmic problems. In addition, some medications, such as antihypertensive drugs and psychotropics, can create an organo-psychogenic sexual dysfunction that also can be debilitating to the couple's relationship. The health care professional will be wise to counsel clients that medications can have different side effects on sexual functioning. (In addition to the *Physician's Desk Reference (PDR)*, which is updated annually, Crenshaw's *Sexual Pharmacology* (1996) is an excellent comprehensive reference source on the sexual side effects of drugs, both positively and negatively.)

HIV/AIDS infection is also an issue for sexually active individuals in middle and late adulthood. HIV infection is the third leading cause of death among all U.S. women ages 25-44 years and the leading cause of death among black women in this age group (CDC, 1996a). Moreover, an estimated 7000 infants are born to HIV-infected women in the United States each year; without intervention, approximately 15% to 30% of these infants would be infected (CDC, 1996a). This imposes a disproportionately high impact on society because of the loss of productive years of life and the loss of parents from families with young children (CDC, 1993). Despite these telling statistics, midlife and older women are not seen by health care professionals, policy makers, and society at large as being at risk for contracting HIV. Midlife and older women have oftentimes been discouraged from considering themselves at risk (Bowman & Wolfe, 1995). Health care professionals often are not adequately prepared to diagnose and treat women in these age groups who normally acquire the disease through heterosexual contact rather than drugs or transfusions. (CDC, 1995)

What makes women vulnerable to HIV/AIDS infection? Anderson, in her report to the American Academy of Nursing HIV/AIDS Nursing Care Summit (AAN, 1994) surmises that there are three main factors:

> First, women are biologically vulnerable due to larger mucosal surface exposed during sexual intercourse. Secondly, women are epidemiologically vulnerable. They tend to have sex with older men who are farther along in their sex lives and hence more likely to have become infected. The third reason is that women are socially vulnerable. Traditional norms, in various ways and intensities, result in sexual subordination, and thus women may have difficulty in protecting themselves from sexual transmission, whether through mutual fidelity or condom use (p. 3).

Generally, the risk of midlife widowhood resulting from AIDS is less than among younger women (ages 30 to 39 years) or among younger males in same-sex relationships (U.S. Bureau of the Census, 1996). However, becoming an AIDS widow during this period carries with it not only the grief and loss of a partner, but the strain of community rejection, whether or not the woman has been infected.

Middle adulthood also is normally the time of perimenopause and menopause (the cessation of menstruation), a normal physiologic and developmental process in a woman's life. The midlife physiologic changes identified with this time of life are slower lubrication and possible vaginitis associated with the cracking and bleeding of atrophic vaginal mucosa. Maintaining satisfying sexual activity, by coitus or by masturbation, will help prevent these problems. Adding a water-soluble lubricant or moisturizer (e.g., K-Y Jelly, Astroglide, Replens) also is helpful, as well as the use of a lubricated condom. Estrogen replacement therapy (ERT) and hormone replacement therapy (HRT) are areas that the health care professional needs to have accurate information about, balancing the increased risks of breast cancer and heart disease with the need to help the menopausal woman deal with hot flashes and vaginal degeneration. Psychologic changes include alterations in body image because of breast atrophy or weight gain and can contribute to the woman's diminished self-concept. There is a debate among women about whether sexuality increases or decreases during "the pause." Increased desire may result from an "empty nest;" having a loving, monogamous partner; and freedom from fear of becoming pregnant, whereas decreased desire can occur if the woman has been physically ill or lacks a sexual partner (Fogel & Lauver, 1990; Lieblum & Rosen, 1988).

For males in the middle years, the physiologic losses are more insidious, manifest in the decline of androgen-dependent tissues and resulting changes in the penis and scrotum. Men in middle years vary greatly in what they consider to constitute a midlife crisis. This time of life for men is associated with erectile dysfunction and ejaculatory retardation, which commonly are concomitant with alcohol ingestion; fatigue; physical illness (such as diabetes, cardiac disease) and the drugs used to treat these chronic diseases; economic losses; or depression resulting from illness or loss of a parent, spouse, or child. Often, the middle years become a "sandwich generation" experience for a couple who now have to care for aging parents as well as older children. Men in the middle years, too, are threatened by HIV/AIDS infection. HIV is the leading cause of death for Americans between the ages 25 and 44 years—particularly among ethnic and racial minorities—with 26% of its cases in men and women in their 40s. HIV/AIDS is sometimes misdiagnosed in older men because its many symptoms mimic other illnesses that affect older persons (Grossman, 1995). Additionally, although in 1995, 42% of the AIDS cases were among men who have sex with men (MSM), its estimated incidence is increasing more rapidly among heterosexuals than among either MSM or intravenous drug users (CDC, 1997a, 1997b).

Whereas maintaining youth and beauty are considered important to a woman's sexual image, money and power are considered important to the male's sexual image; however, stereotypes for both genders are being challenged as the U.S. culture becomes more androgynous.

Older Adult

The aging, persons older than 65 years, are not a homogeneous population. Sexual attitudes and life-style vary greatly according to social class, health status, educational level, and location. The most severe stress on sexual activity for individuals in this phase of life is the growing number of losses that persons in later years experience. Lief and Berman (Lief & Berman, 1981, p. 126) in their classic presentation describe the following four obvious losses particularly distressing for this population's sexual life:

1. Loss due to death, relocation, or simply withdrawal of the people around them who give meaning to their lives (spouses, children, other relatives, and close friends).
2. Loss of role and status with retirement and concomitant loss of income.
3. Some loss of cognitive functioning; less likely with adequate nutrition, social stimulation, and in the absence of severe illness.
4. Loss of physical power or physical health.

In aging men, the most consistent physiologic findings are the need for greater, direct general stimulation to achieve erection; erection is slower; preejaculation seeping may be absent; ejaculatory inevitability may be absent or delayed; seminal fluid is decreased; the refractory period after ejaculation takes longer; and the need and ability to ejaculate at each sexual contact is reduced markedly. It is important for health care professionals to reassure both elderly males and females that the male's orgasmic ejaculation or release is neither necessary nor desirable at each sexual connection and that sexual functioning is negatively affected by age, antihypertensive drugs, and physical illness.

Physiologic changes occurring in the elderly woman are slower lubrication; the need for more direct stimulation; a possibly shorter orgasmic phase; and with low estrogen, possible fragile vaginal tissues and painful clitoral stimulation. Orgasmic response, including being multiorgasmic, remains unchanged for the woman. The principal factor involved in continuing gratifying sexual functioning for women is having an available and interested partner (Lief & Berman, 1981). Masturbation and same-sex relationships may be alternative choices for aging women living alone. The need for intimacy, closeness, and the satisfaction of "skin hunger" continues throughout life. For both elderly men and women, affectionate touching activities, hugging, hand holding, smiling, flirting, and kissing are important aspects of sexual activity, even if the individual is in a nursing home. Helping staff understand sexuality in the aging is essential to health promotion.

The CDC studied women older than 65 years and found that the relatively high proportion of later diagnosis of HIV in this group occurs because postmenopausal women may be less likely to access care in gynecologic settings and that their clinical management is complicated by diseases associated with aging (e.g., dementia) (Fleming, Guina, Ward, Chiasson, & Jones, 1995). The CDC emphasizes the role of the health care professional in reviewing sexual histories and providing safer-sex counseling to all women.

TAKING A SEXUAL HISTORY

Given the prevalence of STDs and the relative increase of HIV infection among women and young adults (U.S. Bureau of the Census, 1996), the need for health care professionals to question their clients sensitively about their sexual lives, assess their risk for STDs and sexual dysfunction, and provide information about prevention measures is a mandate for sexual health promotion. The American Social Health Association (ASHA) (1996), a nonprofit organization that maintains programs in STD education, public policy, and research, feels that the client needs to understand the purpose of the sex history. ASHA recommends that health care professionals explain to their clients the reasons for inquiring about sexual topics and the type of intimate questions that may be asked, clarifying that sexual problems are explored in depth with all clients whenever these problems may have a relationship to other aspects of the clients' lives (Alexander, 1992).

To deal effectively with human sexuality in one's clinical practice, the health care professional must first accept his/her own sexuality. Second, human sexuality must be integrated as a significant component into one's concept of individual development that can be expressed in a wide range of behaviors. The primary need is to deal comfortably with one's own feelings so that the health care professional can then deal effectively with the client's sexual feelings.

Taboos and proscriptions against sexual expression in American society have been largely responsible for the general avoidance of meaningful discussion and understanding of human sexuality. The irony in American society is that although television, computers, and newspaper and magazine stories openly discuss sexual abuse, rape, pornography, extramarital affairs, infidelity, abortion, out-of-wedlock pregnancies, and STDs—the negative aspects of sexuality—they generally do not discuss how to achieve caring, loving, and positive sexual gratification in meaningful sexual relationships. An approachable health care professional needs to deal comfortably with his/her own feelings about sexuality, both negative and positive, which will give permission to the client to express feelings and ask questions openly and comfortably.

The P-LI-SS-IT Model

Jack Annon (1976) developed the widely used "PLISSIT" model of sexual concerns as the method to use for the aforementioned aspect of permission-giving in sexual history taking. Based on learning theory principles, Annon's model provides permission (*P*) by the health care professional first giving reassurance about the sexual behavior and its acceptability. Giving permission is a health promoting intervention but should only be done if the behavior is not physically or emotionally harmful to the individual or the sexual partner (Fogel & Lauver, 1990). In the case of sexuality, permission-giving implies, "You're OK" and "Continue what you're doing" pertaining to sexual thoughts, fantasies, dreams, behavior; feelings of arousal; and pressure to conform.

LI stands for limited information in the PLISSIT model. Information-giving is needed to clarify myths and misinformation and to educate and explain phenomena that may affect significant changes in behavior. For example, giving limited information about phases of the human sexual response cycle and the differences between men and women at different maturational stages of development can be reassuring and enhance self-concept. Another example would be the anticipated changes in desire and libido resulting from illness and fatigue, the aging aspects of sexuality, or the associated sexual dysfunctions related to certain beta blockers for the treatment of hypertension.

SS in the PLISSIT model represents specific suggestions that provide alternative explanations for a problem and offer a framework within which these recommendations can work. These suggestions are specific to the problem presented in the history (e.g., use a lubricant for vaginal dryness associated with postnatal lactation; use a latex condom with water-soluble gel rather than petroleum jelly; for the person with arthritis, take a warm bath before lovemaking). Relaxation techniques, bibliotherapy (specific suggestions about books or articles that provide support or clarification), and movement or positional changes that are specifically tailored to the individual's or couple's needs are part of the health care professional's armamentarium of experience and knowledge to promote sexual well-being.

The health care professional refers clients for intensive therapy (IT) when problems cannot be resolved without a sex therapist. This usually means that sexual problems are ones in which personal and emotional difficulties interfere with healthy sexual expression. Behavioral excesses such as fetishistic behavior, pedophilia, and exhibitionism that elicit inappropriate emotional responses necessitate referral for intensive therapy to a certified sex therapist or mental health professional who has had advanced training in sexology.

SEXUAL AWARENESS & THE HEALTH PROMOTION MATRIX*

Sexual awareness is a healthy behavior. Health care professionals should enter a dialogue with clients concerning sexual awareness as an important part of their interactions and interventions regarding the promotion of client health. The HPM helps guide the dialogue and facilitates a more comprehensive understanding of the client's desired sexual image as well as the patterns that deter and support the client in integrating this image into his/her life-style.

Image Creation

The best way to begin the dialogue is with an understanding of the client's own personal sexual image (i.e., the image the client desires). As the couple may develop their relationship, they may share a mutual image as well. The demeanor of the health care professional is crucial in conveying comfort with and acceptance for the client's desired image. The health care professional offers permission for the client to communicate this image so that both can begin to explore the significance of this image and the factors and forces that may minimize and optimize its realization for the client. The health care professional may ask the client: "When you imagine yourself as a sexual being, how to you appear and behave?" The health care profes-

*Adapted from J. Hott by J. Arnold.

sional communicates how important is it for the client to openly describe a personal image (i.e., to project the image that most closely represents his/her desired sexual self). Often, clients experience discomfort in picturing their sexual image. Perhaps, self-denial, repression, and punishment have prevented clients from authentically conveying their own preferred image. Other clients may simply feel uncomfortable discussing sexuality. Still others may look to this opportunity as a point of liberation, or a door to discovering themselves.

Image Appraisal

A brief sexual history should be included in every total health history. Suggested guidelines for taking a sexual history (ASHA, 1994; Alexander, 1992, p. 41). include the following:

- Health care professionals need to be comfortable with sexual questions and language
- Establish rapport with the client
- Greet the client warmly and with respect
- Use a private location for the interview
- Establish confidentiality
- Use straightforward language the client can understand (may need to suggest multiple terms)
- Identify the purpose of the discussion
- Let clients know the questions may be personal
- Acknowledge that many people find it difficult to discuss sexual issues
- Begin with open-ended questions
- Ask specific questions in a non-threatening, nonjudgmental manner
- Listen carefully and be sensitive to nonverbal cues

Once these suggestions have been acknowledged and acted upon, the health care professional is better able to ask questions and continue the dialogue about the client's actual sexual behaviors and practices. Included in the sexual history are questions about sexual activity and satisfaction with the kind and frequency of sexual activity. To illustrate: "Are you sexually active?" If so: "Are you satisfied with your activity and its frequency?" Deriving an accurate portrayal of the value the client places on sex is important. The health care professional may simply ask, "How important has sex been as a part of your relationship?" The ability to reach arousal is key and must be asked directly: "Do you have difficulty becoming aroused?" This question can be explored in greater depth and with gender specificity. Men can be asked about their ability to attain and maintain an erection and ejaculatory control. Women can be asked whether they have difficulty with arousal or orgasm. Both men and women should be asked about whether they experience pain with intercourse. The appraisal part of the process of health promotion can be augmented by asking the client whether there are questions the health care professional has not asked that the client would like to discuss. It is not unusual for a client to withhold information until the precise question is asked to provoke a response. If the health care professional asks the client what she/he would like to be asked, the health care professional is offering the client permission to discuss sexuality openly and with the acceptance required to facilitate a trusting relationship. Knowledge deficits often limit a full discussion and appraisal. Asking the client whether some aspect of sexuality could be explained opens the door for further clarification, information sharing, and data gathering.

Minimize Health Depleting Patterns

The intent of the Health Promotion Matrix is to assist the client in integrating his/her idealized image of health. This is accomplished through a careful analysis of the data gathered during the image appraisal process. The health care professional and the client identify factors and forces that may be obstacles that limit the internalization of the idealized image.

Questions that identify health depleting patterns and practices attempt to reveal tangible acts that can be altered and minimized to curtail their limiting effect. The health care professional gleans from the appraisal factor the factors and forces that are known to inhibit or minimize sexual activity. Further, the health care professional asks the client whether there is anything that may be interfering with his/her role function as a partner in a relationship. Illness, surgery, medication/drug use, and pregnancy are among the myriad of factors that could deplete or limit sexual activity. Uncovering the clients' perception about sexual activity can be discovered when asking: "Has anything changed the way you feel about yourself as a man or a woman? Again, illness, medical treatment, and surgery are common factors that affect emotional reactions and individual perceptions about sexuality." Another way to uncover practices and patterns with the potential to deplete sexual activity is to ask, "Has anything altered your ability to function sexually?" Fostering patterns and practices that are supportive to health is discussed next.

Optimize Health Supportive Patterns

The health care professional and the client discover the patterns and practices that appear to enhance or optimize sexuality. The health care professional may ask, "What enhances your sexuality?" The health care professional and the client are attempting to discover the practices and patterns that are supportive to the client's idealized sexual image. Once identified, these patterns and practices are supported as factors that strengthen and heighten the client's sexual image. The health care professional asks the client what improves his/her sexual activity and sense of sexual satisfaction. Lastly, the health care professional explores with the client how connected the client's sexual activities are to a sense of general health (i.e., the health care professional and client relate sexuality, sexual awareness, and sexual activities to health and to the promotion of personal health).

Internalize Idealized Image

Achieving sexual awareness is realized in the client's ability to internalize his/her idealized image of sexuality conceived through image creation. Experiencing comfort about one's sexuality is best illustrated in sexual fulfillment and consistency between the creation of an idealized image and the integration of this image in personal actions and behaviors. The client is asked about the fulfillment of his/her idealized image. It is also important to discuss actions that can be taken to enhance one's sexual life and to find deeper meaning in being a sexual human being. The health care professional must be ever mindful of the specific interventions that can be used as sexual awareness grows. Giving permission; providing limited information; offering specific suggestions; and if needed, referring for intensive therapy (based on the PLISSIT model) are areas of intervention that are continuously evaluated as the client reveals needs in moving toward the internalization of his/her/their idealized images of sexuality.

SEXUAL AWARENESS: *A Script**

Image Creation	I'm going to ask you some questions about your sexuality.
	When you imagine yourself as a sexual being, how do you appear and behave?
	How do you envision yourself as a sexual person?
	Is sexuality part of your image of yourself as a healthy person?
Image Appraisal	Are you currently sexually active?
	Often, there are problems that interfere with our sexual satisfaction. Are you satisfied with your sexual activity/response and its frequency?
	Do you use safe sex practices?
	Could you describe these practices to me?
	Share materials and approaches from Helpful Resources section at the end of the chapter.
	Are you sexually fulfilled?
	Do you have any difficulty becoming aroused?

*Adapted from J. Rose Hott by J. Arnold.

SEXUAL AWARENESS: *A Script—cont'd*

	YES **NO**
	Is there any information I have not asked about your sexuality that is important for you to share?
	Do you need information or is there some aspect of sexuality that you would like explained?
	For men: Are you able to attain and maintain erection and ejaculatory control?
	For women: Do you experience difficulty with arousal or orgasm? Do you feel any pain with intercourse?
Minimize Health Depleting Patterns	What has interfered with your being a partner (husband/wife/ mother/father)?
	Has anything changed the way you feel about yourself as a man or a woman?
	Has anything altered your ability to function sexually?
Optimize Health Supportive Patterns	What enhances your sexuality? What improves your sexual activities and satisfaction?
Internalize Idealized Image	Sexuality is a meaningful part of our lives. How do you continue to feel sexually fulfilled?
	How do you continue to enhance your sexuality?
	In what ways do you continue to make sex meaningful to you?

SEXUAL AWARENESS AND GAY, LESBIAN, AND BISEXUAL TEENS

With health care's focus on "safe sex" and "safer sex" to prevent STDs and unwanted pregnancies among heterosexual teens having such prominence in American culture, the teenagers who belong to the sexual minority of gay, lesbian, and bisexual young persons find that rather than entering adulthood with a healthy sense of self and confidence, they are offered one of two equally destructive alternatives: either outright ridicule or denial of their same-sex attraction (Savin-Williams, 1995b). Gay, lesbian, and bisexual teens do not wake up one morning and suddenly realize they are different. They may have known since they were 4 or 5 years old that they did not quite fit in and that something was wrong. By the time they had reached puberty and become aware of their sexual and romantic interest in members of the same sex, they had also learned that the dominant culture discredits same-sex romances and that identifying themselves as gay or lesbian or bisexual is not acceptable to their parents, family, and peers. For a successful adolescence to take place, the teenager has to integrate this sexual identity with the sexual person he/she has always known himself/herself to be. To help gay, lesbian, and bisexual teens, particularly the teen struggling with transsexuality, speak about their sexual identity, the health care professional could apply the Health Promotion Matrix to stimulate discussion. A script (developed from Zuckerman, 1995, pp. 59-61) offering questions to guide interaction with gay, lesbian, and bisexual teens is found on p. 240-241 and was adapted to incorporate the dimensions of the HPM.

By keeping the lines of communication open with gay, lesbian, and bisexual teens, the health care professional can assist these adolescents in coping with whatever is troubling them. This does not mean that this professional caregiver is there for the purpose of "conversion" to heterosexuality. Health care professionals are oftentimes approached by parents who ask how they can broach the subject when they suspect that their child wants to reveal his/her sexual identity at home but just cannot bring himself/herself to do it. Parents can be offered guidance about how to begin such conversations. Instead of directly asking: "Are you gay?" Savin-Williams (1995a) advises the parent to say: "Anytime you'd like to talk about girlfriends or boyfriends, I'd like to do that." "You know, even if it turned out you were gay, that would be OK with me." If the teen denies being gay, parents can leave the subject open by responding: "Whatever you are is fine with me." This then is health promotion (i.e., accepting the teen's sexuality as a healthy dimension of being human).

The following series of questions, developed from Zuckerman (1995) is a guide for health care professionals' interaction with gay, lesbian, and bisexual teens:

Image Creation

- Do you think you really should have been/are of the other gender?
- What sexual identity makes you feel happy and content with your life?
- Have you fantasized about changing your gender?

Image Appraisal

- At what age did you first know you were a boy/girl?
- Did you ever dress in the other gender's clothes/play with their toys?
- For females: Were you a tomboy? Are you still? Do you feel better/more comfortable when you wear masculine clothing?
- For males: Do you ever dress in women's clothes or underclothes or use make-up? When do you do this? How does it make you feel? What do you get from this?
- Did you want to look like someone of the opposite gender?
- Are you aroused sexually by seeing females in the nude?
- Are you aroused sexually by seeing males in the nude?
- Are you sexually aroused by seeing yourself nude?
- Do you look at your genitals when you masturbate?
- Are you aroused sexually by looking at yourself masturbating?
- How many sexual partners have you had? Same sex? Opposite sex? How many have been bisexual?
- Has anyone ever forced you into having sexual intercourse?

Minimize Health Depleting Patterns

- Did you dislike your gender's clothes or body forms?
- Do your genitals (sex organs) disgust you?
- Have you ever tried to injure your genitals?
- Do any of your sexual fantasies distress or frighten you?
- Have you ever forced anyone to have sexual intercourse with you?
- What obstacles (peers, parents, family, religion, school, economics, friends) do you feel get in the way of achieving personal goals of sexual identity?
- Do you feel trapped in a woman's/man's body?

Optimize Health Supportive Patterns

- Do your genitals (sex organs) appear normal to you? Do you like them?
- Do you want to marry a person of your gender?
- What support system and resources (health care professionals, parents, family, school, counselors, religious advisers, friends, community support groups) do you see available to you? Who else is supportive of you?

Internalize Idealized Image

- Can you describe your sense of comfort with yourself sexually?
- Do you feel whole sexually?
- Can you share about your sense of satisfaction with yourself as a sexual being?

Summary

Sexuality is a healthy aspect of human life. Promoting sexual awareness is essential to the healthy functioning of all persons. Sexuality is an activity of daily living and therefore a natural part of life. The health care professional can assist clients in gaining awareness of their sexuality through a detailed understanding of the developmental nature of sexual growth. This chapter explored the healthy development of sexuality from infancy through the later years. Special issues related to each developmental phase were detailed. The health care professional should include data about sexual health patterns and practices in all client assessments and can learn to gain comfort and expertise in taking a sexual history. Becoming comfortable discussing sexual behavior and providing sexual health guidance are important responsibilities that health care professionals must accept.

HELPFUL **RESOURCES**

ORGANIZATIONS AND SERVICES
Intersex Society of North America
P.O. Box 31791
San Francisco, CA 94131
Phone: 415-436-0585
On-line: info@isna.org

Centers for Disease Control and Prevention. Clearinghouse phone number: (800) 458-5231.

Metropolitan King County Council. (1994). *Domestic/dating violence: An information and resource handbook.* Seattle: Author.

continued

HELPFUL **RESOURCES—cont'd**

ORGANIZATIONS AND SERVICES—cont'd

The Planned Parenthood Federation of America, Inc.
810 Seventh Avenue
New York, NY 10019
Phone: (800) 669-0156
Publishes an excellent 25-page booklet called *How to Talk to Your Teen About the Facts of Life*

Emergency Contraception Hotline
Phone: (888) NOT-2-LATE
Provided by Reproductive Health Technologies Project and Bridging the Gap Foundation, Inc.

Adoption services are generally local and can be located through most telephone Yellow Pages directories.

Sexuality Information and Education Center of the United States (SIECUS)
130 W. 42nd St.
Suite 350
New York, NY 10036-7802
Phone: (212) 819-9770
Fax: (212) 819-9776
On-line: SIECUS@siecus.org
Provides its members of the health care professions with a comprehensive annotated bibliography about gender identity through its library

Resolve, Inc.
1310 Broadway
Somerville, MA 02144
Phone: (617) 623-0744
Provides information about fertility support services offered in local communities.

National Center for HIV, STD and TB Prevention, Centers for Disease Control and Prevention, U.S. Department of Health and Human Services, U.S. Public Health Service
Atlanta, GA 30333.

American Social Health Association (ASHA)
P.O. Box 13827
Research Triangle Park, NJ 27709
Telephone: (919) 361-8400
Makes referrals to clinics nationwide and provides general STD information and publications.

The American Association of Sex Educators, Counselors and Therapists
P.O. Box 238
Mt. Vernon, IA 52314
Phone: (315) 895-8407
Fax: (319) 895-6203

READING MATERIALS

Anderson, P.B., de Mauro, D., & Noonan, R.J. (1992). *Does anyone still remember when sex was fun?* (2nd ed.). Dubuque, IA: Kendall/Hunt Publishing.

Anonymous. (1996). Taking a sexual history to help parents prevent STDs. *The Contraception Report, 7*(2), 12-16.

Bennet, J. (1997, January 5). Clinton lauds efforts leading to less teen-age pregnancy. *The New York Times,* 15.

Brody, J.E. (1989, February 28). Who's having sex? Data are obsolete, experts say. *The New York Times,* C1, C10.

Brody, J.E. (1991, October 2). Helping teenagers avoid pregnancy. *The New York Times,* C10.

Brody, J.E. (1996, December 11). Personal health. Sex education made easier for parent and teen-ager. *The New York Times,* C13.

Delgado, V. (1995). *Older women infected or affected by the HIV/AIDS crisis.* Miami: SACE.

Dodd, D.A. (1996, December 18). Seniors get in touch with their sexuality at lecture. *The (Miami) Herald.*

HELPFUL **RESOURCES—cont'd**

READING MATERIALS—cont'd

Doress, P.B., & Siegel, D.L. (1994). *New ourselves, growing older.* Olde Tappan, NJ: Simon & Schuster.

Fay, R.E., Turner, C.F., Klassen, A.D., & Gagnon, J.H. (1989). Prevalence and patterns of same-gender sexual contact among men. *Science, 243,* 338-348.

Frayser, S.G., & Whitley, T.J. (1995). *Studies in human sexuality* (2nd ed.). Englewood, CO: Libraries Unlimited.

Gilbert, S. (1995, October 11). Bias in doctors' offices may harm gay women's health, study finds. *The New York Times.*

Green, R. (Ed.). (1975). *Human sexuality: A health practitioner's text.* Baltimore: Williams & Wilkins.

Goldstein, B. (1976). *Introduction to human sexuality.* New York: McGraw-Hill.

Group for the Advancement of Psychiatry. (1965). *Sex and the college student* (Report No. 60). New York: Author.

Hacker, S.S. (1990). The transition from the old norm to the new: Sexual values for the 1990s. *SIECUS Report, 18*(5), 1-8.

Hammond, D.B. (1987). *My parents never had sex: Myths and facts of sexual aging.* Buffalo, NY: Prometheus Books.

Hatcher, H.A., Sanderson, C.A., & Smith, K. (1990). Sexual etiquette 101. *SIECUS Report, 18*(5), 9.

Herron, W.G., & Herron, M.J. (1996, February). The complexity of sexuality. *Psychology Report, 78*(1), 129-130.

U.S. Department of Health and Human Services, U.S. Public Health Service, Centers for Disease Prevention and Control. (1996). *HIV/AIDS surveillance report.* Atlanta, Ga: Author.

Hott, J.R. (1976). The crisis of expectant fatherhood. *American Journal of Nursing, 76*(9), 1435-1440.

Hott, J.R., Bell, J.L., & Barile, L.A. (1991). Speaking of sex. *American Journal of Nursing, 91*(1), 82.

Kellerman, V. (1995, January 8). Condom lessons upset group of parents. *The New York Times, 9.*

Kerka, S. (1996). *Hearing other voices? Women, human development.* Columbus, OH: ERIC Clearinghouse on Adult, Career and Vocational Education.

Ladas, A., Whipple, B., & Perry, J. (1982). *The G spot: And other recent discoveries about human sexuality.* New York: Dell.

Madaras, L., & Madaras, A. (1983). *The "what's happening to my body?" book for girls: A growing up guide for parents and daughters.* New York: Newmarket Press.

Marshal, J.E., & Konner, L. (1995). *Trouble-free menopause.* New York: Avon Books.

Oaks, W.W., Melchiode, G.A., & Fischer, I. (Eds.). (1976). *Sex and the life cycle.* New York: Gruen and Stratton.

Pomeroy, W.B., Flax, C.C., & Wheeler, C.C. (1982). *Taking a sex history: Interviewing and recording.* New York: Macmillan.

Roberts, S.J. (1996). The sequelae of childhood sexual abuse: A primary focus for adult female survivors. *The Nurse Practitioner, 21*(12), 42-52.

Scharbo-Dehaan, M. (1996). Hormone replacement therapy. *The Nurse Practitioner, 12,* 1-12.

Seidman, S.N., & Rieder, R.O. (1994). A review of sexual behavior in the United States. *American Journal of Psychiatry, 151,* 330-341.

continued

HELPFUL **RESOURCES—cont'd**

READING MATERIALS—cont'd

Simpson, C.C., Pruitt, R.H., Blackwell, D., & Swearingen, G.S. (1997). Preventing pregnancy in early adolescence. *Advance for Nurse Practitioners, 5*(4), 22-29.

Smeltzer, S.C., & Whipple, B. (1991). Women with HIV infection: The unrecognized population. *Health Values, 15*(6), 41-48.

Steinke, E., & Patterson-Midgley, P. (1996). Sexual counseling following acute myocardial infarction. *Clinical Nursing Research, 5*(4), 462-472.

Sutton, R. (1994). *Hearing us out: Voices from the gay and lesbian community.* Waltham, MA: Little Brown.

The Counseling Center for Mental Health, Division of the McKinley Health Center, University of Illinois. (1996). *What is child sexual abuse?* [On-line].

Thompson, S. (1995). *Going all the way: Teenage girls' tales of sex, romance and pregnancy.* New York: Hill and Wang.

Weigel, R. (1994). *Risk-taking is part of growing up for teens.* Plainview, NY: Cornell Cooperative Extension, Nassau County.

Westheimer, R.K. (1995). *Sex for dummies.* Foster City, CA: IDG Books.

Woods, N.F. (1975). *Human sexuality in health and illness.* St. Louis, Mosby.

Zurlinden, J. (1997, January 27). Hormone replacement therapy in menopause. *The Nursing Spectrum, 8.*

References

Alexander, L.L. (1992). Sexually transmitted diseases: Perspectives on this growing epidemic. *Nurse Practitioner: Americal Journal of Primary Health Care, 17* (10), 31, 34, 37-38, 41-42.

American Academy of Nursing (1994). *HIV/AIDS Nursing Care Summit* (p. 3). Washington, DC: Author

American Academy of Pediatrics. (1988). *Child sexual abuse. What it is and how to prevent it.* Elk Grove Village, IL: Author.

American College of Obstetricians and Gynecology. (1997). ACOG practice patterns. Emergency oral contraception, No. 3, December, 1996 (Replaces No. 2, October 1996). *International Journal of Gynecology and Obstetrics, 56*(3), 290-297.

American Medical Association. (1992). Diagnostic and treatment guidelines on domestic violence. *Archives of Family Medicine, 1,* 39-47.

American Social Health Association (1994). *Clinical history form.* Research Triangle Park, NC: Author.

American Social Health Association. (1996). *Women and STDs* (Fact sheet). Research Triangle Park, NC: Author.

Annon, J. (1976). *Behavioral treatment of sexual problems: Brief therapy* (Vol. 1). New York: Harper and Row.

Berger, M.M., Eckardt, M.H., Gilligan, C., Ingram, D.H., Kaplan, H.S., Lief, H.I., Miller, J.B., Olarte, S.W., Quinn, S., & Rendon, M. (1994). *Women beyond Freud: New concepts of feminine psychology.* New York: Brunner/Mazel.

Bowman, J., & Wolfe, L. (1995). *American Association of Retired Persons women's initiative.* Washington, DC: American Association of Retired Persons.

Centers for Disease Control and Prevention. (1993, August 20). Emergency department response to domestic violence—California, 1992. *Morbidity and Mortality Weekly Report, 42*(32), 617-620.

Centers for Disease Control and Prevention. (1995, June). *Providers not diagnosing HIV in older women.* Rockville, MD: National AIDS Clearinghouse.

Centers for Disease Control and Prevention. (1996a, August 30). HIV testing among women aged 18-44 years—United States, 1991 and 1993. *Morbidity and Mortality Weekly Report, 45*(34), 733-737.

Centers for Disease Control and Prevention. (1996b, September 6). Physical violence and injuries in intimate relationships—New York. Behavioral risk factor surveillance system, 1994. *Morbidity and Mortality Weekly Report, 45* (35), 765-767.

Centers for Disease Control and Prevention. (1997a). AIDS cases by age and sex, reported 1981-1996. United States [On-line]. Available: http://www.cdc.gov.nchstp/hiv

Centers for Disease Control and Prevention. (1997b). CDC AIDS information [On-line]. Available: http://www.cdc.gov/nchstp/hiv__aids/hivinfo

Chehrazi, S. (1987). Female psychology: A review. (pp. 22-38). In M.R. Walsh (Ed.), *The psychology of women: Ongoing debates.* New Haven, CT: Yale University Press.

Congressional Caucus for Women's Issues. *Effs of rape* (Monograph). Washington, DC: Author.

Crenshaw, T.L., & Goldberg, J.P. (1996). *Sexual pharmacology,* New York: WW Norton.

Diamond, M., & Karlen, A. (1981). The sexual response cycle. In H. Lief (Ed.), *Sexual problems in medical practice* (pp. 37-51). Monroe, WI: American Medical Association.

Donahoe, P.K., & Schnitzer, J.J. (1996, February 5). Evaluation of the infant who has ambiguous genitalia and principles of operative management. *Seminars in Pediatric Surgery,* 1, 30-40.

Eng, T.R., & Butler, W.T. (Eds). (1996). The hidden epidemic: Confronting sexually transmitted diseases. Washington, DC: The Institute of Medicine.

Finkelhor, D., & Dziuba-Leatherman, J. (1994). Children as victims of violence: A national survey. I. *Pediatrics, 94*(4), 413-420.

Fleming, P.L., Guina, M.E., Ward, J.W., Chiasson, M.A., & Jones, W.K. (1995). *AIDS in older women.* Atlanta: Centers for Disease Control and Prevention.

Fogel, C.I., & Lauver, D. (1990). *Sexual health promotion.* Philadelphia: WB Saunders.

Forrest, J.D., & Singh, S. (1990). The sexual and reproductive behavior of American women, 1982-88. *Family Planning Perspectives, 22,* 206-214.

Furniss, K. (1996). Common clinical problems and issues. In Association of Women's Health Obstetric and Neonatal Nurses (AWHONN) and National Association of Nurse Practitioners and Reproductive Health (NANPRH) (Eds.), *Current practice issues in adolescent gynecology. Contemporary studies in women's health.* Fairlawn, NJ: MPE Communications.

Gadpaille, W.J. (1981). Psychosocial development through the life cycle. In H. Lief (Ed.), *Sexual problems in medical practice* (pp. 17-36). Monroe, WI: American Medical Association.

Gilligan, C. (1982). *In a different voice: Psychological theory and women's development.* Cambridge, MA: Harvard University Press.

Gould, L. (1978). *X, a fabulous child's story.* New York: Daughters Publishing.

Gotwald, W.H., & Golden, G.H. (1981). *Sexuality: The human experience.* New York: Macmillan.

Green, R., & Schiavi, R.C. (Eds.). (1995). Sexual and gender identity disorders. In C.O. Gabbard (Ed.), Treatments of psychiatric disorders, Vols. 1 & 2 (2nd ed., pp. 1837-2079). Washington, DC: American Psychiatric Press, Inc.

Grossman, A.H. (1995). At risk, infected, and invisible: Older gay men and HIV/AIDS. *Journal of the Association of Nurses in AIDS Care, 6*(6), 13-19.

Group for the Advancement of Psychiatry. (1973). *Assessment of sexual function: A guide to interviewing* (Report No. 88). New York: Author.

Hatcher, R.A., Atkinson, A., Cates, D., Glasser, L., & Legins, K. (1993). *Sexual etiquette 101,* Atlanta: Emory University School of Medicine.

Haynes, J.D. (1995). A critique of the possibility of genetic inheritance of same sex relationship orientation. *Journal of Homosexuality, 28*(1-2), 91-113.

Henshaw, S.K. (1997). Teenage abortion and pregnancy statistics by state, 1992. *Family Planning Perspectives, 29*(3), 115-122.

Hogan, R.M. (1980). *Human sexuality: A nursing perspective.* New York: Appleton-Century-Crofts.

Hott, J.R. (1972). *An investigation of the relationship between psychoprophylaxis in childbirth and changes in self-concept of the participant husband and his concept of his wife.* Unpublished doctorate thesis, New York University School of Education.

Kaplan, H.S. (1974). *The new sex therapy: Active treatment of sexual dysfunction.* New York: Brunner/Mazel.

Kinsey, A.C., Pomeroy, W.B., & Martin, C.E. (1948). *Sexual behavior in the human male.* Philadelphia: WB Saunders.

Kirby, D., Short, L., Collins, J., Rugg, D., Kolbe, L., Howard, M., Miller, B., Sonenstein, F., & Zabin, L.S. (1994). School-based programs to reduce sexual risk behaviors: A review of effectiveness. *Public Health Reports, 109*(3), 339-360.

La Freniere, P., Strayer, F.F., & Gautheir, R. (1984). The emergence of same-sex affiliative preferences among preschool peers: A developmental/ethological perspective. *Child Development, 57,* 375-386.

Landau, E. (1986). *Difference drummer: Same sex relationships in America.* New York: J. Messner.

Laumann, E.O., Gagnon, J.H., Michael, R.T., & Michaels, S. (1994). *The social organization of sexuality. Sexual practices in the United States.* Chicago: The University of Chicago Press.

Lief, H., & Berman E.M. (1981). Sexual interviewing throughout the patient's life cycle. In H. Lief (Ed.), *Sexual problems in medical practice* (pp. 119-130). Monroe, WI: American Medical Association.

Levay, A., Sharpe, L., & Kagle, A. (1981). The effects of physical illness on sexual functioning. In H. Lief (Ed.), *Sexual problems in medical practice* (pp. 169-189). Monroe, WI: American Medical Association.

Lieblum, S.R., & Rosen, R.C. (Eds.). (1988). *Principles and practices of sex therapy.* New York: Guilford Press.

Luster, T., & Small, S.A. (1997). Sexual abuse history and number of sex partners among female adolescents. *Family Planning Perspectives, 29,* 204-211.

Masters, W., & Johnson, V.E. (1966). *Human sexual response.* Boston: Brown & Co.

Moore, R. (1996). Overview of developmental and physical milestones and psychosocial issues. Current practice issues in adolescent gynecology. [Monograph]. *AWHONN,* 4-7.

Perry, J.D., & Whipple, B. (1981). Pelvic muscle strength of female ejaculators: Evidence in support of a new theory of orgasm. *Journal of Sex Research, 17,* 22-39.

Pipher, M. (1994). *Reviving Ophelia, saving the selves of adolescent girls.* New York: Ballantine Books.

Ridley, M. (1993). A boy or a girl: Is it possible to load the dice? *Smithsonian, 24*(3), 113-124.

Savin-Williams, R.C. (1995a). Keep lines of communication open with gay, lesbian and bisexual teens. Plainview, NY: Human Development and Family Studies, Cornell Cooperative Extension, Nassau County, New York State College of Human Ecology, Cornell University.

Savin-Williams, R.C. (1995b). Gay, lesbian and bisexual teens need adult help during adolescence. Plainview, NY: Cornell Cooperative Extension, Nassau County, New York State College of Human Ecology, Cornell University.

Sherwen, L.N., Scoloveno, M.A., & Weingarten, C.T. (1991). *Nursing care of the childbearing family* (pp. 165-167). East Norwich, CT: Appleton & Lange.

Shope, D.F. (1975). *Interpersonal sexuality.* Philadelphia: WB Saunders.

SIECUS position statements on human sexuality (1995-96), *SIECUS Report, 24*(3), 21.

Siemens, S., & Brandzel, R.C. (1982). *Sexuality: Nursing assessment and intervention.* Philadelphia: JB Lippincott.

Smith, T.W. (1991). Adult sexual behavior in 1989: Number of partners, frequency of intercourse and risk of AIDS. *Family Planning Perspectives, 23,* 104.

Social Services Law of New York, § 664-412 (1988).

U.S. Bureau of the Census. (1996). *Statistical Abstract of the U.S.* (116th ed.). Washington, DC: Superintendent of Documents.

Whaley, L.F., & Wong, D.L., (1997). *Essentials of pediatric nursing,* St. Louis: Mosby.

Whipple, B., & Ogden, G. (1989). *Safe encounters: How women can say yes to pleasure and no to unsafe sex.* New York: McGraw-Hill.

Zuckerman, E.L. (1995). *Clinician's thesaurus* (4th ed., pp. 59-61). New York: Guilford Press.

CHAPTER

10

Injury Prevention

David A. Sleet and Andrea C. Gielen

Editors' Note

Injury Prevention and the Community Client System.   Injuries in the United States cost billions of dollars each year. These costs include lost wages; medical expenses; motor vehicle damage; fire losses; and administrative costs of police, lawyers, and insurers. Authors David Sleet, PhD, and Andrea Gielen, ScD, discuss injury prevention rather than accidents focusing on avoidable harm. Using an epidemiologic framework, upon which the Health Promotion Matrix also is based in part, Sleet and Gielen outline three generally accepted strategies in injury prevention: education/behavior change, engineering/technology, and legislation/enforcement. They link the education and behavior change strategy to host behavior (e.g., in the use of seat belts). They also discuss how the agent is affected by alterations in engineering and technology (e.g., reflective clothing or smoke detectors), and how the environment is addressed by legislation and enforcement (e.g., the use of highway signs and building codes). The selection of each of these strategies rests on a community needs assessment with consideration of the sitation, the intended target, and local standards, as well as the public's acceptance of various changes needed to reduce injuries. Individuals, families, and groups may carry out injury prevention guidelines, but it is at the community level that injury prevention strategies are recommended to protect the population at large.

Injury Prevention and Internalize Idealized Image.   Sleet and Gielen place injury prevention within the context of the traditional epidemiologic framework, implying the importance of empirical research to better understand the prevalence of injuries across population subgroups, as well as in the assessment of interventions for change. They identify the importance of systematic development of community strategies for injury prevention and emphasize the importance of evaluation of outcomes through modifying host, agent, and environment relationships. They also emphasize the role of reinforcement in long-term client change.

Health Care Professional Dialogue in an Outpatient/Well-Care Setting and the Health Promotion Matrix Script.   Relying on well-developed models of communication, which underpin the Health Promotion Matrix (HPM), Sleet and Gielen provide an example dialogue for the health care professional. In addition to reinforcing change, they emphasize the importance of the health care professional creating a positive atmosphere to talk about injury prevention; eliciting and giving accurate information; asking for feedback; and, as in other health promotion approaches, obtaining client commitment to alter behaviors. This example is coupled with others in the HPM script that follows.

The health of Americans has changed significantly during the last 40 years. Widespread immunization programs have virtually eliminated the threat of infectious diseases such as polio, diphtheria, and measles. Even so, one of the problems that continues to threaten the health of Americans—and is not likely to be eliminated soon—is injuries.

Injury is the third leading cause of death in the United States and is the leading cause of death for children and young adults (National Center for Health Statistics, 1991). Each year, about 149,000 injury-related deaths result in 3.7 million potential years of life lost before age 65 years (Rice & MacKenzie, 1989), whereas less than 3 million potential years of life are lost each for cancer and heart disease and 400,000 each for AIDS and stroke (National Center for Injury Prevention and Control, 1996).

Every year, nonfatal injuries account for 114 million visits to physicians' offices and more than one quarter visits to emergency departments. Injuries are the leading cause of hospital admissions for persons younger than 45 years (Graves, 1993), and this year, one in four Americans will suffer a potentially preventable injury serious enough to require medical attention.

In many respects, injury is today's primary public health problem for Americans younger than 44 years. Injuries among Americans of all ages could be dramatically reduced if health promotion approaches to preventing and controlling them were applied.

INJURY AS A PUBLIC HEALTH PROBLEM

According to the National Academy of Sciences (1988), "Injury is probably the most under recognized major public health problem facing the nation today." In fact, each year, injury is the No. 1 cause of death among school-age children and youths, in virtually every country in the world. Yet until recently, injury prevention was not recognized as a public health issue.

Injury is now recognized as a health problem that can best be understood and controlled by using the same approaches used against other diseases. Injury results from interactions between persons (host factors), energy (agent and vehicle factors), and the environment (environmental factors) (Haddon, 1970). This epidemiologic approach to understanding injury is the foundation upon which health promotion strategies to injury reduction are applied.

Injury can be controlled by reducing the number of times it occurs and by reducing its severity when it does occur. In public health, injury is defined as "unintentional or intentional damage to the body resulting from acute exposure to thermal, mechanical, electrical, or chemical energy or from the absence of such essentials as heat or oxygen" (National Committee for Injury Prevention and Control, 1989). In the case of a sports injury, damage to the host (the person harmed) is brought about through a rapid transfer of kinetic energy. This exchange of energy can be modified in several ways—for instance, by making the host more resistant to it (by increasing injury tolerance) or by separating the host from the kinetic energy exchange (e.g., interposing protective equipment between the host and the energy source. (Haddon, 1970).

Although injury is a public health problem, to solve it, it takes professionals from many disciplines, such as nurses, health educators, school teachers and officials, nursing home and hospital administrators, psychologists, social workers, police, product engineers, highway planners, criminologists, playground designers, sports physicians, coaches, occupational safety scientists, chemists, and surgeons. Injury prevention requires collaboration.

INJURY OR ACCIDENT?

Injury does not happen by accident. Accidents are not predictable or preventable. *The Oxford English Dictionary* defines the term *accident* "as an event without apparent cause . . . unexpected—happening by chance." Typically, accidents" are viewed as random and uncontrollable "acts of fate," unpredictable and unavoidable. This is true even outside public health. For example, in geology, an accident is defined as an irregularity on a surface, the explanation of which is not readily known.

The word *injury* has its root in the Latin term *injurius*, which literally means "unjust" or "not right." The Funk and Wagnalls' Dictionary (1966) defines injury as "harm, damage, or grievous distress inflicted or sustained." Since the term accident implies an unavoidable event, it should not be used when referring to injury, which is a predictable medical outcome. The science of injury prevention teaches that injuries are not accidental or random events—they are predictable, and many are preventable through changes in products, human behavior, and environments. Using terms such as *injury prevention* rather than *accident prevention* helps make clear the potential for preventing these adverse medical outcomes. Former U.S. Surgeon General C. Everett Koop (1989) underscored this distinction in his preface to *Injury Prevention: Meeting The Challenge* (National Committee for Injury Prevention and Control, 1989) when he said:

> We must accept that the injuries associated with motor vehicles are not "accidents" and that much can be done to reduce them. We must realize that violence in the forms of abuse, assault or suicide is not only within the purview of the police and the criminal justice system but also the health system. An informed and aroused public can change the behavior of each of us, but more importantly, it must lead to community outrage and action in regard to unsafe playgrounds, automobiles, highways, work places, toys, homes and use of handguns.

Focusing on prevention of both the event and its medical, social, and economic consequences may help reframe the issue of injury within a disease prevention/health promotion framework.

CAUSES OF INJURY

The specific cause of injury is the transfer of energy to a person at rates and in amounts more than the tolerance of human tissue (De Haven, 1942). The amount of the energy concentration outside the tolerance of tissue usually determines the severity of the injury. The terms *injury* and *trauma* are often used interchangeably.

The two generally recognized categories of injuries are *unintentional injuries* (caused by unintentional means [e.g., a fall, drowning, poisoning, or motor vehicle crash]) and *violence* (intentionally inflicted [e.g., homicide, battery, murder, or suicide]). Domestic violence, particularly to children and youth, is one form of intentional injury in which the health care professional is generally legally obligated to intervene and is discussed in Chapter 9. Homicides and suicides are explored in part in Chapter 11. Unintentional injuries is the focus of this chapter.

Table 10-1

Ten leading causes of death by age group–1994

RANK	AGE GROUPS					
	<1	1-4	5-9	10-14	15-24	25-34
1	Congenital anomalies 6,854	Unintentional injuries 2,517	Unintentional injuries 1,595	Unintentional injuries 1,913	Unintentional injuries 13,898	Unintentional injuries 13,452
2	Short gestation 4,254	Congenital anomalies 714	Malignant neoplasms 543	Malignant neoplasms 510	Homicide 8,116	HIV 12,117
3	SIDS 4,073	Malignant neoplasms 518	Congenital anomalies 241	Homicide 416	Suicide 4,956	Homicide 6,888
4	Respiratory distress syndrome 1,567	Homicide 473	Homicide 156	Suicide 318	Malignant neoplasms 1,740	Suicide 6,354
5	Maternal complications 1,296	Heart disease 285	Heart disease 129	Heart disease 198	Heart disease 992	Malignant neoplasms 5,056
6	Placenta cord membranes 948	HIV 199	HIV 110	Congenital anomalies 193	HIV 641	Heart disease 3,520
7	Unintentional injuries 889	Pneumonia and Influenza 178	Pneumonia and Influenza 57	Bronchitis Emphysema Asthma 86	Congenital anomalies 463	Cerebrovascular 802
8	Perinatal infections 828	Perinatal period 114	Benign neoplasms 54	HIV 72	Bronchitis Emphysema Asthma 232	Liver disease 733
9	Pneumonia and influenza 559	Septicemia 91	Bronchitis Emphysema Asthma 41	Benign neoplasms 47	Pneumonia and influenza 221	Diabetes 682
10	Intrauterine hypoxia 537	Benign neoplasms 79	Anemias 38	Cerebrovascular 46 Pneumonia/ Influenza 46	Cerebrovascular 183	Pneumonia and influenza 647

From *Mortality Data Tapes,* 1996, by National Center for Injury Prevention and Control and National Center for Health Statistics, Atlanta: Centers for Disease Control and Prevention.

		AGE GROUPS		
35-44	**45-54**	**55-64**	**65+**	**TOTAL**
HIV 18,359	Malignant neoplasms 43,588	Malignant neoplasms 89,251	Heart disease 610,330	Heart disease 732,409
Malignant neoplasms 16,843	Heart disease 33,621	Heart disease 69,335	Malignant neoplasms 376,186	Malignant neoplasms 534,310
Unintentional injuries 13,560	Unintentional injuries 8,768	Bronchitis Emphysema Asthma 10,335	Cerebrovas- cular 134,340	Cerebrovas- cular 153,306
Heart disease 13,243	HIV 7,636	Cerebrovas- cular 9,577	Bronchitis Emphysema Asthma 87,048	Bronchitis Emphysema Asthma 101,628
Suicide 6,375	Cerebrovas- cular 5,355	Diabetes 7,784	Pneumonia and influenza 72,762	Unintentional injuries 91,437
Homicide 4,531	Liver disease 5,043	Unintentional injuries 6,432	Diabetes 42,600	Pneumonia and influenza 81,473
Liver disease 3,698	Suicide 4,296	Liver disease 5,530	Unintentional injuries 28,314	Diabetes 56,692
Cerebrovascular 2,717	Diabetes 3,689	Pneumonia and influenza 3,505	Nephritis 19,666	HIV 42,114
Diabetes 1,785	Bronchitis Emphysema Asthma 2,676	Suicide 2,812	Alzheimer's disease 18,217	Suicide 31,142
Pneumonia and influenza 1,508	Pneumonia and influenza 1,985	HIV 2,186	Septicemia 16,439	Liver disease 25,406

Although there are many kinds and causes of injury, the following two main categories prevail:

1. *Acute exposure to energy*—refers to injuries resulting from falls, motor vehicle crashes, firearms, violence, and sports play (kinetic energy); fires and burns (thermal energy); poisonings (chemical energy); electrocution (electrical energy); and radiation (radient energy).
2. *Absence of essentials*—includes lack of oxygen (e.g., as occurs in asphyxiation, strangulation, or drowning) and lack of heat (e.g., as occurs in hypothermia or frostbite).

MAGNITUDE OF THE INJURY PROBLEM

Like diseases, injuries have geographic, socioeconomic, and seasonal variations. Injury also varies according to characteristics among persons (e.g., age, sex, income) and among persons' environment (e.g., neighborhood, workplace, home). Injury epidemiology has developed as a way to understand and explain these variations and as a way to target specific interventions to reduce injuries among persons in specific high-risk populations.

Table 10-1 shows the 10 leading causes of death by age group in 1994. Injury, including unintentional injury, homicide, and suicide, is the leading cause of death for each age group category from ages 1-44 years. Unintentional injuries dominate, with homicide and suicide occupying prominent places as major causes of death for those ages 10-34 years.

Table 10-2 shows the number of deaths caused by injury type and the rates per 100,000 population (including age-adjusted and crude rates) by gender in the United States in 1995. In sheer numbers of injury-related deaths in 1995, motor vehicle crashes

Table **10-2**

Number of deaths caused by injury and rates per 100,000 population by sex, 1995

CAUSE	MALES		FEMALES		TOTAL		
	No.	**RATE**	**No.**	**RATE**	**No.**	**CRUDE RATE**	**AGE-ADJUSTED RATE***
Motor vehicle	29,164	22.7	14,199	10.6	43,363	16.5	16.3
Fall	5,812	4.5	4,671	3.5	10,483	4.0	2.1
Drowning	3,539	2.8	811	0.6	4,350	1.7	1.7
Fire/flames	2,232	1.7	1,529	1.1	3,761	1.4	1.2
Poisoning	6,885	5.4	2,187	1.6	9,072	3.5	3.2
Homicide/legal intervention	17,740	13.8	5,155	3.8	22,895	8.7	9.4
Suicide	25,369	19.7	5,915	4.4	31,284	11.9	11.1
Other	16,239	12.7	9,362	7.0	25,601	9.7	7.1
Total	106,980	83.4	43,829	32.6	150,809	57.4	52.1

*Age-adjusted rate excludes those whose ages are unknown. Standard population is 1940 U.S. all races and both genders.
From 1997 *Mortality Data Tapes,* by National Center for Injury Prevention and Control and National Center for Health Statistics, 1997, Atlanta: Centers for Disease Control and Prevention (CDC).
NOTE: NCHS *Mortality Data Tapes* are used for number of deaths; Demo-Detail postcensal estimates are used for population numbers.

were the leading cause, followed by suicide, homicide, falls, poisonings, drownings, and fires. Violence, when measured by the number of deaths resulting from both suicide and homicide, exceeds the combined total of both motor vehicle- and fall-related deaths. Among males, violent deaths exceeded the combined total of deaths resulting from motor vehicle crashes, falls, drownings, and fires.

Deaths are only a part of the devastating effects of injury on society. Each year, 52,000 persons die from traumatic brain injury (TBI), 300,000 more are hospitalized, and 70,000 to 90,000 are permanently impaired. It is estimated that 10,000 persons are hospitalized each year with spinal cord injury, and about 190,000 persons live their entire lives with the permanent effects from this type of injury (National Center for Injury Prevention and Control, 1996). Although motor vehicle crashes, firearms, falls, poisonings, fires and burns, and drownings account for 80% of deaths resulting from injury each year, they account for only 36% of treated injuries not requiring hospitalization (National Center for Injury Prevention and Control, 1996).

The Epidemiology of Injury

The epidemiologic model developed for infectious and chronic disease can be applied to injury (Gordon, 1949). This model considers the contribution of and interaction between the host (the person getting the disease), the agent (the specific disease-causing element) and vector (the carrier transmitting the agent to the host), and the environment (physical and sociocultural factors influencing transmission and reception) (Haddon, 1980).

Injury results from the interaction between injury-producing agents (e.g., kinetic energy), the environment (e.g., a playground), and a susceptible host (e.g., a young and curious child). Injury can be controlled by preventing its occurrence or minimizing its severity when it does occur. In the case of motor vehicle–related injury, damage to the host is caused by a rapid transfer of kinetic energy when the vehicle stops suddenly. Changing this pattern of energy transfer (either by making the host more resistant to it or by separating the host from the energy exchange) is part of the science of injury control.

An example of the model applied to smoking (Figure 10-1) shows how host factors (amount smoked, depth of inhalation), agent factors (tar and ciliotoxins), and environmental factors (smoking areas, social pressure) each contribute to smoking-related morbidity and mortality. Applying the model to injury control (Figure 10-2) shows how it can be applied to injury morbidity and mortality resulting from traffic crashes. Host factors include age, inexperience at driving, and alcohol or drug use. Environmental factors include road surfaces and signs, and traffic conditions. Agent factors are those factors that affect (1) the amount of energy released, (2) the distribution of that energy, and (3) the transfer of the energy to the host. Examples of agent factors for injury related to motor vehicle crashes are size of vehicle, vehicle speed, force of impact, angle of crash, and type of protective equipment used by the occupants.

Health Promotion and Injury Prevention

Injury prevention has received less coverage than it deserves in the health promotion literature, perhaps because it does not fall within the traditional domain of preventive medicine and public health (Sleet & Rosenberg, 1997). As recently as 1982, injury prevention was not an area of importance in textbooks on principles and clinical applications of health promotion (Taylor, Ureda, & Denham, 1982). This may have been partly due to the way *Healthy People* (U.S. Public Health Service, 1979) had categorized injuries as resulting from

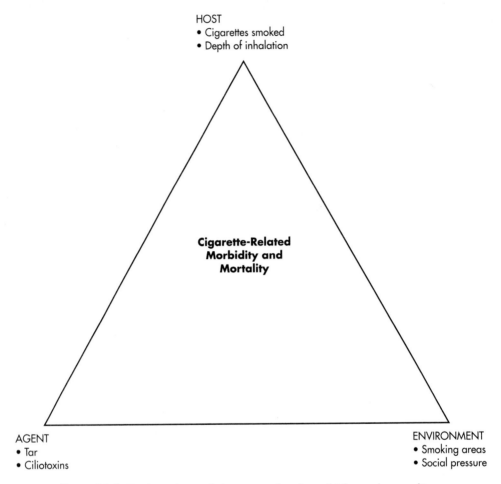

HOST
• Cigarettes smoked
• Depth of inhalation

**Cigarette-Related
Morbidity and
Mortality**

AGENT
• Tar
• Ciliotoxins

ENVIRONMENT
• Smoking areas
• Social pressure

Figure 10-1 Epidemiology of cigarette-related morbidity and mortality.

"accidents" and placed them in the "health protection" category, along with other environmental problems considered to be beyond individual control. Inevitably, as injury prevention and health promotion become closer aligned, the potential benefits of behavior changes as an injury prevention strategy will become clearer and more widely accepted.

Green and Kreuter (1991) define health promotion as "any planned combination of educational, political, regulatory, and organizational supports for actions and conditions of living conducive to the health of individuals, groups, or communities" (p. 432). This widely recognized definition acknowledges the importance of taking a behavioral, environmental, *and* policy approach to the prevention of disease and injury. Client education is only one method within the broader mix of health promotion approaches available.

The immediate goals of health promotion for injury control include the following:

■ Modifying individual risk behaviors.
■ Reducing exposure to hazardous environments.
■ Removing/modifying harmful products.

Individual and community actions are required to succeed in these efforts, which are

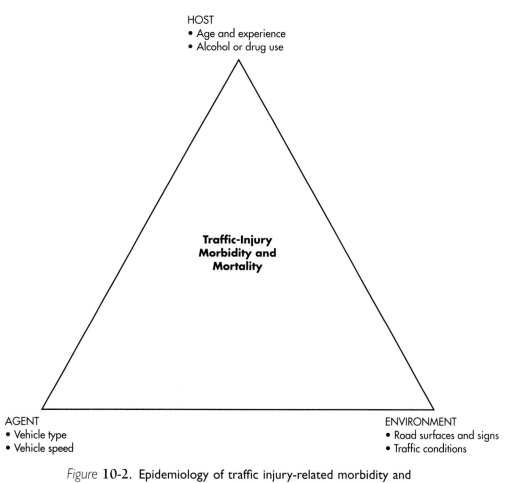

HOST
• Age and experience
• Alcohol or drug use

**Traffic-Injury
Morbidity and
Mortality**

AGENT
• Vehicle type
• Vehicle speed

ENVIRONMENT
• Road surfaces and signs
• Traffic conditions

Figure **10-2.** Epidemiology of traffic injury-related morbidity and mortality.

fostered by education stimulated by social and organizational change and are encouraged through public policy, legislation, and enforcement.

INJURY PREVENTION STRATEGIES

Strategies in injury prevention, which are general plans of action used to reduce injuries, are distinct from *methods,* which are tactics used to implement the strategies. Whereas education is one strategy for preventing burns, clinical counseling is one method of implementing that strategy; another method is a mass media campaign to make the public aware of a burn-related hazard. There are three generally accepted strategies in injury prevention and many distinct methods for implementing each. The three strategies are as follows:

1. Education and behavior change.
2. Engineering and technology.
3. Legislation and enforcement.

A combination of strategies should be selected on the basis of an analysis of the situation, including a needs assessment for the population being served. The strategy mix

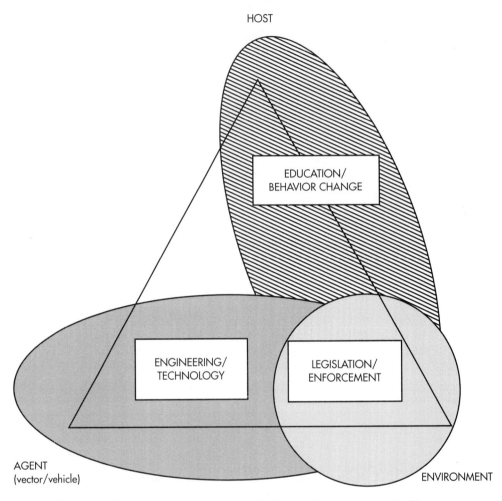

Figure 10-3 Prevention strategies applied to epidemiologic triad of injury causation. *(From "Injury as a Public Health Problem," by D.A. Sleet, G. Egger, and P. Albany, 1991,* Health Promotion Journal of Australia, 1(2), pp. 4-9.)

should also take into consideration local standards and the public acceptability of various behavioral, environmental, or engineering and infrastructural changes necessary to reduce injuries. In general, the three types of strategies interact with the epidemiologic triad of host, agent (vector/vehicle), and environment in a manner described in Figure 10-3.

Figure 10-3 has two implications. First, strategy selection is influenced by the proposed target. Education and behavior change may be used to target the host; legislation and law enforcement may target environmental change; and engineering and technology may target changes in the agent to modify energy transfer. Second, strategies overlap (i.e., one strategy may affect more than one target) (Sleet, Egger, & Albany, 1991).

Education and Behavior Change

Education and behavior change strategies are directed mostly toward decreasing the susceptibility of the host to injury by teaching or motivating persons to behave differently.

Some methods used to implement this strategy (e.g., social marketing) may also affect social norms in the environment, as illustrated by the overlapping circles in Figure 10-3. For example, the designated-driver campaigns aimed at modifying host drinking behaviors also affected attitudes in the community environment, resulting in drinking and driving being socially unacceptable.

Although some controversy still exists about the benefits of educational approaches on injury control (O'Connor, 1982; Pless, 1978), there are numerous examples of successful applications of health education strategies to injury prevention (Athey, 1995; DiGuieseppi, Rivara, Koepsell, & Polissar 1989; Preusser & Blomberg, 1984; Borden, Hall, Levenstein, & Punnett, 1984; Fortenberry & Brown, 1982; Rivara, Booth, Bergman, Rogers, & Weiss, 1991; Frank, Bouman, Cain, & Watts, 1992). Discrepancies in the results of various studies can be attributed to a number of factors, including lack of control groups, use of different methods of education, the absence of theory-based approaches to health education in the design of interventions, poorly designed methods for measuring change, and inadequate "doses" of education.

Behavior change methods, however, have produced more consistently positive results (Roberts, Fanurik, & Layfield, 1987; Streff, & Geller, 1986; Jones, van Hasselt, & Sisson, 1984). Such methods include incentives, social modeling, feedback, rewards, skills training, cognitive rehearsal, and competition to improve injury prevention behavior (Huesmann, Guerra, Miller, & Zelli, 1992; Farrell, Meyer, & Dahlberg, 1996; Geller, Elder, Hovell, & Sleet, 1991; Sleet, Hollenbach, & Hovell, 1986). Behavior change methods can be targeted to change the behavior of one person (e.g., a juvenile's fire-starting behavior), the behavior of a particular group at risk (e.g., that of teenage drivers), or an entire community (e.g., the use of the emergency 911 number).

Behaviors for which behavior change approaches have been successful include the following:

■ Emergency fire safety skills for children in the home
■ Child restraint and child safety belt use
■ Adult safety belt use
■ Worker behavior in hazardous occupations
■ Impaired driving

Education and behavior change approaches can also produce effects on those who make laws and design products, such as legislators and engineers, in ways that ultimately protect whole populations.

For education and behavior change strategies to work, the target audience must:

■ Be exposed to the appropriate information.
■ Understand and believe the information.
■ Have the resources and skills to make the proposed change.
■ Derive benefit (or perceive a benefit) from the change.
■ Be reinforced to maintain the change over time.

Legislation and Law Enforcement

Legislation and law enforcement strategies have their greatest effect by making both the physical environment (e.g., regulated highway signs and building codes) and the sociocultural environment (e.g., social attitudes and policies supporting a safe community) safer. Laws and regulations can be made to require changes in individual behavior or product design or to alter environmental hazards. In each case, there is an opportunity for the legislation and law enforcement strategies to work synergistically with the other two strategies. Laws to discourage individuals from drinking and driving (e.g., laws that permit a maximum of 0.08 g/dL of alcohol in the blood of drivers) can also make persons less tolerant of drinking and boating. Communities that raise the price of alcoholic beverages also stand a good chance of reducing overall alcohol consumption, thereby reducing many alcohol-related injuries.

Legislation can also be aimed at changing the environment, making it less hazardous for everyone. Regulations requiring residential pool fencing, safeguards against workplace hazards, or comprehensive trauma care systems are examples of how these strategies can benefit whole communities. Product safety regulations, such as those affecting toys, home appliances, sports equipment, and playgrounds, are other examples of the application of legislation and law enforcement to benefit multiple targets.

Key factors in making legislation and law enforcement strategies effective appear to be the following:
- The legislation is widely known and understood.
- The public accepts the legislation and its enforcement provisions.
- The probability, or perceived probability, of being caught if one breaks the law is high.
- The punishment is perceived to be swift and severe.

Engineering and Technology

Engineering and technology strategies are likely to have their greatest impact on the agent (vector or vehicle) of energy transfer, but they may also affect environmental factors contributing to injury. Hip pads designed to reduce hip fractures among the elderly by reducing the amount of energy transferred to the host during a fall led to the design of soft flooring materials to reduce environmental risks where risks for falls are high (e.g., nursing homes). Technology and engineering contribute to injury reduction by the development of products that reduce the likelihood of sudden energy release. These strategies can affect the safety of environments as well, and may even lead to safer behavior on the part of the host (e.g., occupants may increase use of safety belts while riding in an air-bag equipped car).

Some of the many technologic and engineering advances that reduce the host's risk for injuries that have also improved environmental safety include reflective clothing, bridged pedestrian paths, child resistant caps on cigarette lighters, household smoke detectors, institutional sprinkler systems, electrical insulation, swimming pool alarms, household fuses, machine guards, break-away bases, air bags, automatic seat belts, tractor rollover protection, and soft playground surfaces.

Successfully implementing engineering and technology solutions that protect large populations, however, requires that the technology:
- Be effective and reliable.
- Be acceptable to the public and compatible with the environment.
- Result in products that dominate in the marketplace.
- Be easily understood and properly used by the public.

Despite advances in technology, however, many protective devices (e.g., swimming pool fences, ignition interlocks, and antilock brakes) have had limited success because one or more of the factors previously listed were ignored (e.g., swimming pool fences were not environmentally aesthetic, the public did not know how to operate antilock brakes).

Combining Strategies

The importance of using a mix of strategies to prevent and control injuries cannot be overemphasized. A good example of combining education and behavior change, engineering and technology, and legislation and law enforcement strategies to reduce injuries is the success in reducing injuries resulting from alcohol-impaired driving in many countries. Legislation controlling young drivers' access to alcohol was combined with legislation to lower blood alcohol concentration (BAC) limits and to impose stiff drunken driving penalties. When the laws were enacted, a widespread public education campaign also began through the news media and grassroots organizations on the reasons for and benefits of the new laws and on the risks of drinking and driving. These strategies and methods were further enhanced through engineering, by the development of more sophisticated alcohol-sensing devices, Breathalyzer and roadside testing devices, and vehicle lockout devices for convicted drunken drivers (Trinica et al., 1988).

These three strategies can help health care professionals develop specific interventions targeted to specific populations in which components of each strategy could be used to design a comprehensive community-based approach to injury prevention.

CLINICAL APPROACHES TO INJURY PREVENTION

Health care professionals have a special role in promoting injury prevention and control. First, they have direct and continuing access to persons whose safety is threatened. Second, standards of practice for most health care professions call for the provision of preventive services, including age-appropriate counseling about safety (American Academy of Pediatrics, [AAP], 1996; U.S. Preventive Services Task Force, 1989, 1996; Murdock, 1994). Health promotion approaches need to consider developmental abilities of young audiences. (Stevenson & Sleet, 1996-97; Schieber & Thompson, 1996). Third, health care professionals are credible and important sources of information for clients and can influence client and parent health behaviors (Eichelberger, Gotschall, Feely, Harstad, & Bowman, 1990; Athey, 1995). The remainder of this section provides examples and principles for promoting injury control in clinical settings, with an emphasis on counseling strategies.

Needs Assessment

Interventions, whether they are directed toward individual clients or a community population, should be developed based on needs assessment. Unless interventions are responsive to the specific needs of the target population, planners risk using limited program resources inefficiently or ineffectively (Green & Kreuter, 1991).

Needs assessment activities can range from simple to complex, depending on the situation. For example, before adding a new brochure on safety to the clinic's client education supply, the material should be tested with a subgroup of the intended audience to be sure that it is readable, understandable, attractive, and useful. Data on the magnitude of the injury problem in the population to be served are needed to determine which types of injuries for which subgroups most need to be addressed. Indicators used depend on the specific setting but can include analyses of injury-related deaths, hospitalizations, emergency department visits, police reports, household or waiting room interviews, and surveys. More qualitative data on persons' perceptions of injury problems, as well as the benefits and barriers to safer behavior, are critically important elements of a needs assessment that are commonly overlooked.

As an example, for a clinic-based needs assessment study of injuries that occurred in the home to infants and toddlers, researchers interviewed mothers in a pediatric clinic waiting room (Gielen, Wilson, Faden, Wissow, & Harvilchuck, 1995). It was found that parents already had favorable beliefs about childproofing but lacked the resources and skills needed to undertake recommended safety measures. These findings and additional information collected through focus groups shaped the subsequent interventions. The needs assessment indicated that safety supplies should be easily accessible to parents and that providing resource information and teaching specific safety skills would be more effective than delivering messages to increase general knowledge and to promote positive attitudes.

Persons responsible for safety education are often under pressure to "do something" to alleviate a perceived or real injury problem, which may make a needs assessment seem unnecessary. However, a needs assessment is important for at least three reasons. First, the data collected helps identify the injury that most needs to be addressed and the interventions most likely to be effective with the population being served, which facilitates efficient use of resources. Second, a needs assessment involves the target audience in program development. This "principle of participation" works well in health promotion (Green & Kreuter, 1991) because when the target population participates in defining its priority problems and in designing solutions, the programs are more likely to be effective. Third, a needs assessment provides baseline data for program evaluation.

Interventions in Clinical Settings

Clinical interventions for injury prevention typically include counseling, providing brochures or audiovisual materials, and rental or low-cost distribution of safety supplies, such as smoke detectors. Miller and Galbrith (1995) found that injury counseling by pediatricians produced a favorable cost-benefit. The Injury Prevention Program (TIPP) of the American Academy of Pediatrics (AAP, 1996) and car seat loaner programs that operate through hospitals are examples of clinical interventions that can have wide application in pediatric settings. The effectiveness of counseling has yet to be evaluated for many safety behaviors (e.g., safety belt use, cardiopulmonary resuscitation training [CPR] training). Bass et al (1993), however, reviewed intervention trials that were conducted in clinical pediatric settings and concluded that these trials had positive educational and behavioral outcomes. They also found that the behavior changes (e.g., increased use of child safety seats in automobiles and smoke detectors in homes) contributed to a decrease in injuries among children. Programs that were more comprehensive (e.g., those that included community outreach or distribution of safety supplies) seemed to be more successful. This conclusion about the superiority of combined interventions is consistent with health behavior change theories and principles (Glanz, Lewis, & Rimer, 1996) as well as recent reports in the injury control literature (Gielen, 1992; Gielen & McDonald, 1996; Sleet, 1984, 1994; Towner, 1995; Downswell, Towner, Simpson, & Jarvis, 1996).

Which combination of interventions will be most effective in achieving safer behavior depends on the target population and the problem being addressed. Programs select which interventions are most appropriate on the basis of the following factors:

- *Knowledge of what works:* Programs should base their intervention strategies on reviews of published reports on injury prevention, descriptions of other successful programs, and an understanding of the theories of behavior change.

- *Availability of resources:* Obviously, the more resources (staff, funds, space) a program has, the more complex it can be.
- *Input from the target population:* For a program to be successful, participation by at least some members of the target population is essential. They can, for example, sit on planning committees or participate in focus groups, surveys, or personal interviews.
- *Access to the target population:* Programs must decide the most suitable method(s) for reaching the target population (e.g., through home visits, in physicians' waiting rooms, or through a mass media campaign).
- *Developmental stages of children:* If children are the target population or affected by the intervention strategy, programs must ensure that the proposed intervention is developmentally appropriate and suitable for the age group targeted.

Evaluation

Program designs should include specific objectives by which to measure success. Program evaluations vary in complexity, from simple counts of persons served by the program (process evaluation) to randomized trials of an intervention's effect on behavior change or injury rates (outcome evaluation). The type of evaluation conducted depends on the specific situation, the availability of resources, and the expectations of those who fund or support the program. Program evaluation theories and methods are beyond the scope of this chapter; interested readers are referred to textbooks (Green & Lewis, 1986; Rossi & Freeman, 1993).

There are unique challenges to evaluating injury prevention programs. First, although injuries are the leading cause of death for children and young adults, evaluating program success solely by measuring decreases in injury-related death rates requires a long time or large samples, or both. Measuring intermediate outcomes, such as changes in safety behaviors (e.g., seat belt use, helmet use), self-reported behavior changes, or improvements in a client's intention to change behavior in the future, may be the most appropriate measures of change in a clinical setting. Whether evaluations rely on participants' self-reported behaviors or whether they involve observations of changes in safety behaviors or skills depends on the program's resources and needs. Some researchers have challenged the validity of self-reported safety behaviors (Robertson, 1994), but recent evidence (Nelson, 1996) indicates that it varies by the prevalence of the behavior in the population. In populations in which the safety behavior is very prevalent (i.e., seat belt use), the validity of self-report was found to be generally high (Nelson, 1996).

Evaluations of health promotion interventions for injury control should also monitor the program's unintended consequences. The unintended hazards to children associated with the deployment of airbags on the passenger side of vehicles underscores the need for ongoing intervention evaluation (Centers for Disease Control and Prevention [CDC], 1993, 1995, 1996). This example also points to the need for accurate and timely communication between those in injury control and the health care professionals who counsel clients and families (CDC, 1997). The approval for installation of airbag on/off switches for certain motor vehicle owners will make risk communication a critical part of the interaction between client and professional (CDC, 1997).

Counseling in the Clinical Setting

Counseling is an important component of any clinically based injury prevention program. In fact, counseling about injury prevention is a recommended component of any preventive service, according to the U.S. Preventive Services Task Force Report (1996). Specifically, the task force recommends the following:

(1) Counsel all patients, and the parents of young patients, to use occupant restraints (lap and shoulder safety belts and child safety seats), to wear helmets when riding motorcycles, and to refrain from driving while under the influence of alcohol or other drugs (p. 643).

The Task Force also recommends the following:

(2) Periodically counsel the parents of children on measures to reduce the risk of unintentional household and recreational injuries. (3) Counsel to prevent household and recreational injuries is also recommended for adolescents and adults. (4) Identify, counsel, and monitor persons with alcohol or drug problems. (5) Counsel elderly patients on specific measures to prevent falls (p. 659).

The American Academy of Pediatrics recommends that pediatricians counsel parents on how to prevent childhood injuries resulting from motor vehicle crashes, falls from bicycles, other types of falls, fires and burns, electrical hazards, poisoning, aspiration, and firearm discharges and on how to prevent children from drowning or suffocating (AAP, 1996). Pediatricians should recommend specific preventive methods (e.g., use child safety seats and bicycle helmets or install a smoke detector in the home). Well-child visits provide a good opportunity to offer such counseling.

The extent to which primary care clinicians provide injury prevention counseling has not been systematically studied. Research published in the 1980s found that pediatricians spend 1 minute on average counseling clients on safety (Reisinger & Bires, 1980). When pediatricians, family physicians, and a sample of the parents of their clients were surveyed (Morrongiello, Hillier, & Bass, 1995), 55% of the physicians reported mentioning safety issues "always" or "most of the time." However, 64% of the parents reported that their physician "rarely" or "never" did so. In a recent analysis of 178 audiotaped well-child visits for children 0 to 4 years old with pediatric residents, Gielen, McDonald, Forrest, Harivilchuck, & Wissow (1997) reported that only 47% of the visits included injury prevention counseling. During the 83 visits that included counseling, an average of 1.96 injury topics were discussed. The average time spent on injury topics was 1.08 minutes per visit, and 33 seconds was spent per injury topic.

As the content of the counseling itself is important, so too is the manner in which health care professionals provide that counseling (Wissow, Roter, & Wilson, 1994). Little is known, however, about physicians' communication skills, although Roter and Hall (1996) consider communication the most basic and most powerful vehicle of health care. They conclude, on the basis of published medical reports, that good communication between medical provider and client is associated with increased client satisfaction and compliance with the physician's instructions.

Compliance improves when health care professionals give adequate information, talk positively, and ask questions about behavioral compliance (Hall, Roter, & Katz, 1988). Because the desired outcomes of injury prevention counseling are behavioral (e.g., compliance with recommendations to install smoke detectors), these communication skills should be used in injury prevention counseling.

Other principles of behavior change also improve compliance when they are used during counseling. The U.S. Preventive Services Task Force (1989) recommends health care professionals use the following principles:

- Develop a therapeutic alliance. Health care professionals should see themselves as expert consultants available to help clients.
- Ensure that clients understand the relationship between behavior and health. Inquire about what clients already know or believe.
- Work with clients to assess barriers to behavior change.
- Gain a commitment from clients to begin the process of change.
- Involve clients in selecting risk factors to change.
- Design a behavior modification plan oriented toward changing clients' behaviors, not merely changing knowledge or attitudes.
- Monitor progress through follow-up contact. Reinforce successes through positive verbal feedback.

Based on these principles, Gielen and others (1997) developed a counseling approach to code audiotapes of pediatric encounters. Eighty-three well-child visits with pediatric residents that included 163 injury prevention counseling episodes were coded for eliciting information, asking for feedback, obtaining a commitment, and reinforcing efforts. Of all the counseling episodes, 22% included only eliciting information and 34% included both eliciting and giving information. Asking for feedback and obtaining a commitment were never done, and reinforcing intentions was done only twice. These findings were shared with pediatric residents during a communication training program (McDonald & Gielen, 1995). The effects are currently being evaluated.

Using a Counseling Framework

Health care professionals' concerns about whether to incorporate new counseling typically have to do with the limited time available during a medical visit. However, through role-playing, McDonald and Gielen (1995) showed that counseling on a single topic takes less than 5 minutes. Research is currently under way to evaluate the effect of injury prevention counseling on parents' practices.

Another concern is the need for health care professionals to have adequate information about the many facets of injury prevention. Health care professionals need specific training in the injury prevention practices being recommended. Experiential training is a useful technique for providing the necessary knowledge and skills (e.g., actually installing a smoke detector and changing its batteries). Health care professionals also should have information on local resources that their clients need to carry out the recommended prevention practice (e.g., how to obtain a bicycle helmet discount coupon).

Finally, incorporating a counseling program into routine clinical practice is a behavior change on the part of the health care professional. Thus, in addition to adequate preparation, knowledge, and skills, health care professionals need incentives and reinforcement for their own behavior change. Adequate administrative support, supplementary client education materials, and ongoing feedback on the effectiveness of their counseling efforts will improve compliance with an injury prevention counseling program.

INJURY PREVENTION & THE HEALTH PROMOTION MATRIX*

Given the counseling guidelines described in this chapter and an empirically based counseling approach developed by Gielen et al (1997), the Health Promotion Matrix may be applied effectively for injury prevention.

In the following example, a health care professional asks mothers about their use of car seats for their children. In the script that follows this example, many more injury topics are included.

Image Creation

Because injury prevention has often neither been embraced as a public health issue nor a clinical issue, the health care professional's questions can bring the topic to the foreground for the client. The health care professional may assist the client to visualize those aspects of his/her life-style or environment that may be injurious and that may need changing.

Image Appraisal

The client's attention is directed to each of the major causes of injury with a set of simple questions designed to elicit information. Although the questions listed in the script that follows cover many topics, the health care professional should choose to assess one particular area at a time, as appropriate to the client's stated interest, stage of life, or unique risks. For example, an individual coming to the health care professional with a burn would be questioned about fire safety. All new mothers, however, can be asked about car seats, as follows:

....

ELICIT INFORMATION

Do you have a car seat for your baby?
Do you use it every time you travel?
Have you heard about the importance of always placing children in the back seat of your car?

....

In regard to injury prevention, field testing by Gielen et al (1997) suggests that the commitment to change, common at this point in the Matrix, may emerge later in the interchange between health care professional and client. The commitment to change may follow the health care professional's sharing information or demonstrating the concrete use of a technique (e.g., installing a smoke detector or putting on a bicycle helmet), as well as asking the client for feedback.

Minimize Health Depleting Patterns

For this dimension, the health care professional gives the client focused information on preventing specific injuries. The health care professional specifies the use of

---

*Adapted from D.A. Sleet and A. Gielen by S. Sheinfeld Gorin.

a particular behavioral approach or tool, such as using seat belts properly or installing and maintaining a smoke detector. She/he may model the use of a tool, such as a childproof latch. After giving concrete information, the health care professional asks the client for feedback to clarify client uderstanding and to better target the intervention.

GIVE INFORMATION

Car seats are very effective for preventing serious injury or death, but they must be used correctly and every time. Air bags are especially dangerous to children, so they should always ride in the back seat when there is a passenger side airbag.

ASK FOR FEEDBACK

What have you heard about how to use a car seat correctly?
What questions or concerns do you have about using a car seat?
What situations might keep you from placing your child in the car seat correctly?

Optimize Health Supportive Patterns

The health care professional supports any positive changes the client has made in his/her injury prevention behavior. She/he gives specific positive feedback to the client, reinforcing the plan to make specific changes, and concludes by obtaining a commitment to change.

OBTAIN A COMMITMENT:

If you don't have a car seat, do you think you can call or stop by the car seat loaner program today? (Give information to client.)
Would you like someone to show you today how to use the car seat correctly?

Internalize Idealized Image

At this step, the health care professional continues to reinforce the client's positive changes and schedules the next appointment. She/he continues to support the client's changed behavior, as she/he did in the previous dimension. As the client's interests, needs, stage of life, and risks change, the health care professional should review the injury prevention script, highlighting different questions, to complete a comprehensive injury prevention intervention.

REINFORCE INTENTIONS OR EFFORTS:

I'm pleased that you're thinking about getting a car seat and using it correctly. We'll talk about your experience with it the next time I see you.

INJURY PREVENTION: *A Script**

The health care professional would ask a series of questions exploring one or more aspects of injury prevention at each session. For example, she/he might ask about water safety during warm weather or poison control as a child becomes mobile. Over time, the health care professional, together with the client would complete the script.

Image Creation — What would a safe environment at home look like?

Can you do anything to improve the safety of your environment at home?

What effect do you see yourself having on the creation of this environment?

Image Appraisal — Do you use *seat belts* when you drive? About how often?

What have you heard about the role *seat belts* and *not drinking* play in reducing traffic accidents?

Do you use a *designated driver* or *refuse to drive* when you have drunk alcohol?

If client has a motorcycle: Do you use a *helmet?*

Do you have a *smoke detector* in your home?

Do you have *fire extinguisher* in your home?

   How often do you *test* or *check* them?

Do you have a *plan* for a fire emergency (e.g., an evacuation plan, a meeting place)?

Is your hot water heater kept *below* 120°F?

Do you know *cardiopulmonary resuscitation* (CPR)? The *Heimlich maneuver?*

If the client has children:
Do you have a *car seat* for your babies and children? Do you use it every time you travel?

Have you heard about the importance of *always* placing children in the back seat of your car?

Do your children wear a *helmet* whenever they ride a bicycle?

Do you have *gates* or *other devices* to block access to stairs by children?

Do you keep *poisons* together in *labeled containers* in a place that is *locked* or *latched* [i.e., out of reach of children and pets]?

*Adapted from D.A. Sleet and A. Gielen by S. Sheinfeld Gorin.

Injury Prevention: *A Script—cont'd*

Do you keep all medications in *labeled, child-proof containers* and in a place that is *locked* or *latched* [i.e., out of reach of children and pets]?

Do you have an *emetic* (such as 1 ounce of syrup of ipecac) in the home? Do you have the *number* of the local poison control center by the telephone?

Do your children sleep in *fire-retardant* clothing?

Do you store matches and lighters in *child-resistant containers?*

Do you *watch* your children when they swim in a pool or other body of water? Do you *watch* your children when they take a bath?

> *If the client lives in a high-rise:* Do you have *window guards* or *locks* to prevent falls?

If an older adult lives in the client's home:
Have you installed *good lighting, hand railings, nonstick traction strips* on floor surfaces to reduce falls? Have you removed *rugs, electrical wires,* and *other items* (such as toys) that promote tripping?

Have you *padded* sharp corners of furniture?

Does the older person wear *sturdy shoes* while at home?

Has the older person been *evaluated* for impaired hearing and/or vision? Has he/she been *evaluated* for changes in walking and balance?

Has *adaptive equipment* been added to the bathroom?

If the client has a pool:
Does a *protective fence* surround your pool and *separate* it from the house? Does it have a *gate* that is kept closed?

If the household lives or vacations near water:
Does everyone in your household know how to swim? Do they use life jackets if they go boating? Do they drink alcohol or use drugs while boating?

Minimize Health Depleting Behaviors

Using the Helpful Resources listed at the end of this chapter, provide information on the effectiveness of reducing serious injury or death through proper use of seat belts while driving; proper placement of children in the car; use of helmets; not drinking and driving; use of window guards, locks, and gates;

continued

INJURY PREVENTION: *A Script—cont'd*

behavior and environmental changes to reduce falls; proper storage and use of poisons and medications; maintenance of smoke detectors; a fire emergency plan; reducing the temperature of tap water; wearing of fire-retardant clothing; proper storage of matches and lighters; not smoking; swimming, bathing, and boating safety; use of CPR and the Heimlich maneuver. Provide the telephone number of the poison control center. For smoking cessation, see Chapter 6, and for substance safety, see Chapter 11.

Ask for Feedback

What situations might keep you from using *seat belts?* From *safe driving?* From wearing *bicycle* and/or *motorcycle helmets? Not drinking and driving?* (See Chapter 11.)

What situations might keep you from *reducing falls?*

What situations might keep you from *placing medications and poisons out of reach?*

What situations might keep you from maintaining a *smoke detector?* A *fire emergency plan?* Having your children sleep in *fire-retardant clothes?* Proper *storage of matches* and *lighters? Not smoking* in the house? (See Chapter 6.)

What situations might keep you from *fencing* and *gating* your pool? Household members *learning to swim?* Household members *learning to use life jackets* while boating? Household members *learning CPR* and the *Heimlich maneuver?*

What might keep you from *supervising* children who are in a pool or other body of water, such as a bath tub, at all times?

List each barrier, one by one, and identify a strategy to overcome it, using the Helpful Resources at the end of the chapter. (Example Strategies include suggesting that the client buckle up after buckling up his/her children, giving the client the name of community agencies that will provide him/her with a car seat, encouraging the client to contact his/her landlord and/or housing authority to install window guards and locks, giving the client a childproof lock for the cabinet where he/she has consolidated all poisons, encouraging the client to purchase an emetic such as syrup of ipecac, encouraging the client to contact the fire department for an emergency plan and the water authority to reduce the temperature of tap water, and encouraging the client to participate in swimming, boating, and CPR and Heimlich maneuver instruction through the American

Injury Prevention: *A Script—cont'd*

Red Cross or the local police or fire department.) Demonstrate the mastery of skills needed to reduce injuries, such as the installation of a battery in a smoke detector; stop, drop, and roll technique; and installation of childproof locks on cabinets and drawers containing harmful substances.

Optimize Health Supportive Patterns

I'm pleased that you're thinking about getting a car seat and using it correctly or using seat belts yourself, encouraging your children to use helmets while riding their bicycles, using a designated driver, making changes in your home to reduce falls, keeping poisons and all medications labeled and out of reach, keeping emergency control telephone numbers near your phone, maintaining a smoke detector, developing a fire emergency plan, storing matches and lighters out of reach, learning to swim, learning to boat safely, and/or learning CPR or the Heimlich maneuver.

Obtain a Commitment

Would you be willing to develop a plan to make your home a safer one by (specify) (e.g., having your children wear helmets while riding their bicycles)?

YES   **NO**

Would you be willing to have someone today show you how to, for example, (install a child safety seat in your car?)

Internalize Idealized Image

How are you and/or your family adapting to these changes?

Reinforce Intentions or Efforts

I'm pleased that you're thinking about or getting a, for example, bicycle helmet.

Would you like to make anymore changes to reduce injuries in your home?

What can I do to help you?

We'll talk about your experience with (specify) (e.g., seat belts) the next time I see you.

Population-Based Injury Prevention Interventions

Health promotion approaches work to reduce injury not only by changing the behavior of individuals, but also by changing the behavior of large populations. In addition to personal counseling, the health care professional, by educating community members about the strategies of injury prevention can empower the community itself. With increased knowledge and skills in using the techniques and tools of injury prevention, individuals may coalesce around unmet needs, such as a community safe swim program and, with the health care professional, build a coalition for change. Two case studies show how health care professionals concerned about injuries used population-based approaches to injury prevention.

CASE #1

Preventing Motor Vehicle-Related Injury in California

The Contra Costa Health Services Department (CCHSD) in California took a long-term approach to reducing motor vehicle-related injuries among children. State law required that children younger than 4 years old be secured in a child safety seat and imposed a fine for noncompliance. The CCHSD, however, believed that the law alone was not enough to motivate parents to put their children in safety seats. Therefore, to find ways of motivating parents, the CCHSD formed a coalition of local civic, government, and business leaders. Represented in this coalition were persons from the local health department, traffic safety department, health care professions, private industry, and community organizations. The coalition worked to have the fine for noncompliance with the state law increased and to have a major portion of the fine go to the health department so that it could fund a program to educate parents about the benefits of using car seats for their children and to subsidize car seats for low-income parents. The coalition was successful. Later, the California state legislature amended the original law and directed law enforcement agencies throughout the state to give a portion of the fine to the local health departments so that they could implement education and subsidy programs for the community (Sleet & Sacks, 1994).

CASE #2

Burn Prevention and Childproof Cigarette Lighters

After seeing many children suffering from burns, Diane Denton, a nurse in Louisville, Kentucky, began asking the children's parents how their tragic injuries occurred. She learned that a large number of cases were the result of children playing with disposable cigarette lighters. The lighters are small enough to fit in the palm of the child's hand, are brightly colored, and become "sparking toys" when moved rapidly along a carpet or mattress. Ms. Denton documented these findings and petitioned the U.S. Consumer Product Safety Commission (CPSC) to investigate the risks posed by disposable cigarette lighters. Others in the burn prevention community joined her effort.

Impressed with the data Ms. Denton and others gathered, the CPSC funded research to examine cases in which children had been badly burned while playing with disposable cigarette lighters. The CPSC found that as many as 200 burn-related deaths among children younger than 3 years could be prevented by a simple and inexpensive childproof device. Ten years after Denton's efforts, with CPSC prompting, the major cigarette lighter manufacturers complied with a CPSC standard, required childproof disposable lighters, and marketed them to the public as safer for the protection of children. In this case, the actions of one nurse changed an entire industry, saving hundreds of lives and preventing thousands of children from being burned (Sleet, 1995).

Summary

Although injury has plagued societies since humans first walked the earth, it has only recently been recognized as an important public health problem. Health promotion can help prevent injuries. Using an epidemiologic approach helps target interventions that modify the host, agent, and/or environment to prevent injury. A focus on behavioral, environmental, and technologic solutions can help public health professionals prevent injuries by reducing or eliminating hazardous energy exchange. Injuries are not random events: they are predictable and preventable. Clinical approaches to injury control are an important health promotion intervention that can be delivered through existing public health and medical settings. Health promotion professionals can be instrumental in implementing individual, family, and population-based interventions for injury prevention.

Reductions in unintentional injuries and associated medical costs can be made by using health promotion and community health approaches. These include using strategies that target host, environmental, and agent factors. The three strategies are education and behavior change, engineering and technology, and legislation and law enforcement. Using multiple strategies is most effective. Injuries affect persons' lives in dramatic ways, and health promotion approaches, including clinical counseling in health care settings, can do much to prevent injuries.

HELPFUL **RESOURCES**

ON-LINE RESOURCES

National Center for Injury Prevention and Control (NCIPC), Centers for Disease Control and Prevention (CDC)
http://www.cdc.gov/ncipc/ncipchm.htm
Resources available include general information on the activities of NCIPC and its divisions, publications, research grants, funding opportunities, "what's new" section, Safe America initiatives, scientific and surveillance data, and links to other CDC centers.

Partnerships against Violence Network Online
gopher//cyfer.esusda.gov:70/11/violence
Offers information about federal resources related to violence prevention; developed by a coalition of federal agencies to improve speedy access to ideas and resources related to violence prevention.

Injury Control Resource Information Network (ICRIN)
http://www.injurycontrol.com/icrin
Provides a comprehensive list of injury control resources throughout the Internet. This Web site was developed by the CDC's Center for Injury Research and Control at the University of Pittsburgh.

Center for Rural Emergency Medicine
http:/www.hsc.wvu/crem/crem.htm
Web site of the CDC's Injury Control Training and Demonstration Center at the University of West Virginia in Morgantown; includes lists of injury mechanisms (similar to E-codes), information on causes of injuries for which persons have sought treatment at the University of West Virginia Emergency Department, hypertext map of West Virginia with extensive injury data by county, and links to other injury research centers.

continued

HELPFUL **RESOURCES—cont'd**

National Program for Playground Safety
http://www.uni.edu/playground
This Web site includes information on playground injury, playground safety inspection, training, and materials distribution.

National SAFE KIDS
http://www.safekids.org
National SAFE KIDS is a nationwide movement to prevent unintentional childhood injury. The Web site has information in Spanish and English language. Subjects include a family safety checklist and a variety of injury topics affecting children.

U.S. Department of Transportation, National Highway Traffic Safety Administration (NHTSA)
http://www.nhtsa.dot.gov
NHTSA is a regulatory agency responsible for reducing deaths, injuries, and economic losses resulting from motor vehicle crashes through setting and enforcing safety performance standards for motor vehicles.

Consumer Product Safety Commission (CPSC)
http://www.cpsc.gov
CPSC is an independent federal regulary agency that helps keep American families safe in their homes by reducing the risk of injury or death from consumer products. The Web site can be used to report unsafe products and find out what consumer products are unsafe or have been recalled.

Children's Safety Network
http://www.edc.org/HHD/csn
The Children's Safety Network fosters the development and inclusion of injury and violence prevention strategies into maternal and child health services.

State and Territorial Injury Prevention Directors Association (STIPDA)
http://www.stipda.org

Resources include state injury projects in member states, news and views on state and local injury initiatives, links to individuals in each state, and state injury World Wide Web sites.

WHO Collaborating Centre on Community Safety Promotion
http://www.ki.se/phs/wcccsp/history.htm
The Centre is the headquarters for the "Safe Community" concept of community injury prevention and safety promotion.

OTHER RESOURCES

Automated Injury Information Telephone Line
Information from the CDC's National Center for Injury Prevention and Control. Receive information on specific injury issues by mail, brief recorded by phone, or documents by fax. There is no charge for any material. (404) 488-4677.

CDC Injury Control Research Centers
CDC administers an extramural grant program of more than $20 million. Grants are awarded to researchers, universities, and health departments. CDC also supports 55 state and community injury prevention programs and 10 comprehensive injury control research centers throughout the United States. In addition to conducting research, surveillance, intervention, and evaluation studies, these centers serve as training centers and resources to the public, the media, and allied health professionals. The following are the 1997 Injury Control Research Centers:

> University of Alabama–Birmingham Injury Control Research Center, (205) 934-7845.
> Harvard Injury Prevention Research Center, Boston, (617) 432-4343.

References

The American Academy of Pediatrics. (1996). *The Injury Prevention Program (TIPP)*. Chicago: Author.

Athey, A.M. (1995). Pediatric injury control: Strategies for the nurse practitioner. *Nurse Practitioner Forum, 6*(3), 99, 167-172.

Bass, J., Christoffel, K.K., Windome, M., Boyle, W., Scheidt, P., Stranwick, R., & Roberts, K. (1993). Childhood injury prevention counseling in primary care settings: A critical review of the literature. *Pediatrics, 92,* 544-550.

Borden, L., Hall, J., Levenstein, C., & Punnett, L. (1984). The impact of health and safety committees. *Journal of Occupational Medicine, 26*(11), 834-844.

Centers for Disease Control and Prevention. (1993, April 16) Warning on interaction between air bags and rear-facing child restraints. *Morbidity and Mortality Weekly Report, 42*(14), 280-281.

Centers for Disease Control and Prevention. (1995, December 13) Air-bag associated fatal injuries to infants and children riding in front passenger seats—United States. *Journal of the American Medical Association, 274*(22), 1752-1753.

Centers for Disease Control and Prevention. (1996, December 13) Update: Fatal air bag-related injuries to children—United States 1993-1996. *Morbidity and Mortality Weekly Report, 45*(49), 1073-1076.

De Haven, H. (1942). Mechanical analysis of survival in falls from heights of fifty to one hundred and fifty feet. *War Medicine, 2,* 586-596.

DiGuiseppi, C.G., Rivara, F.P., Koepsell, T.D., Polissar, L. (1989). Bicycle helmet use by children: Evaluation of a community wide helmet campaign. *Journal of the American Medical Association, 262,* 2256-2261.

Dowswell, T., Towner, E.M.L., Simpson, G., & Jarvis, S.N. (1996). Preventing childhood unintentional injuries—what works? A literature review. *Injury Prevention, 2,* 140-149.

Eichelberger, M.R., Gotschall, C.S., Feely, H.B., Harstad, P., & Bowman, L.M. (1990). Parental attitudes and knowledge of child safety. *American Journal of Diseases of Children, 144,* 714-720.

Farrell, A.D., Meyer, A.L., & Dahlberg, L.L. (1996). Richmond youth against violence: A school-based program for urban adolescents. *American Journal of Preventive Medicine* (Supplement) *12*(5), 13-21.

Fortenberry, J.C., & Brown, D.B. (1982). Problem identification, implementation and evaluation of a pedestrian safety program. *Accident Analysis and Prevention, 14*(4), 315-322.

Frank, R.G., Bouman, D.E., Cain, K., & Watts, C. (1992). Primary prevention of catastrophic injury. *American Psychologist, 47*(8), 1045-1049.

Funk & Wagnalls standard college dictionary (p. 694). (1966). Pleasantville, NY: The Readers Digest Association.

Geller, E.S., Elder, J., Hovell, M., & Sleet, D. (1991). Behavioral approaches to drinking-driving interventions. In W. Ward & F.M. Lewis (Eds.), *Advances in health education and promotion* (Vol. 3, pp. 45-68). London: Jessica Kingsley Press.

Gielen, A.C. (1992). Health education and injury control: Integrating approaches. *Health Education Quarterly, 19*(2), 203-218.

Gielen, A.C., & McDonald, E.M. (1996). The Precede-Proceed planning model. In K. Glanz, F.M. Lewis, & B.K. Rimer (Eds.), *Behavior and health education: Theory, research, and practice* (2nd ed., pp. 359-383). San Francisco: Jossey-Bass.

Gielen, A.C., McDonald, E.M., Forrest, C.B., Harivilchuk, J., & Wissow, L. (1997). Injury prevention counseling in an urban pediatric clinic: Analysis of audiotaped visits. *Archives of Pediatric and Adolescent Medicine,* 151(2):146-151.

Gielen, A.C., Wilson, M.E.H., Faden, R.R., Wissow, L., & Harvilchuck, J.D. (1995). In-home injury prevention practices for infants and toddlers: The role of parental beliefs, barriers, and housing quality. *Health Education Quarterly, 22*(1), 85-95.

Glanz, K., Lewis, F.M., & Rimer, B.K. (1996). *Health behavior and health education: theory, research, and practice* (2nd ed.). San Francisco: Jossey Bass.

Gordon, J.E. (1949). The epidemiology of accidents. *American Journal of Public Health, 39,* 504-515.

Graves, E.J. (1993). *1991 summary: National hospital discharge survey advanced data from vital health statistics* (DHHS Report No. 227). Hyattsville, MD: National Center for Health Statistics.

Green, L.W., & Kreuter, M.K. (1991). *Health promotion planning: An educational and environmental approach* (2nd ed.). Mountain View, CA: Mayfield Publishing.

Green, L.W. & Lewis, F.M. (1986). *Measurement and evaluation in health education and health promotion.* Palo Alto, CA: Mayfield Publishing.

Haddon, W., Jr. (1970). On the escape of tigers: An ecologic note. *Technology Review (MIT), 72,* 44-53.

Haddon, W. (1980). Advances in the epidemiology of injuries as a basis for public policy. *Public Health Reports, 95,* 411-421.

Hall, J.A., Roter, D.L., & Katz, N.R. (1988). Meta-analysis of correlates of provider behavior in medical encounters. *Medical Care, 26,* 657-675.

Huesmann, L., Guerra, N., Miller, L., & Zelli, A. (1992). The role of social norms in the development of aggression. In H. Zumkley & A. Fraczek (Eds.), *Socialization and aggression.* New York: Springer.

Jones, R.T., van Hasselt, V.P., & Sisson, L.A. (1984). Emergency fire safety skills. *Behavior Modification, 8,* 59-78.

Koop, E. (1989). Introduction. In *National Committee for Injury Prevention and Control. U.S. injury prevention: meeting the challenge.* New York: Oxford University Press. Supplement to *American Journal of Preventive Medicine, 5*(3), 1-303.

McDonald, E.M., & Gielen, A.C. (1995, July). *Experiential training to improve pediatric counseling about injury prevention.* Paper presented at Society for Public Health Education, Midyear Scientific Conference, Little Rock, Arkansas.

Miller, T.R., & Galbraith, M. (1995). Injury prevention counseling by pediatricians: A benefit-cost comparison. *Pediatrics, 96,* 1-4.

Morrongiello, B.A., Hillier, L., & Bass, M. (1995). 'What I said' versus 'What you heard': A comparison of physicians' and parents' reporting of anticipatory guidance on child safety issues. *Injury Prevention, 1,* 223-227.

Murdock, M.A. (1994). Injury prevention: A nursing responsibility. *Orthopaedic Nursing, 13*(4), 7-11.

National Academy of Sciences, National Research Council. (1988). *Injury control: A review of the status and problems of the injury control problem at the Centers for Disease Control.* Washington, DC: Author.

National Committee for Injury Prevention and Control. (1989). *Injury prevention: meeting the challenge.* New York: Oxford University Press. Supplement to *American Journal of Preventive Medicine, 5*(3), 1-303.

National Center for Injury Prevention and Control, Centers for Disease Control and Prevention. (1996). *1996 fact book.* Atlanta: Author.

National Center for Health Statistics. (1991). *Vital statistics data tapes.* Hyattsville, MD: Author.

Nelson, D.E. (1996). A validity of self reported data on injury prevention behavior: Lessons from observational and self reported surveys of safety belt use in the U.S. *Injury Prevention, 2,* 67-69.

O'Connor, P.J. (1982). Poisoning prevention: Results of a public media campaign. *Australian Paediatrics Journal, 18,* 250-252.

Pless, I.B. (1978). Accident prevention and health education: Back to the drawing board? *Pediatrics, 62,* 431-435.

Preusser, D.F., & Blomberg, R.D. (1984). Reducing child pedestrian accidents through public education. *Journal of Safety Research, 15,* 47-56.

Reisinger, K., & Bires, J. (1980). Anticipatory guidance in pediatric practice. *Pediatrics, 66,* 889-892.

Rice, D.P., MacKenzie, E.J. et al. (1989). *Cost of injury in the United States: A report to Congress.* San Francisco: University of California Institute for Health and Aging and The Johns Hopkins University Injury Prevention Center.

Rivara, F.P., Booth, C.L., Bergman, A.B., Rogers, L.W., & Weiss, J. (1991). Prevention of pedestrian injuries to children: Effectiveness of a school training program. *Pediatrics, 88,* 770-775.

Roberts, M.C., Fanurik, D., & Layfield, D.A. (1987). Behavioral approaches to preventing childhood injuries. *Journal of Social Issues, 43*(2), 105-118.

Robertson, L.S. (1994). Self-reports yield invalid results on seat belt use. *American Journal of Public Health, 84,* (9), 1521-1526.

Rossi, P.H., & Freeman, H.E. (1993). *Evaluation: A systematic approach.* Newbury Park, CA: Sage.

Roter, D.L., & Hall, J.A. (1996). Patient provider communication. In K. Glanz, F.M. Lewis, & B.K. Rimer (Eds.), *Health behavior and health education: theory, research, and practice* (2nd Ed., pp. 206-226). San Francisco: Jossey-Bass.

Schieber, R.A., & Thompson, N.J. (1996). Developmental risk factors for childhood pedestrian injuries. *Injury Prevention, 2*(3), 228-236.

Sleet, D.A. (Ed.). (1984). Occupant protection and health promotion. [Whole issue]. *Health Education Quarterly, 11.*

Sleet, D.A. (1994). Injury prevention. In P. Cortese & C. Middleton (Eds.), *The comprehensive school health challenge* (pp. 443-489). Santa Cruz, CA: ETR Associates.

Sleet, D. (1995). *Injury control 594.* [Course text material, teaching learning group (distance education)]. Perth, Australia: Curtin University of Technology.

Sleet, D.A., Egger, G., & Albany, P. (1991). Injury as a public health problem. [Special issue on injury prevention]. *Health Promotion Journal of Australia, 1*(2), 4-9.

Sleet, D.A., Hollenbach, K., & Hovell, M. (1986). Applying behavioral principles to motor vehicle occupant protection. *Education and Treatment of Children, 9*(4), 320-333.

Sleet, D.A., & Rosenberg, M.L. (1997). Injury control. In D.F. Scutchfield & C.W. Keck (Eds.), *Principles of public health practice.* New York: Delmar Publishers.

Sleet, D., & Sacks, J. (1994). Partnerships for reducing unintentional injuries. In U.S. Public Health Service (Ed.), *For a healthy return on investment* (pp. 31-33). Washington, DC: U.S. Department of Health and Human Services.

Stevenson, M.R., & Sleet, D.A. (1996-1997). Which prevention strategies for child pedestrian injuries? A review of the literature. *International Quarterly of Community Health Education, 16*(3), 207-217.

Streff, F.M., & Geller, E.S. (1986). Strategies for motivating safety belt use: The application of applied behavior analysis. *Health Education Research, 1,* 47-59.

Taylor, R.B., Ureda, J.R., & Denham, J.W. (1982). *Health promotion: Principles and clinical applications.* Stamford, CT: Appleton & Lange.

Towner, E.M.L. (1995). The role of health education in childhood injury prevention. *Injury Prevention, 1,* 53-58.

Trinca, G.W., Johnston, I.R., Campbell, B.J., Haight, F.A., Knight, P.R., Mackay, G.M., McLean, A.J., & Petrucelli, E. (1988). *Reducing traffic injury—A global challenge.* Melbourne, Australia: Royal Australasian College of Surgeons.

U.S. Preventive Services Task Force. (1989). *Guide to clinical preventive services: An assessment of the effectiveness of 169 interventions.* Baltimore: Williams & Wilkins.

U.S. Preventive Services Task Force. (1996). *Guide to clinical preventive services* (2nd ed.). Baltimore: Williams & Wilkins.

U.S. Public Health Service. (1979). *Healthy people: The Surgeon General's report on health promotion and disease prevention* (PHS Publication No. 79-55071). Washington, DC: U.S. Department of Health Education and Welfare.

Wissow, L.S., Roter, D.L., & Wilson M.E.H. (1994). Physician interview style and mothers' disclosure of psychosocial issues. *Pediatrics, 93,* 289-295.

CHAPTER

11

Substance Safety

Edith S. Lisansky Gomberg and Kristen Lawton Barry*

*Edith S. Lisansky Gomberg wrote pp. 276 to 288, and Kristen Lawton Barry wrote pp. 289 to 291.

Brief Intervention With a Mother Who Has Experienced Substance Abuse and a Script.
Within a developmental framework spanning the phases of adulthood, Lisansky Gomberg
identifies the importance of cutting down alcohol use and stopping substance use for clients
who are drinking or using drugs at hazardous levels. Using the Health Promotion Matrix
(HPM), Lawton Barry provides explicit guidance to the health care professional in screening
and working with a client to reduce her drinking. Lawton Berry's empirically tested intervention is integrated with the HPM script.

Substance safety is a major public health concern. Social interaction in American society is characterized by the use of substances such as alcohol. This chapter begins with
a discussion of the differentiation of the classes of drugs, focusing specifically on alcohol
and banned substances, and then outlines health promotion through substance safety for
special groups. Specific criteria for recognizing levels of risk and problem use are identified, and an effective brief intervention is detailed.

SUBSTANCE CLASSES

In dealing with health promotion related to substance use and abuse, the complexity of
the issues is manifest in the different classes of drugs, which are assumed under the term
"substances."

Prescribed and Over-the-Counter Drugs

The purpose of prescribed and over-the-counter drugs is to foster health or at the very
least to minimize symptoms of discomfort and ill health. The major health promotion issues concerning these drugs in general are related to prescribing practices and Food and
Drug Administration (FDA) monitoring of drugs sold over-the-counter. Health care professionals are often concerned about medication compliance (i.e., the client following the
instructions), but that is an ambiguous issue because accurate follow-up is difficult; over-
the-counter drugs are taken largely as self-medication. Further, prescribing practices are
influenced by differences in medical education, practice norms, and pharmaceutical marketing approaches.

Banned Substances

Banned substances are drugs that appear on the Schedule list of the FDA, as defined
under the Controlled Substances Act (1970). The medicinal value of these drugs is
disputed, and these illegal substances are generally obtained for recreational usage.
Banned substances include marijuana, cocaine, heroin, morphine, lysergic acid diethyl-
amide (LSD), and phencyclidine (PCP). Although there are obvious sociocultural
influences in declaring some drugs off-limits—and the battle for the legalization of
marijuana and all other banned substances goes on—one can only conclude that
avoiding such substances is a factor in health promotion. Preoccupation with illegal
drug use leads to a particular life-style—one that is not conducive to good health.
Although the rationality of the bans may be argued, the fact remains that these drugs
are illegal, are obtained through unlawful channels for recreational use, and produce a
life-style that is not healthy.

Social Drugs

There are also so-called "social drugs," which are used by large segments of the population and include caffeine, nicotine, and alcohol. These drugs are readily available—at least, by law, to adults—and are widely used. Caffeine, the most widely used psychoactive drug in the world, is a relatively mild stimulant, and it is consumed by most persons within reasonable limits (Greden & Walters, 1992). There has been a shift in recent decades in which Americans consume caffeine more from soft drinks than from coffee. The amount of caffeine consumed in coffee, tea, and soft drinks produces relatively limited stimulant effects when compared with amphetamines and cocaine. Caffeine is also the only stimulant not forbidden by the Olympic Committees. Despite unclear evidence linking caffeine to benign breast disease and coronary disease and except for the occasional case of "caffeinism" and the mild discomfort of caffeine withdrawal, the linkage between health depleting behaviors and caffeine is limited, provided one consumes it moderately (Lamarine, 1994).

Nicotine is another matter, and there is clear evidence of long-term consequences of smoking. Chapter 6 deals with health promotion through smoking cessation, and although persons may continue to choose to use nicotine, the relationship between nicotine and health consequences have been clearly established for many decades. The first clear evidence of a relationship between smoking and lung cancer appeared in the 1950s, and the first Surgeon General's report that defined nicotine as a "health hazard" was issued decades ago (Ray & Ksir, 1996).

The use and abuse of alcoholic beverages is an area in which there is a good deal of information and there is some work on health promotion via prevention (Miller & Nirenberg, 1984; Gerstein, 1984; Morrissey, 1986; Nirenberg & Gomberg, 1993). Because of the widespread use of alcohol and some of the consequences that follow—both for the individual user and for society—alcohol is treated separately in this text as a challenge to health promotion.

Alternative Medicines

Alternative medicines include herbs and vitamins. Sales of "natural herbal remedies" have increased during the last decade. In 1993, the FDA issued a notice that regulation of these medicines was needed; this was followed by a well-organized program of writing-to-Congress, as a result of which Congress issued the Dietary Supplement and Health Education Act of 1994. Herbal remedies were declared to be "supplements" and exempt from FDA investigatory rules. Whereas prescription and over-the-counter drugs must be proved safe and effective and meet standards of safety, the plant products touted to produce medicinal effects are exempt. Manufacturers are not required to test these products or to engage in quality control. Eventually, the FDA probably will specify minimal quality controls, and the relationship of these alternative herbal remedies to health promotion will become clearer.

ALCOHOL AND HEALTH PROMOTION

Alcohol abuse includes a far higher percentage of the U.S. population than does abuse of other substances. The use of alcohol by age group and gender is described in Table 11-1 (Substance Abuse and Mental Health Services Administration [SAMHSA], 1995). Although not of legal drinking age, more than 40% of adolescents ages 12- to 17-years report that they have consumed alcohol.

Women report comparatively less alcohol use than men. It should be noted that for women, the 26-to-34 age group had the largest percentage of alcohol consumers and for men, the older-than-35 group had the highest rate of drinkers. In the 1993 figures report (SAMHSA, 1995), there was little change from 1992 to 1993. Generally, alcohol use is relatively more common among men, whites, adults ages 26 to 34, and those who attended college; heavy alcohol use is relatively more common among young adults 18 to 25 years old, those who did not graduate from college, and unemployed persons. The gender gap in relation to alcohol use appears to widen with increasing age.

Racial and ethnic comparisons show whites reporting more lifetime, past-year, and current alcohol use than blacks or Hispanics (Table 11-2). The overall figures for Hispanics are close to those of blacks, and Hispanic males report higher levels of lifetime and past-year use than black males or females and Hispanic females. Adult white males (18 years and older) report greater current alcohol use than females of the same age in any racial/ethnic group. Additionally, white adult females (18 years and older) report greater current alcohol use than black or Hispanic females of the same age. A Michigan Indian Health Task Force report pointed out an estimated 80% to 85% alcoholism rate among American Indian men and a 35% to 55% rate among females (Hayman & Copeland, 1989). Estimates of apparent per capita alcohol consumption by state note the following seven states with heaviest consumption: Nevada, New Hampshire, District of Columbia, Alaska, Wisconsin, Delaware, and Arizona (U.S. Secretary of Health and Human Services, 1993).

The latest figures available in the 8th Special Report to Congress show that 32% of American male adults and 53% of American female adults abstain from alcohol consumption (U.S. Secretary of Health and Human Services, 1993). Heavy drinkers include 18% of American male adults and 7% of female adults, approximately a 3:1 ratio.

Data from the Epidemiologic Catchment Area Study (Robins & Regier, 1991) show a peak of alcohol abuse/dependence for both men and women in the age group 18 to 29 years, followed by declines in the age groups 30 to 44, 45 to 65, and 65 and older. The epidemiologic data gathered from black respondents show a different age trajectory: there is a much smaller proportion of abuse/dependence diagnoses in the age group 18 to 29 years than among whites, but starting with age 30, the reported percentages of abuse/dependence are higher than among whites—this is true for both men and women. Among men, the most striking differences between blacks and whites occur in the age group of 45 to 64; for women, the most notable differences are found in the 45 to 64 age group. When all ethnic/racial groups are combined—as they are usually are in tables—these differences are obscured. No explanation has been offered for these ethnic/racial variations.

The epidemiologic literature provides targets for prevention and health promotion programs and details differences that exist between genders, age groupings, and ethnic/racial groupings in the U.S. population. Some interventions have proved to be ineffective. As history demonstrates, Prohibition (the 18th Amendment) was not a spectacular success in deterring Americans' fondness for alcoholic beverages. Recommending abstinence from alcohol also is not an effective or accurate health education strategy. Furthermore, there are some apparent health benefits from small or moderate amounts of alcohol. The recent nutritional guidelines issued by the federal government list not only the medical consequences of drinking but also note that moderate drinking is associated with lower risk for coronary heart disease (U.S. Department of Health and Human Services

Table 11-1

Alcohol use by sex within age group for total population in 1994

RATE ESTIMATES (PERCENT)

Age/Sex	Ever Used		Used Past Year		Used Past Month	
	Observed Estimate	95% CI	Observed Estimate	95% CI	Observed Estimate	95% CI
12-17	41.7	(39.9-43.5)	36.2	(34.5-37.9)	21.6	(20.2-23.2)
Male	42.9	(40.3-45.6)	36.2	(33.8-38.7)	22.1	(20.1-24.3)
Female	40.4	(37.9-43.0)	36.1	(33.7-38.7)	21.1	(19.1-23.3)
18-25	86.3	(84.5-87.9)	78.5	(76.3-80.6)	63.1	(60.5-65.6)
Male	87.9	(85.4-90.0)	82.3	(79.3-85.0)	70.9	(67.6-74.0)
Female	84.8	(82.7-86.6)	74.8	(72.1-77.3)	55.3	(52.1-58.6)
26-34	91.8	(90.7-92.8)	78.8	(76.8-80.6)	65.3	(63.1-67.5)
Male	94.6	(93.2-95.7)	83.7	(81.3-85.9)	73.9	(70.9-76.7)
Female	89.1	(87.6-90.4)	74.0	(71.8-76.1)	57.1	(54.7-59.4)
≥35	89.0	(87.2-90.5)	66.2	(63.3-68.9)	54.1	(51.2-56.9)
Male	95.4	(93.8-96.5)	72.5	(68.4-76.2)	60.9	(57.1-64.6)
Female	83.4	(80.5-85.9)	60.7	(56.9-64.4)	48.1	(44.2-51.9)
Total	84.2	(83.0-85.3)	66.9	(65.1-68.7)	53.9	(51.9-55.8)
Male	88.4	(87.3-89.4)	71.8	(69.3-74.2)	60.3	(57.9-62.7)
Female	80.3	(78.6-81.9)	62.4	(60.0-64.7)	47.9	(45.4-50.5)

POPULATION ESTIMATES (IN THOUSANDS)

		(95% CI)		(95% CI)		(95% CI)
12-17	9,079	(8,695-9,468)	7,880	(7,507-8,260)	4,711	(4,398-5,040)
Male	4,780	(4,489-5,075)	4,035	(3,765-4,313)	2,466	(2,241-2,706)
Female	4,300	(4,027-4,577)	3,845	(3,585-4,113)	2,246	(2,032-2,476)
18-25	24,186	(23,691-24,631)	22,010	(21,381-22,594)	17,673	(16,943-18,383)
Male	12,188	(11,844-12,480)	11,421	(11,000-11,792)	9,838	(9,383-10,265)
Female	11,997	(11,703-12,262)	10,588	(10,202-10,949)	7,835	(7,375-8,288)
26-34	33,584	(33,174-33,949)	28,816	(28,118-29,472)	23,895	(23,088-24,679)
Male	16,935	(16,686-17,136)	14,987	(14,543-15,383)	13,232	(12,693-13,733)
Female	16,649	(16,372-16,896)	13,829	(13,409-14,227)	10,663	(10,225-11,095)
≥35	109,441	(107,239-111,369)	81,415	(77,897-84,793)	66,524	(62,964-70,050)
Male	54,788	(53,886-55,470)	41,635	(39,299-43,776)	34,995	(32,819-37,097)
Female	54,653	(52,770-56,308)	39,779	(37,280-42,196)	31,529	(29,012-34,061)
Total	176,290	(173,820-178,619)	140,121	(136,285-143,852)	112,804	(108,675-116,907)
Male	88,691	(87,620-89,683)	72,079	(69,518-74,507)	60,531	(58,079-62,932)
Female	87,599	(85,727-89,356)	68,042	(65,457-70,564)	52,273	(49,466-55,093)

CI, Confidence intervals.

From *1994 National Household Survey on Drug Abuse, New Questionnaire Data (1994-B Sample)* by Substance Abuse and Mental Health Services Administration, 1994, Washington, DC.

Table 11-2

Alcohol use by age group and sex for whites, Hispanics and blacks in 1994

ALCOHOL USE BY AGE GROUP AND SEX FOR WHITES

AGE/SEX	EVER USED		USED PAST YEAR		USED PAST MONTH	
	OBSERVED ESTIMATE	95% CI	OBSERVED ESTIMATE	95% CI	OBSERVED ESTIMATE	95% CI
	RATE ESTIMATES (PERCENT)					
Age						
12-17	45.3	(43.1-47.6)	39.6	(37.4-41.9)	23.9	(22.0-25.9)
18-25	91.6	(89.7-93.1)	84.0	(81.4-86.2)	68.2	(65.1-71.2)
26-34	95.5	(94.3-96.5)	82.3	(80.0-84.4)	68.6	(65.9-71.2)
≥35	91.1	(89.0-92.8)	68.3	(64.8-71.7)	56.2	(52.7-59.6)
Sex						
Male	90.5	(89.3-91.6)	73.4	(70.3-76.4)	61.7	(58.7-64.7)
Female	84.8	(82.7-86.7)	66.5	(63.5-69.4)	51.9	(48.7-55.2)
Total	87.6	(86.2-88.8)	69.8	(67.5-72.1)	56.7	(54.2-59.1)

ALCOHOL USE BY AGE GROUP AND SEX FOR HISPANICS

AGE/SEX	EVER USED		USED PAST YEAR		USED PAST MONTH	
	OBSERVED ESTIMATE	95% CI	OBSERVED ESTIMATE	95% CI	OBSERVED ESTIMATE	95% CI
	RATE ESTIMATES (PERCENT)					
Age						
12-17	39.1	(35.6-42.8)	33.0	(29.6-36.6)	18.3	(15.3-21.7)
18-25	76.7	(73.2-79.8)	68.3	(63.8-72.4)	53.6	(49.4-57.7)
26-34	83.4	(80.5-85.9)	71.6	(68.2-74.9)	56.6	(52.8-60.3)
≥35	84.2	(81.4-86.7)	65.8	(62.3-69.2)	50.0	(46.3-53.6)
Sex						
Male	86.3	(84.2-88.1)	73.8	(71.2-76.3)	60.0	(57.0-62.9)
Female	66.3	(63.7-68.8)	52.2	(49.4-54.9)	35.4	(32.8-38.1)
Total	76.2	(74.3-78.1)	63.0	(61.0-64.9)	47.7	(45.6-49.7)

CI, Confidence intervals.

From *1994 National Household Survey on Drug Abuse, New Questionnaire Data (1994-B Sample)* by Substance Abuse and Mental Health Services Administration, 1994, Washington, DC.

Table 11-2

Alcohol use by age group and sex for whites, Hispanics and blacks in 1994—cont'd

	ALCOHOL USE BY AGE GROUP AND SEX FOR BLACKS					
	EVER USED		USED PAST YEAR		USED PAST MONTH	
AGE/SEX	OBSERVED ESTIMATE	95% CI	OBSERVED ESTIMATE	95% CI	OBSERVED ESTIMATE	95% CI
	RATE ESTIMATES (PERCENT)					
Age						
12-17	32.9	(29.1-36.9)	27.9	(24.5-31.4)	18.2	(15.3-21.5)
18-25	74.8	(70.8-78.4)	67.2	(63.1-71.1)	51.5	(47.0-56.0)
26-34	83.0	(79.8-85.7)	70.2	(66.5-73.7)	59.2	(55.5-62.7)
≥35	80.8	(77.1-84.0)	54.2	(50.1-58.3)	42.4	(38.5-46.4)
Sex						
Male	78.7	(75.6-81.4)	61.1	(57.3-64.8)	51.5	(47.7-55.3)
Female	70.1	(66.8-73.3)	51.5	(48.5-54.6)	37.7	(34.5-41.0)
Total	73.9	(71.4-76.3)	55.8	(53.4-58.2)	43.8	(41.4-46.3)

[USDHHS], 1988; Rimm, Klatsky, Grobbee, & Stampfer, 1996); there is a good deal of medical evidence to support that association (Renaud & DeLorgeril, 1992). Alcohol is a substance that when consumed in heavy amounts, however, produces all sorts of negative consequences. Heavy drinking is bad for the health status of any individual.

Whatever the guidelines might suggest concerning sensible or reasonable drinking, it is imperative that the gender difference be emphasized. Because women tend to weigh less than men and because their bodies contain a lower proportion of water (resulting in higher tissue concentration of alcohol), it is recommended by all authorities that the limits of sensible drinking be lower for women than for men. This presents a challenge to prevention work and health promotion.

Finally, there are lobbying groups working to influence public policy concerning alcohol consumption. These lobbies include the distilled beverage, beer, and wine industries and groups that share the mantle of the Anti-Saloon League and the Women's Christian Temperance Union, which seek to abolish alcohol production and consumption.

Any health promotion program concerning alcohol use must take into account differences in the lifespan. Not only are the patterns and attitudes toward the use of alcoholic beverages different among young persons, adults, the middle-aged, and the elderly, it is likely that the physiologic and neurologic impacts of alcohol differ as well.

Health care professionals must recognize the relationship between heavy/problem drinking—consumption of large quantities of alcohol that inevitably produces health, social, and legal problems—and the diagnosable conditions of alcohol abuse and alcohol dependence. After drinking one beer, glass of wine, or mixed drink (about ½ ounces of alcohol), an individual's blood alcohol concentration (BAC) is .02, and he/she feels relaxed and loosened up. With 2½ beers, glasses of wine, or mixed drinks, the BAC rises to .05, judgement is impaired, and inhibitions are decreased. The legal limit for blood alcohol concentration under Driving While Intoxicated (DWI) laws is .10 grams per 100 milliliters. This amounts to about 5 beers, glasses of wine, or mixed drinks (2½ ounces of alcohol). At 10 beers, glasses of wine, or mixed drinks (5 ounces of alcohol), the BAC is .20, and the individual experiences slowed reflexes and erratic changes in feelings. Fifteen beers, glasses of wine, or mixed drinks (7½ ounces of alcohol) yields a BAC of .30, a stupor, complete loss of coordination, and little sensation. At 20 beers, glasses of wine, or mixed drinks (10 ounces of alcohol) (BAC of .40), one may be comatose, and breathing may cease (Edlin & Golanty, 1992; Boston Women's Health Care Collective, 1992). The criteria for diagnoses are further described in the *Diagnostic and Statistical Manual of Mental Disorders, IV* (American Psychiatric Association, 1994).

Some Causes of Substance Abuse

According to the traditional models of etiology and prevention, high risk groups for alcohol/drug abuse among men and women include: (1) alcoholism/drug abuse in a family member; (2) disruptive early family experiences; (3) membership in peer groups with heavy alcohol/drug use; (4) depression or antisocial personality factors; (5) life crises; (6) use of alcohol/drugs to relieve stress; (7) sociocultural factors (e.g., neighborhood, community distribution of consumption); and (8) the degree of heavy drinking/drug use in the society. The Health Promotion Matrix adds a final critical factor: the person's representation of health. The Matrix assists the health care professional in determining the client's idealized picture of health—an important influence on substance use. A number of experimental studies of the concept of *expectancy* (i.e., what individuals expect to happen) posit that the individual's *view* of the effect of the alcohol/drug when it is ingested is an important aspect of his/her attraction to it (Oei & Young, 1987; Brown, Millar, & Passman, 1988; Jaffe & Lohse, 1991; Christiansen, Goldman, & Brown, 1985). Alcohol, for example, is often perceived as "a magic elixir" that promotes sociability, sexual pleasure, confidence, and power (Marlatt, 1987). Children apparently have expectations about alcohol effects long before drinking actually occurs (Miller, Smith, & Goldman, 1990). The media present images of drinkers as problem-free, mature, sexual, and engaged with others; these images pervade the culture and predispose children to view drinking as an escape from the turmoil of their stage of development.

Healthy Substance Use

Does healthy behavior mean total abstinence from alcohol and drugs? Again, the distinction must be made regarding the different classes, or categories, of drugs. Obviously, prescribed and over-the-counter drugs that are taken for therapeutic purposes need not be included in this discussion. The issue of healthy behavior arises only when an individual is considering compliance or noncompliance. While, overall, the safety of therapeutic drugs is limited and monitored by the FDA and recommended dosages are well-codified, these drugs may be misused. Persons are admitted to emergency rooms with drug-related diagnoses including those from therapeutic medications (Substance Abuse and Mental Health Services Administration, 1996).

Healthy behavior does mean abstinence from banned substances. Not only are there negative effects of recreational use of drugs such as cocaine, heroin, and marijuana, but there are also legal and medical/psychologic consequences. Use of the "social drugs" caffeine and nicotine raises other questions. Healthy behavior does apparently mean abstinence from nicotine, but caffeine consumed in moderate amounts, does not appear to be a major health hazard. As pointed out earlier, there has been some writing documenting the relationship between caffeine and benign breast disease and coronary disease, but the evidence is ambiguous and most persons do not seem to suffer ill effects from small to moderate amounts of caffeinated beverages (Lamarine, 1994).

The consumption of alcoholic beverages is a controversial area in health promotion. There are still active prohibition groups in the United States, and several church denominations encourage abstinence from alcohol. Much of the alcohol education in the school system depicts it as being linked to negative consequences (e.g., cirrhosis, accidents, cancer, birth defects, and violence). For years, however, findings have shown that individuals who drink small to moderate amounts of alcoholic beverages have less coronary disease than those who abstain from alcohol. The antithetical view about alcohol is entrenched in history, and the debate between prohibitionists and those who make health claims about alcohol is long-standing.

The British government is so convinced of the benefits of moderate drinking that it recommends middle-age and older abstainers to drink in moderation (Shiflett, 1996). World Health Association statistics for 1989 show the U.S. death rate from cirrhosis at 17 per 100,000, compared with cardiovascular disease death rates of 464 per 100,000. The cirrhosis death rate in France, where per capita consumption of alcohol is considerably higher than in the United States, is almost double—31 per 100,000—but cardiovascular disease death rates are lower—310 per 100,000 (WHO, 1995; Embland, 1995; Renaud & DeLorgeril, 1992). The view that small-to-moderate amounts of alcoholic beverages may have beneficial health effects has now appeared in the U.S. nutritional guidelines. This makes the question of whether substance safety means total abstinence from alcohol a difficult one.

With what is known so far, it can be concluded that substance safety in regard to alcohol indicates that the consequences of heavy, immoderate consumption are clear—it is risky behavior. The problem that remains is how to define small, moderate, and heavy amounts of alcohol consumption. The generally accepted criteria for heavy drinking is 5 or more drinks per occasion; it should be noted that the criteria for the heavy drinking differs from country to country. There are further complexities in that it is generally agreed that the criteria of moderate and heavy drinking for women should be fewer drinks than that for men. There also is the question of whether women should drink at all during pregnancy. The U.S. Surgeon General has issued a recommendation that women avoid drinking while pregnant (USDHHS, 1988). This recommendation is directed at least in part to the prevention of fetal alcohol syndrome, a confluence of clinical symptoms including growth retardation, central nervous system deficits, and altered facial features that has been associated with moderate to heavy drinking by women during pregnancy (Centers for Disease Control and Prevention, 1997). Some women who drink during pregnancy give birth to an impaired infant—but questions remain about quantity, frequency, and the trimester in which the drinking occurs.

A HEALTH PROMOTION MODEL FOR SUBSTANCE ABUSE

The model used most frequently in public health work encompasses the agent, environment, and host (Gomberg, Breslow, Hamburg, & Noble, 1980).

Agent

The health promotion measures that deal with the agent (alcohol/drugs) include licensing regulations; taxation of alcoholic beverages; and regulations governing the number and places of outlets that sell alcohol, beverage ingredients, minimum purchase age, and labeled health warnings. These are policies that are determined by politics and social usage.

Environment

Health promotion measures may start with the mass media and advertising by groups such as Partnership for a Drug-Free America. The educational system is a major arena for health promotion efforts in relation to the use and abuse of alcohol and drugs, and there are many reported studies of the effectiveness and ineffectiveness of using such an approach (Bangert-Drowns, 1988). A major environmental concern is directing health promotion/prevention measures toward families in which alcohol and/or drug abuse is manifested by parents and older siblings. Although the genetic etiology of addiction is well-documented, not all families in which a parent or parents use alcohol or drugs abusively produce children who also become alcoholics or drug abusers. Such families and the variables that contribute to next-generation alcohol/drug abuse have been studied in a number of ways (Wolin, Bennett, Noonan, & Teitelbaum, 1980). The workplace is another environmental area to be considered in health promotion/prevention—there is a sizable amount of literature that reports on employee assistance programs, and there are earlier studies that show differences in drinking problems among the employed, the unemployed, and shift workers (Smart, 1979). Finally, the community itself can be a powerful focus for the development of health promotion/prevention strategies. These measures may take the form of the removal of billboards advertising liquor, community campaigns against drunken drivers, laws that affect liquor stores and bartender training, the policing of communities plagued by drug dealers, and the formation of school-community partnerships for substance safety.

Host

Most efforts at health promotion have been directed toward the individual. This seems to be a by-product of the value Americans place on individualism, including in health care. This approach is not a problem as long as agental and environmental factors are also part of a general health promotion program.

Considerations in health promotion campaigns begin with host factors (i.e., should high-risk groups be targeted first?). High-risk groups might include children in alcoholic families or adolescents who are already using drugs. Host considerations might lead to the development of biochemical diagnoses of alcohol/drug abuse so that early detection and early intervention can be fostered. More information is needed about the relationship of life stressors, social supports, and coping mechanisms and their role in the onset and development of substance abuse. There are a number of screening methods for alcohol/drug problems (e.g., the Michigan Alcohol Screening Test [MAST]) that are suitable for a wide range of age groups (Herrington, Jacobson, & Benzer, 1987). Again, early detection is an advantage in treatment.

Research on socialization, family dynamics, and parenting shows that basic attitudes, values, and expectancies about alcohol or drug effects develop in the early years of life. Parents view their role in alcohol education as transmitting information and modeling positive behaviors. Health-compromising behaviors may also be modeled and unfortunate lessons learned in a family where drinking immoderately, smoking, and questionable drug use occurs. Parents who are moderate drinkers, nonsmokers, and abstain from using marijuana and other drugs convey health-promotive values to their children. Children also are influenced by messages conveyed by the ethnic/religious/neighborhood community of which the family is part (i.e., normative attitudes toward sensible or immoderate drinking and/or the use of recreational drugs). Promoting healthy attitudes about alcohol consumption and drug usage begins with making distinctions between normative behaviors, individual vulnerability, and individual response to alcohol and drugs.

MINIMIZING HEALTH DEPLETING PATTERNS RELATED TO SUBSTANCE USE

Minimizing the negative health consequences of various classes of drugs will differ. When prescribed medication and over-the-counter drugs are considered, depletion of negative health consequences lie in both physician and client roles. Physicians are trained to prescribe but inadequately trained to counsel the client; a conservative attitude in prescribing medication would go a long way to minimize adverse drug reactions. The client's role in minimizing negative effects is reasonable compliance with the drug regimen prescribed. These principles of physician and client action are even more important for those groups who are likely to receive a disproportionate number of prescriptions (e.g., women and the elderly).

As for "street" drugs or illegal substances, there is no way to minimize their potential negative health effects. It must be remembered that it is not only the pharmacologic effects of banned substances that are relevant but also the life-style that inevitably accompanies sustained use. Some illegal substances create more havoc with health than others (e.g., cocaine used regularly has swift and complex negative health effects; animal experiments have borne this out) (Bouknight & Bouknight, 1988; Woods, 1977; Billman, 1995; Thadani, 1995). Additionally, some individuals, due to genetic predisposition or developmental stage, are more sensitive and susceptible than others to the effects of these drugs (Morse, Erwin, & Jones, 1995). Some of the banned substances do have medical uses, (e.g., the use of marijuana in glaucoma treatment or the alleviation of chemotherapy response); however, this discussion pertains to recreational uses.

As for the legal drugs caffeine and alcohol, the key is moderation. The use of caffeinated or alcoholic beverages in modest amounts does little harm to most adults, although there are persons who have genetic, familial, and/or personality vulnerability and probably should avoid such drugs (Simmons, 1996; Hinds, West, Knight, & Harland, 1996; USDHHS, 1988; Ozkaragoz, Satz, & Noble, 1997). Although there are persons who believe that any alcoholic beverage is toxic and should be obliterated, the strength of the evidence does not support such a view. As stated previously, the key is *moderation,* which is usually defined by the family, social groups, and community to which an individual belongs. Moderation may also be characterized as "low-risk drinking," or alcohol use that does not lead to problems. Low-risk drinkers do not engage in binge drinking—more than 2 and 4 drinks per occasion for women and men, respectively—or in excessive regular drinking—more than 7 drinks a week for women and 14 drinks a week for men (National Institute of Alcohol Abuse and Alcoholism, 1995a, 1995b). With tobacco, there is little ambiguity—the safest course is abstinence, and there is no substance safety in any tobacco alternative.

SUBSTANCE-RELATED HEALTH PROMOTION FOR SPECIAL GROUPS

While the course and consequences of alcohol abuse and alcohol dependence may be about the same for all persons (Schuckit, 1991), the importance of tailoring the health promotion scripts to specific populations cannot be overemphasized.

Gender

In the field of alcohol studies, it has been clearly demonstrated that women are more vulnerable to some of the consequences. They are, for example, more likely to develop medical problems related to heavy alcohol intake, particularly liver disorders. The exact mechanism and process remains unclear; however, one explanation for the difference between genders is related to a difference in gastric enzymes involved in the metabolism of alcohol (Frezza et al., 1990). Another explanation concerns the combined effect of estrogen and alcohol (Johnson & Williams, 1985). Women who are problem drinkers are at greater risk of alcoholic cardiomyopathy than are men who are problem drinkers (Urbano-Marquez et al., 1995). There are also problems associated with drinking during pregnancy and issues regarding double-standard social attitudes toward heavy drinking and intoxication in men and women.

Minorities

Too little is known about ethnic/religious/social class differences in the use and abuse of substances. One clear fact, however, has emerged: age trajectories are different among racial/ethnic groups. For the white population, the youthful years are the most risk-laden; for blacks and other minority groups, the pattern is different. Black youngsters, for example, are less likely to be alcohol/drug abusers than white youngsters (Wallace, 1994), but as the percentage of problem alcohol/drug users among whites declines slowly through the adult years, it rises for blacks. A study of black and white elderly alcoholics (Gomberg, 1995) indicates that black men drink more heavily, manifest more negative health and community consequences, and are more likely to use a variety of substances. All of these factors must be considered in prevention and health promotion strategies.

Age

It is obvious that alcohol and drug use patterns vary at different stages of the lifespan. It is also clear that health promotion strategies need to be designed for adolescents, for young adults, for the middle-aged, and for the elderly; health promotion strategies are not a case of one-size-fits-all. Specific campaigns need to be developed for young persons and adolescents; the traditional educational approach has had very limited value (Bangert-Drowns, 1988). Health strategies for adults must address the issues of marriage, occupation, and parenting. The middle-age and elderly years present some particular issues, too; for example, for older persons, the question of medication/alcohol interactions is a major issue, and there are issues surrounding the lifespan of women (Gomberg, 1996).

Older adults. Older adults present special concerns when setting criteria for drinking and medication use. Compared with younger adults, the elderly have an increased sensitivity to alcohol and over-the-counter and prescription medications (Finch & Barry, 1992). In addition, there is an age-related decrease in lean body mass compared to total volume of fat, and the resultant reduction in total body volume increases the total distribution of alcohol and other mood-altering chemicals in the body. Central nervous system sensitivity increases and liver enzymes that metabolize alcohol and certain other drugs are less efficient with age.

The potential interaction of medication and alcohol is of great concern with this age group. For some clients, any alcohol use at all combined with the use of specific over-the-counter or prescription medications can result in problematic consequences. Therefore alcohol use recommendations are generally lower than those for adults younger than 65 and are usually made on a case-by-case basis.

To determine the prescription and over-the-counter medication use of older clients, the health care professional can use the "brown bag" approach: Ask clients to bring to their next office visit a brown paper bag that contains every medication they take. This will provide an opportunity to better determine potential medication problems.

CATEGORIES OF SUBSTANCE USE

Psychoactive drugs may be sanctioned medically to modify or control moods; however, any use of a psychoactive substance to change the state of mind that is harmful to oneself or others is considered abuse. *Abuse* and *dependence* pertain to both alcohol and drugs. Definitions for adults regarding low risk, at-risk, and problem use focus primarily, but not exclusively, on alcohol (Barry, 1997). To determine whether a client could benefit from drinking less or needs to stop entirely, it is necessary to use operating definitions of varying levels of alcohol and drug use.

Low-risk drinking is alcohol use that does not lead to problems. Persons in this category can set reasonable limits on alcohol consumption and do not drink when pregnant or trying to conceive, driving a car or boat, operating heavy machinery, or using contraindicated medications. As stated earlier, they do not engage in binge drinking—more than 2 or 4 drinks per occasion for women and men, respectively—or in excessive regular drinking—more than 7 drinks a week for women and 14 drinks a week for men (NIAAA, 1995a). Low-risk use of medications/drugs would include using an antianxiety medication for an acute anxiety state according to the physician's prescription (Trachtenberg & Fleming, 1994). Low-risk clients can benefit from prevention messages but do not need interventions. Prevention messages follow this format:

> *"Our goal is to prevent future health problems. Your exercise program looks good and your weight has remained stable. Since you have no family history of alcohol or drug problems and are taking no medication to interfere with alcohol, not exceeding a glass of wine a few times a week should not cause any additional problems for you."* (Barry, 1997, p. 354).

Alcohol consumption that increases the chances for a person to develop problems and complications is called *at-risk drinking*. Women who consume more than 7 drinks per week, men who consume more than 14 drinks per week, or persons who drink in risky situations are considered to be at-risk drinkers. Although these individuals do not currently have a health problem caused by alcohol, they may be experiencing family and social problems, and if this drinking pattern continues over time, health problems could result. These clients can benefit from brief interventions based on the Health Promotion Matrix.

Clients who engage in *problem drinking* consume alcohol at a level that has already resulted in adverse medical, psychologic, or social consequences. Potential consequences can include accidents and injuries, legal problems, sexual behavior that increases the risk of HIV infection, and family problems (Barry & Fleming, 1994). It is important to note that some persons who drink small amounts of alcohol may experience alcohol-related problems, such as elderly individuals (see the Older Adults section) or those persons with severe medical or psychiatric problems. With special populations, the presence of consequences, rather than quantity and frequency of alcohol use, should drive the need for intervention using the Health Promotion Matrix.

Alcohol or drug dependence refers to a medical disorder characterized by loss of control, preoccupation with alcohol or drugs, continued use despite adverse consequences, and physiologic symptoms such as tolerance and withdrawal (American Psychiatric Association, 1994). A wide range of legal and illegal substances can be addictive. The Health Promotion Matrix can be especially helpful with this group of clients in defining the problem and assisting them to engage in more structured treatment, as necessary.

ALCOHOL-RELATED INTERVENTIONS

Alcohol interventions were developed based on original work in smoking cessation. Scripts for reducing alcohol use are very similar to smoking cessation scripts. The main difference between the two areas is the focus of the intervention. Smoking scripts are designed with the ultimate goal of smoking cessation; drinking scripts are often designed to assist the client to *cut down* rather than to stop drinking. If cutting down is ineffective, abstinence then becomes the goal.

All of the alcohol-related brief interventions, like the smoking cessation interventions, include assessment and direct feedback, contracting and goal-setting, behavioral modification techniques, and the use of written materials such as self-help manuals. A number of trials, conducted primarily in Europe, have examined the efficacy of brief advice in reducing alcohol use. Although there are several ongoing studies of brief alcohol interventions for older adults, no reports are in the literature at this time.

Kristenson, Ohlin, Hulten-Nosslin, Trell, & Hood (1983) reported the results of a trial conducted in Malmo, Sweden, in the late 1970s in which the subjects were advised in a series of health education visits to reduce their alcohol use. They subsequently demonstrated significant reductions in gamma glutamyl transferase levels and health care utilization up to 5 years after the brief interventions. Wallace, Cutler, and Haines (1988), in the Medical Research Council (MRC) trial conducted in 47 general practitioners' offices in Great Britain, found significant reductions in alcohol use by the intervention group, as compared with the control group 12 months after the intervention. The World Health Organization Trial, conducted in 10 countries, found similar differences in alcohol use between the study and control groups (Babor & Grant, 1992).

Most recently, a brief alcohol intervention trial was conducted in the United States, with 67 community-based primary care physicians serving as intervenors. A total of 392 at-risk or problem drinkers younger than 65 received a physician-delivered brief advice protocol (382 were controls). The main outcome variables of the Trial for Early Alcohol Treatment (Project TrEAT) were decreased alcohol use, emergency department visits, and hospital days. At baseline, the study and control groups were comparable on alcohol use, age, socioeconomic status, smoking status, rates of depression or anxiety, frequency of conduct disorders, lifetime drug use, or health care utilization. At the time of the 12-month follow-up, there was a significant reduction in 7-day alcohol use ($t = 4.33$, $p < .001$)*, episodes of binge drinking ($t = 2.81$, $p < .001$)*, and frequency of excessive drinking ($t = 4.53$, $p < .001$)* in the experimental group compared with that of the control group. Chi-square tests of independence revealed a significant relationship between group status and lengths of hospitalization over the study period for men only ($p < .01$)†. Project TrEAT provided the first direct evidence that physician intervention with at-risk and problem drinkers decreases alcohol use and health resource utilization in a community-based U.S. health care system.

The basic design of most brief intervention studies is a randomized controlled trial of individuals with at-risk or problem drinking patterns who are assigned either to an experimental condition, ranging from 1 to 10 sessions, or to 1 or more control conditions (Kristenson et al. 1983; Chick, 1988; Heather, Campion, Neville, & MacCabe, 1987; Wallace et al, 1988; Persson & Magnusson, 1989; Harris & Miller, 1990; Anderson & Scott, 1992; Babor & Grant, 1992; Fleming, Barry, Manwell, Johnson, & London, 1997). Overall, 8 of the nine studies found significantly greater improvements in drinking outcomes for the brief intervention group compared with the control group.

Studies of Strategies to Change Drinking Behavior

Studies of brief interventions for alcohol problems have used various approaches to change drinking behaviors. Strategies have ranged from relatively unstructured counseling and feedback to more formal structured therapy and have relied heavily on concepts and techniques from the behavioral self-control training (BSCT) literature (Miller & Taylor, 1980; Miller & Hester, 1986; Miller & Munoz, 1976; Miller & Rollnick, 1991). Drinking goals of brief treatment interventions are flexible, allowing the individual to choose drinking in moderation or abstinence. The overall goal of brief counseling is to motivate the problem drinker to change his/her behavior, not to assign self-blame.

Most brief alcohol intervention studies have explicitly excluded dependent drinkers with significant withdrawal symptoms. The rationale for this has been that alcohol-dependent individuals, or those affected most severely by alcohol, should be referred to formal specialized alcoholism treatment programs because their conditions are not likely to be amenable to a low-intensity intervention (Institute of Medicine, 1990; Babor, Ritson, & Hodgson, 1986). One study addressed the validity of that assumption. Sanchez-Craig, Neumann, Souza-Formigoni, & Rieck (1991) found that there were no significant differences in rates of abstinence or moderate drinking when comparing the 12-month treatment outcomes of severely dependent and nonalcohol-dependent men receiving brief treatment in Toronto and Brazil. Additionally, rates of spontaneous remission of alcoholism suggest that there is a portion of the most severe alcoholic population who will reduce or stop drinking without formal intervention (Institute of Medicine, 1990).

---

*A p value of $<.001$ means that there is less than a 1 in 1000 probability that this result would have occurred by chance alone.

†A p value of $<.01$ means that there is less than a 1 in 100 probability that this result would have occurred by chance alone.

SUBSTANCE SAFETY & THE HEALTH PROMOTION MATRIX*

The following section and the script that follows on pp. 295-297 provide the basic tools for the health care professional to assess and intervene with an at-risk drinker. Other drug/medication use can be assessed using this same model. Following the script and adapting it to the client's drinking level and gender, as in the case example, will provide the framework to assist clients in managing their alcohol intake. The recommendations for the client based on the definitions found earlier in this chapter are described in the proceding case example.

This case involves a 34-year-old mother of two daughters, ages 8 and 10. She is a secretary at a large marketing firm and was recently divorced. She shares child custody with her ex-husband. She has been experiencing stomach pain, difficulty in sleeping, mild hypertension, and stress at work and at home. She recently tripped and fell while getting out of the shower.

Image Creation

The health care professional works with the client to discuss his/her idealized picture of health. This image may include a drink, as alcohol is an ever-present social drug. In the case of the 34-year-old woman, the image that she holds with a drink in her hand—relaxed and confident—influences her subsequent behavior, in that she may see herself as healthier with than without alcohol. The image the client holds in her own mind as healthier while drinking may be reinforced by the media, thus solidifying her idealized positive view of herself. To begin, the health care professional accepts the client's picture. As they move through the HPM dimensions and the script, however, the health care professional collaborates with the client to modify the image to make it more reflective of the positive and negative consequences of drinking and other risky substance use.

> Q. *Tell me what you see when you picture yourself as a healthy person.*
> *What kinds of activities do you see yourself doing?*
> *How would you feel physically? Emotionally?*

Image Appraisal

This dimension includes several subelements: screening questions, discussing the client's current health status, the types of drinkers in the United States, and the client's reasons for drinking. The health care professional begins by asking a set of screening questions related to drinking patterns and other health habits (this often includes smoking and nutrition [see Chapters 6 and 7]). Questions about alcohol use are generally part of an overall health assessment. The responses to these queries enable the health care professional to determine whether the client is at-risk and to customize the client feedback.

The health care professional then discusses the client's health status, including physical and emotional functioning. Some examples of problems resulting from risky drinking behaviors include difficulties with stress, sleep, family, stomach pains, depressed feelings, and accidents or injuries.

*Adapted from K. Lawton Barry by S. Sheinfeld Gorin.

This element is followed by a discussion of the types of drinkers in the United States or elsewhere, as geographically appropriate. The health care professional places the client's drinking pattern into the population norms for her age group. Using principles of motivational interviewing, the health care professional is somewhat directive, attempting to move the client toward a commitment to change.

The dimension ends with a discussion of the client's reasons for drinking. This is particularly important because the health care professional needs to understand the role of alcohol in the context of the client's life.

From the screening questions you completed as part of your health assessment, you indicated that you walk 3 times a week for ½ to 1 hour. Do you have friends who walk with you? Where do you walk?

Client's answer: I walk with another woman in my neighborhood.

That's great. I'm glad to hear that you are getting some good exercise. Your weight has stayed the same for quite a while now. You said that you stopped smoking 4 years ago? I know that was hard to do, but it's one of the best things you could do for your health.

On the screening, you indicated that, on average, you drink alcohol (6) days a week and drink (2 to 3) drinks at a time.

Tell me, how do you see your current health status?

What kinds of issues are causing you the most stress at this time?

How do you feel physically? Emotionally?

National guidelines recommend that women your age drink no more than 7 drinks per week. Your pattern of alcohol use fits into the at-risk drinking category.

We've spent some talking about your sleep problems, your stomach pains, the fall you took in the bathroom, and your loneliness since your divorce.

Minimize Health Depleting Patterns

At this point, the health care professional discusses the consequences of the client's heavy drinking pattern to encourage the client in her motivation to change. Often, myriad physical, psychologic, social, and economic aspects of the client's life have been affected by drinking. These are addressed by the health care professional to move the client toward change.

You are drinking at a risky level at this time. I know that you have been experiencing a lot of stress. Sometimes people use alcohol to help in coping with stressful situations. I am concerned about some of the health problems you've had and your loneliness, and I think your alcohol use may be making these other problems even worse, rather than helping you cope with them.

Optimize Health Supportive Patterns

The reasons to cut down or to quit drinking are emphasized at this point, and a drinking agreement is negotiated and summarized. Maintaining good work and family relationships are often important reasons to control alcohol intake, and families may serve as primary supports for change.

During the discussion of the drinking agreement, the client may negotiate for a higher level of drinking that is still within the national guidelines. Some clients are not willing to decrease consumption to the recommended levels of use. In this instance, the health care professional should negotiate the lowest temporary limit possible and note that changing behavior is an ongoing process and that drinking limits, as well as other issues, can be discussed at subsequent visits.

Negotiated, written drinking agreements that are signed by the client and the health care professional are particularly effective in changing drinking patterns. The script contains an example of a drinking agreement.

It is important to summarize expectations and to set a follow-up appointment in 1 month.

....

Remember your drinking limit for the next month is (specify) beverages. (State agreement).

Think of an activity you do frequently every day. Whenever you do that activity, think of your reasons to cut down on drinking.

Every time you are tempted to drink more than allowed in the agreement and can resist, congratulate yourself on breaking an old habit and helping yourself. One follow-up visit is important to assess any ongoing problems. I'll see you in 1 month on (specify date).

....

Internalize Idealized Image

Strategies that are useful for cutting down or quitting include developing social opportunities that do not involve alcohol, getting reacquainted with hobbies and interests, and pursuing new activities unrelated to alcohol use.

The health care professional gives heed to the social isolation, boredom, and negative family interactions that can present special problems to those who drink and works with the client to develop strategies to deal with these issues. Role-playing specific situations can be helpful.

Any progress toward the goal needs to be rewarded. Risky situations need to be assessed to develop coping strategies.

....

From your drinking diary cards, it looks like you did a very good job working toward your goal.

Congratulations! The only times you drank more than 1 drink a day were Sundays. What was happening on those days?

Let's look at some ways to cope with days that are more stressful.

....

Substance Safety: *A Script**

Image Creation	Tell me what you see when you picture yourself as a healthy person.
	What kinds of recreational activities do you see yourself doing? Is drinking alcohol or taking other substances part of this image?
Image Appraisal	The screening questions can be administered on a form or by interview.

Screening Questions

Do you drink alcohol?

YES   **NO**

        Is that a change?

About how many days a week do you drink alcohol?

On a day when you drink, how much do you drink?

How many days a month do you drink 4 or more drinks?

Screening positive for adult men is drinking more than 14 drinks/week; for adult women, more than 7 drinks/week; and for adult men or women, any single occasion when they have consumed more than 4 drinks in the past month. Guidelines for older adults recommend no more than 7 drinks/week, or 1 per day.

Do you use more than the recommended or prescribed amount of prescription or over-the-counter medications?

YES   **NO**

        Is that a change?

What medications are you using?

Do you use any nonmedical drugs?

YES   **NO**

        Is that a change?

What drugs are you using?

*Adapted from K. Lawton Barry by S. Sheinfeld Gorin.

continued

SUBSTANCE SAFETY: *A Script—cont'd*

> An individual screens positive if he/she uses any prescription or over-the-counter drugs in excess of the directions or uses any banned drugs.

From the screening questions you completed as part of your health assessment, you indicated that you (*specify behavior, including drinking patterns and other health habits to customize client feedback*).

Tell me how you see your current health status.

What kinds of issues are causing you the most stress at this time?

> National Guidelines recommend that women your age drink no more than 7 drinks per week (no more than 1 per day) (or) that men your age drink no more than 14 drinks per week (no more than 2 per day). Your pattern of alcohol use fits into a(n):

| At-risk category | Low-risk category |

Our goal is to prevent future health problems. Your exercise program looks good and your weight has remained stable. Since you have no family history of alcohol or drug problems and are taking no medication to interfere with alcohol, not exceeding a glass of wine a few times a week should not cause any additional problems for you.

Minimize Health Depleting Patterns

How do you feel about drinking at a level that is considered risky?

Have you ever thought about cutting back on your alcohol use?

What prevents you from cutting back on your drinking?

Optimize Health Supportive Patterns

What reasons would you have to cut back?

Have you ever tried to cut down on your drinking?

> I would recommend that you cut back to drinking no more than 4 days a week, no more than 1 (2 for men) drink per occasion.

How do you feel about that level of alcohol use?

Substance Safety: *A Script—cont'd*

> Negotiate a drinking limit consonant with national guidelines. Complete the drinking agreement (Figure 11-1).

Remember that your drinking limit for the next month is (specify).

> State agreement.

Think of an activity you do frequently every day. Whenever you do that activity, think of your reasons to cut down on drinking.

Every time you are tempted to drink more than the agreement and can resist, congratulate yourself on breaking an old habit and helping yourself.

Our follow-up visit is important to assess any ongoing problems. I'll see you in 1 month on (specify date).

Internalize Idealized Image

> Reassess strategies for cutting down or quitting. Use the Helpful Resources at the end of the chapter for assistance. Continue to work with the client to develop strategies to deal with issues such as social isolation and negative family interactions. Role-playing specific stressful situations can be helpful.

From your drinking diary cards, it looks like you did a very good job working toward your goal. Congratulations! Let's look at some ways to cope with days (or situations) that are more stressful.

Date _____

Agreement: *No more than 1 drink a day, no more than 5 days/week.*

Follow-up: *Return visit in 4 weeks.*

Client signature: _____

Practitioner signature: _____

Figure **11-1** Drinking agreement.

Summary

Potentially unsafe substances may be classified as prescribed and over-the-counter drugs; banned "street" drugs, such as marijuana, cocaine, and heroin; alternative medicines, such as herbs and vitamins; and "social drugs," such as nicotine, caffeine, and alcohol. Alcohol is among the more widely used risky substances. Because the rates and effects of immoderate drinking differ by age, gender, and minority/racial status, strategies to promote moderate drinking should be customized. Each client should be screened by the health care professional for at-risk use of alcohol. A brief, focused script, designed for an adult outpatient population, may be effectively used to reduce drinking through direct feedback, a behavioral contract, goal-setting, and social reinforcement. Clients may be encouraged to reduce their drinking, rather than to eliminate it entirely.

HELPFUL **RESOURCES**

ON-LINE

National Directory of Drug Abuse and Alcoholism Treatment and Prevention Programs
(http://www.health.org)
This site offers the opportunity to search for local treatment programs by facility function (e.g., substance abuse treatment services, methadone treatment, primary prevention, or other nontreatment services); facility type (e.g., detoxification, outpatient, or residential); subpopulation (e.g., youth, dually diagnosed); specific addictions (e.g., alcohol, cocaine), and payment type (e.g., Medicare, Medicaid).

National Clearinghouse for Alcohol and Drug Information
(http://www.health.org/index.htm)
The PREVLINE, or Prevention Online, allows access to databases and substance abuse prevention materials that pertain to alcohol, tobacco, and illegal drugs.

National Institute on Alcohol Abuse and Alcoholism (NIAAA)
(http://www.niaaa.nih.gov)

The NIAAA, a part of the U.S. Department of Health and Human Services, lists publications and databases that provide information on alcohol problems, as well as referrals and links to other organizations and associations.

Alcoholics Anonymous (AA)
(A.A. World Services, Inc.)
(http://www.alcoholics-anonymous.org)
This web site provides information and resources on AA programs in English, Spanish, and French.

AL-ANON/ALATEEN
(http://www.al-anon.alateen.org)
The web site describes the Twelve Steps, Twelve Traditions, and Twelve Concepts of Service adapted from AA for families and friends of alcoholics. It also lists local groups.
Information from Al-ANON Family Group Headquarters, Inc. is also available at: 1600 Corporate Landing Parkway, Virginia Beach, VA 23454-1655. Phone: (757) 563-1600. FAX: (757) 563-1655.

References

American Psychiatric Association. (1994). *Diagnostic and statistical manual of mental disorders—fourth edition (DSM-IV)*. Washington, DC: Author.

Anderson, P., & Scott, E. (1992). The effect of general practitioners' advice to heavy drinking men. *British Journal of Addiction, 87,* 891-900.

Babor, T.F., & Grant, M. (1992). *Project on identification and management of alcohol-related problems. Report on phase II: A randomized clinical trial of brief interventions in primary health care.* Geneva, World Health Organization.

Babor, T.F., Ritson, E.B., & Hodgson, R.J. (1986). Alcohol-related problems in the primary health care setting: A review of early intervention strategies. *British Journal of Addiction, 81,* 23-46.

Bangert-Drowns, R. (1988). The effects of school-based substance abuse education. *Journal of Drug Education, 18,* 243-264.

Barry, K. (1997). Alcohol and drug abuse. In M. Mengel, & W. Holleman (Eds.), *Fundamentals of clinical practice: A textbook on the patient, doctor, and society.* New York: Plenum Press.

Barry, K.L., & Fleming, M.F. (1994). The family physician. *Alcohol Health and Research World, 18*(1), 105-109.

Billman, G.E. (1995). Cocaine: A review of its toxic actions on cardiac function. *Critical Reviews in Toxicology, 25*(2), 113-132.

Boston Women's Health Care Collective. (1992). *Our bodies, ourselves.* New York: Simon & Schuster.

Bouknight, L.G., & Bouknight, R.R. (1988). Cocaine: A particularly addictive drug. *Postgraduate Medicine, 83*(4), 115-116.

Brown, S.A., Millar, A., & Passman, L. (1988). Utilizing expectancies in alcoholism treatment. *Psychology of Addictive Behavior, 2*(2), 59-65.

Centers for Disease Control and Prevention (1997, April 25). Alcohol consumption among pregnant and childbearing-aged women—United States, 1991 and 1995. *Morbidity and Mortality Weekly Report* (MMWR), *46*(16), 346-350.

Chick, J. (1988). Early intervention for hazardous drinking in the general hospital setting. *Australian Drug Alcohol Review, 7*(3), 339-343.

Christiansen, B.A., Goldman, M.S., & Brown, S.A. (1985). Differential development of adolescent alcohol expectancies may predict adult alcoholism. *Addictive Behaviors, 10*(3), 299-306.

Controlled Substances Act, 21 U.S.C. §§ 13-801 *et seq.,* 1970.

Dietary Supplement and Health Education Act, 21 U.S.C. 321, 1994.

Edlin, G., & Golanty, E. (1992). *Health and wellness.* Boston: Jones & Bartlett.

Embland, H. (1995). What would happen in the world if "sensible drinking" was adopted as a reasonable concept and advertised universally? *Addiction, 90*(2), 169-171.

Finch, J., & Barry, K. (1992). Substance use in older adults. In M. Fleming & K. Barry (Eds.), *Addictive disorders: A practical guide to treatment.* St. Louis: Mosby.

Fleming, M.F., Barry, K.L., Manwell, L.B., Johnson, K., & London, R. (1997). Brief physician advice for problem alcohol drinkers: A randomized controlled trial in community-based primary care practices. *Journal of the American Medical Association, 277*(13), 1039-1045.

Frezza, M., DiPadova, C., Pozzato, G., Terpin, M., Baraona E., & Lieber, C.S. (1990). High blood alcohol levels in women: The role of decreased gastric alcohol dehydrogenase activity and first-pass metabolism. *New England Journal of Medicine 322*(2), 95-99.

Gerstein, D.R. (1984). *Toward the prevention of alcohol problems. Government, business and community action.* Washington, DC: National Academy Press.

Gomberg, E.S.L., Breslow, L., Hamburg, B.A.M., & Noble, E.P. (1980). Prevention issues. In National Academy of Sciences (Ed.). *Report of a study: Alcoholism and related problems: Opportunities for research* (pp. 103-138). Washington, DC: National Academy of Sciences.

Gomberg, E.S. (1995). Older women and alcohol. Use and abuse. *Recent Developments in Alcoholism, 12,* 61-79.

Gomberg, E.S.L. (1996). Womens' drinking practices and problems from a lifespan perspective. In J.M. Howard et al (Eds.), *Women and alcohol: Issues for prevention research* (NIH Publication No. 96-3817, pp. 185-214). Bethesda, MD: National Institute on Alcohol Abuse and Alcoholism.

Greden, J.F., & Walters, A. (1992). Caffeine. In J.H. Lowinson, P. Ruiz, R.B. Millman, & J.G. Langrod (Eds.), *Substance abuse* (2nd ed., pp. 357-369). Baltimore: Williams & Wilkins.

Harris, K.B., & Miller, W.R. (1990). Behavioural self-control training for problem drinkers: Components of efficacy. *Psychology of Addictive Behaviour, 4*(2), 90-92.

Hayman, C.R., & Copeland, L. (1989). Insights on American Indians. *EAPA Exchange, 19*(10), 42-45.

Heather, N., Campion, P.D., Neville, R.G., Mac-Cabe, D. (1987). Evaluation of a controlled drinking minimal intervention for problem drinkers in general practice (the DRAMS scheme). *Journal of the Royal College of General Practitioners, 37*(301):358-63.

Herrington, R.E., Jacobson, G.R., & Benzer, D.G. (1987). *Alcohol and drug abuse handbook* (pp. 449-450). St. Louis: Warren H. Green.

Hinds, T.S., West, W.L., Knight, E.M., & Harland, B.F. (1996). The effect of caffeine on pregnancy outcome variables. *Nutrition Reviews, 54*(7), 203-207.

Institute of Medicine. (1990). *Broadening the base of treatment for alcohol problems.* Washington, DC: National Academy Press.

Jaffe, A., & Lohse, C.M. (1991). Expectations regarding cocaine use: Implications for prevention and treatment. *Addiction and Recovery, 11*(3), 9-12.

Johnson, R.D., & Williams, R. (1985). Genetic and environmental factors in the individual susceptibility to the development of alcoholic liver disease. *Alcohol and Alcoholism, 20*(2), 137-160.

Kristenson, H., Ohlin, H., Hulten-Nosslin, M., Trell, E., & Hood, B. (1983). Identification and intervention of heavy drinking in middle-aged men: Results and follow-up of 24-60 months of long-term study with randomized controls. *Alcoholism, Clinical and Experimental Research, 7*(2): 203-209.

Lamarine, R.J. (1994). Selected health and behavioral effects related to the use of caffeine. *Journal of Community Health, 19*(6), 449-466.

Marlatt, G.A. (1987). Alcohol, the magic elixir: Stress, expectancies, and the transformation of emotional states. In E. Gottheil, K.A. Druly, S. Pashko, & S.P. Weinstein (Eds.), *Stress and addiction* (pp. 302-322). New York: Brunner/Mazel.

Miller, P.M., & Nirenberg, T.D. (1984). *Prevention of alcohol abuse.* New York: Plenum Press.

Miller, P.M., Smith, G.T., & Goldman, M.S. (1990). Emergence of alcohol expectancies in childhood: A possible critical period. *Journal of Studies on Alcohol, 51*(4), 343-349.

Miller, W.R., & Hester, R.K. (1986). *Treating addictive behaviors: Processes of change.* New York: Plenum Press.

Miller, W.R., & Munoz, R.F. (1976). *How to control your drinking.* Englewood Cliffs, NJ: Prentice-Hall.

Miller, W.R., & Rollnick, S. (1991). *Motivational interviewing.* New York: The Guilford Press.

Miller, W.R., & Taylor, C.A. (1980). Relative effectiveness of bibliotherapy, individual and group self-control training in the treatment of problem drinkers, *Addictive Behaviors, 5,* 13-24.

Morrissey, E.R. (1986). Of women, by women or for women? Selected issues in the primary prevention of drinking problems. In National Institute on Alcohol Abuse and Alcoholism (Ed.), *Women and alcohol: Health-related issues* (Research Monograph No. 16). DHHS Publication No. (ADM) 86-1139, pp. 226-259). Washington, DC: U.S. Government Printing Office.

Morse, A.C., Erwin, V.G., & Jones, B.C. (1995). Pharmacogenetics of cocaine: A critical review. *Pharmacogenetics, 5*(4), 183-192.

National Institute of Alcohol Abuse and Alcoholism. (1995a) *NIAAA Physician Intervention Guide, 1995.* Rockville, MD: Author.

National Institute of Alcohol Abuse and Alcoholism (NIAAA). (1995b). *The Physicians' guide to helping patients with alcohol problems* (NIH Publication No. 95-3769). Bethesda, MD: National Institutes of Health.

Nirenberg, T.D., & Gomberg, E.S.L. (1993). Prevention of alcohol and drug problems among women. In E.S.L. Gomberg & T.D. Nirenberg (Eds.), *Women and substance abuse* (pp. 339-359). Norwood, NJ: Ablex Publishers.

Oei, P.S., & Young, R.M. (1987). Roles of alcohol-related self-statements in social drinking. *International Journal of the Addictions, 22*(10), 905-915.

Ozkaragoz, T., Satz, P., & Noble, E.P. (1997). Alcohol neurophysiological functioning in sons of active, alcoholic, recovering alcoholic and social drinking fathers. *Alcohol, 14*(1), 31-37.

Persson, J., & Magnusson, P.H. (1989). Early intervention in patients with excessive consumption of alcohol: A controlled study. *Alcohol, 6*(5), 403-408.

Ray, O., & Ksir, C. (1996). *Drugs, society and human behavior.* St. Louis: Mosby.

Renaud, S., & DeLorgeril, M. (1992). Wine, alcohol, platelets, and the French paradox for coronary heart disease. *The Lancet, 339*(8808), 1523-1526.

Rimm, E.B., Klatsky, A., Grobbee, D., & Stampfer, M.J. (1996). Review of moderate alcohol consumption and reduced risk of coronary heart disease: Is the effect due to beer, wine, or spirits? *BMJ, 312*(7033), 731-736.

Robins, L.N., & Regier, D.A. (1991). *Psychiatric disorders in America: The epidemiologic catchment area study.* New York: Free Press.

Sanchez-Craig, M., Neumann, B., Souza-Formigoni, M., & Rieck, L. (1991). Brief treatment for alcohol dependence: Level of dependence and treatment outcome. *Alcohol and Alcoholism,* (Suppl. 1), 515-518.

Schuckit, M.A. (1991). Importance of subtypes in alcoholism. *Alcohol and Alcoholism,* (Suppl. 1), 511-514.

Shiflett, D. (1996, October). Here's to your health. *The American Spectator,* 26-30.

Simmons, D.H. (1996). Caffeine and its effect on persons with mental disorders. *Archives of Psychiatric Nursing, 10*(2), 116-122.

Smart, R.G. (1979). Drinking problems among employed, unemployed and shift workers. *Journal of Occupational Medicine, 21*(11), 731-736.

Substance Abuse and Mental Health Services Administration, Office of Applied Studies. (1995) *National household survey on drug abuse. Main finding 1993.* Washington, DC: U.S. Department of Health and Human Services.

Substance Abuse and Mental Health Services Administration, Office of Applied Studies. (1996). *1996 DAWN (Drug Abuse Warning Network) Survey.* [On-line]. Available: http://www.health.org/pubs/95dawn

Thadani, P.V. (1995). Biological mechanisms and perinatal exposure to abused drugs. *Synapse, 19*(3), 228-232.

Trachtenberg, A., & Fleming, M. (1994, Summer). Diagnosis and treatment of drug abuse in family practice [Monograph]. *American Family Physician,*

Urbano-Marquez, A., Estruch, R., Fernandez-Sola, J., Nicolas, J.M., Pare, J.C., & Rubin, E. (1995). The greater risk of cardiomyopathy and myopathy in women compared with men. *Journal of the American Medical Association, 274*(2), 149-154.

U.S. Department of Health and Human Services, Public Health Service (1988). *The Surgeon General's Report on nutrition and health* (DHHS Publication No. (PHS) 88-50210). Washington, DC: Author.

U.S. Department of Health and Human Services, Public Health Service. (1995). *Healthy people 2000: Midcourse review and 1995 revisions.* Washington, DC: Superintendent of Documents.

U.S. Secretary of Health and Human Services. (1993). *Alcohol and health, 8th special report to Congress (1994).* Washington, DC: U.S. Government Printing Office.

Wallace, J. (1994). Race differences in adolescent drug use. *African American Research Perspectives, 1*(1), 31-36.

Wallace, P., Cutler, S., & Haines, A. (1988). Randomized controlled trial of general practitioner intervention in patients with excessive alcohol consumption. *BMJ, 297*(6649), 663-668.

Wolin, S.J., Bennett, L.A., Noonan, D.L., & Teitelbaum, M.A. (1980). Disrupted family rituals. A factor in the intergenerational transmission of alcoholism. *Journal of Studies on Alcohol, 41*(3), 199-214.

Woods, J. (1977). *Behavioral effects of cocaine in animals. Cocaine: 1977.* (NIDA Research Monograph No. 13, pp. 63-95). Washington, DC: U.S. Government Printing Office.

World Health Organization (WHO). (1995). Alcohol—Less is better. European Action Plan. *WHO Regional Publications, European Series (70).* Geneva, Switzerland: Author.

CHAPTER

12

Oral Health

Barbara J. Steinberg, Joan I. Gluch, and Susanne Kozich Giorgio

EDITORS' NOTE

Oral Health Promotion and the Community Client System   Oral health is an optimal behavior from which to view the community as the client system in the Health Promotion Matrix (HPM). Co-authors Barbara J. Steinberg, DDS, Joan I. Gluch, PhD, RDH, and Susanne Kozich Giorgio, RDH, identify the various barriers to accessing dental care among different subpopulations. They identify particular groups in the community who may have difficulty gaining access to oral health care because of poverty, age, depleted health, geographic isolation, fear, lack of knowledge, and the relative importance of other survival concerns. The issue of access is a critical one in health promotion. Further, many vulnerable subpopulations have a great need for oral health promotion because their general health is so compromised or depleted for the same reasons they experience limited access. Oftentimes, this process is further impeded by the lack of attention to oral health promotion at the policy level.

Oral Health and Image Creation   The issue of access requires that health care professionals reach out to vulnerable groups and communities to engage them in considering integrating oral health as part of a healthy image. Health care professionals are instrumental in facilitating the creation of an image that includes oral health and in linking clients with dental professionals for preventive dental care and treatment.

Dialogue with a Pregnant Woman and the Health Promotion Matrix Script   The authors' script explores the dynamics of health promotion intervention between a dental health care professional and a pregnant woman. Together, the health care professional and the client focus on image creation. The client is assisted to picture her smile, teeth, gums, breath, and mouth as important aspects of her health. Pregnant women who are not receiving prenatal care are often difficult to engage in health promotion. Even among those who are receiving prenatal care, oral health promotion is often not considered. The HPM Script therefore becomes an important means for promoting oral health with every client.

This chapter provides health care professionals with an overview of the importance of oral health as an essential component of total health care. The inclusion of oral health as one of the nine positive healthy behaviors in the Health Promotion Matrix emphasizes its importance in health promotional activities with individual clients, families, and community groups. Proper oral health care is essential to ensure the optimal health status for an individual. Although oral health care professionals provide specialized care to treat oral diseases, all health care professionals should include oral health promotional activities and referrals as an integral component of their care.

This chapter is designed to help health care professionals recognize common oral diseases and describes health conditions that place clients at risk for periodontal diseases, dental decay, and oral cancer. Emphasis is placed on symptom recognition of these oral diseases through clinical assessment and/or evaluation of clients' reported concerns. Specific primary and secondary preventive health activities are provided for health care professionals to assist in preventing new disease and in reducing the severity of existing disease.

THE ROLE OF ORAL HEALTH IN GENERAL HEALTH CARE

Health care professionals must realize the critical, interrelated role of oral health care within general health care and health promotion. The HPM places the client's image of health at the central core of health promotion activities, and oral health issues often take a primary role in the creation of an ideal health image. For example, oral health concerns (e.g., having a nice smile, physical attractiveness, the ability to eat and swallow, and freedom from mouth pain) are normally reflected in the client's discussion of ideal health status, appearance, and function. Even when oral health concerns are not identified by the client as a separate issue, health care professionals can initiate these discussions by emphasizing the interrelationships of oral health and the other eight positive healthy behaviors.

Health care professionals should include oral health as an integral component of their health promotion advice with clients. For example, any discussion of medication compliance with clients should include the possible side effect of dry mouth and specific suggestions for optimizing health supportive patterns when little saliva is present in the client's mouth. Reducing the negative effects of decreased salivary flow and related root decay often associated with dry mouth are ways to minimize health depleting patterns that clients may develop to compensate for the feeling of a dry mouth. This chapter provides health care professionals with specific examples of health promotion interventions to promote optimal oral health for clients at risk for oral diseases resulting from their specific health condition or life stage.

Clinical preventive oral health care represents a strong success story in health promotion activities (Harris & Christen, 1995; White, Caplan, & Weintraub, 1995). Community water fluoridation, school-based prevention programs, and use of oral hygiene products and fluoride home products have resulted in a declining trend in prevalence of dental decay (Bowen & Tabak, 1993; Newbrun, 1992). In the United States, rates of dental decay for children have been decreasing steadily, with current statistics revealing that more than half of children 5 to 17 years are caries-free in their permanent teeth (Frazier & Horowitz, 1990; White et al., 1995). However, not all children have shared equally in access to these proven preventive measures. Of the youngsters who have experienced dental decay, non-Hispanic African-American and Mexican-American children and adolescents have higher percentages of decayed surfaces than non-Hispanic Caucasian youth. Closer examination of the data illustrates that most of the decayed surfaces in the permanent teeth occur in a relatively small number of children. (Statement of Coalition, 1993; Oral Health Coordinating Committee [OHCC], 1993).

Dental decay continues to be a major oral health problem in adults (Bowen & Tabak, 1993; White et al., 1995). Root decay, which is more commonly seen in older adults, is strongly associated with age and the loss of periodontal (gum) attachment, which accompanies periodontal diseases (Burt & Eklund, 1992; OHCC, 1993).

Like dental decay, periodontal diseases will affect most adults some time in their lives, and the consequences, including pain, dysfunction, tooth loss, and treatment costs, can be high (OHCC, 1993; White et al., 1995; Marcus, Drury, Brown, & Zion, 1996). Approximately 40% of adults have gingivitis, which is the mildest form of periodontal disease. Early to moderate periodontitis is seen in approximately 70% of adults. However, the most severe forms of periodontal disease are seen in only 13% of the adult population, although a much higher prevalence rate has been documented among senior citizens (Brown, Brunelle, & Kingman, 1996; White et al., 1995).

Oral health promotion is the connecting link between primary preventive regimens and their acceptance and use by the client, family, and community. The combined efforts of health care professionals and individual clients are needed to ensure that everyone has access to the information and services needed for appropriate oral health behaviors (Gift, Drury, Nowjack-Raymer, & Selwitz, 1996).

Lack of access to dental care has become a major health issue for many individuals and is reflected in the uneven distribution of the prevalence of both caries and periodontal diseases (White et al., 1995). In 1989, more than 40% of Americans did not visit a dentist in the preceeding year (Statement of the Coalition, 1993). Financial barriers represent the major reason for decreased access to care, as limited health care resources have caused dental benefits to be reduced and in many cases eliminated in both government and employer-based insurance programs (Dolan & Atchison, 1993). Socioeconomic status has been documented to have a strong influence in determining the caries status of a community, with lower rates of decay found in groups with higher socioeconomic status (Burt & Eklund, 1992; Statement of Coalition, 1993).

In addition, there are many nonfinancial barriers individuals face in receiving dental care (Burt & Eklund, 1992). Fearful clients may postpone dental care, which inevitably complicates the care needed and increases the cost. Many individuals lack geographic access to a dentist or lack transportation to get to a dental office; for example, more than half of the homebound elderly have not seen a dentist for 10 years (Statement of the Coalition, 1993). In addition, many individuals do not visit a dentist because they do not perceive the need to receive routine preventive care to keep their mouths healthy (Strauss & Hunt, 1993). This is a special problem among older individuals who may not have experienced the benefits of modern preventive dentistry (Dolan & Atchison, 1993).

Negative attitudes and misinformation about oral health among both clients and some health care professionals can limit access to both preventive and restorative oral health care. The general perception of dental care as a discretionary, cosmetic service was reflected in the omission of oral health care as an essential primary care service in the health care reform political discussions and is also reflected in the greater number of individuals who lack dental insurance (approximately 150 million) as compared with those who lack health insurance (37 million) (Statement of Coalition, 1993). Health care professionals need to develop strategies at the community and public policy levels to reposition oral health as a critical element of a healthy image.

However, current trends in health promotion have increased the scope of health care, so many policy makers and health care professionals have begun to include oral health as an integral part of general health care. The *Healthy People 2000* document included oral health as an essential component of the health protection objectives, and 16 specific oral health objectives have been developed to guide and measure health promotion activities. Seven objectives focus efforts on the reduction of prevalence of gingivitis, periodontitis, dental caries, and oral cancer among specific population groups at risk; four objectives define risk reduction activities, including community water fluoridation and sealants; and five objectives guide efforts in service provision, including examination utilization rates. These objectives provide guidance for this chapter during discussion of each specific component of oral health promotion (U.S. Department of Health and Human Services [USDHHS], 1991a).

COMMON ORAL HEALTH PROBLEMS
Dental Caries

Recent research into the mechanism and causes of dental decay has shed considerable light on the safest and most effective preventive measures (Bowen & Tabak, 1993; Harris & Christen, 1995). Although traditional efforts to prevent dental decay have focused on reducing the consumption of sweets and thorough plaque removal through brushing and flossing, the latest research findings reveal that these activities are less effective than traditionally believed (Burt & Eklund, 1992; Nowak & Anderson, 1990). More effective health promotion efforts to reduce dental decay focus on optimizing health supportive patterns, such as combining the use of water fluoridation, fluoride products, dental sealants, and prompt professional care to reduce the risk of decay and reverse early areas of decay inside the tooth (Burt, 1992; Frazier & Horowitz, 1990; Newbrun, 1992). Through a combination of these preventive oral health strategies, most decay can be prevented or treated early; national caries prevalence rates have declined because of this availability of preventive oral health care (Burt & Eklund, 1992; White et al., 1995).

Although many consumers may report that they have soft teeth, the mineral content of mature enamel composes about 85% of the tooth by volume and 95% of tooth by weight, and this does not vary greatly among individuals (Shore, Robinson, Kirkham, & Brookes, 1995). Soon after tooth eruption, minerals in the tooth begin a dynamic exchange with the surrounding fluids in the oral cavity. Current research into the causes of dental decay reveals a complex, constant battle in which the tooth enamel is continuously in a process of losing minerals from the crystalline prisms (demineralization) and repairing these crystalline prisms (remineralization) (Bowen & Tabak, 1993). Although the surface of the tooth appears quite hard, there are microscopic channels through which acid produced by oral bacteria can penetrate and erode the spaces between the enamel prisms. Demineralization occurs first below the surface of the enamel and cannot be detected until it becomes moderately advanced and a white chalky area appears on the tooth surface. At these early stages, the decay process can be reversed when fluoride is applied to the tooth. Although the exact mechanism is still unknown, fluoride and other minerals appear to be deposited in these demineralized areas and serve to recrystallize the enamel, reversing the decay process (Shore et al., 1995). It is only when the demineralization has advanced and the surface of the tooth has been undermined and broken that dental care is needed to remove the decay and fill the tooth to restore function (Bowen & Tabak, 1993; Harris & Christen, 1995).

Fluoride is essential to promote remineralization of the subsurface tooth enamel broken down by bacterial acids (USDHHS, 1991b). Fluoride can be applied topically to the tooth through fluoridated toothpaste, mouth rinses, and professional gel treatments

Table 12-1

Fluoride recommendations for home use	
CLIENT	**RECOMMENDATION**
All clients	Fluoride toothpaste
Children age 6 months to 16 years who do not drink fluoridated water	Sodium fluoride liquid drops or tablet supplementation at 0.25 mg, 0.5 mg, or 1.0 mg concentration, prescribed based on age and amount of fluoride naturally occurring in the water
Children older than 6 years and adults at moderate risk for dental decay	0.05% sodium fluoride mouth rinse used once a day
Adults at high risk for dental decay	0.4% stannous fluoride gel or 1.1% sodium fluoride gel used once or twice daily

(Darby & Walsh, 1995; Newbrun, 1992). Table 12-1 summarizes the clinical guidelines for topical fluoride products that health care professionals can use to optimize oral health supportive activities. All clients should use at least one source of topical fluoride each day, preferably a fluoridated toothpaste. Daily use of sodium fluoride mouth rinses (0.05% concentration) can be helpful for clients who are at a moderate risk for dental decay. Clients with orthodontic appliances or who have experienced dental decay within the last year can use these fluoride rinses, which are readily available as over-the-counter products.

For clients at higher risk for dental decay, oral health care professionals can prescribe home gel treatments, which provide intensive levels of fluoride to remineralize teeth. Both 1.1% neutral sodium fluoride or 0.4% stannous fluoride can be prescribed to reduce the risk of dental decay (Harris & Christen, 1995; Wilkins, 1994). For example, any client who is taking a medication that produces dry mouth should be using additional sources of fluoride to reduce the high risk for dental decay. Clients who have completed radiation therapy to the head and neck have impaired salivary gland function with little to no saliva and are also at high risk for dental decay. With these clients, health care professionals' use of the HPM should focus on image creation and appraisal based on the clients' new oral health status. The best treatment for these clients is a twice daily application of 1.1% sodium fluoride gel placed in a tray designed to fit over the teeth to ensure that an intensive amount of fluoride reaches all the vulnerable teeth without salivary dilution (Harris & Christen, 1995). Without the buffering and cleansing effects of saliva, decay can proceed rapidly, especially in the vulnerable narrow part of the tooth where the gingival tissues interface with the crown. This area, known as the *cervical portion* or *neck* of the tooth, contains a thin layer of enamel covering the dentinal portion of the root and is more readily demineralized than other parts of the tooth.

Fluoride treatments can also be provided by oral health care professionals and include both 2.0% sodium and 1.23% acidulated phosphate fluoride, used either as a foam, gel, or a varnish placed in a tray or painted directly onto the teeth for 1 to 4 minutes (Newbrun, 1992; Wilkins, 1994). These professional fluoride treatments are popular among oral health care professionals and provide high amounts of fluoride on a low-frequency basis, especially if given every 6 months to 1 year at the dental recall visit. The most effective regimens for increasing remineralization and preventing decay include the low-dosage products (toothpastes and mouth rinses) used at least daily on a high-frequency basis (Bowen & Tabak, 1993). These frequently used products provide a constant source of fluoride for remineralization and help to reduce the initiation and progression of dental decay (Harris & Christen, 1995; Woodall, 1993).

Two objectives in the oral health section of *Healthy People 2000* describe goals for fluoride usage to prevent decay. One objective sets the goal for the inclusion of fluoride in community water systems for at least 75% of the nation's population, and the other objective identifies the need to increase the use of professionally and self-administered fluoride products for at least 85% of individuals who are not drinking optimally fluoridated water. Although topical application of fluoride through a variety of products provides a direct source for remineralization, this primary preventive procedure requires the client's cooperation in purchasing and using the product. Since 1945, fluoride has been added to many community water supplies at very low levels (1 part per million) to increase access to this proven preventive measure for all children, despite economic and nonfinancial barriers to oral health care. Early studies completed in the 1950s documented that children who drank fluoridated water experienced a reduction in dental decay, with ranges from 30% to 60% (Burt & Eklund, 1992; Newbrun, 1992). More modern studies, which account for the widespread distribution of fluoride in toothpaste and other products, indicate decay reductions from 20% to 40% for children and 15% to 35% for adolescents (Burt, 1992; Harris & Christen, 1995). Adults who have been lifelong residents of communities with fluoridated water supplies show a reduction in dental decay as much as 35% (Burt & Eklund, 1992).

Unfortunately, political controversy regarding the appropriateness and safety of fluoride as a community preventive agent has detracted from the adoption of fluoridation in all community water supplies. In 1992, 62.1% of all community water systems were fluoridated, with a majority of the Western and Southern states without this critical preventive service (Gift et al., 1996). In 1995, California passed a mandatory water fluoridation bill that will allow it to meet the *Healthy People 2000* goal of 75% of persons consuming fluoridated water.

The critical opposition has cited a number of key arguments that have consistently surrounded this issue since Grand Rapids, Michigan, was the first city to fluoridate its water supply in 1945. Claims of forced medication usage, ineffective preventive activity against dental decay, carcinogenic effects, chemical safety in storing and adding the fluoride product to the water, and other toxic effects have been argued by antifluoridationists, often in an emotional context that is quite compelling to politicians and consumers unfamiliar with scientific principles and practices (Burt & Eklund, 1992). Multiple studies have documented the safety and effectiveness of fluoride as a caries-preventive agent, and a recent summary report from the U.S. Public Health Service, the Review of Fluoride Benefits and Risks, 1991, confirmed both human safety issues and caries reduction when fluoride is added to public water systems.

Health care professionals should be prepared for the few clients who may state objections to fluoride recommendations because of concerns related to safety and effectiveness. A list of oral health promotion resources is included at the end of the chapter to provide clients with accurate information from credible, reliable sources, particularly in relation to the safety and efficacy of water fluoridation in reducing dental decay. The issue of fluoridation emphasizes the necessity of targeting health promotion efforts at the four levels specified in the HPM: individual, family, group, and community.

When the community water is not fluoridated, health care professionals should recommend and prescribe fluoride supplementation for children between ages 6 months and 16 years. This systemic fluoride supplementation, either in the form of liquid drops (sometimes combined with other vitamin supplementation) or tablets, provides a source of fluoride for the developing permanent teeth (Burt, 1992; Harris & Christen, 1995).

In addition to fluoride, dental sealants have been documented as a highly effective means to prevent decay by blocking the penetration of demineralizing acids into the enamel grooves of the teeth (Woodall, 1993). The molar and premolar teeth in the posterior region of the mouth contain narrow and uneven grooves and fissures on the occlusal (chewing) surface so that these teeth may function well to chew and grind food properly. However, the grooves are often smaller than a single bristle of a toothbrush, and frequently trap small pieces of food and retained acids from bacteria, which produce decay. Through the application of plastic resin material that is bonded to the enamel, the dental sealant serves to seal and block the grooves so that food particles can be easily brushed from the tooth. Dental sealants have been shown to reduce virtually all decay when the sealant is retained in the occlusal surface of the tooth (Harris & Christen, 1995).

The *Healthy People 2000* guidelines also outline the goal to increase to at least 50% the proportion of children who have received sealants—a large increase from the current number of children (11%) who had received sealants in 1986. Current recommendations are for all children to have their first and second permanent molars sealed as soon as the teeth erupt (Darby & Walsh, 1995). The first permanent molars (often called 6-year-old molars) erupt between the ages of 5 and 7 years; the second permanent molars (often called the 12-year-old molars) erupt between the ages of 11 to 14 years. Sealants can be used only on the chewing surfaces of teeth that have not been previously restored with a filling material, so it is important to seal the teeth as soon as they erupt to prevent decay. Adults should consult with their dentist to determine the appropriateness of sealing their unfilled teeth, depending on their risk for decay. Clients who are taking medications that produce dry mouth, who have experienced dental decay in the past, and who have difficulties in completing their own oral hygiene should be evaluated carefully for sealant placement (Harris & Christen, 1995).

Although early studies identified the consumption of high-sugar snacks as causing dental decay, modern research has presented a far more complex picture regarding the role of diet and the initiation of dental decay (Harris & Christen, 1995). Simple and complex carbohydrates can be used by oral bacteria to form destructive acids that begin the demineralization process within the tooth. The term "fermentable carbohydrates" has been used to describe all sugars and cooked starches that can be used by bacteria (mainly *mutans streptococci*) to form acid that initiates the demineralization process (Bowen & Tabak, 1993). Although some clients may select honey, fresh fruit, or fruit juices without added sucrose in the belief that these natural products are healthy, oral bacteria do not distinguish from natural or processed sugar and use all fermentable carbohydrates to initiate the caries process (Harris & Christen, 1995). Clients and families should be counseled to minimize health depleting factors, such as limiting the frequency and duration of these fermentable carbohydrates and to avoid the constant use of mints, gum, or candy that contain sucrose and other sugars. Although some oral health care professionals recommend that clients avoid retentive foods, research shows that even fermentable carbohydrates that are not perceived by clients as "sticky," such as corn chips, crackers, and pancakes, can produce acid for demineralization (Harris & Christen, 1995). The optimal time to eat fermentable carbohydrates is during a meal, when salivary volume is the greatest to clear the food from the mouth quickly and to buffer any acids. Foods that have been found to promote little decay include cheese, nuts, popcorn, and sugarless chewing gum, which has the added benefit of increasing saliva to serve as an additional source of remineralization (Harris & Christen, 1995).

Because of the complex nature of the dental caries process, there is no single preventive agent that will control dental caries (Gift, 1991). Fluoride applied to the tooth either topically or ingested systemically will provide a source of minerals to help reverse the decay process through remineralization. Fluoride has its greatest anticaries effect on the smooth surfaces of teeth. Dental sealants can be used to physically block the minute grooves from acid penetration but can only be used on the chewing (occlusal) surfaces of premolars and molars of teeth that have not been restored. Current research has highlighted the critical and highly effective role both fluoride and sealants have in reducing decay. All clients with teeth should use at least one source of fluoride and should be evaluated for sealant placement with all unrestored teeth. Dietary reductions in sugars and cooked starches can help reduce the frequency and duration that oral bacteria can form destructive acids; however, dietary changes are notoriously difficult to change, particularly in an American culture that enjoys sweetened products and where sugar consumption has continued to rise (Frazier & Horowitz, 1990). Although toothbrushing is often cited by most clients as the major method they use to prevent decay, toothbrushing alone is not effective in removing all microbial plaque, which may hide between the teeth and in small grooves and fissures. The major caries reduction benefit in toothbrushing involves the application of fluoridated toothpaste, which will increase remineralization of enamel prisms (Burt & Eklund, 1992; Harris & Christen, 1995).

Periodontal Diseases

Periodontal diseases are a collection of diseases of the gum (gingiva) and supporting bone structure of the teeth (periodontium) and are predominantly caused by a collection of bacteria, commonly referred to as *bacterial plaque.* Bacterial plaque is a soft deposit on the tooth consisting of a salivary glycoprotein matrix to which colonies of bacteria and food debris adhere. Bacterial plaque is found on surfaces of the teeth and gingival tissues and in the space between the gum and the tooth, which is called the *sulcus,* or *gingival crevice.* Mineralization of undisturbed or inadequately removed plaque results in hard deposits known as *tartar (calculus).* These deposits make it more difficult for cleansing, and the result is that more plaque will accumulate. Most persons are affected by one or more of the periodontal diseases at some time in their lives, and the consequences in terms of treatment costs and tooth loss can be high. Periodontal diseases are largely preventable (Greene, Louie, & Wycoff, 1990).

Two of the most common periodontal diseases are gingivitis and periodontitis. Gingivitis is inflammation of the gum (gingiva), resulting in a redder appearance of the gum and edema in the points of gum (papillae) between the teeth. The most common sign of gingivitis is bleeding, although many clients may perceive that overzealous brushing is the cause of blood on their toothbrush or after rinsing (Brown et al., 1996; Gift, 1988). As part of their activities in image appraisal, health care professionals should explain to clients that healthy gum tissue does not bleed and that any bleeding, even if minor, should be investigated during an examination visit with the oral health care professional. There is usually no pain involved with gingivitis except in severe acute conditions. Gingivitis can be found in children from the time teeth erupt.

As the tissue becomes more inflamed and swollen (edematous), the accumulation of bacterial plaque increases. As the tissues swell, the space between the gum and tooth increases, and the bacterial plaque in this space under the gum tissue shifts to gram-negative anaerobic bacteria. These gram-negative anaerobic microorganisms are mediated by host factors and are destructive, causing recession of soft tissue and loss of bone support around the tooth. The tooth becomes mobile and eventually is lost. This destructive periodontal disease is called *periodontitis*. A number of studies have shown that although periodontitis is preceded by gingivitis, not all sites with gingivitis progress in a predictable manner to periodontitis (Brown et al., 1996; Greene et al., 1990).

Because the primary cause of periodontal diseases is bacterial plaque, early and thorough plaque removal is the most important treatment both clients and health care professionals can complete. Interrupting the destruction caused in periodontitis requires professional scaling and root planing by oral health care professionals to remove calcified deposits and to control the subgingival bacterial flora. However, professional removal of plaque and calculus without daily removal of supragingival plaque will permit the bacteria to recolonize the gingival crevice and reinstate the periodontitis. Thus neither supragingival plaque control nor professional care alone will effectively limit the progress of periodontitis (Greene et al., 1990).

The challenge for the client comes in keeping the teeth plaque-free because this demands time, good dexterity, and motivation to brush thoroughly and clean between the teeth with dental floss. Health care professionals can emphasize to clients the positive benefits of a clean, healthy mouth to internalize the clients' idealized image of health. Surfaces between the teeth (interproximal surfaces) cannot be cleaned with a standard toothbrush. Dental floss, small interproximal brushes, or appropriately shaped wooden picks are necessary to clean these difficult-to-reach places. The thoroughness of plaque control is more important than the frequency of cleaning. Plaque should be disrupted thoroughly at least once a day, preferably at night and more often if possible (Greene et al., 1990).

Oral Trauma

Traumatic injuries that cause damage to the face and teeth can create long-term dilemmas in terms of clinical diagnosis and treatment in oral health. After an injury, clients will need assistance in reevaluating their idealized image of oral health in relation to their current status. Traumatic injuries manifest in many ways and most commonly involve fracturing of the maxilla or mandible or damage to the temporomandibular joint. Teeth may be fractured, knocked out of alignment (occlusion), or lost. Repairs to teeth injuries are unlike the usual repair process of other areas in the body and heal slowly. For example, it may take up to 5 years to determine whether a treated tooth will survive an injury (Kaste, Gift, Bhat, & Swango, 1996; Greene et al., 1990).

The prevention of trauma to the face and teeth is addressed in *Healthy People 2000* and is underscored in two objectives: one dealing with unintentional injury and the other with oral health. These objectives call for extending requirements for the use of orofacial protective devices (head, face, eye, and mouth protection) in sporting and recreation events that present risks of injury. Clients seeking school or sports physicals may need guidance in determining ways to keep their face and mouth intact and not altered by injury. Health care professionals can encourage these clients to visualize positive health images by counseling them in the use of mouthguards, helmets, face shields, and seat belts.

Baseball players do not look upon the sport as a high-risk activity with heavy contact, yet a high percentage of injuries (41%) are to the head, face, mouth, and eyes (Nowjack-Raymer & Gift, 1996).

The National Collegiate Athletic Association (NCAA) in 1974 implemented mandatory mouth protector wear for its players (Greene et al., 1990). It has estimated that up to 200,000 injuries to the mouth from football contact are prevented annually through the use of mouth guards (American Dental Association, 1984). Other athletic associations involved in contact sports have followed the NCAA's direction, thus the number of prevented dental injuries is rising. However, interviews with national athletics associations report inconsistencies in philosophy, enforcement, and regulations in many child and youth sports.

Clients and their families should be directed to obtain one of the following three types of mouth guards readily available today: the ready-made and the mouth-formed appliances, which can be purchased at any athletic store and are often available through the coach and/or school administration, and the custom-fit athletic mouthguard, which can be fabricated by a dental professional for the athlete and is recommended for athletes participating in high-contact sports and those unable to use the other types of mouth guards.

The facial region is the most commonly injured body area in automobile accidents (Huelke & Compton, 1983). Encouraging seat belt usage will greatly reduce these injuries. Two investigations report a decrease in facial injuries by 50% and 72% after the implementation of seat belt laws (Greene et al., 1990).

Health care professionals can promote clients' use of helmets when biking and skateboarding by conducting helmet decorating contests and bicycle and skateboarding rodeos in elementary schools and recreation centers. These activities of optimizing health supportive patterns extend to both families and to advocacy at the community and public policy level. There has been a decrease in head injuries in states that have implemented mandatory helmet use for bicyclers of a certain ages, which varies by state (Greene et al., 1990).

Common Oral Lesions

Two of the most common disorders of the mouth, causing discomfort and annoyance to millions of persons, are fever blisters (herpes simplex) and canker sores (aphthous stomatitis) (American Academy of Oral Medicine, 1993). Fever blisters are highly contagious and frequently spread by kissing. Most persons infected with fever blisters of the Type 1 herpes simplex virus become infected before age 10 years. As a way to minimize health depleting patterns, health care professionals can counsel their clients who have fever blisters not to kiss young children when blisters are present. Reactivation of this latent virus can be triggered by the following factors: fever, stress, exposure to sunlight, trauma, and hormonal alterations (National Institutes of Health, 1994). Visualizing a face free of fever blisters could be one way of encouraging a client to use lip sunscreen as a health supportive pattern.

Canker sores are not contagious and are an altered immune response to certain precipitating factors, including stress, trauma, allergies and endocrine alterations, some acidic foods and juices, and foods that contain gluten. In addition, individuals who are anemic, have diabetes mellitus or inflammatory bowel disease, or are immunocompromised may also report frequent aphthous ulcers (National Institutes of Health, 1994). Health care professionals should counsel these clients not to eat abrasive foods, which could traumatize the mouth; to use care when cleaning the mouth to prevent trauma; and to avoid acidic or spicy foods as ways to minimize common health depleting patterns.

Dry mouth (xerostomia) and yeast infections (candidiasis) are two common oral conditions that often lead to a client's complaint of burning mouth syndrome. Dry mouth is most commonly induced by the anticholinergic properties of most medications and is seen in a number of autoimmune disorders, particularly among women. Oral candidiasis is associated with immunocompromised status and is commonly seen in older clients because of prolonged wearing of dentures. Oral candidiasis is best treated with a wide range of antifungal medications; however, there is no clear-cut treatment for dry mouth, with symptom relief forming the basis for recommendations for clients (American Academy of Oral Medicine, 1993). Health care professionals should encourage clients to frequently sip water to keep the mouth moist and to use artificial saliva, which is sold as an over-the-counter gel or liquid, as ways to optimize supportive patterns to maintain health. Clients can also help to stimulate the salivary glands by sucking on sugarless lemon drops or mints. Additional health supportive patterns include keeping the lips moisturized and using a humidifier in the sleeping area to decrease skin and lip chapping and to promote hydration in the oral facial region (American Academy of Oral Medicine, 1993).

Oral Cancer

Healthy People 2000 identifies the reduction of deaths resulting from cancer of the oral cavity and pharynx as a priority objective within oral health care. Although oral facial cancers comprise approximately 3% to 4% of total cancers, the morbidity and mortality rates are high (Swango, 1996). One objective of the *Healthy People 2000* document identifies the goal of reducing deaths resulting from oral and pharyngeal cancer to no more than 10.5 per 100,000 men and 4.1 per 100,000 women. Currently, the death rate among males is 13.6 per 100,000 and women, 4.8 per 100,000 (Gift, Drury, Nowjack, Raymer, & Selwitz, 1996).

The tragedy of oral and pharyngeal cancers is that most of them can be prevented because about 75% of these cancers are attributable to tobacco and alcohol use (Swango, 1996). Health care professionals should encourage their clients to complete a variety of health promotional activities to prevent oral cancer (Horowitz, Goodman, Yellowitz, & Nourjah, 1996). Tobacco cessation, particularly smokeless tobacco, is an important, life-saving intervention that health care professionals can complete with their clients. Limiting exposure to the sun, always using a sunscreen and lip protection, and limiting alcohol ingestion are specific behaviors that decrease the risk of oral and pharyngeal cancers.

Early detection of any cancerous lesions can be critical to ensure prompt care, and clients can be taught to examine their face, mouth, and neck for common signs of early oral lesions and to assess their status against their visualized ideal oral health image. Any growth or swelling that is tender and firmly bound to the head or neck area should be investigated. Any mixed red and white lesion in the mouth that does not heal within a week should be examined by a dentist, especially when the lesion is located on the lips, in the floor of the mouth, or on the posterior lateral border of the tongue—common sites for oral cancer. Clients who are at risk for oral cancer include men older than 45 years, clients who smoke or use smokeless tobacco, and clients who drink alcohol. All adults, especially those at high risk for oral cancer, should visit the dental office at least once a year for head and neck examinations and to receive information and motivation to optimize health supportive patterns and to minimize health depleting patterns.

HEALTH RISK FACTORS WITH ORAL HEALTH IMPLICATIONS

The following section describes the oral health implications of several health risk factors or conditions. Table 12-2 provides a summary of this discussion along with relevant health promotion strategies.

Diabetes

Diabetes increases the risk of both the incidence and severity of periodontal disease progression by approximately two- to three-fold (Grossi, 1993; Haber, 1991). The presence of bacterial pathogens, as well as dysfunction of neutrophils and host response; increased production of inflammatory mediators; and connective tissue alterations all contribute to the severity of periodontal disease.

Most diabetic clients whose disease is controlled respond well to conventional periodontal treatment, so frequent dental visits for examination, periodontal therapy, and good oral hygiene home care are required for all diabetic clients (Bay, Ainaimo, & Gad, 1974). The frequency and scope of recommended dental treatment takes into account the diabetic status of the client, whether controlled or uncontrolled; the presence of any health complications; and the degree of periodontal disease.

Cardiovascular Disease (Valvular Heart Disease)

One of the main concerns of individuals with valvular heart disease is the possibility that endocarditis will develop. Oral infection and dental procedures involving manipulation of soft tissue resulting in bleeding can produce transient bacteremia. Blood-borne bacteria may lodge on damaged and abnormal heart valves in the endocardium or in the endothelium near congenital anatomic defects, resulting in bacterial endocarditis. Since it is not possible to predict which clients will develop this infection, all individuals with the following cardiac conditions (endocarditis risk factors) should be very scrupulous in oral hygiene self-care and should visit their dentist for frequent evaluation to ensure they are free of oral infection (Dajani et al., 1997).

- Prosthetic cardiac valves, including bioprosthetic and homograft valves
- Previous bacterial endocarditis, even in the absence of heart disease
- Most congenital cardiac malformations
- Rheumatic and other acquired valvular dysfunction even after valvular surgery
- Hypertrophic cardiomyopathy
- Mitral valve prolapse with valvular regurgitation.

Antibiotic prophylaxis per American Heart Association guidelines (Dajani et al., 1997) is recommended for clients at moderate or high risk for endocarditis before those dental procedures that are likely to cause a significant bacteremia, including professional cleaning. Health care professionals should educate these clients to the necessity of complying with the antibiotic prophylaxis regimen to prevent endocarditis.

Organ Transplants

The dentist should participate in the treatment planning for clients about to undergo elective organ transplantation. Active and potential sources of oral infection should be

Table 12-2

Oral health promotion for clients with health risk factors

HEALTH RISK FACTOR	ORAL IMPLICATIONS	HEALTH PROMOTION
Diabetes	Increased incidence and severity of periodontal disease Poor healing and slow response to care	Encourage thorough daily oral hygiene Encourage regular dental examinations and cleanings Complete dietary counseling to reduce decay promoting patterns
Cardiovascular diseases (valvular diseases)	Potential for endocarditis Risk of transient bacteremia	Encourage thorough daily oral hygiene Encourage compliance with antibiotic premedication schedule, when necessary
Organ transplant	Oral infection may be life-threatening Immunosuppressant medications cause gingival enlargement and can mask signs of oral infections	Refer for dental treatment before transplant, when possible Encourage frequent dental examinations and cleanings Encourage thorough daily oral hygiene
Acute leukemia	Gingival hemorrhage Oral discomfort and pain Loss of appetite	Encourage gentle, thorough daily oral hygiene Recommend use of chlorhexidine mouth rinse Refer for emergency care during acute phase Refer for dental examination and care during remission phase
Thrombocytopenia	Purpura Gingival hemorrhage	Refer for dental consultation Recommend oxidizing mouth rinses Encourage gentle, thorough daily oral hygiene
Hemophilia	Spontaneous gingival hemorrhage Hemarthrosis	Encourage gentle, thorough daily oral hygiene
HIV infection and AIDS	Oral candidiasis Oral hairy leukoplakia Kaposi's sarcoma (KS) Gingivitis and periodontitis	Refer for dental evaluation and frequent cleanings Refer for early treatment with antifungal medications Recommend chlorhexidine mouth rinses Encourage thorough daily oral hygiene Complete dietary counseling

Table **12-2**

Oral health promotion for clients with health risk factors—cont'd		
HEALTH RISK FACTOR	**ORAL IMPLICATIONS**	**HEALTH PROMOTION**
Chemotherapeutic agents	Mucositis Oral ulcerations	Encourage only minimal dental care during oral chemotherapy Use therapeutic mouth rinse as needed Encourage comprehensive dental care after active chemotherapy

eliminated and necessary dental care should be accomplished whenever possible before the transplant. After the transplant, recipients are maintained on an immunosuppressive drug regimen for life. All of the immunosuppressive agents may mask early manifestations of oral infection. Oral mucosal lesions suggestive of herpes simplex, candidiasis, or other fungal infections should be evaluated by cytologic examination, culture, and/or biopsy, when indicated. The infections may lead to severe or disseminated disease in immunosuppressed clients and must be detected early so that antimicrobial therapy can be instituted. In addition, the medication cyclosporine, which is commonly given to transplant patients, can cause gingival enlargement, which complicates plaque removal and may lead to increased severity of periodontal diseases (American Academy of Oral Medicine, 1993).

Acute Leukemia

It has been reported that there are oral lesions in more than 80% of clients with acute monocytic leukemia, in 40% of clients with acute myeloid leukemia, and in more than 20% of those with lymphoid leukemia. Acute leukemia commonly causes a massive infiltration of leukemic cells into the gingival tissues. Because of this, the gingiva appears as if it has lost its normal contour and texture and becomes hyperplastic, edematous, and bluish red, with blunting of the interdental papillae. Varying degrees of gingival inflammation, ulceration, and necrosis have been noted in clients with leukemia, depending on their health status (Burkett, 1944; Lindhe, 1983; Wentz, Anday, & Orban, 1949). Oral mucosal ulcers are also a common finding in clients with leukemia.

Complications that occur during leukemia (e.g., gingival hemorrhage, marked discomfort and pain, and loss of appetite) may cause considerable difficulty for clients. During the acute phase of the disease only those dental procedures that are necessary to alleviate the pain, discomfort, and hemorrhaging should be performed. Oral hygiene procedures should be completed daily in a gentle manner with a very soft toothbrush to remove plaque but not to provoke hemorrhage. Soft gauze wipes and chlorhexidine rinses can provide additional assistance in plaque control. When the disease is in a period of remission, every attempt should be made to achieve a state of periodontal health, and dental care procedures can be performed in consultation with the health care team. Health promotion activities should stress oral comfort and function, with referral to oral health care professionals for consultation in managing oral complications and any necessary dental care.

Thrombocytopenia

The oral manifestations of thrombocytopenia (decrease in the number of blood platelets) may represent the initial signs of the disease. *Purpura*, the most common oral sign, is defined as any escape of blood into subcutaneous and/or submucosal tissues and includes petechiae and ecchymoses, which are often seen on the tongue, lips, and occlusal line of the buccal mucosa secondary to minor trauma. Other oral signs include spontaneous gingival hemorrhage and prolonged bleeding after trauma, toothbrushing, extractions, or periodontal therapy.

Spontaneous gingival bleeding usually can be managed by oxidizing mouth washes, such as glyoxide, but platelet transfusions may be required to stop the bleeding. Good oral hygiene and conservative periodontal therapy will help in the removal of plaque and calculus, which potentiate the bleeding. Accidental trauma can be avoided by having the dentist replace ill-fitting partial and full dentures and remove all orthodontic appliances. These clients should be cautioned not to sleep with any prostheses in place. Definitive dental treatment should be delayed until normal platelet function returns. Platelet levels greater than 50,000 millimeters are desired before dental treatment, and further transfusions are given as needed postoperatively to maintain hemostasis.

Hemophilia

Episodic, prolonged bleeding—either spontaneous or traumatic—is the most common oral presentation of hemophilia. Bleeding from the nose, mouth, and lips may be severe. Hemarthrosis, which may lead to ankylosis and erosion of the temporomandibular joint surface, is incapacitating and painful for clients, who will need support and referral for specialized oral care.

The health care professional should encourage clients to continue daily oral hygiene in a gentle, thorough manner to aid in the reduction of gingival bleeding. Frequent dental care visits should be recommended because oral prophylaxis can generally be accomplished without factor replacement. Factor replacement is necessary, however, preceding deep scaling, curettage, and surgery.

Acquired Immunodeficiency Syndrome (AIDS)

Oral manifestations are common early signs of symptomatic HIV infection, and more than 95% of AIDS clients have oral changes during the course of their illness (Muzyka, 1993). Health care professionals should evaluate their clients with AIDS and recommend frequent dental care visits, which can be very helpful in locating, monitoring, and treating orofacial conditions that can become life-threatening in the severely immunocompromised client. In addition, health care professionals can teach these clients the oral self-examination procedure to identify any early signs indicating the need for prompt oral health care. The most common of the HIV-related oral diseases include candidiasis, hairy leukoplakia, Kaposi's sarcoma, oral warts, HIV-associated periodontal lesions, xerostomia, herpes simplex, varicella zoster, bacterial infections, and recurrent aphthous stomatitis.

In HIV-infected clients, oral candidiasis is the most common early oral manifestation. There are four major types of oral candidiasis in conjunction with HIV infection: pseudomembranous (thrush), hyperplastic, erythematous (atrophic), and angular cheilitis. The pseudomembranous type is characterized by the presence of creamy white plaques that can be removed to reveal a bleeding surface. This type of candidiasis may involve any part of the oral mucosa but most commonly affects the palatal, buccal, and labial mucosa and dorsum of the tongue. Hyperplastic candidiasis is characterized by white plaques that cannot be removed by scraping and are most commonly located on the buccal mucosa. The erythematous (atrophic) type is characterized by a red appearance, commonly located on the palate and dorsum of the tongue or as spotty areas of the buccal mucosa. Angular cheilitis is characterized by fissures radiating from the angles of the mouth and is often associated with small white plaques.

Oral candidiasis is best treated early with antifungal medications to reduce infection and related oral complications, such as sore mouth and difficulties in eating and swallowing. Twice daily use of chlorhexidine mouth rinse has been used for clients with AIDS as an effective preventive measure to provide antimicrobial support to reduce infections, particularly candidiasis.

Hairy leukoplakia almost always indicates HIV seropositivity. The lesion is characterized by a white patch, usually occurring on the lateral margins of the tongue, often bilaterally. The surface is irregular and may be characterized by upward prominent folds or projections, sometimes so marked that it resembles hairs. Current evidence suggests that the Epstein-Barr virus is the etiologic agent. Although usually asymptomatic, the lesion may occasionally cause discomfort if superinfected with candida. Because the lesion may be extensive, bothersome, and unaesthetic, the client should be referred to the medical and/or dental health care professional who may prescribe medications.

Kaposi's sarcoma (KS) remains the most common tumor associated with AIDS. KS may first appear anywhere in the oral cavity; however, the palate has most often been the first area involved. The lesions may appear as bluish, blackish, or reddish macules that are flat in the early stages. In later stages, the lesions may become darker, elevated, lobulated, and ulcerated. Suspicious lesions in a client in whom a diagnosis of AIDS has not been made should be biopsied. Treatment depends on the location, size, and number of lesions and severity of symptoms. The client should be referred to the appropriate medical and/or dental health care professional for evaluation and treatment.

Oral warts are caused by the human papillomavirus and may be sexually transmitted. Evaluation for removal by a medical and/or dental health care professional is recommended.

Unique forms of periodontal disease have been discovered in individuals infected with HIV. HIV-gingivitis (HIV-G), presently called linear gingival erythema, and HIV-periodontitis (HIV-P), now called necrotizing ulcerative periodontitis (NUP), have microbiologic profiles similar to conventional adult periodontitis, although the lesions are different clinically. Linear gingival erythema can manifest clinically either as an erythematous linear banding, usually 2 mm wide, or a diffuse or petechial redness along the gingival margin. This subtle lesion, which may go unnoticed by an untrained examiner, is an early indicator of HIV infection not associated with T4 cell counts. Necrotizing ulcerative periodontitis is associated with low T4 cell counts and has the following clinical characteristics: severe, deep pain; extensive soft tissue necrosis; severe loss of periodontal attachment; and rapid onset and progression. Clients infected with HIV can safely receive periodontal care and should be referred to a dentist for this treatment. Before initiating periodontal treatment, the dentist should consult the client's physician to establish the client's current status and determine the most appropriate course of action for therapy. Dental care for clients with HIV combines frequent scaling and debridement with a strong emphasis on client participation in thorough daily oral hygiene care.

Systemic antiviral therapy (acyclovir) in high doses has been found to be effective in the treatment of orofacial varicella zoster in immunocompromised clients. In addition, unusual bacterial infections sometimes occur in the oral cavity of clients infected with HIV. Treatment should be based on culture and sensitivity testing performed by the medical or dental health care professional.

In addition to health conditions as risk factors for oral diseases, many medications that clients take for these conditions pose additional challenges for clients in maintaining optimal oral health. The following sections explain the interrelationship between selected medications and oral health status.

Three drugs that exhibit gingival overgrowth are phenytoin, cyclosporine, and calcium channel blockers. Clients using these medications should be encouraged to complete daily thorough oral hygiene and self-care. In addition, these clients should visit a dental professional on a regular basis since the research has shown that meticulous plaque control combined with professional care will prevent or significantly decrease the severity of the hyperplasia.

Gingival overgrowth occurs in about one half of individuals who ingest phenytoin as their sole antiepileptic medication on a long-term basis. However, the prevalence of gingival overgrowth is much higher when phenytoin is taken in combination with other antiepileptic agents. Gingival overgrowth often becomes clinically apparent during the first 6 to 9 months of therapy and has a clinically similar appearance to the tissue enlargement seen with the antirejection medication cyclosporine, which is used with transplant clients, and the cardiac drugs classified as calcium channel blockers.

Chemotherapeutic Agents

Health care professionals should strongly recommend a referral to a dentist before the onset of chemotherapy so that all oral sources of infection (e.g., periodontal disease and infected teeth) can be eliminated. Only minimal necessary dental intervention should be provided to control acute oral problems that occur during the active phases of myelosuppression secondary to chemotherapy. After chemotherapy is completed, comprehensive dental care may be provided for the client after consultation with the oncologist.

Frequent recall examinations, symptomatic support (for mucositis or ulcerations), and aggressive preventive intervention should be part of the medical/dental care of clients receiving chemotherapy. A 0.12% chlorhexidine mouth rinse (Peridex or Periogard) to reduce fungal and bacterial overgrowth and assist in oral hygiene care is strongly recommended. Topical analgesia contained in an oral suspension may be prescribed to provide relief from painful mucositis or ulceration. Viscous lidocaine 2%, lidocaine ointment 5%, dyclonine 1% and diphenhydramine 0.5% mixed with milk of magnesia suspension, Kaolin (Kaopectate), or other topical analgesics can be applied frequently to areas of painful mucositis or ulceration.

ORAL HEALTH PROMOTION THROUGHOUT THE LIFESPAN

In addition to specific service objectives, the *Healthy People 2000* document included emphasis on specific health concerns identified at each stage of the lifespan. As in all areas of health, oral health promotion activities should be targeted based on the specific at-risk factors for each age group. Table 12-3 provides a summary of oral health promotion activities for the following groups: infants and children, adolescents, adults, women, and older adults. Women's health issues are also addressed in a separate section to underline the importance of providing targeted oral health promotion activities to meet the special needs of women.

Infants and Young Children

Currently in dentistry there is much interest in dental decay seen in children younger than 3 years. Although still labeled *baby bottle tooth decay* (BBTD), many oral health researchers are using the term *early childhood caries* (ECC) to more accurately describe this type of decay (Harris & Christen, 1995). BBTD is characterized by multiple areas of dental decay on the primary teeth, generally affecting the anterior teeth but also sometimes the posterior teeth. Research has shown that the bacteria that cause early childhood caries come primarily from mothers or caregivers who have active untreated decay in their mouths. Through salivary contact via kissing or food sharing, the bacteria are passed from mother to child and serve to initiate decay. The traditional etiologic explanation for BBTD has included the child's habit of falling asleep with a bottle in his/her mouth so that any liquid, including formula, milk, juice, or sweetened drinks, when allowed prolonged contact with the primary teeth (most often the maxillary anterior teeth) causes dental decay (Wilkins, 1994).

Health care professionals should examine all infants for evidence of early decay and teach parents proper image appraisal of their child's oral health. White spot lesions on the surface of the tooth represent the earliest signs of decay, which progress to small white and brown or gray depressions in the tooth, which then continue to enlarge until portions of the tooth are lost because of fracture. Parents should be taught to cleanse the child's teeth as soon as the first tooth erupts, usually between 6 to 8 months of age. Health care professionals can assist parents to create a positive oral health image for their baby as soon as the first tooth erupts. Teeth can be cleaned by using a washcloth or cloth wipe, and a small toothbrush can be used when comfortable for the child. A small smear of toothpaste should be used during infancy, with no more than a pea-size amount of toothpaste placed on the brush for children up to 6 years of age.

Health care professionals should also teach parents to discontinue bottle feeding at 1 year of age and to promote mealtime drinking from a trainer cup until the child can master drinking from a glass. If parents allow the child to continue sleeping with the bottle, *only water* should be used in the bottle. For many parents and caregivers, the health depleting aspects of bottle feeding on erupting teeth are poorly understood. Health care professionals can use resource information from the American Dental Hygienists' Association and the American Dental Association to illustrate to parents the critical nature of oral health promotion regarding BBTD (DeBiase, 1991).

The Academy for Pediatric Dentistry recommends that all children visit the dentist by 1 year of age (Wilkins, 1994). Parents should take the time to speak with oral health care professionals about appropriate care for children's teeth and should be encouraged to use fluoride tablet supplementation with their children if the community drinking water does not contain fluoride (Harris & Christen, 1995).

Table 12-3

Oral health issues throughout the lifespan		
AGE GROUP	**SPECIFIC ORAL HEALTH CONCERNS**	**ORAL HEALTH PROMOTIONAL ADVICE**
Infants and children	Baby bottle tooth decay (BBTD) Dental decay	Evaluate child's teeth as soon as eruption occurs Teach parents oral care with infant and child Encourage cessation of bottle at 1 year of age Refer for dental visits at 1 year of age Recommend fluoride supplements beginning at 6 months when drinking water is not fluoridated
Adolescents	Dental caries Tobacco use Periodontal diseases Oral facial injury	Refer for frequent dental visits and dental sealants Recommend topical fluoride products Recommend fluoride supplements when drinking water is not fluoridated Encourage use of protective devices, such as mouth guards, helmets, seat belts Encourage thorough daily oral hygiene
Adults	Dry mouth Dental caries Periodontal diseases Specific conditions based on health risk factors Alcohol use Tobacco use Oral facial injury	Recommend use of salivary substitutes and other means to hydrate mouth Refer for frequent dental visits Recommend topical fluoride products Encourage consultations with dentist for specific health risk factors
Women	Increased gingivitis resulting from increased progesterone Aphthous ulcers Herpetic lesions Dry and burning mouth	Refer for dental evaluation and frequent cleanings Encourage thorough daily oral hygiene Recommend salivary substitutes and other means to hydrate mouth Complete dietary counseling Recommend topical fluoride

Table **12-3**

Oral health issues throughout the lifespan—cont'd		
AGE GROUP	**SPECIFIC ORAL HEALTH CONCERNS**	**ORAL HEALTH PROMOTIONAL ADVICE**
Older adults	Root caries Periodontal diseases Candidiasis	Encourage thorough daily oral hygiene Recommend intensive topical fluoride Complete dietary counseling Refer for dental evaluation and frequent cleanings Teach denture care Encourage caretakers to complete thorough daily oral hygiene and denture care

Adolescents

Because adolescents are in one of the highest risk groups for dental decay, special efforts should be made to ensure that all adolescents visit the dental office at least once a year (White et al., 1995). All adolescents should use fluoride toothpaste, and fluoride rinses either at home or school are recommended if even one area of decay has been noted recently. Supplemental fluoride tablets should be continued to at least age 16 years if the drinking water is not fluoridated. All adolescents should have dental sealants placed on the first and second molars, and these sealants should be evaluated each year and reapplied if necessary. Other preventive measures, such as proper toothbrushing and dietary counseling, should be included as appropriate oral health supportive patterns.

It is often during adolescence that sports injuries occur, so the health care professional should provide education and referral to the dental office to ensure proper protection is available for the oral-facial region. Unfortunately, many coaches and other individuals are unaware of the need for mouth guards and eye protection, and injuries may occur that need prompt treatment (American Dental Association, 1984). When teeth are avulsed from the mouth, they may be successfully replanted within 12 hours, depending on the type of injury. Parents should be taught to bring the teeth with the child to the dental office or emergency room and to preserve the teeth in milk or saliva without cleaning or brushing the avulsed teeth in any way. When some fibers or cells are retained on the teeth, they can be replanted more successfully.

Adults

Many adults are at risk of dental decay because of the common medications they take for a variety of health conditions (Dolan & Atchison, 1993). Many medications have anticholinergic properties that produce xerostomia. When saliva is reduced or absent, its protective buffering properties are also decreased; food is retained longer in the mouth; and bacteria can more readily produce acid, which increases the demineralization process (Bowen & Tabak, 1993). In addition, dental decay can proceed more quickly, especially around the gum line and between teeth. Health care professionals should warn their clients about these dangerous effects and should recommend that these clients drink more water to lubricate the mouth. Artificial saliva products (e.g., Optimoist) provide temporary relief for many clients and contain fluoride to promote remineralization. Unfortunately, many clients keep sugar-containing hard candy or gum in their mouth to increase saliva and provide a fresh taste to their breath. The use of sugar mints or candy only increases the risk for decay by providing more nutrients for oral bacteria to produce additional acid for demineralization.

Clients who have undergone radiation therapy to the head and neck lose their ability to produce saliva because of the effects of radiation on the salivary glands. All clients with xerostomia should use artificial saliva and frequently use intensive fluoride products, applied either by brush or mouth tray, to increase remineralization. These clients should also visit an oral health care professional at least every 3 months to be evaluated for any early sign of dental decay (Wilkins, 1994).

Bad breath, or halitosis, affects most adults and many children during their lifetime. Most individuals view an ideal oral image as one of fresh breath and clean teeth. Halitosis can occur occasionally, regularly, or chronically and at specific times of the day or month. Breath freshness is a major cause of concern for most adolescents and adults, especially in social situations. Oral malodor can be caused by certain medications; dry mouth; respiratory infections; and certain foods, such as garlic, onion, or spicy foods. At times, certain diseases, such as tumors of the upper respiratory and gastrointestinal track or liver and/or kidney failure, can cause halitosis, which usually occurs late in the disease process, with rapid onset and progressive intensity (Richter, 1996).

Volatile sulphur compounds have been suggested to be the cause of halitosis in the absence of any of the previously mentioned factors. Volatile sulphur compounds are formed from anaerobic bacterial activity on sulphur-containing amino acids derived from degraded proteins present in the saliva. These compounds can be removed by thorough oral hygiene, particularly tongue brushing and scraping, and use of antimicrobial and oxidizing mouth rinses (Richter, 1996).

Health care professionals can recommend that clients minimize health depleting factors, such as decreasing ingestion of culprit foods, using salivary substitutes and other products to hydrate the mouth, and completing thorough daily oral hygiene, to prevent halitosis. Thorough brushing of all mouth structures, including the cheeks and tongue—especially the posterior portion—helps remove any food particles and microorganisms that may be causing the offending odor. All clients should receive a dental referral to rule out existing dental disease or other infections.

It is often during the adult years that periodontal diseases are initiated and progress in their destructive pattern (White et al., 1995). Although the major etiologic factor for periodontal diseases is microbial plaque, many health conditions present risk factors that complicate oral hygiene and exacerbate the inflammatory patterns of periodontal diseases (American Academy of Oral Medicine, 1993).

Older Adults

The expanding population of older individuals has begun to provide oral health care professionals with many challenges and opportunities. Although 1 in 8 Americans is currently older than 65 years, the most recent projections from the U.S. Census Bureau predict significant increases by the year 2020 and beyond. In 2020, 1 in 6 Americans, approximately 53 million individuals, will be older than 65, and by the year 2050, the overall population of older individuals will reach 80 million, or 1 of every 5 Americans. These demographic projections provide the challenge for all health care professionals to increase their knowledge and develop their skills to provide appropriate and sensitive care to older adults (Gluch-Scranton & Sheridan, 1996).

In addition to living longer, healthier lives, older individuals are keeping their teeth longer and need specialized dental care to continue in optimal oral health. As documented in progress reports regarding the oral health objectives in *Healthy People 2000*, complete tooth loss has continued to be limited to approximately one third of older adults (Gift et al., 1996). However, root caries and periodontal diseases are still proportionately higher in older individuals (Burt & Eklund, 1992; White et al., 1995). Since this age cohort has not had the benefits of modern dental care or preventive dentistry, health care professionals have many challenges in persuading older adults to engage in frequent dental care and oral health promotional activities.

Older individuals experience a significantly higher rate of root caries, primarily seen in the exposed root areas, because of loss of tissue and bone attachment associated with periodontal diseases, which also increase with age. Root caries can be prevented with thorough daily oral hygiene and use of intensive topical home fluoride gels (Gluch-Scranton & Sheridan, 1996). Root caries should be treated early because these lesions are more difficult to treat as they progressively enlarge. Dry mouth associated with many medications increases the risk of root decay, so older clients, many of whom take medication, must use salivary substitutes. They should also receive dietary counseling, especially since many older clients may choose a softer diet that is higher in fermentable carbohydrates (Ettinger & Kambhu, 1992).

Health care professionals may recommend modifications in oral hygiene techniques, depending on whether the older client has any disabilities (Wilkins, 1994). For example, powered toothbrushes are often easier for a client with arthritis and can prove easier for a caretaker who cleans the client's mouth. If the older client wears dentures, these should be cleaned thoroughly after eating; should always be soaked overnight, preferably in a commercially available cleansing solution; and should never be left in the mouth overnight. Older individuals should clean their mouth tissues with a soft toothbrush or washcloth and complete an oral facial self-examination at least once a month to locate any suspicious lesions or sores (Wilkins, 1994).

Unfortunately, candidiasis is often a problem for clients when dentures are improperly cleaned or left in the mouth overnight, and it often manifests as a client's complaint of a "denture sore." "Denture sores" should receive careful evaluation from an oral health care professional who can determine whether the denture has been fractured or is ill-fitting or whether a candida infection is present. Treatment with antifungal medications should also be applied to the denture to remove any residual sources of infection. In addition, the perception of a dry mouth will also affect the comfort of denture wear, so clients taking medications that produce dry mouth should be cautioned to sip water frequently and use a salivary substitute to reduce any denture discomfort.

Women's Oral Health Issues

Women have special oral health needs and considerations that men do not have. Women often report aesthetic concerns in their ideal oral health image, and motivational strategies are often effective when framed as supporting the transition to the client's idealized aesthetic oral image. Hormonal fluctuations have a surprisingly strong influence on the oral cavity. Puberty, menses, pregnancy, and menopause all influence women's oral health and the way in which oral health care is provided.

Puberty. During puberty, an increased level of sex hormones, such as progesterone and possibly estrogen, in a young woman's maturing system causes increased blood circulation to the gingiva, which leads to a greater sensitivity and susceptibility for gingivitis. Localized enlargement of the gingival tissue is most commonly seen in young women, most often a result of the interaction of local irritants (microbial plaque and tartar) with fluctuating hormone levels. Health care professionals should alert girls and their parents to these phenomena and stress that proper treatment involves both careful and thorough oral hygiene and professional scaling and root planing to remove all microbial irritants. Image assessment should include teaching self-examination of gingival tissues and explaining health supportive patterns to control and eliminate the transient gingivitis. Continued attention to thorough brushing and flossing is necessary, or the swelling will return.

Menses. Gingivitis is also prevalent during menstruation because of the combination of increased levels of progesterone with microbial plaque. Menstruation gingivitis usually occurs right before a woman's period and clears up once menses has started. As always, good home oral hygiene care, including brushing and flossing, is important to maintain oral health, especially during hormonal fluctuations. In addition, more frequent dental visits for cleanings may be indicated, and an antimicrobial mouth rinse may need to be prescribed for more thorough plaque removal.

Occasionally during menses, some women may experience aphthous ulcers in the mouth or herpetic lesions on the lips. They may appear 3 or 4 days before menses begins and heal after menstruation. Palliative treatment, such as topical anesthetic agents and/or systemic analgesics, may be necessary for the discomfort associated with aphthous ulceration and herpetic lesions. Topical corticosteroids also may be indicated for severe aphthous ulcers.

Pregnancy. During pregnancy many women experience increased gingivitis beginning in the second or third month that increases in severity through the eighth month and begins to decrease in the ninth month. This condition, called *pregnancy gingivitis,* is marked by an increased amount of swelling, bleeding, and redness in the gum tissue in response to a very small amount of plaque or calculus and is caused by an increased level of progesterone that occurs during pregnancy.

If the gingival tissues are in a state of good health before pregnancy occurs, a woman is less likely to have any gum problems during her pregnancy. Pregnancy gingivitis usually affects areas of previous inflammation—not healthy gum tissue. If a woman experiences some swelling and bleeding of the gums before pregnancy, she might be at increased risk for pregnancy gingivitis. Just like any other type of gingivitis, if left untreated, pregnancy gingivitis can have damaging effects on the gums and bone surrounding the teeth, resulting in tissue (bone and gum) loss. Occasionally, the inflamed gum tissue will form an enlarged growth, called a *pregnancy tumor,* as an extreme inflammatory response to any local irritation. These areas of enlargement vary in size and usually appear by the third month of pregnancy but may occur at any time during the pregnancy. A pregnancy tumor is usually painless; however, it can become painful if it interferes with chewing or becomes further inflamed by local irritants.

Health care professionals should encourage their pregnant clients to seek professional dental care when signs of either pregnancy gingivitis or tumors occur. Dental care usually involves conservative periodontal therapy and oral hygiene instructions, with further treatment or removal generally delayed until after delivery. Pregnancy gingivitis and pregnancy tumors usually diminish after pregnancy, but they may not go away completely. Because of this, it is of utmost importance after the completion of the pregnancy, that a dental examination be performed to assess periodontal health. Any treatment that might be needed can be determined at this time.

Any woman contemplating pregnancy should see her dentist to make sure her mouth is in a good state of health and that any source of infection is eliminated before pregnancy. During pregnancy it is important that the woman seek more frequent professional cleanings for the removal of irritants and to maintain a diligent daily home oral care routine, including brushing and flossing. If tender, swollen, and bleeding gums, as well as any other dental problems, occur at any time during the pregnancy, a dentist must be contacted immediately. The pregnant client can be treated safely as long as the dentist is aware that the client is pregnant so that modifications can be made in the proposed treatment, if necessary.

A script is included at the end of this chapter to assist the health care professional in facilitating oral health promotional activities pertinent to pregnant clients. This script also includes relevant information regarding oral care of infants and young children. Based on the Health Promotion Matrix, this script contains questions that guide health care professionals' activities through each of the five dimensions for intervention.

Oral contraceptives. Women taking oral contraceptives may be susceptible to the same oral health conditions that affect pregnant women as a result of the documented effects of progesterone on the gingival tissues. Treatment of gum inflammation exaggerated by oral contraceptives should include establishing an excellent oral hygiene home care program and ongoing dental examinations and cleanings to eliminate all predisposing factors. More definitive periodontal therapy may also be indicated. Antimicrobial mouth washes may also be prescribed as part of the home care regimen.

Menopause. For the most part, menopause does not directly cause any oral problems. Estrogen supplements have little effect on oral health status; however, progesterone supplements may increase the gingival response to local irritants, causing redness, bleeding, and swelling of the tissues. On rare occasions a woman may experience a condition called *menopausal gingivostomatitis*. This condition is marked by gingival tissues that are dry and shiny, bleed easily, and range in color from abnormally pale to deep red.

Additional oral symptoms that women may experience during menopause include a dry or burning sensation in the mouth and abnormal taste sensations, especially salty, peppery, or sour tastes. In some women, oral symptoms and complaints respond favorably to estrogen supplement therapy. Professional scaling and root planing in combination with daily thorough oral hygiene care can relieve symptoms by controlling the inflammatory response and any enlargement of the gingival tissues. In addition, there is some empirical evidence to show that nutritional supplements in the form of vitamin B complexes and vitamin C are somewhat successful. Saliva substitutes and use of sugarless candy and mints may also be prescribed to reduce mouth dryness.

ORAL CARE

Numerous clinical trials have shown that effective oral self-care can control plaque and gingivitis in most individuals (Burt & Eklund, 1992; Harris & Christen, 1995). Other studies have shown, however, that proper client teaching and reinforcement of oral hygiene care is critical to ensure adherence to recommended oral hygiene practices (Gift, 1991; Schou & Blinkhorn, 1993). Health care professionals can initiate oral health promotional activities by encouraging clients to visualize clean and healthy teeth, fresh breath, and the ideal appearance of their smile (Matthias, Atchison, Lubben, DeJong & Schweitzer, 1995). Health care professionals should encourage visits to the dental office for oral prophylaxis, oral hygiene instructions, and examinations on a frequent basis, as necessary. Health care professionals can recommend one or more of the oral hygiene techniques described in the following section as ways to optimize the client's current oral health supportive techniques.

Brushing

Soft toothbrushes are recommended because they help avoid damage to gum tissue and enamel. Both manual and powered toothbrushes are considered acceptable, based on the client's preference and needs. Powered toothbrushes provide additional assistance to clients with physical or other disabilities that limit the effectiveness of their brushing technique. If the cost of a powered brush is a deterring factor, a variety of hand grips can be improvised to help the client brush; these include a rubber ball with the toothbrush inserted in the center, a large wad of tin foil wrapped around the handle of the toothbrush, or a rubber bicycle grip with the toothbrush inserted into the end.

Although oral health care professionals recommend at least a 3-minute period for thorough toothbrushing, most individuals brush for 30 seconds or less—an inadequate amount of time to ensure thorough cleansing. Reminders, such as using an egg timer or brushing the length of one radio song, can encourage clients to spend more time brushing, especially children. The following two brushing techniques are most commonly recommended and are often combined to most thoroughly clean the mouth:

Rolling stroke brushing method—Place the bristles of the brush at a 45-degree angle to the gum line. Sweep the brush away from the gum toward the chewing surface of the tooth. Continue throughout the mouth, covering each tooth. Brush the chewing surfaces of the teeth next by holding the brush flat on the chewing surface and gently scrubbing. With paste still on the brush, gently sweep the brush with several strokes along the tongue from the back of the throat to the front. After brushing the tongue, gently sweep the brush along the inside of the cheeks (Harris & Christen, 1995; Wilkins, 1994). (Figure 12-1.)

Bass (sulcular) brushing method—Place the thoroughly rinsed brush at a 45-degree angle to the gum line. Direct the bristles of the brush under the margin of the gum so that a slight pressure is felt. Vibrate the brush and slightly rotate in small circles under the gum line to clean the sulcular space between the gum and the tooth. As each area is cleaned, withdraw the brush from under the gum and reposition the brush to the next tooth under the gum (Harris & Christen, 1995; Wilkins, 1994). (See Figure 12-2.)

In young children or older adults with dexterity problems, a circular or scrub brushing technique is considered an acceptable alternative to these two traditional brushing techniques. However, older adults should be cautioned to use a gentle stroke and an extra soft toothbrush to avoid excessive abrasion, especially around exposed root surfaces (Harris & Christen, 1995; Wilkins, 1994).

Interproximal Cleansing

The anatomy of the teeth make it very difficult for toothbrushing alone to be sufficient for cleansing the entire tooth surface. Additional products, such as dental floss, small ta-

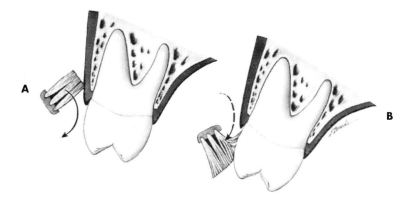

Figure 12-1 Rolling stroke brushing method. **A,** Place bristles pointing apically on gingiva. **B,** Sweep bristles over teeth from gingiva toward incisal or occlusal surface. *(From Woodall, I.R. (1993). Comprehensive dental hygiene care (4th ed.). St. Louis: Mosby.)*

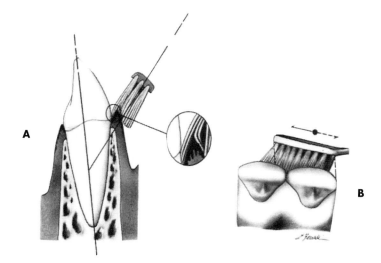

Figure 12-2 Bass brushing method. **A,** Place bristles pointing apically at 45-degree angle to long axis of tooth. First row of bristles will approximate sulcus, and adjacent row will touch gingival margin. **B,** Activate brush with a short back-and-forth vibration to disorganize plaque at entry to sulcus. After this step, complete rolling stroke to clean clinical crowns (modified Bass method). *(From Woodall, I.R. (1993). Comprehensive dental hygiene care (4th ed.). St. Louis: Mosby.)*

pered brushes, and wooden picks, are necessary to maneuver between the teeth to disrupt the bacterial plaque. Although there are a number of acceptable techniques for using dental floss, the following procedures are most commonly recommended: pull about 18 inches of floss from the dispenser and wrap the ends around the middle fingers; hold the floss firmly, using the fingers to gently guide the floss between the teeth; curve the floss snugly around the sides of the tooth, and gently slide the floss under the gum until a slight pressure is felt; keeping the floss adapted around the tooth, scrape the floss several times on the tooth surface to remove the bacterial plaque; after cleansing that one side of the tooth, slide the floss up to the tight contact area and readapt the floss to the side of the other tooth in that area; repeat the flossing procedure on each tooth, upper and lower, using a clean segment of the floss on each area (Harris & Christen, 1995; Wilkins, 1994).

Antimicrobial Rinses

Many clients will report using mouth rinses for fresh breath and clean teeth. Although most over-the-counter mouth rinses provide a temporary fresh taste, only two products (essential oils and chlorhexidine) are accepted for the control of gingivitis, but neither of these products has been shown to reduce periodontitis. Since most over-the-counter mouth rinses contain alcohol, clients taking medications that produce dry mouth should not use these rinses because the alcohol content will exacerbate the symptoms of a dry mouth (Harris & Christen, 1995).

The essential oil rinse (sold as Listerine and as generic equivalents) has a potent antimicrobial effect and has been shown to reduce gingivitis (Darby & Walsh, 1995). However, the antimicrobial effect is short term because the essential oil rinse lacks substantivity, or staying power. In addition, ethyl alcohol is used to increase the solubility of the essential oils (Eucalyptus oils, oil of wintergreen) in the mouth rinse. The concentration of alcohol could be as much as 24% to 27%, which could create problems for clients taking medications or clients recovering from alcohol abuse (Wilkins, 1994).

Chlorhexidine mouth rinse is the most effective antiplaque and antigingivitis mouth rinse currently available. Chlorhexidine has been used in many randomized, controlled studies since the mid-1960s, and there is strong evidence to support its use to prevent gingivitis (Wilkins, 1994). However, because clients commonly report uncomfortable side effects, such as alterations in taste perception, unpleasant taste, tooth staining, and tartar formation, chlorhexidine is not recommended for routine use. Instead, this prescription drug is recommended for use in a controlled situation for managing acute gingivitis, for controlling periodontal involvement in immunocompromised clients, and for promoting healing after periodontal treatment. Most oral health care professionals recommend that chlorhexidine be prescribed in a limited, conservative manner, rather than for routine use for either symptom relief or simplified oral hygiene, because of its ability to mask existing periodontal conditions (Wilkins, 1994).

Professional Care

Professional dental care is necessary to control subgingival bacteria, remove calcified deposits, and reinforce personal oral hygiene techniques. Neither supragingival plaque control alone nor professional care alone will effectively limit the progression of periodontitis or maintain periodontal health, but the combination of the two is effective for the majority of clients (Brown et al., 1996). The appropriate frequency for professional therapy depends on the client's medical history, medical status, age, risk factors, and the state of the dentition. Most oral health care professionals recommend that periodontal and high-risk clients be evaluated every 3 months and nonperiodontally involved clients every 6 months to 1 year. Frequent reevaluation assists the client in continued appraisal and internalization in his/her ideal image of oral health.

Health care professionals need to be aware of clients who are at high risk for periodontal diseases. High-risk clients include immunocompromised individuals; diabetic patients; longtime users of antiepileptic drugs; pregnant women; alcoholics; tobacco users; individuals receiving radiation therapy; or individuals with certain blood dyscrasias, Down syndrome, or Sjögren's syndrome (Greene et al., 1990). Health care professionals counseling these high-risk individuals should promote oral health interventions that both optimize health supportive patterns and minimize health depleting patterns. Table 12-2 provides a summary of the health risk factors that affect oral health care, which should be considered during activities related to image creation and image appraisal.

ORAL HEALTH PROMOTION & THE HEALTH PROMOTION MATRIX

Oral health promotion is generally the province of a specially trained professional, such as a dentist or dental hygienist. More general health care professionals, such as nurses, however, may use the Health Promotion Matrix to enhance the client's image of health and to encourage the client to view oral health as part of healthy patterns. The Matrix that follows contains example statements for the health care professional to encourage oral health promotion for a woman who is pregnant and has other children, as many women begin to be concerned about their special health care needs and the needs of the developing baby at this time. The health care professional may begin a discussion with a pregnant woman with a question that frames the need for oral health promotion at this stage of life, such as: "Did you know that there are many oral health care issues for both you and your baby? You may have heard some old wives' tales about teeth and pregnancy, but most of those stories are not true. For example, some people believe that you lose a tooth with each baby, or that the baby steals calcium from your teeth, and they decay. These tales are not true, yet there are some changes in the mouth commonly seen in pregnancy."

Image Creation

This dimension addresses the woman's image of her own healthy teeth and gums, as well as those of her baby. The health care professional may address a series of questions to the woman that target her *through* the image of the baby.

How do you picture your baby's ideal smile? Do you see your baby with clean, healthy teeth and gums? Do you envision your baby as a child with straight teeth? Does your picture include a baby becoming a child with a comfortable bite and able to chew easily? Does the child in your image have fresh breath? Does this imagined baby visit the dentist on a regular basis?

Image Appraisal

At this dimension, the woman would be queried about changes in oral health unique to pregnancy. The expected physical and psychologic changes associated with pregnancy are assessed. Any nutritional approaches, drugs, herbs, or supplements she may be using are examined for their effects on oral health.

An important aspect of the assessment process is the relationship between the client, the health care professional, and the community. The health care professional asks the client about existing community resources that can promote oral health, such as fluoridation of the water, as well as the client's access to clinics and other affordable treatment sites. Through compiling multiple Image Appraisals, the health care professional may uncover unmet community needs and thus may begin to work with the community to address them.

The dimension ends with a plan for the client to see a dental professional to have her teeth, as well as her child's teeth, cleaned and examined.

Have you noticed any changes in your gums or teeth since you have been pregnant?

Have you noticed any blood on your toothbrush when you rinse?

Have you experienced any morning sickness or nausea during your pregnancy?

Have you noticed a bad taste in your mouth?

Have you changed your diet since you have been pregnant?

Have you postponed a visit to the dentist since you have been pregnant?

Do you sometimes have problems chewing food?

Do you drink tap water or bottled water that is not fluoridated?

Have you changed your mouth care routine at home?

Do you plan to use a bottle to feed your baby?

Do you need information on how to care for your baby's new teeth?

NO
|
Would you like to receive more information about caring for your mouth or your baby's mouth?

YES
|
What changes have you seen in your gums or teeth?

When you have morning sickness or nausea, what do you do to calm your stomach and to clean your mouth?

What kind of dietary changes have you made during your pregnancy?

Are you snacking more?

Do you use sugar-containing candy, gum, or mints frequently?

When was your last dental visit?

What was done?

When was the last time you had your teeth cleaned?

What kind of oral hygiene procedures were you taught?

How do you take care of your teeth at home?

What kind of water do you drink?

Is the water in your town fluoridated?

Do you know when the baby should get his/her first tooth?

Do you know how to clean a baby's mouth?

Do you know when a baby should visit a dentist?

Do you know how feeding patterns affect a baby's teeth?

Are you interested in an educational program about taking care of your teeth during pregnancy?

Are you interested in an educational program about taking care of your baby's mouth and teeth?

Would you be willing to see a dental professional to have your oral hygiene techniques customized to your needs?

Would you be willing to see a dental professional to have your teeth cleaned and examined?

Would you be willing to develop and complete a plan to promote the best oral health for you and your baby?

Minimize Health Depleting Patterns

With this dimension of the Health Promotion Matrix, the health care professional is interested in discussing brief, targeted approaches for oral health. The health care professional would recommend approaches to maintaining healthy gums and teeth consistent with eating well and substance safety, such as sucking on sugar-free mints to reduce nausea. These approaches are reinforced through the use of educational booklets or videotapes, often available in Spanish as well as English. (Booklets may be obtained from the sources listed in the Helpful Resources section at the end of this chapter.) In addition, the health care professional may give the client toothbrushes, dental floss, and toothpaste to overcome minimal barriers to oral health. If appropriate, she/he could suggest dental clinics that accept clients for little or no charge.

Have you changed your diet since you have been pregnant?

When you have morning sickness or nausea, what do you do to calm your stomach and to clean your mouth?

What kind of dietary changes have you made during your pregnancy?

Are you snacking more?

Do you use candy, gum, or mints frequently?

How do you take care of your teeth at home?

Would you like to receive more information about caring for your mouth?

Would you be willing to see a dental professional to have your teeth cleaned and examined?

What problems could you see as barriers for you to have a clean, healthy mouth?

Are you limiting usage of sugar products?

Do you know how to clean a baby's mouth?

Do you know how feeding patterns affect a baby's teeth?

Would you like to receive more information about caring for your baby's mouth?

Would you be willing to have your child see a dental professional to have his/ her teeth cleaned and examined?

What problems could you see as barriers to your child having a clean, healthy mouth?

Are you limiting your baby's usage of sugar products?

Optimize Health Supportive Patterns

The health care professional is most interested in encouraging the client to rely on existing strengths in her community and family. The health care professional would encourage the drinking of fluoridated water and visiting local dentists or clinics. She/he would reinforce the importance of a familial trip to the dentist to review proper brushing and flossing techniques and the habit of regular check-ups.

Have you changed your diet since you have been pregnant?

Have you scheduled a visit to the dentist since you have been pregnant?

Do you and your family use tap water or bottled water that is fluoridated?

Have you changed your mouth care routine at home?

Would you like to receive more information about caring for your mouth?

When you have morning sickness or nausea, what do you do to calm your stomach and to clean your mouth?

What kind of dietary changes have you made during your pregnancy?

What kind of oral hygiene procedures were you taught?

How do you take care of your teeth at home?

Are you interested in an educational program about taking care of your teeth during pregnancy?

Would you be willing to see a dental professional to have your oral hygiene techniques customized to your needs?

Would you be willing to see a dental professional to have your teeth cleaned and examined?

Are you using something to clean your tongue every day?

Do you clean in between your teeth every day?

Are you using a soft toothbrush at least twice a day?

Are you using a fluoridated toothpaste?

Do you plan to use a bottle to feed your baby?

Do you need information on how to care for your baby's new teeth?

Would you like to receive more information about caring for your baby's mouth?

Is the water in your town fluoridated?

Do you know how to clean a baby's mouth?

Do you know when a baby should visit a dentist?

Do you know how feeding patterns affect a baby's teeth?

Are you brushing the baby's teeth with a soft toothbrush at least twice a day?

Are you using a small dab of fluoridated toothpaste on the brush when you clean the baby's teeth?

Are you interested in an educational program about taking care of your baby's mouth and teeth?

Internalize Idealized Image

Often, change is slow, so the health care professional would continue to ask about the modifications necessary to the client's oral hygiene program. A customized program would continue to encourage compliance, as well as increase the pace of change.

What factors have helped you to continue this customized oral care program?

What factors have detracted from your ability to complete this program?

Since you have been completing this customized oral care program, what kinds of changes have you noticed in your mouth?

What kinds of changes have you made in your oral hygiene program?

How frequently have you been able to visit a dental professional?

Have you changed your eating patterns based on our discussions?

A woman's oral health needs change once she delivers the baby. How can I help you keep your mouth healthy now that the baby is born?

Since you have been completing this customized oral care program, what kinds of changes have you noticed in your baby's mouth?

What kinds of changes have you made in your child's oral hygiene program?

How frequently has your child been able to visit a dental professional?

Have you changed your child's feeding patterns based on our discussions?

A baby's oral health needs change as they grow and as their teeth erupt from 6 months to 2 years. How can I help you keep your child's mouth healthy as he/she grows?

The following script directs many of the same questions to a generic client. The health care professional may easily customize the script by adding queries unique to *one* client's oral health.

ORAL HEALTH PROMOTION: *A Script**

Oral health promotion is important to your overall health.

Image Creation	How do you picture yourself with an ideal smile?
	Do you see yourself with clean, healthy teeth and gums?
	Do you envision yourself as maintaining healthy teeth and gums throughout your lifetime?
	Does your picture include a comfortable bite and an ability to chew easily?
	Does your image of yourself include fresh breath?
	Do you want to keep your teeth?
	Do you want a clean, healthy mouth?
	Do you see yourself having your teeth cleaned regularly?
Image Appraisal	Have you been able to set aside time to complete thorough oral hygiene each day?
	Have you been able to thoroughly look in your mouth each day?
	Have you noticed any blood on your toothbrush or when you rinse your mouth?
	Have you noticed a bad taste in your mouth?

*Adapted from B.J. Steinberg, J.I. Gluch, and S. Kozich Giorgio by S. Sheinfeld Gorin.

ORAL HEALTH PROMOTION: *A Script—cont'd*

Do you sometimes have problems chewing food?

Do you feel comfortable smiling and talking to people?

Do you feel as if you have an acceptable smile?

Do you feel as if you have a comfortable bite and can chew easily?

Do you feel as if you have fresh breath?

When was your last dental visit? What was done?

Were you pleased with your smile after your dental visit?

Do you drink tap water or bottled water that is not fluoridated?

Would you be willing to develop and to complete a plan to promote your oral health?

YES   **NO**

Minimize Health Depleting Patterns

YES	NO
Provide more detailed information and skill teaching.	Provide brief information to promote awareness.
Identify barriers to adoption of new behaviors (e.g., suggest local dentists, clinics; self-efficacy; brushing skills; give toothbrush, floss).	Ask whether client is willing to attempt gradual change in health behaviors.
Make referral to a dental professional.	

Optimize Health Supportive Patterns

Try to drink more tap water if it is fluoridated.

Try to brush with fluoridated toothpaste.

Suggest cleaning the tongue every day.

Suggest cleaning between the teeth every day.

Suggest using a soft toothbrush at least twice a day.

For some: advise the client use a fluoridated mouth wash.

Internalize Idealized Image

What kinds of changes have you noticed in your mouth?

What kinds of changes have you made in your self-care program?

continued

ORAL HEALTH PROMOTION: *A Script—cont'd*

Have you been able to visit a dental professional?

Have you changed your eating patterns based on our discussions?

YES

Congratulations! A beautiful smile is ageless! Remember to visit the dental office on a regular basis.

NO

Can we discuss any obstacles in your way to making these changes?

Is there anything more I can do to help? Do you need a dental referral?

Summary

Oral health, one of the nine positive healthy behaviors, is essential to ensure optimal general health. The oral health educational information and activities presented in this chapter allow the health care professional to explore different methods of encouraging the client to visualize, identify, and incorporate oral health promotion as an integral part of his/her health behaviors. All of us, professionals and clients, need continuous reinforcement to meet the challenges of staying healthy and to integrate all nine positive healthy behaviors to reach an optimal level of wellness.

HELPFUL RESOURCES

PROFESSIONAL ASSOCIATIONS

American Dental Hygienists' Association
444 N. Michigan Ave.
Chicago, IL 60611
(800) 243-ADHA
Publishes educational catalogue, posters, pamphlets; established Dental Hygiene Week

American Dental Association
Order Department, Suite 1430
211 E. Chicago Ave.
Chicago, IL 60611
(800) 621-8099
Publishes educational catalogue, posters, pamphlets, videos, slide programs; sponsors Children's Dental Health and Senior Smile Program

American Academy of Periodontology
737 N. Michigan Ave.
Suite 800
Chicago, IL 60611-2690
(312) 787-5518
Publishes pamphlets

American Society of Dentistry for Children
875 N. Michigan Ave.
Suite 4040
Chicago, IL 60611
(800) 637-ASDC
Produces children's dental health materials, posters, pamphlets, videos

HELPFUL RESOURCES—cont'd

American Society for Geriatric Dentistry
"OBRA Dental Manual"
C/O South Texas Geriatric Education Center
7703 Floyd Curl Drive
San Antonio, TX 78284-7921
(210) 567-3370
Publishes resource book *How to Develop, Implement, & Manage a Nursing Facility Dental Program to Meet OBRA Requirements*

National Dairy Council
120 W. 44th St., Room 730
New York, NY 10036
(212) 764-4060
Produces nutrition educational materials

American Cancer Society
19 W. 56th St.
New York, NY 10019
(212) 586-8700
Produces posters, pamphlets, and videos regarding oral cancer, smoking cessation and smokeless tobacco

American Lung Association
432 Park Avenue South
New York, NY 10016
(212) 889-3370
Produces posters, pamphlets, and videos regarding smoking cessation and smokeless tobacco

GOVERNMENTAL AGENCIES

U.S. Department of Health and Human Services
Public Health Service
National Institute of Health
Building WW, Room 522
9000 Rockville Pike
Bethesda, MD 20892
Produces posters and pamphlets

Texas Department of Health
State Health Department
Bureau of Dental and Chronic Disease Prevention
1100 W. 49th St.
Austin, TX 78756
(512) 458-7323
Produces "Toothtown II Oral Health" curriculum for kindergarteners through 12th-graders

COMPANIES

Colgate's Bright Smiles, Bright Futures
C/O JMH Communications
1133 Broadway
New York, NY 10160-1573
(800) 334-7734
Produces school educational information, including videos, activity sheets, and guidebooks

Colgate Oral Pharmaceuticals
One Canton Way
Canton, MA
(800) 2-COLGATE
Produces educational information and oral hygiene products

Health Edco, Inc.
P.O. Box 21270
Waco, TX 76702
Produces educational catalogue and audiovisual aids

Practicon
102 Station Court, Suite D
Greenville, NC 27934
(800) 334-0956
Produces educational catalogue and audiovisual aids

References

American Academy of Oral Medicine. (1993, Fall). *Clinician's guide to treatment of common oral conditions* (3rd ed.). Chicago.

American Dental Association, Bureau of Health, Education, and Audiovisual Services, Council on Dental Materials, Instruments, and Equipment. (1984, July). Mouth protectors and sports team dentists. *Journal of the American Dental Association, 109,* 84-87.

Bay, I., Ainaimo, J., & Gad, I. (1974). The response of young diabetics to periodontal disease. *Journal of Periodontology, 45,* 806-816.

Bowen, W.H., & Tabak, L.A. (1993). *Cariology for the nineties.* Rochester, NY: University of Rochester Press.

Brown, L.J., Brunelle, J.A., & Kingman, A. (1996, February). Periodontal status in the United States, 1988-1991: Prevalence, extent, and demographic variation. *Journal of Dental Research [Special issue], 75,* 672-683.

Burkett, L.W. (1944). Histopathologic explanation for the oral lesion in the acute leukemias. *American Journal of Orthodontics Oral Surgery, 30,* 516.

Burt, B.A. (1992). The changing patterns of systemic fluoride intake. *Journal of Dental Research* [Special issue], *71,* 1228-1232.

Burt, B.A., Eklund, S.A. (1992). *Dentistry, dental practice and the community* (4th ed.). Philadelphia: WB Saunders.

Dejani, A.S., Taubert, K.A., Wilson, W., Bolger, A., Bayer, A., Ferrier, P., Gewitz, M.H., Shulman, S.T., Nouri, S., Newburger, J.W., Hutto, C., Pallasch, T.J., Gage, T.W., Levison, M.E., Peter, G., & Zuccaro, Jr., G. (1997). Prevention of bacterial endocarditis. Recommendations by the American Heart Association. *Journal of the American Medical Association, 277*(22), 1794-1201.

Darby, M.L., & Walsh, M.M. (1995). *Dental hygiene theory and practice.* Philadelphia: WB Saunders.

DeBiase, C.B. (1991). *Dental health education.* Philadelphia: Lea & Febiger.

Dolan, T.A., & Atchison, K.A. (1993). Implications of access, utilization and need for oral health care by the non-institutionalized and institutionalized elderly on the dental delivery system. *Journal of Dental Education 57,*(16), 876-87.

Ettinger, R.L., & Kambhu, P.P. (1992). Selected issues on care and management of the aging patient. II. Prevention and treatment. *Dental Update, 19*(6), 246-254.

Frazier, P.J., & Horowitz, A.M. (1990). Oral health education and promotion in maternal and child health: A position paper. *Journal of Public Health Dentistry,* [Special issue] *50*(6), 390-395.

Gift, H. (1988). Awareness and assessment of periodontal problems among dentists and the public. *International Dental Journal, 38,* 147-153.

Gift, H. (1991). Prevention of oral diseases and oral health promotion. *Current Opinion in Dentistry, 1,* 337-347.

Gift, H.C., Drury, T.F., Nowjack-Raymer, R.E., Selwitz, R.H. (1996). The state of the nation's oral health: Mid-decade assessment of Healthy People 2000. *Journal of Public Health Dentistry, 56*(2), 84-91.

Gluch-Scranton, J., & Sheridan, O. (1996). Oral health promotion with older patients. *Compendium of Continuing Education in Oral Hygiene, 3*(2), 3-11.

Greene, J.C., Louie, R., & Wycoff, S. (1990). Preventive dentistry. II. Periodontal disease, malocclusion, trauma, and oral cancer. *Journal of the American Medical Association, 263* (3), 421-425.

Haber, J., Watts, J., Crawley, R., Mandell, R., Joshipura, K., & Kent, R. (1991). Assessment of diabetes as a risk factor for periodontitis. *Journal of Dental Research, 70,* 414.

Grossi, S.G., Zambon, J.J., Norderyd, C.M., Dunford, R.G., Ho, A.W., Machtel, E.E., Preus, H., & Genco, R.V. (1993). Microbiological risk indicators for periodontal disease. *Journal of Dental Research, 72,* 206.

Harris, N.O., & Christen, A.G. (1995). *Primary preventive dentistry* (4th ed.). Norwalk, CT: Appleton & Lange.

Horowitz, A.M., Goodman, H.S., Yellowitz, J.A., & Nourjah, P.A. (1996, Fall). The need for health promotion in oral cancer prevention and early detection. *Journal of Public Health Dentistry, 56*(6), 319-330.

Huelke, D.F., & Compton, C.P. (1983). Facial injuries in automobile crashes. *Oral Maxillofacial Surgery, 41*(4), 241-244.

Kaste, L.M., Gift, H., Bhat, M., & Swango, P.A. (1996, February). Prevalence of incisor trauma in persons 6 to 50 years of age: United States, 1988-1991. *Journal of Dental Research* [Special issue], *75,* 696-705.

Lindhe, J. (1983). *Textbook on clinical periodontology.* Philadelphia: WB Saunders.

Marcus, S.E., Drury, T.F., Brown, L.J., & Zion, G.R. (1996, February). Tooth retention and tooth loss in the permanent dentition of adults: United States, 1988-1991. *Journal of Dental Research* [Special issue], *75*, 684-695.

Matthias, R.E., Atchison, K.A., Lubben, J.E., DeJong, F., & Schweitzer, S.O. (1995). Factors affecting self-ratings of oral health. *Journal of Public Health Dentistry, 55*(4), 197-204.

Muzyka, B.C. (1993, July/August). Diagnosis and treatment of common oral manifestations associated with HIV disease. *Pennsylvania Dental Journal, 60*(4), 30-31.

National Institutes of Health, National Institutes of Dental Research. (1994, February). *Fever blisters and canker sores* (revised). Bethesda, MD: U.S. Department of Health and Human Services.

Newbrun, E. (1992). Current regulations and recommendations concerning water fluoridation, fluoride supplements and topical fluoride agents. *Journal of Dental Research, 71*(5), 1255-1265.

Nowak, A.J., & Anderson, J.L. (1990, January/February). Preventive dentistry for children: A review from 1968-1988. *Journal of Dentistry for Children, 57*(1), 31-37.

Nowjack-Raymer, R.E., & Gift, H. (1996, January/February). Use of mouthguards and head gear in organized sports by school-aged children. *Public Health Reports, III*(1), 82-86.

Oral Health Coordinating Committee (OHCC), Public Health Service. (1993). Toward improving the oral health of Americans: An overview of oral health status, resources and care delivery. *Public Health Reports, 108*(6), 657-672.

Richter, J. (1996, April). Diagnosis and treatment of halitosis. *Compendium of Continuing Education in Dentistry, 17*(4), 370-386.

Schou, L., & Blinkhorn, A.S. (1993). *Oral health promotion.* Oxford, NY: Oxford University Press.

Shore, R.C., Robinson, C., Kirkham, J., & Brookes, S.J. (1995). *Structure of mature enamel in dental enamel: Formation to destruction.* Boca Raton, FL: CRC Press.

Statement of the Coalition. (1993). *Journal of Dental Education, 57*(4), 273-282.

Strauss, R.P., & Hunt, R.J. (1993, January). Understanding the value of teeth to older adults: Influences on the quality of life. *Journal of the American Dental Association, 124*, 105-110.

Swango, P.A. (1996). Cancers of the oral cavity and pharynx in the United States: An epidemiologic overview. *Journal of Public Health Dentistry, 56*(6), 1996.

U.S. Department of Health and Human Services, U.S. Public Health Service. (1991a). *Healthy people 2000: National health promotion and disease prevention objectives.* USDHHS Publication No. (PHS91-50213). Washington, DC: U.S. Government Printing Office.

U.S. Department of Health and Human Services, U.S. Public Health Service. (1991b). *Review of fluoride benefits and risks.* Washington, DC: U.S. Government Printing Office.

Wentz, T.M., Anday, G., & Orban, B. (1949). Histopathologic changes in the gingiva in leukemia. *Journal of Periodontology, 20*, 119.

White, B.A., Caplan, D.J., & Weintraub, J.A. (1995). A quarter century of changes in oral health in the United States. *Journal of Dental Education, 59*(1), 19-57.

Wilkins, E. (1994). *Clinical practice of the dental hygienist* (7th ed.). Philadelphia: Williams & Wilkins.

Woodall, I. (1993). *Comprehensive dental hygiene care* (4th Ed.). St. Louis: Mosby.

CHAPTER

13

Self-Development

Penelope Buschman Gemma and Joan Arnold

EDITORS' NOTE

Self-Development and the Family Client System.   Co-authors Penelope Buschman Gemma, MS, RN, CS, FAAN, and Joan Arnold, PhD, RN, focus on the development of self as an interactive process. Development is a complex process. Individuals, families, groups, and communities each have their own developmental course and dynamics. The individual is the essential element of all these systems. Among the various systems with which the individual affiliates and in which the individual is nurtured, the family is surely the most significant. The support of families and the promotion of healthy family life is essential to self-development.

Families prepare members to move into the outside world and to function beyond the familiar interrelationships within the family system. Yet families are often at risk and inadequately prepared or unable to enrich their members with needed survival skills. Many individuals suffer from the absence of family unity and sustenance and find themselves isolated, alienated, and poorly prepared to enter and to find successful ties in larger systems. These are overwhelming obstacles that thwart the development of healthy families and hence the developed self.

Self-Development and Internalizing the Idealized Image.   The family can sustain its members and equip them to engage in the everexpanding circles of interaction outside the family. Healthy families support the development of healthy individuals, as well as contribute to healthy group and community development. Individual members incorporate the family's image of health and the practices and beliefs that support it. Through the process of internalizing this image of health, the family serves as educator and advocate for its members and informs groups and communities about the individual as client systems interact. The health care professional, working with the family as a system, can assist it in developing a positive image of health.

Dialogue for for Expressing Grief and a Script.   Inherent in growth is loss. Grieving is viewed as an important aspect of self-development. Buschman Gemma and Arnold provide health care professionals with a suggested means for facilitating the grieving process by integrating loss into a client's life and thereby assisting with development, as well as a more general Health Promotion Matrix-based script.

The importance of self-development to health cannot be denied. Individuals, families, groups, and communities possess a self-identity that shapes and influences the actualization of their health potential. Identity is a composite of factors and forces that make up the essence of the individual, the family, the group, and the community. The lifespan provides a continuum along which health is defined and monitored. Measurements of how proximate or distal one is to a healthy norm have been a constant source of investigation and wonder in trying to understand the uniqueness of each individual, as well as more general patterns of human development. Families can create an atmosphere that is positive to the health of their individual members. Families also have developmental types and phases that characterize their identity. The group and community are the contexts that allow families and individuals to grow. Whereas a group is defined as two or more persons and a community as a larger system and place, both are interactional systems with identities and discernible styles of leadership. Each individual, family, group, and community has a lifetime. A lifetime may be limited or elongated, but regardless of its duration, the life of each individual, family, group, and community can be viewed from the perspective of its development along an ongoing, dynamic continuum. Self-development is an interactive process of actualizing the potential for health across the lifespan.

Development of the self—the essence of being, whether individual, family, group, or community—is the focus of this chapter. Because human systems are dynamic, they require connectedness to each other and the nurturance found in relationships to sustain themselves. Just as the individual self requires the family to envelop and sustain it, so does the family require its individual members to contribute to its functions and join other members to shape and create it. Individuals and families depend on the larger system of groups and community for their resources and support while contributing to their identify and participating in their organizational structure and function. The interconnectedness of human systems facilitates growth and development. The dynamic exchanges between and among these systems reflect the uniqueness of each. Thwarted self-development, as well as factors that contribute to the replenishment and sustenance of the healthy self, are also explored in this chapter.

THE DYNAMIC PROCESS OF DEVELOPMENT

Development is a dynamic, lifelong process. Development, by its nature, is never complete. It is a process that unfolds within the context of every individual, family, group, and community, and it is molded by its interaction with environment and culture.

Individual Development

Self-development of the individual is a gradually unfolding, dynamic process. No one theory has been constructed to encompass all aspects of growth. There are as many developmental theories as there are theorists. Theorists, as they strive to build frames of reference in which to order and interpret the facts and patterns of human development, differ in their views of the origin of behavior. Old arguments, based on the philosophies of John Locke (1964) and Jean Jacques Rousseau (1962), such as nature versus nurture, and heredity versus environment, continue to influence thinking and theory formation regarding individual development. More recently, the notion of self-generativity (i.e., the individual's ability to actively shape the self within the context of heredity and environment) has taken hold in developmental thinking (Schuster & Ashburn, 1992). Development also has been considered within the context of culture. Selected theorists whose work address development of the individual over the lifespan and whose theories support the Health Promotion Matrix are discussed in this chapter.

Beginning with conception and ending with death, the development of the individual evolves over a lifetime. The first theorist to build upon the psychodynamic view of development postulated by Sigmund Freud (1935) was Erik Erikson (1963), who extended this theory to cover the lifespan of the individual. Erikson (1963) identified eight stages of development, each posing an essential task for growth. In each task are opposing dispositions that must be brought into balance for the individual to achieve the basic and necessary strength to move ahead. Erikson viewed each stage, or step, as a potential crisis (i.e., a turning point or crucial period of vulnerability and potential) and as "the ontogenetic source of generational strength and maladjustment" (Erikson, 1968, p. 96).

Erikson proposed that development itself is an orderly process that is determined biologically and occurs within the context of family and community. Erikson described the healthy individual as one who actively masters his/her environment, demonstrates a unified personality, and is able to perceive himself/herself accurately in the world (Erikson, 1968).

> Personality, therefore, can be said to develop according to the steps predetermined in the human organism's readiness to be driven toward, to be aware of, and to interact with a widening radius of significant individuals and institutions (Erikson, 1968, p. 93).

Robert Havighurst (1972), who was greatly influenced by Erikson's (1963) theory of psychosocial development, identified tasks crucial to the individual's growth. According to Havighurst, a developmental task arises in a certain time period in an individual's life. Successful completion of these tasks of life phases leads to satisfaction and future success, whereas failure leads to unhappiness, lack of future achievement, and ultimate social disapproval. Havighurst postulated that all human beings demonstrate a readiness to master life-phase–related tasks and that this readiness is based on a unique confluence of physical, psychologic, and social factors.

Havighurst (1972) proposed that development is a cognitive learning process. Tasks develop out of a combination of pressures arising from physical development, cultural expectations, and individual values and goals. He postulated the occurrence of "teachable moments" when a special sensitivity or readiness to learn a task arises from the unique combination of physical, social, and psychic preparedness.

Many other theorists have contributed to an understanding of development in highly specific areas and during defined time periods. Piaget's seminal work in the study of cognition (Piaget, 1963; Piaget & Inhelder, 1969); Chess' and Thomas' (1986) and Kagan's (1984, 1989) studies of temperamental patterns in young children; Gilligan's (1984) extensive research on gender-specific developmental issues; Piaget's (1965), Kohlberg's (1981), Gilligan's (1987), and Coles' (1997) contributions to moral development; and Maslow's (1968) description of self-actualization all address areas of development that significantly influence the health and well-being of the individual and the ease with which a person and family within the context of the community can make truly healthy decisions.

Individual development is a process that is complex to identify and analyze. Many forces contribute to a healthy developmental process. Among these are genetic, physiologic, physical, emotional, social, cultural, moral, and spiritual factors which, taken together, form the dimensions of the self. Each individual is constructed out of a genetic history that greatly affects the potential of the individual to achieve a standard of health. Genetic influences predetermine the potential for health, illness, disability, and death and contribute to accelerated risk for health depleting conditions. Patterns of family risk for illness are found in repeated incidence of illness from one generation to the next. The profound impact of genetics on human growth and development is yet to be realized as research advances.

The idea that persons are whole makes it difficult to break down the individual into component parts. When examining the parts, the health care professional must be mindful that this vantage point is myopic in nature. This microscopic view must be mediated by the more expansive perspective of the whole system, but a holistic perspective alone is difficult to substantiate because of the lack of holistic indicators. It is possible to understand the smallest unit of human matter in all its intricacies, yet it is impossible to fully comprehend a particular human action. The whole being is also difficult to comprehend; therefore guideposts are used to set parameters for what appears to fall within the range of normal. Hence, normal blood values for human biochemistry are available, just as behavioral manifestations are used to determine socially acceptable responses. These ranges of normal, or expected patterns, for behavior are termed *milestones* and have become markers for human development. The "outliers" may also be "normal," even though they fall beyond the parameters set; it must be remembered that the characteristic most valued in a person is, in fact, individuality. Each individual is appreciated for the extent to which his/her individuality is manifested and is unique while also sharing common bonds and characteristics with other human beings.

Tracing the developmental process from conception to death has been well-explicated in the human growth and development literature (Erikson, 1963; Havighurst, 1972; Maslow, 1968; Schuster & Ashburn, 1992). Underlying the concept of growth is the idea of a lifespan that traverses the life process and extends to death. No individual is guaranteed long life, but each person has a lifetime (Mellonie & Ingpen, 1983). For some, the lifetime is quite limited. Prenatal, infant, and child death (Arnold & Gemma, 1994) are exquisitely painful losses that deepen the respect for the realization that lifetimes can be short. With this realization comes the awareness that each life, regardless of its length, is powerful and affects the everexpanding circles of significant others connected to it. Many anticipate an extended lifetime, as the average lifespan has increased and persons older than 75 years have become the fastest growing segment of the population (Schuster & Ashburn, 1992).

The individual develops and is nurtured in relationships. These relationships are critical to survival and growth. The infant is a competent and multitalented human being yet dependent on parents and other caregivers for his/her existence. In the earliest phases of development, the infant depends on the caregiver for nurture and safety. As development proceeds, the child grows in independent competencies and becomes more able to sustain himself/herself and to meet his/her own needs. In addition, the child's connections to others are expanded beyond the immediate caregivers to significant others, from whom the child also derives nurturance. As growth continues, the individual enters into interdependent relationships and into a dynamic exchange, balancing need and want, as the recipient as well as the provider. As aging continues, the individual learns to continue to develop through disconnections and even solitude as support systems die and allow new growth through memory and reminiscence.

Family Development

The family, or cluster of persons living with and relating to one another, is the essential unit in which development occurs. Families grow and diminish as members are born or adopted, move away, and die. Families move through stages of development as the configuration and relationships among members change and grow (Carter & McGoldrick, 1989). The family is the system that challenges and nurtures the individual and provides the context that supports the healthy development of the self. The family is both a source of strength as well as a source of stress (Fogarty, 1985). Dysfunctional family interactions can support the potential for thwarted self-development. Development is dependent on the nature and consistency of support the family can give its members. The family identifies and responds to the needs of the members with its inner resources. When the family is depleted of its own resources, members' needs may be unmet unless alternate sources of support outside the family system can be located. The family milieu involves this kind of "give and take," and members quickly learn the capacities of the family to respond to their needs. The exchanges among members can be viewed much like the steps of a dance, as members come together and then pull apart in an effort to maintain connectedness with and to disengage from each other (Haley, 1980). Family life is a profound determinant of self-development; each member is affected individually by the myriad factors and forces found in the family.

Each family is held together by ties of history and experience that bind the members to each other and the family as a whole (Carter & McGoldrick, 1989). Family ties are deep and longlasting, regardless of the stress and strife within the unit, and they influence the development of family members. Each family has a unique history, which traverses generations of members. Family history not only influences family values and beliefs, but also the health potential of each member, as generational patterns are transmitted from one to the next.

Within functional families there is a tendency for the unit to operate as an open system (Bowen, 1978). The boundaries that identify and define the family allow for mutual exchange with the larger environment of the community and society. The boundaries also regulate input and output by filtering the amount and type of interchange with the environment. This kind of system regulation provides stability and enables the members of the family to experience constancy and predictable patterns, which facilitates a sense of security. Members derive satisfaction from the safety net provided by the unit's ability to navigate its way through the daily challenges of family and community life. The family that adheres to its values and beliefs while also exhibiting flexibility provides a dependable structure for its members.

Families are the primary educators of their members. Families prepare their members to move ultimately outside the system yet remain connected to it. They teach their members survival skills, including norms, values, roles, and communication and decision-making patterns. In addition, the transmission of family history and traditions, culture, religion, and spirituality provides members with a strong sense of family beliefs. It is the family belief system that provides the framework for the moral, ethical, and spiritual aspects of self-development. The individual forms self-defined boundaries, inner principles, and beliefs that govern patterns of living and relating.

The functional family is goal-directed; goals are transmitted through the family's actions and efforts. Additionally, individual members learn to establish goals that are self-enhancing, and hopefully, attainable. Among these is the goal of health. The healthy patterns and practices of the family are discernible. Families provide for the needs of daily life (i.e., food, shelter, and safety) and thus promote the developing self.

Family roles and expectations contribute to the identity of individual members (Walsh, 1989), and are often carried on in contexts and relationships outside the family of origin. Roles are the expected behaviors that members assume to help support the functions of the family. Roles permit orderly social interaction, as well as balance and stability in the family. Roles that are flexible and reciprocal allow for growth, whereas roles that limit transactions and bind members to fixed behaviors limit growth and personal development.

Family communication patterns provide the foundation for the individual member to relate to others in the family and to the world. When communication is functional, the receiver gets the same message that the sender intended. Members are able to state their case; clarify and qualify the meaning of the message; ask for feedback; exhibit receptivity to the feedback; and accept responsibility for personal thoughts, feelings, and actions. Communication becomes a mutual process when clarity is the aim. Effective communication skills will support the member in all interactions and broaden the opportunities for gaining social support and a network of significant others (Watzlawick, 1978). Communication patterns that block, confuse, or manipulate interactions limit authentic interactions with others and result in lack of support, distortion, and alienation, thereby reducing the chances of maintaining a network of colleagues and social support.

Family norms provide the developing self with rules that guide and regulate family behavior, whereas family values provide the inner convictions of what is right and wrong, good and bad, and desirable and undesirable. These family dynamics provide the developing self with guidelines to follow in deciphering the external world, evaluating the behavior of others, and reacting to observed behavior. The family also conveys values and beliefs concerning health and illness to its individual members. These shape the way the individual perceives and values health and its promotion. If the expectation for health is constrained by a lack of expectation for well-being, the individual will image positive health as unattainable.

Family decision-making patterns provide skills in negotiating and methods for finding agreement in and demonstrating a commitment to a particular course of action (Minuchin, 1974). Families that allow decisions to be processed and arrive at decisions by consensus provide a rich foundation for their members in this area of skill development. Families who decide through compromise, unilaterally, or by indecision confine the individual to "giving-up," rather than "gaining," from the perspective of others and the reformulation of personal thoughts. Effective decision-making enables the individual to make choices about health and health care, thus fostering the development of the healthy self.

Self-care rests in the ability of individuals to meet their own needs, maximize their personal strengths, and become autonomous. The family supports the individual's development of personal boundaries and achievement of separation in order to become a distinct self (Minuchin & Nichols, 1993). Self-care enables members to identify and seek their own health agenda. Individuals possess personal health strengths that assist in coping with health depleting threats. The individual who learns dependency rather than self-care is more likely to turn control over to health care professionals rather than to negotiate and participate actively in decisions about his/her health.

Evelyn Millis Duvall (1985) focused on the family as a dynamic system whose individual members progress developmentally. Changes in one member necessitate changes in others and most certainly in the entire family system. Duvall maintains that as families develop, responsibilities remain constant but the focus shifts according to the specific stages. Duvall (1985) looks at the dynamics of development occurring in stages across the lifespan of the family. Each stage presents opportunities for individual members and families to make decisions, act on readiness, grow, and change.

In conclusion the family provides an important context in which individuals learn and grow; the family is generally the primary context for individual development. The family nurtures and educates its members, providing a vital system of support that is identifiable by its own style and integrity. The family is also a stressful social and emotional system. Development is supported and thwarted as the family and its members interrelate. The individual is influenced by a multitude of family dynamics, which affect self-development and prepare the individual for the larger world of the community.

Group Development

The family is a type of group. Groups have their own organizational structure and dynamics. Individuals affiliate with myriad groups throughout their lives and grow and develop through and in these group relationships. Groups have a life of their own and not only significantly influence their members but also the larger circle of community. Groups are a rich resource for individuals, families, and communities. Groups vary according to their intended purpose, style of leadership, phase of development, longevity, and interactional patterns. Each group is unique and balances the needs of the individual members with its own particular focus (Clark, 1994).

Groups can be informal or formal in their organization, depending on the type of group and its leadership process. Friendships and a variety of other affiliations result as individuals bond together and form groups. These informal groupings may last throughout a lifetime or may be connected to developmental phases or purposefully short-lived goals. Groups serve to foster development beyond the family and to strengthen connections to schools, agencies, religious institutions, and other persons. They protect against isolation and enable individuals to identify special interests and skills. There are at least four types of formal groups: task, teaching, support, and psychotherapy. A task group focuses on the accomplishment of a given task and emphasizes decision-making and problem-solving. In most task groups there is pressure to complete the task in an allocated time period; the outcome is key. Examples of task groups include a parent-teacher association, a committee to form a library, and volunteer community service groups. A teaching group is concerned with the processing of information and the teaching-learning exchange. Teaching groups abound and include scouting organizations, 4-H clubs, and health education groups. Support groups are commonplace in most communities. These groups assist their members in dealing with emotional stress and focus on the expression of thoughts and feelings. The members often serve as living examples of effective coping survivorship since many support groups deal with loss and adjustment. These groups may be self-help or led by professionals. Support groups include Alcoholics Anonymous and Alanon, bereavement groups, and coalitions such as the Alliance for the Mentally Ill. Psychotherapy groups deal with intrapersonal and interpersonal aspects of personality (Ormont, 1992; Yalom, 1985). Psychotherapy groups may subscribe to a particular psychologic theory or paradigm. These groups serve persons with diverse needs, such as families, partners, children, and those with common psychiatric problems.

Leadership is best described as a process that occurs within groups. This process may be shared among the members or reside with a particular leader, either someone identified by the group or someone who emerges from the group. When the leadership process is directed by an identified leader, it is considered to be authoritarian or leader-centered. If group process is shared, the leadership style is considered democratic, or group-oriented. When the process is less active, the style is thought of as laissez-faire; in this case, consultation may be offered, information provided at timely interludes, and less activity expected from the leadership process.

Groups, as living systems, have a lifespan. Some groups may be intentionally short lived, whereas others may extend for months or years. Longevity influences the development of a group. Some groups may exist for a particular purpose and meet only once. Other groups may unfold and grow into different types for other purposes, taking on new form over time because of changing needs of the members. Groups generally begin with an orientation phase in which common issues are discussed, namely, identity; control and power; the balancing of individual needs with group needs; and finally, acceptance and intimacy. Each of these issues are revisited again and again as the group develops. To move into working phase, many of these issues must be dealt with and assumptions stated so that members are clear about what the group stands for and what they believe. To arrive at the working phase, the group must learn to work together cooperatively toward its intended purpose—accomplishing a given task, imparting knowledge, gaining support, or enabling intrapsychic analysis. As groups move toward closure, they evaluate and summarize the group experience.

A group is characterized by its dynamics, which include communication, conflict, decision-making, bonding, and role identification and are influenced by the individual members who comprise the group, as well as the forces from outside the group that impinge on its development. *Communication* within a group occurs through not only what is said but also through behaviors, including body language and tone of voice (Watzlawick, 1978). Tension and anxiety exist in every group and reflect unexplained feelings of discomfort, especially when members' expectations are not being met. *Conflict* is a normal and necessary group dynamic that signifies opposing forces within a group. Conflict may be restricted to individual members, occur in subgroups, or take place for the entire group. Subgroups are subsystems of a group. These subgroups, referred to as *coalitions,* may occur when individual needs supersede the group so that small groups or pairs within the group compete and split off from the group as a whole. *Decision-making* is another important dynamic that every group experiences. Groups can make decisions through consensus (when all members agree), by accommodation (when members come to agreement through compromise), or by a defacto process (when members simply lack dissent). Groups make decisions and carry out their intended purpose with a strong orientation to shared norms, which are the rules that govern group behavior. Another dynamic, group *bonding,* creates a sense of belonging to something beyond the self and thus helps create the group's own identity. Cohesiveness, the attraction of group members for each other, is necessary for bonding to occur. Members of groups also experience *role identification.* Roles are expected behaviors of members. Members generally assume task roles, which help the group function through the accomplishment of group goals, or maintenance roles, which serve to keep members connected to each other and to keep the group functioning. In addition to these healthy roles, there are self-serving roles that impede group process. Some groups experience the dynamic of *apathy,* which occurs when the group is unable to mobilize energy to continue. Indifference and boredom are characteristic of group apathy.

Community Development

The community comprises the wider circles of interaction that support the family, other groups, and the individual members. The community supports the tangible resources that individuals use to grow and develop beyond the family and groups. Resources include schools, houses of worship, recreational facilities, health and social services, communication networks, safety and protective agencies, transportation, and political and economic structures (Anderson & McFarlane, 1996). Each community has its own particular identity and style of leadership (Warren, 1977; Loomis, 1957). Communities provide the broader context of living in which individuals, families, and groups may learn to become consumers and participants.

A community refers to "people in the context of their environment as they continuously interact with each other and the environment" (Arnold, 1997, p. 107). Communities can be viewed from a variety of perspectives to gain a fuller understanding of the nature of the community and the interactions that characterize it. A simple way to look at a community is through its structure and function. The structure of a community includes the persons who comprise it and its physical characteristics. The function of a community includes the use of community resources by its members and the linkages between persons and the resources, as well as members' unique patterns of living in their environment. Other definitions of a community relate to the alignment or misalignment of resources and the nature of intimacy in it (Loomis, 1957). Typologies (Warren, 1977) of community life have been shaped to reflect the nature of leadership, cohesiveness, self-sufficiency, and ties to the larger society. Communities can also be viewed by their functional capacity to undertake responsibilities such as space utilization, livelihood, protection, education, participation, productivity, and linkages to other systems (Higgs & Gustafson, 1985). Communities, like groups, are formed through affiliations as persons come together through common union, which may be a geographical locale or a shared culture or value system. Some communities are created through memberships or common experiences or causes. Communities are capable of self-care through effective partnerships (Anderson & McFarlane, 1996) or alliances (Klainberg, Holzemer, Leonard, & Arnold, 1997). Communities also possess caring capacities that enable them to be the providers of care and nurture for their members. Communities, to a great extent, define themselves. Each community forms its own image that is appreciative of its unique components, including the population of the community and its resources, culture, economics, and geography. A community is a system that develops and grows through the interaction of these component forces.

Within the community context, the individual develops and grows. The community provides multiple opportunities for socialization; the individual relates to neighbors, makes friendships, and forms acquaintances through routine tasks such as food shopping and obtaining necessary services. Through these tasks, the individual becomes known and is afforded opportunities to participate in community life. Commitments, such as volunteering at the local hospital, fire department, library, or athletic events, enable the individual and family to develop larger networks for socialization and to develop and use skills that may assist others and deepen involvement in the life of the community. Development is also fostered by the ability of individuals to locate work and earn a living within the community context. Working provides the individual with a means of livelihood and the ability to support an independent life-style. The development of self through work or professional identify expands the defining qualities of the self and fosters role assumption. The community, by providing the context for means of livelihood through employment, establishes an economic foundation to support community services.

The community is an educator, informing its members about resources and support systems that promote development. The community can protect its members through its resources, individuals, families, and social agencies. Its resources also can nurture and support growth in individual members, as illustrated by an excerpt from Jonathan Kozol's work. Jonathan Kozol (1995), writing of children living in the crime and drug-ridden community of Mott Haven in the South Bronx, describes Anthony, a bright, reflective 12-year-old who presents himself as a "writer of novels." Befriended by the pastor of his community church, Anthony is introduced to Juan Castro, a poet and true intellectual who has lived in the South Bronx for more than 50 years, writing, teaching, and translating the works of Milton into Spanish. Under the protective wing of Castro, Anthony's image of himself as a writer is nurtured. He brings his work to Castro, who reads it carefully, responds to it, and introduces Anthony to the great writers and poets of the Western world. Castro says to Kozol:

> The solitary figure of this child touches me tremendously. His mentality, as you have noticed, is not organized and that is part of his attraction. When he rings my bell, it pleases me. He reminds me by his earnestness of Don Quixote. He told me once, 'If I could not write, I would go crazy.' Children long for this—a voice, a way of being heard—but many sense that there is no one in the world to hear their words, so they are drawn to ways of malice (Kozol, 1995, p. 239).

Anthony is a rare child whose spirit and talent are nurtured by a significant adult in his community. Kozol describes this situation as a "little miracle" that happens infrequently as certain children create safe spaces for themselves that help them transcend the dreariness and danger of their lives (Kozol, 1995, p. 160). These safe spaces can be filled with teachers, clergy, caregivers, and neighbors within a community who offer nurture and protection to the child and his/her hopes and dreams in absence of family or family support. The nurture, protection, and support of a community can be life saving for both the individual and family.

Some communities are depleted of resources and have little to offer their members. Increased crime, limited services, insufficient leadership, and natural disasters contribute to the demise of communities. Withdrawal of governmental funding and private investment drains communities of the means to support services for members, thereby abandoning them. As publicly funded health and social services diminish and the public health infrastructure disappears, communities become at great risk. Communities may become so depleted and chaotic that members cannot access even limited services. Persons who live in poverty; who are homeless; and who suffer chronic illness and disability and recently arrived immigrant populations are severely affected by the lack of community supports for individuals and families. Communities also become alienated from their members when they lose their unique flavors or identities, giving way to large, impersonal commercial areas.

The community's development is influenced by the availability of resources beyond it, as well as the needs and contributions of families and individuals within it. Communities form, grow, die, or transform as their members and institutions change. There is potential in communities for transformation. For instance, surviving agencies and organized groups in communities depleted of most resources often open their doors to serve community needs. For example, a local house of worship may temporarily house a vulnerable member of the community and become a shelter as the need grows and others seek assistance. In many communities, nonhealth care agencies and groups of individuals and families united by common bonds are extending their missions and boundaries and are becoming the community's social service agencies.

THWARTED AND NONACTUALIZED DEVELOPMENT

The complex and dynamic process of development beginning at conception and ending at death can be viewed as a trajectory moving through space and time. There is a convergence of factors and events that affect development at any time along this trajectory. These include genetic, physiologic, and intrapersonal factors; interpersonal connections; societal patterns; cultural traditions and variations; and the occurrence of significant life events and stressors. Separately and in combination, these events and factors may adversely affect development, resulting in a nonactualized self. The nonactualized self may be recognized in the person who does not reach his/her potential; whose options are perceived to be or are in fact limited; and who views himself/herself as unworthy, unhealthy, or abnormal.

Recent advances in the complex and evolving field of genetics reveal linkages between specific genes or genetic patterns and the presence of illness—both mental and physiologic. Because of this, a new area for exploration and understanding is unfolding, contributing to a broader appreciation of the origins of some human conditions and behaviors. The affective, addictive, and psychotic disorders, which normally begin in adolescence and adulthood, are debilitating chronic mental disorders with genetic underpinnings that are not well understood. These conditions severely impair a person's perception of himself/herself and his/her ability to make plans and choices for the present and future. Physical illnesses with strong genetic bases, such as cystic fibrosis, Huntington's chorea, and sickle cell disease, can adversely affect development in childhood, adolescence, and throughout adulthood, depending on severity, age of onset, availability of treatment, and family and community support.

Substance abuse, poor nutrition, and lack of prenatal care during pregnancy separately and in combination influence the growth of the fetus in utero and affect the health and well-being of the newborn, which has lasting effects on development as the infant evolves into a child, adolescent, and adult. Children born to substance-abusing mothers, including those born with fetal alcohol syndrome, are affected throughout their lives in areas of cognition and social and emotional development. Infants born of HIV-infected mothers who themselves become infected, as well as children who acquire or develop life-threatening illness during infancy and early childhood, risk interference in normal development imposed by their disease, treatment, frequent hospitalizations, and separation from families.

The death of a parent or sibling deeply affects the developing child, especially the young or adolescent child. Interference in early relationships with parents and siblings because of mental or physical illness also adversely affects the child's development. Indeed, relationships—the connections between and among human beings—when broken or altered significantly throughout the lifespan thwart or delay development at any age or at any stage and thus impede learning and growth.

There are external factors that can impinge on the developing individual, family, and community. Societal patterns, including poverty, violence, racial discrimination, and oppression, contribute adversely to development. Violence within families, groups, and communities severs the trust between persons and erodes the foundations upon which development is built. Violence within families and communities may result in placement of children in foster care agencies or other homes; incarceration of adults; death; or emotional injury to members, young and old. Violence can alter the ability of the family and community to protect and care for its members. Violence, as a negative force, limits options and opportunity.

A social and political climate that devalues and does not support education and health care for its population deprives individuals and families of opportunities to learn, grow, and maintain health. External events, including natural disasters, wars, and violent conflicts, contribute to the deprivation of all affected individuals, families, and communities by interfering with development by limiting opportunities for decision-making and growth.

The individual, family, group, or community may be more vulnerable to certain stressors than others at specific times along the developmental trajectory. Consider the infant or young child dependent on parents and adult caretakers for nurturance, sustenance, protection, and care who is orphaned and set adrift with hundreds of refugee children. Without care, nurturance, and love, the young child will most certainly die. Consider the young adolescent sold into prostitution for a meager sum to support her family, moved from rural to urban surroundings away from known supports of family and community. Consider the elderly man or woman abandoned by family and placed without warning in a residential setting, deprived of loved ones and personal possessions. In these three situations, the stressors are so overwhelming (the individuals are deprived of external supports) that development and actualization of self are quite literally halted. Consider families left homeless by massive flooding and devastation. Consider groups and communities robbed of their resources and inhabitants in the wake of war or natural disaster. In these cases, mere survival or the wish to die becomes the goal of existence. Without intervention, the effect of these stressors on the developing self at any stage can be profound. The loss of potential in the individual, family, group, and community cannot be measured; development can be thwarted, altered, or halted temporarily or forever.

Replenishing and Sustaining Development

There is within every human being, family, group, and community the potential for fullness of development. This potential is realized as the person, family, group, and community participate in directing their development. Actualizing the image of the healthy self rests in the capacity for projecting a personal image of health and in doing so, choosing actions that reduce health risks and optimize health strengths, making informed decision and choices, and assuming responsibility for self-care. This process occurs at both the micro-level for individuals and families and the macro-level for communities and larger systems. Development is not a steady, measured process. The healthy person, family, group, and community grow and develop through self-sustaining efforts.

Effective strategies to promote self-development, family growth, and group and community strength focus on partnership and participation. Social support is a recognized vehicle for promoting the healthy self. Individuals who receive little support from others have lower positive well-being, which is one aspect of health (Schaefer, Coyne, & Lazarus, 1981). Longitudinal research has shown that individuals who occupy few social roles, particularly those in a family; have little interaction with others; and have no close contacts have higher mortality rates than others (Berkman & Syme, 1979; Blazer, 1982). The impact of social support on health, particularly mental health, either buffers or protects from the effect of stress (review in Cohen & Willis, 1985; Sheinfeld Gorin, 1995).

There are actions that can be taken to replenish and sustain the self as it develops. These actions for the individual include the following:

1. Maintenance of relationships that provide nurture, support, and the opportunity for reciprocity.
2. Participation in purposeful activity in the form of working, producing a product, obtaining satisfaction, and providing income and support.

3. Provision of adequate nutrition, physical exercise, and rest.
4. Participation in educational and recreational activities.
5. Enjoyment of aesthetic and cultural experiences.
6. Enhancement of spirituality.
7. Experiencing necessary losses and expressing grief.
8. Introspection and self-examination.

Families develop and grow through the accomplishment of tasks and functions that sustain and strengthen them. Some families grow through the need to separate or divorce. These actions are self-preserving and often serve to protect the members of the family. Divorce leads to the possibility of blending or reconstituting a family with others (Carter & McGoldrick, 1989). The new family survives with the hope of creating its own identity and to become a healthier support for its members.

Groups change as their intended purposes are fulfilled and as phases of group development meld into each other and move toward termination with the establishment of new ties outside the group. Groups are replenished through the introduction of new members, as members leave, and as groups reshape their purpose. Groups expand and contract through the interactional process of membership, desired affiliations, and inner dynamics.

Communities are replenished as they transform and develop, as populations and cultural groups enter and leave, as resources open and close, and as industrialization and housing expansion alter the structure and function. Communities also change as their populations and resources shift; when resources are linked to human need, the community's development is enhanced. Communities are strengthened through crises, as members pull together to support each other and rebuild.

Change is often an introspective process. The healthy self must undergo self-examination. The process of growth encompasses times of triumph, as well as struggle; challenges are met, adversity is translated into meaning, stressors are coped with, and pride is taken in valued choices. Inherent in change is loss and a resultant reexamination of the self. This reexamination often calls upon the inner sources of strength derived from spiritual beliefs and values. Spirituality provides hope in the time of adversity and affirms an inner core of support. Development also necessitates the integration of loss, as well as gains, so that unmet challenges, adversity, and stress do not result in paralysis and apathy. Grieving assists in the healthy process of integration of loss and gains.

The significance of spirituality and grieving to health and health promotion cannot be overestimated. Special attention must be directed to each as powerful processes for replenishing and sustaining the healthy self.

Spirituality

Spirituality is a self-sustaining force as well as a domain of the individual, family, group, and community. As such, spirituality nurtures the development of self and is a reflection of the health of the self. Schuster and Ashburn (1992) describe the spiritual domain as encompassing all the transcendental aspects of self. It is the center of awareness of existence. It is also the hopefulness within the self, the family, and community that sustains life in the face of adversity and loss.

Erikson, Erikson, and Kivick (1986) traced the early development of the spiritual domain in the emergence of trust and hope in infancy. This essential strength matures over the lifespan and sustains the development of all subsequent strength.

At the end of life, we may find that some rudimentary hope has blossomed into a mature faith in being that is closely related to essential wisdom. (Erikson, Erikson, & Kivick, 1986, p. 218)

All of the basic virtues, including hope, will, purpose, competence, fidelity, love, care, and wisdom, that emerge from a successful resolution of the developmental tasks described by Erikson are components of the spiritual domain (Schuster & Ashburn, 1992).

Spirituality as a life force in the individual, family, group, and community is less well-understood. Persons confronting dependencies and addictions often find strength through spiritual awakening during the struggles of detoxification and recovery. Spirituality is the life force that might help to explain the resilience and courage of a grandmother as she realizes the task of raising her grandchildren bereft of their mother while she grieves for her daughter. Groups and communities hold to their spiritual beliefs and values in the face of poverty, oppression, and victimization, finding perseverance, emancipation, and repudiation possible. Spirituality, as a life force (Coles, 1990), contributes to the self-esteem and strength of the individual; to the courage and resilience of the family; and to the energy, hope, and steadfastness of groups and the community.

Grief and Loss

Grief is a vital function of human experience that facilitates healing and the potential for personal growth and development through the integration of loss into the self (Arnold, 1995). The facilitation of grief assists individuals, families, and even communities to live with losses inherent in the life process. Some losses are part of the natural experience of development (e.g., losing the innocence of childhood for the realizations of adolescence or losing one's youth as aging ensues). Other losses are unexpected, such as sudden death, losing employment, or having to move to another home. Some losses are sadly expected (e.g., those that occur after a terminal diagnosis is given or after disease progresses and health is diminished). It is not uncommon for the grief associated with the myriad losses in life to be unacknowledged. Grieving can be a solitary experience and one that many persons try to put away and leave unattended because the pain of their loss may be unbearable and difficult to experience. Loss may become a family secret or be denied. There are many reasons for grief being unacknowledged. For some, time simply increasingly separates them from the loss and therefore the opportunity to grieve. The health care professional will often encounter clients, whether individuals, families, or communities, who have experienced loss but have not had the opportunity to grieve or to recognize their need to grieve. Consider the impact of one person's death. This person may have been the partner of another who is now dealing with the pain of loss and emotional separation. This person may have had a family that now feel unwhole without this member. This person may have been part of a community which experiences the loss and seeks to protect its members from a similar death. Each individual touches others and thus everexpanding circles of affected individuals are left to experience the emotions of loss through grief.

Life is filled with loss. Losses may be minor, almost imperceptible, or they may be significant and overwhelming. Individuals grieve as they leave childhood and move through adolescence into middle adulthood and old age. Individuals grieve as relationships change and end and when separation and divorce occur. Individuals grieve for jobs lost and positions changed. Individuals grieve at graduations, birthdays, celebrations of the new year, the changing seasons, and events marking a passage of time never regained. Individuals also grieve in their dying, and their survivors grieve for them (Arnold, 1996).

The grieving process, although a universal response to loss, becomes individualized as each person reacts and copes using his/her own sources of strength and comfort. In this way, each person forms a unique mosaic of responses that become a pattern of grieving (Arnold, 1995). Some pieces of the mosaic are internal, whereas others reflect religion, culture, family belief systems, and traditions.

Memory fuels grief and helps to maintain the connection with the lost object, experience, or person. Grief is not a tragic episode, nor a pathologic state, and it cannot be equated with illness. On the contrary, grief is a healthy process in which one integrates loss and maintains a connection to the lost person or object and learns to live without (Arnold, 1995).

Facilitating the grieving process assists individuals, families, and communities to learn to live with and integrate loss. It is never too late to acknowledge grief or to facilitate the expression of grief. Facilitation of grief is a therapeutic intervention that fosters-self development and growth. The script that follows serves to guide the health care professional through an example conversation about loss and grief. Statements and questions are given that help move the interaction closer to the feelings of loss, which allow for the expression of grief. Throughout this interaction, the health care professional is a careful, active listener. The client is not pushed to answer; the health care professional thoughtfully waits for the client to choose a response. Each response is acknowledged for its importance and the inherent difficulty that can be experienced in uncovering unacknowledged loss. If the client chooses to not respond or replies, "No" to questions about a loss, then the health care professional accepts this response, recognizing with the client that this is something the client does not wish to speak about or put into words.

SELF-DEVELOPMENT & THE HEALTH PROMOTION MATRIX

Clients often seek out a health care professional expecting to be able to let go of a loss and detach from the relationship and are often troubled by their inability to do so. When the grieving person has incorporated the concepts of abnormality or pathology into his/her notion of grief, the internal imaging is of illness or disability. For example, a middle-age woman seeks the assistance of the health care professional at her family's urging because they are worried about her emotional health, fearing she is preoccupied with her mother's death and becoming depressed. The woman indicates to the health care professional that she cannot "get over" the death of her mother. Recognizing that her mother died about 1 year ago, the client believes that something is wrong because she continues to grieve for her mother. She continues to think about her mother, and recently she has been experiencing more thoughts of her mother, which started to increase around the time of the anniversary of her mother's death. Recognizing this association between the more intense expressions of her grief and the anniversary date only made the client wonder whether she was "losing her mind." The client finds little solace in her recollections of her mother; rather these memories provoke anxiety and fear. The client expected her grief to diminish. It became difficult for the client to share her anxiety and fears, believing that once admitted, these expressions would prove her emotional instability. Her family's concern served to validate her fears.

Image Creation

....

Client: I cannot seem to get over the death of my mother. She died more than 1 year ago, and I find myself thinking about her more than ever.
Health care professional: How had you expected to feel now more than 1 year after her death?
Client: I had not expected to be thinking about her so much.
Health care professional: What do you think about and remember of your mother?
Client: Not so much of her dying but of the many times we were together— when I was a child and an adult with her.
Health care professional: It sounds as if so many of those memories are good.
Client: Oh, very good. I do enjoy them, as I miss her.
Health care professional: What you are experiencing in your grief is both sadness and healing. Your many memories provide a connection between you and your mother. Your expectation of getting over your grief was based on a misconception of extended grief as being abnormal.
Client: I would like to feel better. I want to feel connected to my mother and not be so sad and afraid of my feelings.

....

The client's communication to the health care professional conveys an image of pathology, which provides an opportunity for intervention. The health care professional can interpret for the client that what she is experiencing in her grief is both sadness and healing. The health care professional indicates that memories can provide a link (i.e., an important connection between the client and her mother) and clarifies an expectation the client holds about getting over her grief, which is based on a misconception that extended grief is abnormal. Rather, healthy grieving has no bounds and serves as a connection, thereby enabling healing through the integration of the loss into the self. This client will feel better (her desired image) by feeling connected to her mother and not so sad or afraid to allow herself to grieve.

Grief is experienced and integrated into the life of the person experiencing a loss. During image creation, the health care professional validates that the client's grief is a healthy expression of her sadness in being separated by death from her mother. The expressions of her grief are her way of keeping connected to her mother and healing (i.e., learning to live without her mother). Expressions of intense grief are often associated with anniversary dates, birthdays, and other occasions of particular importance to the individual and family. The health care professional can also ask this client whether she would like to ask her family members to join her for a subsequent appointment so that her grief experience could be shared and understood with her family. Members of the family will also be experiencing grief, each in his/her own way.

Image Appraisal

Image appraisal offers an opportunity for the client and health care professional to examine the client's experience of grief both in relation to her current loss and past experiences with loss. It is not uncommon for childhood and even adult experiences of loss to go unrecognized and unattended. Individuals often grieve in a solitary way. Families can become emotionally splintered when a death occurs. Members may not communicate with each other or as a whole family. Individual family members can isolate themselves, feel misunderstood, and disconnected. Each person grieves in his/her own way. The health care professional can be instrumental in bringing family members together to listen and understand each other, as well as to appreciate each person's differences.

During image appraisal the health care professional is able to delve with the client into past experiences with loss and grief. These past expressions, often denied, may emerge and become intertwined with the current loss. It is often useful to learn about the client's prior experiences with loss, how that loss was dealt with, whether emotions were expressed, and if a support network was in place. The health care professional assists the client to learn about prior experiences of loss and grief as a context for understanding current experiences and concerns.

Minimize Health Depleting Patterns

The health care professional and client explore the conditions that seem to have limited the client in expressing grief. Recalling how expressions of grief were treated in the past is informative. The client may have been taught that emotions are to be supressed or reduced so that self-control is maintained. This expectation may have resulted in the capacity to hide emotions and not share them. The client may have learned to bury emotions in favor of appearing unaffected. As expressions of grief break through, the client has learned to repress them. Reoccurring expressions of grief may alarm the client, because a past "successful" strategy is no longer effective. Together the health care professional and client identify the many ways that grief has been limited in its expression.

Optimize Health Supportive Patterns

Sharing expressions of grief can often be a way to validate a loss and to gain support from others. Identifying a client's natural support system and learning how and when the client is comfortable to call upon that support system is therapeutic. In this way, the client will not feel so alone and will locate the capacity to call upon others during times of sadness and aloneness. Simply identifying a supportive person or network helps the client not feel so alone. It may be helpful for clients to set the parameters for the support they seek, since others may be uncomfortable discussing loss and grief. The client must learn to ask for what is needed and what is helpful. For example, it may be necessary for the client to be able to say; "It helps me to share memories of my mother—sharing helps me remember the good times and that helps me feel better. It means so much to me that you want to listen."

Internalize Idealized Image

The client begins to learn to live with loss as he/she becomes more aware of its presence and power. Each client will find some way to feel satisfaction and comfort in the experience of loss and learning to live without. Writing in a journal is an example of a tangible means for self-expression. Some will find visits to a cemetery are therapeutic because they allow for private time and the expression of private thoughts. Others will volunteer or engage in some kind of unfinished business. Each person can find comfort in personal expressions that enable grief to become more a part of the self. The health care professional prepares the client for the ongoing nature of grief, which changes in depth and intensity over time. Periods of greater intensity may occur predictably at special events (e.g., birthdays, anniversaries) or quite unexpectedly. The client learns about the complexities of grief, how to find solace in memories, and to recognize that feelings of happiness can mingle with feelings of sadness and loss. The health care professional invites the client to make follow-up appointments at times the client wants to return. If other referrals (e.g., grief therapist, family therapist) are indicated, these can be planned with the client and expedited. Lastly, the health care professional recognizes the sense of satisfaction the client may experience in learning about the process of grief, gaining self-understanding, and living with loss.

GRIEF AND LOSS: *A Script*

Image Creation	How had you expected to feel at this time?
	When you think about your loss, what do you think about and remember?
	I'd like to know more about your loss. Can you share more?
	It sounds as though many of your memories are good ones. Is this so?
	Is it possible to think that your grief is your way of keeping connected?
Image Appraisal	Every person experiences loss. Some losses are never expressed.
	Can you remember a loss that you have experienced and perhaps have never talked about?
	Can you talk about that loss?
	When did this loss occur?
	How old were you at the time?
	Do you remember where you were when the loss occurred?
	How did this loss affect you?
	Can you remember how you felt?

continued

GRIEF AND LOSS: *A Script—cont'd*

As we talk about the loss, do those feelings surface?

Can you describe the feelings now?

Where have those feelings been?

Minimize Health Depleting Patterns

Would your life have been changed or different if you had been able to express your loss?

Is there anything now that you can do with those feelings?

What do you want to do?

How do these feelings connect to what you are experiencing now?

Optimize Health Supportive Patterns

Is there someone you would like to tell about your feelings?

Would you be able to write down your feelings?

Is there a way you can express them?

Internalize Idealized Image

Can you search for ways to express your grief that provide self-satisfaction and comfort?

Can you create a special way to remember?

The health care professional assists the client in identifying the various ways that feelings can be expressed (e.g., writing in a journal, creating a service, planting a tree, creating a plaque, planning a family or community meeting, seeking counseling, completing something left undone.

When you find yourself feeling very sad or alone, do you think you will find solace in the memories you have created?

Feelings of happiness will mingle with grief. Can you allow these feelings of happiness and pleasure to be experienced?

Times of more intense grief can recur. Will you call for a follow-up appointment to talk about your feelings and concerns at these times?

The health care professional contracts with the client for follow-up (e.g., another appointment, a referral) so that a plan can be fulfilled. The health care professional recognizes the satisfaction the client may experience—satisfaction felt at last.

SELF-DEVELOPMENT AND THERAPEUTIC INTERACTION

Problems That Hamper Therapeutic Interaction

The following reactions limit a health care professional's interventions in facilitating the grieving process:

- Avoidance: The health care professional may experience discomfort with discussing personal loss and may discourage or avoid, rather than encourage, authentic communication because the pain of the client provokes the health care professional's own sense of loss and pain.
- Depletion: The health care professional may experience emotional exhaustion and feel unable to give of herself/himself. Therapeutic communication about grief rests in the health care professional's ability to share by giving of the self for therapeutic purpose. Health care professionals need to find ways to refuel themselves, particularly when their work immerses them in the experience of others' grief.
- Anxiety: Painful areas of discussion are often difficult to sustain. The health care professional may exhibit anxiety during such times in the communication. Talking, rather than active listening, may be a sign that the health care professional is experiencing anxiety. Supervision and thoughtful analysis of the interaction is essential to give the health care professional a greater understanding of other means to meet personal needs and how to sustain a client-centered focus.
- Forced resolution: The health care professional is careful not to seek resolution since grief is often experienced as an ongoing process, rather than a event that must be resolved. Forcing resolution is often done because the health care professional is uncomfortable with the emotions of the client and hopes the situation can end. Rather than offering reassurance, the health care professional offers acceptance and validation of the pain of the expression. This is experienced by the client as acceptance and validation of the self.

Efforts that Facilitate Therapeutic Interaction

The following actions enhance a health care professional's interventions in facilitating the grieving process:

- Supervision: Health care professionals benefit from opportunities for reflection and introspection that are available in an organized and consistent fashion through supervision. Supervision can be contracted with colleagues or through case conferences. The intent is to allow the health care professional the opportunity to objectively analyze the case material and her/his own interactions.
- Case finding: Health care professionals who are willing to recognize the importance of loss and grief as human experiences that facilitate growth and personal development are more likely to be open and available to clients for these discussions. The health care professional listens for experiences of loss and is particularly attuned to the possibility of unacknowledged grief. The health care professional also recognizes that losses are experienced not only by individuals but also by families and communities. Family meetings and group meetings are just as feasible as a session with an individual client.
- Expanding the comfort zone: As the health care professional becomes astute in listening for experiences of loss and responding to them, she/he becomes more comfortable in dealing with loss. It is possible to become more comfortable in interacting with loss through clinical experience and with clinical supervision.

■ Continuing education: Health care professionals may desire to pursue education about loss and grief through clinical literature and conferences and through seeking certification in the field of grief counseling and grief education.

■ Shifting paradigm of grief: The health care professional views grief as an integrative life process that continues throughout the lifespan and enables the client to gain insight as well as to grow as personal development is enhanced. Closing the door on grief or containing it only serves to limit the potential for personal growth.

■ Tool development: Assessment tools for patterns of health and risk often neglect to include incidence of loss and death in the individual and family health components. Use of the genogram (Pendagast & Sherman, 1973-1978) as a graphic representation of family connectedness can also reveal deaths and health problems, which should prompt the health care professional to explore with the client the meaning and significance of these losses in the client's history and family life. Further development of inventories of loss and the creation of clinical guidelines for attending to loss will enhance clinical practice.

Summary

Each individual, family, group, and community possesses a self-identity that shapes and influences the actualization of its health potential. Self-development is an interactive process of actualizing the potential for health across the lifespan. Development of the self traverses all ages and times in the lives of human beings. Individuals grow and contribute to the development of themselves, their families, groups they affiliate with, and communities in which they live. Likewise, families, groups, and communities each have developmental processes and dynamics. Individuals, families, groups, and communities all possess self-identities that affect and are affected by the interactive nature of these dynamic human systems.

HELPFUL **RESOURCES**

BOOKS ON GRIEF

Arnold, J.H., & Gemma, P.B. (1994). *A child dies: A portrait of family grief.* Philadelphia: The Charles Press.

Borg, S., & Lasker, J. (1989). *When pregnancy fails: Families coping with miscarriage, ectopic pregnancy, stillbirth, and infant death.* New York: Bantam Books.

Grollman, E.A. (1990). *Talking about death: A dialogue between parent and child.* Boston: Beacon Press.

Grollman, E.A. (1993). *Straight talk about death for teenagers.* Boston: Beacon Press.

Gunther, J. (1949). *Death be not proud: A memoir.* New York: Harper and Row.

Klass, D., Silverman, P.R., & Nickman, S.L. (Eds.). (1996). *Continuing bonds: New understandings of grief.* Bristol, PA: Taylor and Francis.

Moffat, M.J. (Ed.). (1992). *In the midst of winter: Selections from the literature of mourning.* New York: Vintage Books.

Worden, J.W. (1996). *Children and grief: When a parent dies.* New York: Guilford Press.

ON-LINE

GriefNet
http://www.griefnet.demon.co.uk
http://rivendell.org/about.html

References

Anderson, E.T., & McFarlane, J.M. (1996). *Community as partner: Theory and practice in nursing* (2nd ed.). Philadelphia: Lippincott.

Arnold, J. (1995). *A reconceptualization of the concept of grief for nursing: A philosophical analysis.* Unpublished doctoral dissertation, New York University.

Arnold, J. (1996). Rethinking grief: Nursing implications for health promotion. *Home Healthcare Nurse, 14*(10), 777-783.

Arnold, J. (1997). The community as client. In M. Klainberg, S. Holzemer, M. Leonard, & J. Arnold. *Community health nursing: An alliance for health.* New York: McGraw Hill.

Arnold, J.H., & Gemma, P.B. (1994). *A child dies: A portrait of family grief* (2nd ed.). Philadelphia: The Charles Press.

Berkman, L.R., & Syme, S.L. (1979). Social networks, host resistance, and mortality: A nine-year follow-up study of Alameda County residents. *American Journal of Epidemiology, 109,* 186-204.

Blazer, D.G. (1982). Social support and mortality in an elderly community population. *American Journal of Epidemiology, 115,* 684-694.

Bowen, M. (1978). *Family therapy in clinical practice.* New York: Jason Aronson.

Carter, B., & McGoldrick, M. (Eds.). (1989). *The changing family life cycle: A framework for family therapy* (2nd ed.). Boston: Allyn & Bacon.

Chess, S., & Thomas, A. (1986). *Temperament in clinical practice.* New York: Guilford.

Clark, C.C. (1994). *The nurse as group leader* (3rd ed.). New York: Springer.

Coles, R. (1990). *The spiritual life of children.* Boston: Houghton Mifflin.

Coles, R. (1997). *The moral intelligence of children.* New York: Random House.

Cohen, S., & Willis, T.A. (1985). Stress, social support, and the buffering hypothesis. *Psychological Bulletin, 98,* 310-357.

Duvall, E.R.M. (1985). *Marriage and family development* (6th ed.). New York: Harper and Row.

Erikson, E.H. (1963). *Childhood and society* (2nd ed.). New York: Norton.

Erikson, E.H. (1968). *Identity, youth and crisis.* New York: Norton.

Erikson, E.H., Erikson, J.M., & Kivick, H.Q. (1986). *Vital involvement in old age.* New York: WW Norton.

Fogarty, T.F. (1985). On stress. *The Family, 12*(2), 15-19.

Freud, S. (1935). *A general introduction to psychoanalysis* (authorized English translation of the revised edition by J. Riviere). New York: Liveright.

Gilligan, C. (1984). *In a different voice.* Cambridge, MA: Harvard University Press.

Gilligan, C. (1987). Remapping the moral domain. In T.C. Keller et al (Eds.). *Reconstructing individualism: Autonomy, individuality, and the self in Western thought.* Stanford, CA: Stanford University Press.

Haley, J. (1980). *Leaving home.* New York: McGraw-Hill.

Havighurst, R.J. (1972). *Developmental tasks and education* (3rd ed.). New York: McKay.

Higgs, Z.R., & Gustafson, D.D. (1985). *Community as a client: Assessment and disgnosis.* Philadelphia: FA Davis.

Kagan, J. (1984). *The nature of the child.* New York: Basic Books.

Kagan, J. (1989). *Unstable ideas: Temperament, cognition, and self.* Cambridge, MA: Harvard University Press.

Klainberg, M., Holzemer, S., Leonard, M., & Arnold, J. (1997). *Community health nursing: An alliance for health.* New York: McGraw-Hill.

Kohlberg, L. (1981). *The philosophy of moral development.* San Francisco: Harper & Row.

Kozol, J. (1995). *Amazing grace.* New York: Crown Publishers.

Locke, J. (1964). Some thoughts concerning education (abridged). In P. Gay (Ed.), *John Locke on education.* New York: Bureau of Publications, Teachers College, Columbia University.

Loomis, C.P. (Ed.). (1957). *Tönnies: Community and society (Gemeinschaft und Gesellschaft).* East Lansing, MI: Michigan State University Press.

Maslow, A.H. (1968). *Toward a psychology of being* (2nd ed.). Princeton, NJ: Van Nostrand.

Mellonie, B., & Ingpen, R. (1983). *Lifetimes.* New York: Bantam Books.

Minuchin, S. (1974). *Families and family therapy.* Cambridge, MA: Harvard University Press.

Minuchin, S., & Nichols, M. (1993). *Family healing.* New York: Free Press.

Ormont, L.R. (1992) *The group therapy experience: From theory to practice.* New York: St. Martin's Press.

Pendagast, E.G., & Sherman, C.O. (1973-1978). *A guide to the genogram. The Family Compendium I. The Best of the family 1973-1978.* (pp. 101-112). Washington, DC: Georgetown University Family Center.

Piaget, J. (1963). *The origins of intelligence in children.* New York: WW Norton.

Piaget, J. (1965). *The moral judgment of the child.* New York: Free Press.

Piaget, J., & Inhelder, (1969). *The psychology of the child.* New York: Basic Books.

Rousseau, J.J. (1962). Emile (W. Boyd Trans.). In W. Boyd (Ed.), *The Emile of Jean Jacques Rousseau.* New York: Bureau of Publications, Teachers College, Columbia University.

Schaefer, C., Coyne, J.C., & Lazarus, R.S. (1981). The health-related functions of social support. *Journal of Behavioral Medicine,* 4(4), 381-406.

Schuster, C.S., & Ashburn, S.S. (1992). *The process of human development* (3rd ed.). Philadelphia: JB Lippincott.

Sheinfeld Gorin, S. (1995). Relationship enhancement intervention: Social support program for women survivors of breast cancer. *1995 Program/Proceedings of the American Society for Clinical Oncology, 236.*

Walsh, F. (1989). The family in later life. In B. Carter & M. McGoldrick (Eds.), *The changing family life cycle: A framework for family therapy* (2nd ed., pp. 312-327). Boston: Allyn & Bacon.

Warren, D.I. (1977). Neighborhoods in urban areas. In R.L. Warren (Ed.), *New perspectives on the American community: A book of readings.* Chicago: Rand McNally.

Watzlawick, P. (1978). *The language of change: Elements of therapeutic communication.* New York: Basic Books.

Yalom, I. (1985). *The theory and practice of group psychotherapy.* New York: Basic Books.

Productivity

Diane J. Powell

EDITORS' NOTE

Productivity and the Group Client System.   The United States has long valued rugged individualism and working hard. Even as the structure of work is changing, these values remain embedded in the culture. Productivity is often discussed in terms of efficiency (i.e., in a ratio that relates inputs [e.g., staff time, costs, or number of customers] to outputs [e.g., number of products meeting quality standards or number of products sold] and that forms a standard of success). Both the individual's and the work group's performance are evaluated in relation to this standard of success or past work efforts and the organization's mission and goals. A worker's satisfaction with his/her productivity is often related to these objective measures, as well as his/her own image of "success." If productivity changes at work or a job is lost entirely, the effects may be felt strongly in other sectors of one's life (e.g., in one's sense of contributing to family life as bread winner, child care provider, or household manager), thus affecting self-worth. In this sense, productivity is a measure of the total ability to negotiate the environment and to produce goods, services, or activities.

Author Diane Powell, RN, MA, MBA, explores organizational programs—the corporate wellness and the clinical disability rehabilitative—designed to both assess and to change the factors that may affect productivity. These programs rely on modifying the behavior of clients in organizations, particularly through change in work groups. The existing work group is used to change behavior through programs such as "stretch breaks" so that the norms are altered to establish more healthy behaviors. Groups are also formed to introduce more specific changes (e.g., corporate-sponsored weight loss or smoking cessation programs). Often, these are coupled with behavioral counseling to reduce disease risk factors (Gomel, Oldenburg, Simpson, Chilvers, & Owen, 1997). These programs may affect productivity of both the work group and the individual employee and consequently their health.

Productivity and Image Appraisal.   Powell explores the relationship between the client's image of productivity and his/her present behavior. She also describes employees in the "gray zone"—a state in which employees are too well to be absent from work yet too sick to perform at peak levels. Powell highlights the importance of obtaining a comprehensive assessment using multiple sources of data, including a risk appraisal and a measure of perceived pain, to understand clients' capacity for work and their quality of life.

Exploration of an Employee in the "Gray Zone" and a Script. Powell examines the use of the Health Promotion Matrix to assess a client's current health status in the workplace. Health care professionals may have particular influence on improving the productivity of clients within the "gray zone" and thus enhance their sense of empowerment.

Variations in a person's productivity may be intertwined with many behaviors (e.g. smoking, obesity, poor nutrition, drug abuse; these behaviors were discussed in earlier chapters). Evaluation of productivity is not an isolated activity nor something to be left to the vocational counselors or the efficiency experts, for in its broadest sense, productivity is the total measure of the client's ability to negotiate the environment and produce goods, services, or activities. An individual's evaluation of his/her productivity, as well as an organization's evaluation of that worker's productivity, needs to be considered by all health care professionals as a component of every client assessment, because productivity is both a predictor and a powerful indicator of the overall state of the client's health.

Productivity can bolster health or impede it. Similarly, productivity can be promoted through healthy behaviors. Certain alterations in health can limit or eliminate productivity altogether. Although it is often difficult to measure productivity, there are some tools to help health care professionals assess it in relation to the client's health. This chapter is based on the assumption that health promotion, through facilitating clients to attain their highest level of wellness, has a positive effect on productivity. In turn, the achievement of a desired productivity level will help the client achieve and maintain health and wellness.

Two models of promoting health and addressing productivity in relation to health are proposed and examined in this chapter: the corporate wellness model and the clinical disability rehabilitative approach. A script using the the Health Promotion Matrix (HPM) that enables health care professionals to assess the client's productivity level and to determine how it is affecting health and how the client's health, in turn, is affecting productivity is presented. Through application of an organized frame of reference—the HPM—health care professionals and clients may work together to develop a plan to initiate and monitor changes in behavior to enhance productivity and health in an interactive way.

DEFINITIONS OF PRODUCTIVITY

Productivity has been studied on a formal level by many corporations to measure the output of workers. A baseline is established as the level at which workers should perform certain tasks, produce certain items, or put together certain products in relation to the resources (e.g., time or money) consumed. Productivity gains and losses are measured against this baseline.

Productivity is also measured in terms of absenteeism and time lost from work. If the worker is not on the job, he/she obviously cannot be productive in that capacity. Although this measure seems simple and clear-cut, it does not take into account the person who continues to work but does not feel well because of an accident or injury or someone who has a chronic illness or condition that impairs full productivity. These clients are in what might be called, for purposes of this chapter, the *gray zone*—too well to take sick time or disability leave but too sick to perform at peak level on the job or at home (Figure 14-1). These persons represent a vast number of health care professionals' clients in the outpatient setting; if only asked the right questions, these clients would provide a wealth

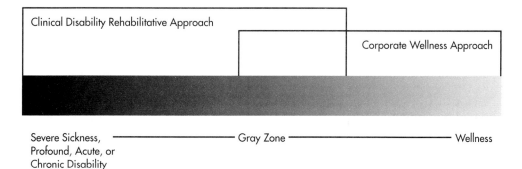

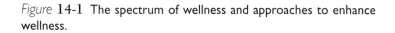

Figure **14-1** The spectrum of wellness and approaches to enhance wellness.

of information pointing to their need to improve their health status. Unfortunately, many times health care professionals, both within the corporate setting and the health system, are rushed for time or are not attuned to the more subtle cues the client may give to express a health deficit and its accompanying effects on productivity.

THE CORPORATE WELLNESS APPROACH

Corporations strive to maximize productivity and their ability to be competitive in a fast-paced market. One way they can increase competitiveness is to decrease costs, including medical costs. Corporations pay an estimated 30% to 40% of national health expenditures (Stokols, Pelletier, & Fielding, 1995). In 1994, U.S. health care costs were an estimated $1 trillion (Greenberg, Finkelstein, & Berndt, 1995). The national average costs for health benefits per employee rose from $1,724 in 1985 to $3,741 in 1994 (*Business and Health,* 1995). Studies have shown that companies are spending about one half of their after-tax dollars on medical care for their employees (Pelletier, 1993), and some predict that this figure will increase to more than 60% by the year 2000 (Herzlinger & Schwartz, 1985).

Companies can reduce medical costs and improve productivity in two major ways: (1) through participation in a variety of managed care or similar programs and (2) by keeping employees healthier through health promotion activities (Holzbach et al., 1990). Comprehensive worksite wellness programs can reduce health risks and promote healthy life-styles (Fielding, 1986) as between 10% and 30% of health care costs are the result of unhealthy behavior (Mandelker, 1993). In the early 1990s, the American Medical Association released a study revealing that unhealthy behaviors, such as abusing drugs and alcohol, account for more than $171 billion of the overall $666 billion spent per year on health care in America. In another study, the most costly life-style factor—stress—was found to generate more than $35 million in medical costs at Union Pacific Railroad, which is based in Omaha, Nebraska (Leutzinger, Goetzel, Richling, & Wade, 1993).

Early interest in employer-sponsored health promotion activities grew out of a concern to reduce the toll of worksite injuries. Among the first large employers to develop comprehensive programs in the 1970s and early 1980s were Kimberly Clark, Control Data Corporation, Tenneco, AT&T, and Johnson & Johnson (Breslow, Fielding, Herrman, & Wilbur, 1990). In 1984, 22 major corporations, including Amdahl, Apple, ARCO, AT&T, Bank of America, Chevron, Hewlett-Packard, IBM, Johnson & Johnson, Levi-Strauss,

Lockheed, Shaklee, Syntex, and Xerox, joined with Stanford University in a collaborative research effort to form the Stanford Corporate Health Program within the Stanford Center for Research in Disease Prevention at the Stanford University School of Medicine (Pelletier, 1993). Many more companies have since recognized the impact of all aspects of health on the productivity of its workers and have created corporate climates that encourage wellness in the workplace.

The National Survey of Work Site Health Promotion Activities (1989) identified approximately two thirds of companies with more than 50 employees as having some sort of health promotion activity that assesses worker life-style behaviors through methods including health risk appraisals; screening activities directed at hypertension, cancer detection, fitness, and diabetes mellitus; and programs for smoking cessation, blood pressure control, nutrition education, exercise weight control, and stress management (Fielding & Piserchia, 1989). By 1992, 81% of private worksites had one or more health promotion activities. Programs are generally more common in larger firms (more than 750 employees) (Guidotti, 1996). Participation in worksite wellness programs does not in itself constitute a change in health status, but "it is an important preliminary step on a continuum from awareness to participation to behavior change to ultimate risk reduction" (Sorensen, Stoddard, Ockene, Hunt, & Youngstrom, 1996, p. 200).

Corporate wellness approaches may include activities such as worksite wellness, employee assistance programs (EAPs), and risk management/accident prevention programs; this chapter deals mainly with corporate wellness programs, although they may actually incorporate elements of the latter two programs, as well. Corporate wellness programs can be as simple as providing health risk appraisals, information, and education or as elaborate as the construction and operation of large fitness centers or the creation of comprehensive corporate programs linking the employer's image and identification with health and vitality (Russell, 1993). Health screening and early disease detection, as well as risk reduction and health promotion, are part of many programs (Gehlbach & Mundt, 1994). If an employee, with the help of a corporate/wellness program, recognizes unhealthy behaviors, he/she can address and improve them with the support of health care professionals in the corporation. The company and the employee both stand to gain in terms of cost control and better health and productivity. Although their benefits are often difficult to measure and their health care cost savings indeterminate, corporate wellness programs have gained recognition as a way to help both employees' health and the corporate bottom line. These programs are designed to maintain health for those who are already healthy and to improve the level of health of those in the "gray zone."

One of the better-known comprehensive health promotion programs, which is specifically designed to improve employee health by encouraging healthful life-styles, is Johnson & Johnson's Live for Life (LFL) Program (Holzbach et al., 1990). In 1978, Johnson & Johnson offered its employees an opportunity to be "the healthiest in the world" (J.E. Burke, corporate communication, 1978). Many employees who participated in this pioneer wellness program found it both interesting and reinforcing.

Much has been learned about corporate wellness programs and their impact on health and productivity since the time Johnson & Johnson employees first completed a physical examination and an evaluation form, were given health profile ratings, and embarked on a program of running, weight training, and aerobic exercises. At that time, the late 1970s, the tangible reward for fulfilling a required number of activities, miles run, or hours in the gym was a T-shirt or a new gym bag. Wearing the colorful Live for Life T-shirt made employees feel part of a club, but the physiologic and psychic rewards were even greater:

feeling fit; looking good; and knowing that when they saw one another at the indoor company track, they were trying to stay fit for themselves. In addition to the use of the gym, employees were offered nutrition classes, smoking cessation programs, and stress reduction programs. Today, almost 20 years later, the Johnson & Johnson tradition of corporate wellness promotion continues with a more sophisticated program combined with simple interventions, such as the occasional "stretch and fitness" break, in which employees are encouraged to get up from their desks and stretch at regular intervals. Employee inducements to become part of the program and to address high-risk factors have been expanded to include a $500 discount on insurance premiums. Now, 96% of the company's 35,000 employees have reportedly completed health assessments, up from 40% before the discounts were offered (Jeffrey, 1996).

In October 1992, Johnson & Johnson's Live for Life worksite health care program was one of eight companies' programs to be awarded the first C. Everett Koop National Health Award (the other programs were those of Blue Shield of California, Coors, DuPont, Southern California Edison, Tenneco, The Travelers, and Ventura County, California). In addition, Johnson & Johnson has benefited from its Live for Life program: the reduced medical and absenteeism costs resulting from the program provided a 1.7:1 return on investment, and the program reportedly resulted in productivity increases as well (Johnson & Johnson Health Management, 1992). Many corporations have modeled their comprehensive programs after the Johnson & Johnson programs.

In the early 1990s, Duke University in North Carolina began a corporate wellness program using Johnson & Johnson's model, including health screenings and life-style improvement programs, such as smoking cessation, weight control, stress management, nutrition education, fitness, and blood pressure interventions. A 4-year study of 4972 Duke University hourly employees showed that program participants experienced an average of 4.6 fewer absentee hours in the third year of the program's availability compared with nonparticipants. Baseline absenteeism, gender, race, education, and age were all controlled. The results suggest that employer-sponsored health promotion initiatives can have a favorable influence on absenteeism (Knight et al., 1994).

In Britain, the Department of Health started a 10-year Health at Work initiative in 1992 in the National Health Service (NHS), which involves everything from offering healthy food for employees; promoting sensible drinking; and developing supportive work environments, including no-smoking policies, on-site exercise classes, and instruction in stress reduction. In at least eight sites, including hospitals within the NHS, programs have been put into place directing preventive services, such as the National Back Exchange, to nurses and other health employees (Snell, 1995).

Fitness programs, which normally are less comprehensive than the Johnson & Johnson approach, are the most popular type of corporate wellness programs and often expand into more elaborate programs. For example, Union Pacific decided to seek out health management strategies in the early 1990s to contain the nearly $6000 in medical costs it was paying per employee. "Life-style claims analyses suggest that Union Pacific was likely to realize significant benefits by expanding its program of promoting health and preventing disease and injuries" (Leutzinger, Goetzel, Richling, & Wade, 1993, p. 42). Between 1987 and 1993, Union Pacific's health promotion program grew "from a single exercise facility in corporate headquarters, to more than 59 sites, or system health facilities, provided either on-site or through contracted local vendors," (Leutzinger, Goetzel, Richling, & Wade, 1993, p. 40) serving more than 20,000 employees, 71% of the company's 28,000 workers at that time. In 1993, the company was awarded the Health

Promotion Leadership Award by the Washington Business Group on Health for meeting the health needs of its workforce. In addition to the fitness program, the company screens employees for blood pressure, cholesterol, body fat, and life-style habits in areas such as exercise, nutrition, and stress. The company also assists employees in becoming smart consumers of health care services by providing a direct mail program on medical self-care, which consists of a videotape and booklet to teach employees how to get the most from their health benefits (Leutzinger, Goetzel, Richling, & Wade, 1993).

Union Pacific has stated that its future goal is to "manage its complex employee health care system through a partnership with employees, labor organizations, third party health care providers, and its insurer" (Leutzinger, Goetzel, Richling, & Wade, 1993, p. 44). This initiative includes managed care networks to ensure high quality care at reasonable prices, employee education programs to encourage informed health care purchasing decisions, and the integration of prevention programs into the company's overall focus on quality (Leutzinger, Goetzel, Richling, & Wade, 1993). Eventually, even home-based businesses may benefit from membership in such a program. In fact, during the next decade, employee wellness could become the dominant product in the health care industry (Busbin, 1990); already, hospitals have begun to offer fitness, aerobics, and other specialty programs to the general public (Blair, 1995).

Many other corporations have targeted their employees' needs by analyzing data in workers' health claims forms. Claims data are difficult to analyze and may be unreliable when cross company comparisons are effected; yet more obvious diagnoses, such as cardiac disease, are easier to identify. Using the claims analysis approach, Sky Chef, an airline food company, found that 63% of all claims dollars for 8000 employees were related to life-style factors such as smoking and eating poorly. Sky Chef adopted an approach to changing employee behavior through a health risk appraisal, coupled with targeted communications. For example, if an individual is identified as having high blood pressure or not wearing a seat belt on a regular basis, the company may send him/her a letter explaining that his/her risk profile is higher because of this and encourage him/her to make an appointment with the health center professional to discuss the situation (Mandelker, 1993).

Evaluation of the Corporate Wellness Approach

Between 1980 and 1993, 48 studies were conducted to evaluate the health and cost benefits of comprehensive health promotion and disease prevention programs in the worksite. One half of these took place between 1990 and 1993, indicating the rate at which interest in these types of programs is growing. Of the 48 studies, all but 1 demonstrated evidence of positive health outcomes, and all but 1 indicated a positive return on cost-effectiveness, or cost benefits (Pelletier, 1993). In contrast, a leadership group entitled the Health Project Consortium identified only 8 out of 200 studies reviewed as demonstrating convincing documentation of savings, despite reductions in sickness absence, outpatient costs, and hospitalization (Fries, Koop, Beadle, Cooper, et al, 1993; Russell, 1993). Because of these equivocal reports, measuring the amount of savings that wellness programs generate is considered difficult, particularly on a short-term basis (Jeffrey, 1996). *Healthy People 2000* specifies the need for research to prevent illness and injury at the worksite (Lusk & Kerr, 1994). In particular, it identifies occupational health and safety problems in the worksite that need further research (U.S. Department of Health and Human Services, 1991). Additionally, to convince corporations to invest in wellness programs, cost-effectiveness data are critical.

Generally, those who participate in worksite wellness programs tend to be middle class, younger, more physically fit, and more aware of health risk factors. Questions remain about the factors affecting participation by blue-collar workers, ethnically or linguistically isolated workers, or those who are most at risk for certain conditions such as heart disease (Rost, Connell, Schechtman, Barzilai, & Fisher, 1990). Overall employee participation rates at the outset of many worksite health promotion programs have been only about 15% to 20% (Baker, Israel, & Schurman, 1994). Although there is a need to increase participation in programs, the question of *how* to do this may be different for each company. A variety of marketing approaches, including using competitions, incentives, the corporate culture, networking, and special events, all have a role (Wilson, 1990). A well-planned marketing strategy that serves the needs and wants of a target group should be able to define the benefits employees need to become involved and also should be able to capitalize on this information to promote the program in such a way that it appeals to these employees. For example, if the majority of employees want to "look good" and that is why they would join the program, then it is important to highlight this benefit, along with the fitness benefits, when trying to "sell" the program.

Worksite research needs to be reviewed with a critical eye, because many studies contain weaknesses such as less rigorous designs, bias in subject recruitment, and conflicts of interest between the investigator and his/her corporate sponsor (Witherspoon & Wilson, 1990). There is little consensus on the definition of either what constitutes a "program" or participation in a program. Further, early methodologies were less rigorous in the appropriateness of control groups and their use of prospective designs (Sheinfeld Gorin, personal communication, December 10, 1997).

When innovative strategies are implemented to increase participation, many times they are not recorded, so it is difficult for others to use the information (Wilson, 1990). There are obviously many opportunities for health care professionals to study the issues surrounding participation in wellness programs, since different groups of employees seem to be attracted to different types of health promotion activities (Mavis, Stachnik, Gibson, & Stoffelmayr, 1992).

One direction for research is the relationship between employee health programs and attitudes toward organizational commitment, supervision, working conditions, job competence, pay and fringe benefits, and job security. The exact mechanism relating program participation and attitude change is unknown (Holzbach et al., 1990).

Another direction for this research is viewing the goal of both corporate wellness programs and occupational safety and health interventions as the improvement of health and the prevention of illness/injury. For example, occupational health nursing, according to the American Association of Occupational Health Nurses (AAOHN), includes the "promotion, protection and restoration of workers' health . . . with an emphasis on optimizing health, preventing illness and injury, and reducing health hazards" (Lessure & Griffith, 1995, p. 72). Often, companies have corporate wellness and occupational health programs working in isolation from one another, with different intervention targets, methods, and personnel. An "overarching model of work and health" (Baker et al., 1996, p. 175), called the *integrated model*, suggests that "such a narrow view, regardless of its focus, will be less effective than programs that attend to the multiplicity of psychosocial and contextual factors that affect the health outcome of interest" (Baker et al., 1996, p. 181). This model suggests that no single intervention to improve health in the worksite is likely to be the answer and that health care professionals from a multitude of disciplines are required to create necessary worksite changes. The integrated model also suggests that expertise exists in both the corporate wellness and occupational safety areas, and together they should work to consider "long-term, rather than short-term, definitions of change and intervention effectiveness" (Baker et al., 1996, p. 187).

Further, in examining health outcomes for employees, retirees need to be considered. It has been estimated that some companies provide employer-supported health care plans to nearly one half of their full-time employees after retirement (Clark & Kreps, 1989). Southern California Edison's Generation program, a clinic-based program designed to provide cost-effective geriatric health care services for 9000 retired employees and their dependents, includes as its objectives the enhancement of its members' well-being and the improvement of their social functioning; both of these objectives may ultimately reduce the need for use of high-cost health care services (Scharlach, Mor-Barak, & Birba, 1994).

THE CLINICAL DISABILITY REHABILITATIVE APPROACH

The clinical disability rehabilitative approach to health promotion is complementary to the corporate wellness approach, although both the clients and the setting for intervention differ. Both approaches seek to help the individual achieve his/her highest level of wellness, but for purposes of this chapter, the corporate model addresses the needs of persons who are "basically well" and working more than does the clinical disability rehabilitative approach. The clinical disability rehabilitative model addresses persons in the gray zone—the middle of the spectrum—and those at the "lower" end of the health spectrum, where there is identifiable, or diagnosable, serious illness and/or profound disability.

Clients who end up in the formal health care system—most obviously those who enter a hospital or clinic—probably need some form of "rehabilitation," or change in living, to help them become healthier and thus more productive. If health care professionals broaden their definition of those who could benefit from "rehabilitation," many clients would learn how to better control their diabetes, allergies, and asthma conditions; to move more freely with their osteoarthritis; to prevent headaches through better stress management, and to express a rehabilitative need.

If health care professionals looked at rehabilitation in this broadened scope, then every client would be in need of some form or level of rehabilitation. Although many persons, including some health care professionals, think of rehabilitation as something that benefits only those who require physical or occupational, speech/language pathology, or assistance recovering from addiction to drugs or alcohol, this author views rehabilitation in a much broader sense, one that permeates all aspects of every level of care (from intensive care to the outpatient setting). In addition, a relatively new field, called *trauma rehabilitation,* pertains to individuals who have been salvaged from injury in an accident and begins the instant the first health care services are provided to the client who has experienced a trauma. Rehabilitation in this sense is essential to any health care professional in any setting, from the emergency room and critical care unit, to rehabilitation facilities, to transitional and home care and beyond (Cardona, Hurn, Mason, Scanlon-Schilpp, and Veise-Berry, 1988).

Rehabilitation has been defined in many ways. In the physical, musculoskeletal sense, rehabilitation means "changing the habit of the muscles to allow for a return to normalcy in function and/or pain and discomfort, by training them and their habits through manual or exercise methods" (R. Henderson, personal communication, May 1, 1997). Another definition of rehabilitation, which incorporates the components of the HPM, states: "Rehabilitation is the process of maximizing the use of an individual's capabilities or resources to foster optimal growth and functioning. It recognizes the uniqueness and wholeness of each individual and views each person and his (or her) environment as interdependent systems" (Sayles, 1981, p. 3). Rehabilitation also has been defined clinically as the "evaluation and treatment of patients who have pain, disability or diminished function" (B. Root, personal communication, December 18, 1996).

There are also many settings in which rehabilitation is provided, including centers devoted to physical medicine and rehabilitation, such as the Rusk Institute at the New York University Medical Center in New York City, the Kessler Institute in New Jersey, and the Burke Rehabilitation Center in Westchester, New York. These institutions were established with the primary mission of rehabilitating clients, whether broadly or narrowly defined.

Registered nurses have traditionally been concerned with the rehabilitation plan for their hospitalized and home care clients, and they are taught that planning for the hospital-based client's discharge begins the moment the client enters the hospital (Kelly, 1991).

Capitalizing on the traditional involvement that nurses have had in the rehabilitation of clients, the Stanford University School of Medicine focused on beginning rehabilitation for hospitalized clients as soon as possible during recovery and had nurses follow up with the clients by telephone after discharge from the hospital. The goal was to get clients back to work sooner, with a higher level of activity and fewer problems at a much lower cost. Research indicates that this approach may be working (Dennis, et al., 1988; Picard, et al., 1989; Pilote, et al., 1992).

The clinical disability rehabilitative approach targets those persons who may be struggling to regain their level of health or health equilibrium after an accident, injury, or illness; who are cared for in the hospital, rehabilitation center, outpatient or even at-home setting and who seek acute, subacute, or long-term care; and whose productivity has been affected by a variety of physical, psychologic, economic, and social factors. In contrast, the corporate wellness approach targets the "basically well" employee who is trying to improve his/her health status through a variety of measures by polishing up certain weak areas of his/her health profile and by trying to stay well or maintain high-level wellness, with the goal of sustaining or enhancing productivity levels.

It is to the person who is trying to regain his/her level of health or health equilibrium that the next part of this discussion on health and productivity is addressed, for it is with this person that many health care professionals have the opportunity to do case-finding, triaging, direct care, and follow-up referral and consultation. It is this person who may fall through the cracks of the health care system unless health care professionals are ready to work together to screen vigilantly for those who may have a diagnosis that affects productivity. How successful health care professionals are in supporting the overall health and well-being of each person depends in part on the diagnostic cues (both verbal and nonverbal) that the health care professional picks up, especially the subtle ones, and how much the health care professional believes in the value of rehabilitation toward wellness. Although much of this success relies on the health care professional's acute observational and interpersonal skills, there are also physiologic and psychologic measures that can help determine the client's level of impairment and need (see the Assessment Tools for Productivity section). By doing a baseline assessment, health care professionals can help determine how much they will need to empower clients to help them get better, stay better, and be well at their maximal level. Such assessments can also determine which clients are in the "gray zone"—that area in which clients are somewhere between health and wellness and in which their productivity is affected in ways that are sometimes difficult to measure.

After identifying these clients, the next wave of rehabilitative care is to work with clients to control, alleviate, and prevent disability, with the goal of greater productivity. The aim is to focus not only on the direct, out-of pocket costs of health care, but to also consider the indirect effects and costs of illness, from workers' inabilities to function fully on the job to their absenteeism. Although direct treatment cost is usually of greatest interest in the corporate setting, the full effects of illness are not measured this way alone. Indirect costs of a worker's health problems can cause the individual's functioning and well-being to be impaired, and this reduces overall quality of life (Greenberg et al., 1995).

Common illnesses that may impair persons, yet not take them off the job completely, are ailments such as depression, asthma and allergies, sinusitis, back and neck problems, diabetes, and arthritis. Depression is a good example of an illness that, if identified early in the worksite by the alert health care professional, can save the individual and the company a heavy toll. It has been estimated that diminished performance of workers with depression (e.g., employee incapacitation while at work or employee absenteeism) costs companies $24 billion, or 55% of the total financial cost of depression. If not identified early in the worksite setting, depression can eventually incapacitate individuals to the point at which they can no longer function effectively on the job, sometimes necessitating inpatient psychiatric care or a leave of absence and resulting in many major upheavals in the work and home environments. Unfortunately, once the employer finds out that a worker has taken time off to be treated for depression, he/she may face what seems like a far worse situation when he/she returns to work. In some cases, individuals have even been fired after taking a medical leave of absence for acute treatment of depression and subsequent rehabilitation. (Although the legality and humanitarianism of this is highly questionable, it does happen, even in major corporations.) This represents yet another opportunity for the health care professional to intervene during the rehabilitation process, or even earlier, in the worksite setting before the problem reaches acute clinical proportions.

Many individuals with symptoms of conditions that affect productivity remain on the job but do not function at their full potential and may affect the productivity of others, as well. Unfortunately, "when workers are unhealthy, their diminished performance can dramatically affect co-workers. For example, if ill health results in more accidents or increased errors, all who explicitly or even implicitly interact with unhealthy employees can become less productive" (Greenberg et al., 1995, p. 36). Opportunities exist for health care professionals to do an early assessment of these problems through employee worksite wellness programs and if those checkpoints fail, to assist the individual to return to work as quickly as possible through an efficient approach of rehabilitation and disability management.

INTEGRATING THE CORPORATE WELLNESS APPROACH AND THE CLINICAL DISABILITY REHABILITATIVE APPROACH

Some corporations have instituted a new system called *integrated disability management* (IDM), which is the application of managed care principles and activities without regard to the source of the event to provide quality health care and to return the individual to work as early as practical. IDM seeks to address the needs of clients through available resources and more coordinated care. It combines all the various coverages and systems relative to the employee (e.g., worker's compensation, short-term disability, long-term disability, and health insurance) to treat the person as a whole rather than subdividing him/her by the illness categories of care and payment schedules. Health care professionals and employers expect that IDM will, through a system of case management, do the following:

- Improve quality of care
- Improve efficiency of medical care to reduce costs
- Return employees to work at appropriate times (disability management)
- Allow fair disability ratings
- Minimize litigation

Disability management uses a case manager to act as the account coordinator for the employee who is ill or injured, the health care professional and the company. Working with the case manager, the employee is exposed to a system that emphasizes appropriate return to work, manages disability through transitional work, facilitates work-station modification for return to work, and minimizes residual disability. Some of the services that might be coordinated are inpatient hospital certification and ambulatory care certification, including outpatient surgery, diagnostic testing, physical medicine (rehabilitation), home health, home intravenous (IV) therapy and durable medical equipment, all with the goal of providing medically necessary and appropriate care.

One company that used the system, Wausau, found that IDM reduced work-related injuries/illnesses; nonwork-related injuries/illness; disability claims costs; disability litigation costs; severity and frequency of injuries/illnesses; and lost time. IDM also improved productivity, loss ratios, employee relations, morale and enhanced safety procedures (M. Voyvodich, personal correspondence, 1996).

Case management is pushing along the rehabilitative process to help persons recover faster and to return to work sooner. Using an IDM approach, many companies are becoming self-insured, forming buying coalitions, and putting case management to work through cost-effective, individualized medical, emotional, and vocational services (Mullahy, 1995). Case managers are beginning to offer personalized employee wellness programs, as corporations look at total health care-disability management (or "24-hour coverage") to maintain quality care while managing costs, particularly for a disease such as AIDS (Mullahy, 1995). Some vendors sell corporations the services to enable HIV-positive individuals to take responsibility as their own case managers, thereby helping persons with the disease to work and live as fully as possible.

Other firms help individuals and their families deal with all aspects of head trauma and spinal cord injury, including community reentry, worker's compensation, rehabilitation, job reentry, job placement, and disability services (Mullahy, 1995). A firm that specializes in life care planning does a systematic appraisal of individual needs at a given time, then broadens the review to encompass projected financial and medical requirements as the individual progresses through his/her life course (Jensen, 1993). Another company, Champion International, offers on-site physical therapy to enable workers at its paper and pulp mills to recover faster without leaving the worksite (Jeffrey, 1996).

Taking this concept one step further, DRI, a hospitality company with 1,000 employees, set up the Wellness Center on its premises in September 1995. Staffed by two nurse practitioners and a receptionist, the Wellness Center offers health assessments, episodic care, health counseling, family planning, allergy injections, and laboratory services free of charge to employees. The goals of increasing employee satisfaction and reducing absenteeism while remaining cost neutral have been fulfilled. DRI has avoided lost productivity resulting from employees going to outside health care professionals' offices and has saved an estimated $100,000 during the first 6 months of the center's operation. In addition, 93% of customers surveyed by the Wellness Center are satisfied, and clients have rated the nurse practitioners and care at the center as excellent and exceeding their expectations (Lugo, 1997).

Even greater savings, an estimated $250,000 yearly, are being reported in the Suffolk County (New York) Department of Health, where nurse practitioners staff and run a freestanding employee health service and clinics for the 10,500 Suffolk County employees, including Suffolk County Police Officers and health personnel. While conducting physical examinations, the nurse practitioners emphasize health promotion and disease prevention through effective counseling tailored to client needs (L. Peterson, personal communication, April 30, 1997), an approach emphasized in the Health Promotion Matrix.

ASSESSMENT TOOLS FOR PRODUCTIVITY

Many assessment tools have been used by organizations in their worksite wellness programs to determine health risk factors.

Health risk appraisals (HRAs) look at personal medical and life-style factors but also identify the likelihood of preventable or chronic disease within a specific time period, with the purpose of motivating persons to change their life-styles for the better (Turner, 1995; Peterson & Hilles, 1992). Health risk appraisals are common features of worksite health promotion programs. It has been noted that there are more than 50 recognized HRAs, including those developed originally to aid physicians in doing preventive counseling; the one developed by and for the Centers for Disease Control and Prevention (CDC) employees (originally in 1978); and those developed by private corporations to meet the needs of their own employees or those of their corporate clients (Turner, 1995; De Friese & Foster, 1990). One important area assessed through the Johnson & Johnson survey and others like it is the employee's nutritional intake. Workers' productivity closely depends on their nutritional intake (Fogel, 1994; Foster, 1995).

Another health risk appraisal form was developed for the Harvard Nurses' Health Study and is available to worksite wellness centers. Initially, the study's appraisal form asked questions that would shed light on the relationship among the variables: use of oral contraceptives, cigarette smoking, and major illness. The study has broadened over time to include the evaluation of the health consequences of certain life-style practices such as diet, physical activity, and specific forms of estrogen replacement therapy (Colditz, 1995).

The Medical Outcomes Study (MOS) 36-Item Short Form Health Survey (SF-36) form views health more broadly, with measures of physical functioning and role limitations as well as mental health, social functioning, vitality, and general health (McHorney, Ware, & Raczek, 1993). As a "quality of life" form, it is an indicator of the client's overall sense of well-being. Knowing the client's response to certain SF-36 questions can lead the health care professional to continue to explore related issues with the client, some of which may lead to the identification of concerns about productivity resulting from some underlying physical or psychologic concern. The SF-36 may serve to "red flag" certain clients as needing more in-depth history taking or physical review and may also be used to measure the health outcomes of corporate wellness or clinical disability rehabilitative programs.

In the clinical disability rehabilitative model, the most basic assessment tools are the standard health history and physical assessment. The health history includes questions about the individual's social habits (e.g., smoking, alcohol use, drug use or abuse); medication history; work and work-related risk factors; family history; previous illnesses and injuries; allergies; and other factors that might seem pertinent during the interview, which is usually conducted by a physician or nurse practitioner. Health history forms are widely available in medical and nurse practitioner textbooks (e.g., Bates, 1995).

Some physiatrists (medical physicians with a specialty in physical medicine and rehabilitation), neurologists, orthopedists, and chiropractors use a form that helps determine a baseline of pain and dysfunction, both of which may affect productivity. On this form, the client draws on a body outline to indicate where he/she has the most pain and by using different shape figures (e.g., $>>$ or $\backslash\backslash\backslash$) indicates what kind of pain he/she has. One of the most common tools of this type is the Neck Pain Disability Index Questionnaire (Figure 14-2). This questionnaire is self-administered and is specific to certain parts of the body (e.g. neck, back). On the front side, it asks questions such as age and occupation. It shows a diagram of the body upon which the client locates pain. The client can identify different types of pain using different letters (i.e., A = ache, P = pins and needles, B = burning, S = stabbing, N = numbness, and O = other). On the back of the questionnaire, clients can specify the limiting effects of their pain by circling the choice indicating the level that each of the following categories is affected: pain intensity, personal care, lifting, reading, headaches, concentration, work, driving, sleeping, and recreation. This information helps enable the health care professional to understand how much a client's low back pain, for example, has affected his/her ability to manage everyday activities. If the client has pain in two areas, (e.g. neck and low back), he/she completes two questionnaires—one for each affected area of the body. These forms may then be used as baselines for the evaluation of the client after he/she has started a course of pharmaceutical, physical rehabilitative, and/or psychologic therapy.

PRODUCTIVITY & THE HEALTH PROMOTION MATRIX*

Productivity enhancement is, to a great extent, dependent on both the healthy behaviors already explored in Chapters 6 to 13, as well as changes in organizations (see Chapter 4). The script and discussion that follow are based on an organization that has developed a health promotive environment, including the formation of an Employee Assistance Program (EAP). Because the health care professional using the script may be employed or contracted by the same organization for which the employee works and because the discussion is highly sensitive, confidentiality is paramount to the development of trust necessary to obtain truthful information. At the start of the discussion, the health care professional should tell the client what information, if any, will be shared; with whom; and under what conditions. If the information could be shared with the employee's organization in an *undisguised form,* so that the employee could be identified, the health care professional must state this clearly to the client so that he/she understands that the information is *not confidential.* When the interchange takes place in a group setting, each member must be informed that all discussions are to be held in absolute and complete confidence. The health care professional is directive and firm in stating this principle and in obtain-

Text continued on p. 379

*Adapted from D.J. Powell's clinical case by S. Sheinfeld Gorin.

NECK PAIN
DISABILITY INDEX QUESTIONNAIRE

BACKGROUND

The Neck Pain Disability Index Questionnaire provides a reliable and valid means to quantify the effect of neck pain on a person's daily living activities.(1-2)

The term "disability" is used generically and the questionnaire should not be confused with a formal disability evaluation or impairment rating. The information provided, however, is useful in reporting the effect of pain on a patient's quality of life compared to their pre-illness state.(2,3)

REPORT USAGE

A typical example of report language would be: "The pain interferes with the patient's daily living activities (e.g., lifting, walking, standing, social life, sleeping, etc.) by 40% as assessed by the Neck Pain Disability Index Questionnaire." Further, individual sections of the questionnaire relative to the patient's condition could be summarized and compared, if follow-up questionnaires are available.

ADDITIONAL INFORMATION

For comprehensive information on the Neck Pain Disability Index Questionnaire, you may order the following references from the D.D. Palmer Health Sciences Library at 1-319-326-9896 from 8:00 AM to 4:00 PM (CST).

REFERENCES

1) Vernon H, Mior S. The neck disability index: a study of reliability and validity. *J Man Physiol Ther* 1991;14(7):409-15

2) Deyo RA. Measuring the functional status of patients with low back pain. *Arch Phys Med Rehabil* 1988;69:1044-53

3) Triano JJ. The subluxation complex: outcome measure of chiropractic diagnosis and treatment. *Chiropractic Technique* 1990;2(3):114-20

Scoring:

Within each section, choices are scored as follows:
$$A = 0 \quad B = 1 \quad C = 2 \quad D = 3 \quad E = 4 \quad F = 5$$

Sum the score for all sections, divide by the total possible (50 points if all sections are completed). Deduct 5 points from the total for each uncompleted or missed section and then multiply by 100%.

Example:
16 (total points) / 50 (total possible) x 100% = 32%

Disability Rating:

0-9%	None
10-29%	Mild
30-49%	Moderate
50-69%	Severe
70%+	Complete

Figure 14-2 Owestry Scale for Neck Disability. Available in an Outcome Assessment Package from Activator Methods, Inc., P.O. Box 80317, Phoenix, AZ 85060-0317. For more information or to order forms for this index or other disability indexes, call (602) 224-0220 or (800) 598-0224.

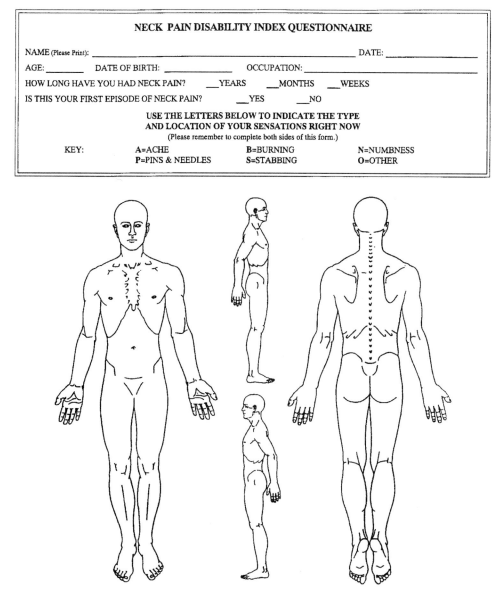

OVER PLEASE

Figure 14-2, cont'd. For legend, see opposite page.

NECK PAIN DISABILITY INDEX QUESTIONNAIRE

Please Read: This questionnaire is designed to enable us to understand how much your neck pain has affected your ability to manage your everyday activities. Please answer each section by circling the **ONE CHOICE** that most applies to you. We realize that you may feel that more than one statement may relate to you, but **PLEASE, JUST CIRCLE THE ONE CHOICE WHICH MOST CLOSELY DESCRIBES YOUR PROBLEM RIGHT NOW.**

Section 1 — Pain Intensity
A I have no pain at the moment.
B The pain is very mild at the moment.
C The pain is moderate at the moment.
D The pain is fairly severe at the moment.
E The pain is very severe at the moment.
F The pain is the worst imaginable at the moment.

Section 2 — Personal Care (Washing, Dressing, etc.)
A I can look after myself normally without causing extra pain.
B I can look after myself normally, but it causes extra pain.
C It is painful to look after myself and I am slow and careful.
D I need some help, but manage most of my personal care.
E I need help every day in most aspects of self care.
F I do not get dressed, I wash with difficulty and stay in bed.

Section 3 — Lifting
A I can lift heavy weights, without extra pain.
B I can lift heavy weights, but it gives extra pain.
C Pain prevents me from lifting heavy weights off the floor, but I can manage if they are conveniently positioned, for example, on a table.
D Pain prevents me from lifting heavy weights, but I can manage light to medium weights if they are conveniently positioned.
E I can lift very light weights.
F I cannot lift or carry anything at all.

Section 4 — Reading
A I can read as much as I want to with no pain in my neck.
B I can read as much as I want to with slight pain in my neck.
C I can read as much as I want with moderate pain in my neck.
D I cannot read as much as I want because of moderate pain in my neck.
E I cannot read as much as I want because of severe pain in my neck.
F I cannot read at all.

Section 5 — Headaches
A I have no headaches at all.
B I have slight headaches which come infrequently.
C I have moderate headaches which come infrequently.
D I have moderate headaches which come frequently.
E I have severe headaches which come frequently.
F I have headaches almost all the time.

After Vernon & Mior, 1991
Reprinted by permission of the Journal of Manipulative and Physiological Therapeutics

Section 6 — Concentration
A I can concentrate fully when I want to with no difficulty.
B I can concentrate fully when I want to with slight difficulty.
C I have a fair degree of difficulty in concentrating when I want to.
D I have a lot of difficulty in concentrating when I want to.
E I have a great deal of difficulty in concentrating when I want to.
F I cannot concentrate at all.

Section 7 — Work
A I can do as much work as I want to.
B I can only do my usual work, but no more.
C I can do most of my usual work, but no more.
D I cannot do my usual work.
E I can hardly do any work at all.
F I cannot do any work at all.

Section 8 — Driving
A I can drive my car without any neck pain.
B I can drive my car as long as I want with slight pain in my neck.
C I can drive my car as long as I want with moderate pain in my neck.
D I cannot drive my car as long as I want because of moderate pain in my neck.
E I can hardly drive at all because of severe pain in my neck.
F I cannot drive my car at all.

Section 9 — Sleeping
A I have no trouble sleeping.
B My sleep is slightly disturbed (less than 1 hour sleepless).
C My sleep is mildly disturbed (1-2 hours sleepless).
D My sleep is moderately disturbed (2-3 hours sleepless).
E My sleep is greatly disturbed (3-5 hours sleepless).
F My sleep is completely disturbed (5-7 hours sleepless).

Section 10 — Recreation
A I am able to engage in all of my recreational activities, with no neck pain at all.
B I am able to engage in all of my recreational activities, with some pain in my neck.
C I am able to engage in most, but not all of my usual recreational activities because of pain in my neck.
D I am able to engage in a few of my usual recreational activities because of pain in my neck.
E I can hardly do any recreational activities because of pain in my neck.
F I cannot do any recreational activities at all.

REVISED January 1, 1995

Comments: _____

Patient Signature: _____ Date: _____

Figure 14-2, cont'd. For legend, see p. 376.

ing the group's commitment to it. The client should be encouraged to ask the health care professional questions to clarify the nature of the confidentiality assurances. Some organizations have clients sign a written understanding of this, as well. Once the health care professional feels that the client understands the nature of their relationship, the interchange may begin.

Image Creation

This dimension of the Matrix allows the health care professional and the client to understand the image a client holds of himself/herself as healthy and productive. Oftentimes, the connection between satisfying work and physical activity, for example, is not realized in the client's picture of himself/herself.

A health care professional working with middle managers from different areas of a large, successful software company who have been referred to an EAP, for example, may help them to develop an image for themselves. In a group setting, this discussion may take place between the health care professional and the client, either one at a time or in a general discussion. One of the members, a middle-age female who suffers from intermittent, chronic severe pain in the neck and back because of an automobile accident works full time for the company but is often absent. She is in the "gray zone," neither too sick nor optimally well for productive work. The health care professional may ask her the following questions:

What do you see if you try to picture yourself as healthy? Do you see yourself running? Jumping? Dancing? Playing volleyball? Skiing? Playing golf? Playing tennis? Traveling? Having sexual relationships without pain? Lifting a child? Biking? Riding a roller coaster? Commanding a high salary in a demanding job? Resting comfortably in a chair without pain?

Image Appraisal

During this phase, the health care professional is seeking to match the client's image of himself/herself as a healthy and productive individual with his/her daily life at present and then to formulate a plan for change. Throughout, the health care professional must remain aware that the organization's own effectiveness has a considerable effect on both the individual's health and his/her productivity. Tools to assess the organization's effectiveness, as well as its approaches to creating safe work environments, are beyond the scope of this chapter (see Chapter 10). Yet, in assessing the practicality of the client's plan, both assessment perspectives—the individual's and the organization's (oftentimes derived from the work group and/or the supervisor)—should be considered. A group may be helpful in sharing common concerns and in assisting one member in formulating a more realistic assessment of himself/herself. As part of a general discussion, the health care professional may ask the following question:

Health care professional: What kinds of things are preventing you from achieving your image(s) of being productive and healthy?

Client: I have chronic back pain. I will share a sample week to detail my difficulties. I experienced limited productivity because of 3 appointments with a physical therapist, which, including travel time and treatment, take 3 hours for each visit. In addition, my condition requires one half hour of home exercises per day. I have difficulty working on the computer at work because of pain and stiffness, and I take analgesics with antiinflammatory medications, as needed. I also take time off from work to go to the chiropractor, orthopedist, and exercise physiologist, as needed. I missed 4 hours of work this week and had difficulty figuring out a "bug" in a program because of my pain.

Minimize Health Depleting Patterns and Optimize Health Supportive Patterns

These two dimensions are combined in the healthy behavior of productivity because the interventions are similar for both and rely heavily on the previous chapters in Part Two. The health care professional uses the information derived from the Image Assessment to isolate each of the specific factors inhibiting or supporting productivity. Group members, too, may join in this process. In particular, by juxtaposing the client's responses to his/her image and the responses to the assessment tools, the health care professional may prompt the client to examine aspects of the relationship between health and productivity not formerly seen. Although the health care professional will have a critical role in prompting the client, it is the client's idealized view of himself/herself that will drive the implementation of the care plan. The health care professional may share information on programs designed to manage time, for example, or clinical disability rehabilitative settings that may be available to the client.

To assist with this problem-solving process in a group setting, often the other members will share common approaches to overcoming barriers that one member may not have considered. As joint problem-solvers, group members may develop alternative strategies, examine their consequences, and validate member choices. Both the health care professional and other group members may assist the client to decide on a program and/or to advocate for the development of organizational changes, such as implementation of a broad corporate policy of acceptance of the differentially abled.

Health care professional: What factors might interfere with your plan to be more productive?

Client: My supervisor is very accepting of my difficulties, as I have always exceeded my productivity targets from the previous quarter. I am concerned, however, that I may not be able to continue to maintain this level if I need to take so much time off from work.

Health care professional: A supportive supervisor is a real plus. Are you also aware that your company has a flexible time program that allows you to attend an excellent local rehabilitation program 2 mornings a week, with transportation to and from work? Your company's insurance plan covers the cost. Since your company has a well-developed productivity management system and you have an accepting supervisor, I understand that your goals for this quarter can be officially changed while you take part in rehabilitation.

Internalize Idealized Image

The health care professional should establish a means for following up with the client, particularly if he/she has been referred to a rehabilitative setting. With the client's explicit (oftentimes written) consent, the health care professional could contact the Department of Human Resources/Personnel to assess whether the client's record has been updated to reflect changes, such as a modification of productivity baselines or targets. The health care professional should remain apprised of general changes in the organization's approaches to productivity assessment, connections to Employee Assistance Plans, and coverage for various health problems, as well as other relevant policy changes so that she/he may remain a usable resource.

Health care professional: May I call you in about 1 month to see how the plan we have worked out is going? After you talk with your supervisor, would you like me to contact the Director of Human Resources to ensure that your productivity targets are modified for this quarter? If so, please sign this form giving me your permission to request a change only in the quarterly targets.

	PRODUCTIVITY: *A Script**
Image Creation	What do you see if you try to picture yourself as healthy?
	What do you envision when you see yourself as productive?
	When you imagine a productive environment for you, what does it look like?
	How productive do you think you are?
Image Appraisal	How satisfied are you with the work you do (e.g., pay, benefits, promotions; the work itself in its level of challenge, routinization, autonomy, control, safety; relationships with supervisors, co-workers, clients, staff, suppliers, distributors; organizational decision-making structure, culture)?
	How is productivity measured in your present work environment?

*Adapted from D.J. Powell by S. Sheinfeld Gorin.

continued

PRODUCTIVITY: *A Script—cont'd*

How does your own work compare to the standards in place at this time?

What may be preventing or facilitating your joining these two?

> Administer the SF-36, health risk appraisal, and Neck Pain Disability Index Questionnaire

Do you participate in any wellness activities (e.g., smoking cessation, eating well, physical activity, sexual awareness, injury prevention, substance safety, oral health promotion, and/or self-development)?

Do you feel that your health may prevent you from being fully productive?

> Review SF-36, health risk appraisal, Neck Pain Disability Index Questionnaire, stated image. Identify barriers to health stated or not stated by client.

Would you be willing to develop a plan to enhance your productivity?

Minimize Health Depleting Patterns and Optimize Health Supportive Patterns

YES	**NO**
Can we examine these factors one by one to think about developing a plan?	What would prevent you from developing this plan?

Productivity: *A Script—cont'd*

	What would you need to do to be more productive?
	Explore scripts in Chapters 6 to 13. Examine results of health risk appraisal, SF-36, Neck Pain Disability Index Questionnaire to isolate particular *productivity* impediments and supports. Assess available Employee Assistance, stress management, team building, communication, decision-making, safety enhancement, and organizational culture-building programs, among others, for suitability. Discuss these, as appropriate, with the client.
Internalize Idealized Image	What changes have you seen in your own productivity? How may I continue to assist you in implementing changes to enhance your productivity?

Summary

Productivity measures the output of workers and generally relates changed behavior to a given baseline. Two models of wellness programs designed to enhance productivity—the corporate wellness approach and the clinical disability rehabilitation approach—are discussed in this chapter. Trends in employee wellness programs and disability-rehabilitative services have been identified, with specific guidelines for all health care professionals to consider in evaluating the health and productivity of their clients. Most corporate wellness programs enhance other healthy behaviors such as physical activity or eating well to increase productivity and to reduce costs. The clinical disability rehabilitation approach, by engaging individuals who are not "well," seeks to increase productivity *directly, by assisting these individuals to return to work*. Systematic evaluations of these burgeoning programs, particularly in corporate settings, have demonstrated some efficacy. A script designed for counseling individuals in healthy behaviors related to productivity and incorporating some specific tools for image appraisal is detailed. Health care professionals need to remember that each client's potential for productivity is unique to him/her and that by helping clients enhance their productivity, they are enriching the development of health.

HELPFUL **RESOURCES**

ASSESSMENT TOOLS

Activator Methods Inc.
PO Box 80317
Phoenix, AZ 85060-0317
Phone: (602) 224-0220
Fax: (602) 224-0230
Provides Oswestry forms (Neck Pain Disability Index Questionnaire) and other disability indexes.

The Health Institute
Box 345
New England Medical Center
750 Washington St.
Boston, MA 02111
Phone: (617) 636-8098
Fax: (617) 636-8077
Provides the Medical Outcomes Study (MOS) Short Form and the General Health Survey (SF-36; SF-20)

Nurses' Health Study (Brigham & Women's Hospital/Harvard Medical School)
Channing Lab
181 Longwood Ave.
Boston, MA 02115
Phone: (617) 525-2279
Fax: (617) 525-2008

US Public Health Service, Office of Disease Prevention and Health Promotion, Washington, D.C.
Phone: (202) 401-6295
On-line: http:\\www.healthfinder.gov
Publishes *Health finder: Health risk appraisals,* no date.

Wellsource, Inc.
15431 SE 82nd Drive
Clackamas, OR 97015
Phone: (503) 656-7446
Fax: (503) 650-0880

Association for Worksite Health Promotion
60 Revere Drive
Suite 500
Northbrook, IL 60062
Phone: (847) 480-9574
Fax: (847) 480-9282

Johnson & Johnson Health Care Systems Inc.
Piscataway, NJ 08855
Phone: (800) 443-3682
Fax: (908) 562-2297

References

Baker, E.A., Israel, B.A., & Schurman, S.J. (1994). A participatory approach to worksite health promotion. *Journal of Ambulatory Care Management, 17*(2), 68-81.

Baker, E., Israel, B.A., & Schurman, S. (1996). The integrated model: Implications for worksite health promotion and occupational health and safety practice. *Health Education Quarterly, 23*(2), 175-190.

Bates, B. (1995). *A pocket guide to physical examination and history taking* (2nd ed.). Philadelphia: JB Lippincott.

Blair, J.E. (1995). Social marketing: Consumer focused health promotion. *AAOHN Journal, 43*(10), 527-531.

Breslow, L., Fielding, J., Herrman, A.A., & Wilbur, C.S. (1990). Worksite health promotion: Its evolution and the Johnson & Johnson experience. *Preventive Medicine, 19*(1), 13-21.

Burke, J.E. (1978). Johnson & Johnson internal communication.

Busbin, J. (1990). Marketing evolutions in health care and the emergence of employee wellness as a new product category. *Health Care Marketing, 11*(4), 22-30.

Cardona, V.D., Hurn, P.D., Mason, P.J., Scanlon-Schilpp, A.M., & Veise-Berry, S.W. (1988). *Trauma nursing: From resuscitation through rehabilitation.* Philadelphia: WB Saunders.

Clark, R.L., & Kreps, J.M. (1989). Employer-provided health care plans for retirees. *Research on Aging, 11,* 206-224.

Colditz, G. (1995). The nurses' health study: A cohort of U.S. women followed since 1976. *JAMWA, 50*(2), 40-63.

Dennis, C., Houston-Miller, N., Schwartz, R., Ahn, D., Kraemer, H., Gossard, D., Juneau, M., Taylor, C., & DeBusk, R. (1988). Early return to work after uncomplicated myocardial infarction: Results of a randomized trial. *Journal of the American Medical Association, 260,* 214-220.

De Friese, G.H., & Fielding, J.E. (1990). Health risk appraisal in the 1990s: Opportunities, challenges and expectations. *Annual Review of Public Health, 11,* 401-418.

Fielding, J. (1986). Evaluations, results and problems of worksite health promotion programs. In M. Cataldo & T. Coates (Eds.), *Health and industry: A behavioral medicine perspective.* New York: John Wiley & Sons.

Fielding, J.E., & Piserchia, P.V. (1989). Frequency of worksite health promotion activities. *American Journal of Public Health, 79*(1), 16-20.

Fogel, R.W. (1994). Economic growth, population theory and physiology: The bearing of long-term processes on the making of economic policy. *The American Economic Review, 84,* 369-389.

Foster, A.D. (1995). Household savings and human investment behavior in development: Nutrition and health investment. *AEA Papers and Proceedings, 85*(2), 148-152.

Fries, J.F., Koop, C.E., Beadle, C.E. et al. (1993). Reducing health care costs by reducing the need and demand for medical services. *New England Journal of Medicine, 329*(5), 321-325.

Gehlbach, S.H., & Mundt, K.A. (1994). Evaluating worksite health programs. *Journal of Ambulatory Care Management, 17*(2), 82-91.

Gomel, M.K., Oldenburg, B., Simpson, J.M., Chilvers, M., & Owen, N. (1997). Composite cardiovascular risk outcomes of a worksite intervention trial. *American Journal of Public Health, 87*(4), 673-676.

Greenberg, P.E., Finkelstein, S.N., & Berndt, E.R. (1995, Summer). Economic consequences of illness in the workplace. *Sloan Management Review,* 26-38.

Guidotti, T.L. (1996). Providing preventive care at the worksite. In S.H. Woolf, S. Jonas, & R.S. Lawrence (Eds.), *Health promotion and disease prevention in clinical practice* (pp. 511-518). Baltimore: Williams & Wilkins.

Herzlinger, R., & Schwartz, J. (1985, July-August). How companies tackle health care costs. I. *Harvard Business Review,* 69-81.

Holzbach, R.L., Piserchia, P.V., McFadden, D.W., Hartwell, T.D., Herman, A., & Fielding, J.E., (1990). *Journal of Occupational Medicine, 32*(10), 973-978.

Jeffrey, N.A. (1996). 'Wellness plans' try to target the not-so-well. *The Wall Street Journal,* Thurs, June 20.

Jensen, D. (1993). Moving with the market. *The Case Manager, 4*(1), 60-69.

Johnson & Johnson Health Management, Inc. (1992, October 23). *Johnson & Johnson's LIVE FOR LIFE program, seven other health promotion programs, receive C. Everett Koop national health award; serve as cost-effective models for the nation.* [Press Release]. Author.

Kelly, L. (1991). *Dimensions of professional nursing* (6th ed.). New York: Permanon Press.

Knight, K.K., Goetzel, R.Z., Fielding, J.E., Eisen, M., Jackson, G.W., Kahr, T.Y., Kenny, G.M., Wade, S., Duann, S. (1994). An evaluation of Duke University's LIVE FOR LIFE health promotion program on changes in worker absenteeism. *JOM, 36*(5) 533-536.

Lessure, L.J., & Griffith, H.M. (1995). Putting prevention into clinical practice. *AAOHN Journal, 43*(2), 72-75.

Leutzinger, J., Goetzel, R., Richling, D., & Wade, S. (1993, mid-March). Projecting the impact of health promotion on medical costs. *Business and Health,* 39-44.

Lugo, N.R. (1997). Nurse-managed corporate employee wellness centers. *The Nurse Practitioner, 22*(4), 104-113.

Lusk, S.L., & Kerr, M.J. (1994). Conducting worksite research: Methodological issues and suggested approaches. *AAOHN Journal, 42*(4), 177-181.

Mandelker, J. (1993, mid-March). Using claims data to expand a health promotion program. *Business and Health,* 32-35.

Mavis, B.E., Stachnik, T.J., Gibson, C.A., & Stoffelmayr, B.E. (1992). Issues related to participation in worksite health promotion: A preliminary study. *American Journal of Health Promotion, 7*(1), 53-60.

McHorney, C., Ware, J., & Raczek, A. (1993). The MOS 36-item short form survey (SF-36). II. Psychometric and clinical tests of validity in measuring physical and mental health constructs. *Medical Care, 31*(3), 247-263.

Mullahy, C. (1995). *The case manager's handbook.* Gaithersburg, MD: Aspen Publishers.

Pelletier, K.R. (1993). A review and analysis of the health and cost-effective outcome studies of comprehensive health promotion and disease prevention programs at the worksite: 1991-1993 update. *American Journal of Health Promotion, 8*(1), 50-62.

Peterson, K.W., & Hilles, S.B. (Eds.). (1992). *The Society of Prospective Medicine: Directory of health risk appraisals.* Indianapolis: Society of Prospective Medicine.

Picard, M., Dennis, C., Schwartz, R., Kraemer, H., Berger, W., III, Blumberg, R., Heller, R., Lew, H., & DeBusk, R. (1989). Cost-benefit analysis of early return to work after uncomplicated acute myocardial infarction. *American Journal of Cardiology, 63,* 1308-1324.

Pilote, L., Thomas, R., Dennis, C., Goins, P., Miller, N., Kraemer, H., Leong, C., Berger, W., III, Lew, H., Heller, R., Rompf, J., & DeBusk, R. (1992). Return to work after uncomplicated myocardial infarction: A randomized clinical trial of practice guidelines in the community setting. *Annals of Internal Medicine, 117,* 383-389.

Rost, K., Connell, C., Schechtman, K., Barzilai, B., & Fisher, E.B., Jr. (1990). Predictors of employee involvement in a worksite health promotion program. *Health Education Quarterly, 17*(4), 395-407.

Russell, L.B. (1993). The role of prevention in health reform. *New England Journal of Medicine, 329,* 352-354.

Sayles, S.M. (Ed.). (1981). Rehabilitation nursing: Concepts and practice. A core curriculum. Evanston, IL: Rehabilitation Nursing Institute.

Scharlach, A.E., Mor-Barak, M.E., & Birba, L. (1994). Evaluation of a corporate-sponsored health care program for retired employees. *Health and Social Work, 19*(3), 192-198.

Snell, J. (1995). Health at work. *Nursing Times, 91*(25), 48-51.

Sorensen, G., Stoddard, A., Ockene, J.K., Hunt, M.K., & Youngstrom, R. (1996). Worker participation in an integrated health promotion/ health protection program: Results from the WellWorks project. *Health Education Quarterly, 23*(2), 191-203.

Stokols, D., Pelletier, K.R., & Fielding, J.E. (1995). Toward an integration of medical care and worksite health promotion. *Journal of the American Medical Association, 273,* 1136-1142.

Turner, C. (1995). Health risk appraisals. *AAOHN Journal, 43*(7), 357-467.

U.S. Department of Health and Human Services, U.S. Public Health Service. (1991). *Healthy people 2000.* (PHS Publication No. 91-50213). Washington, DC: U.S. Government Printing Office.

Wellness programs pay dividends. (1995). *Business and Health, 13,* Suppl. 3A, 23-27.

Wilson, M.G. (1990). Factors associated with, issues related to, and suggestions for increasing participation in workplace health promotion programs. *Health Values, 14*(4), 29-36.

Witherspoon, D., & Wilson, B.R.A. (1990). Evaluating research in worksite health promotion. *Health Values, 14*(4), 22-28.

POLITICAL and ECONOMIC CONSIDERATIONS in HEALTH PROMOTION

CHAPTER

15

Economic Considerations in Health Promotion

Wendy Dahar and Duncan Neuhauser

To understand the large changes rapidly occurring in the delivery of care, it is important to understand their history. Knowing these historical trends is essential to understand economic influences on health promotion and disease prevention.

MEDICAL CARE ORGANIZATIONS IN THE RECENT PAST

To greatly oversimplify a complex reality, up until recently, health care in the United States was made up of a mix of federal, state, and local government programs and private, nonprofit, and for-profit organizations. Most of the health care dollars spent were for services provided by independent hospitals (largely private and nonprofit); physicians, dentists, and other health care professionals (mostly those in fee-for-service private practice); nursing homes (mostly small for-profit organizations) and for drugs. The four major sources of payment were private insurers, including Blue Cross/Blue Shield; Medicare, mostly for persons older than 65 years; Medicaid, for the poor; and individuals, who paid out-of-pocket. Private insurance usually was purchased through employers and covered employees and their families. Medicare, a federal program, was funded by Social Security payroll deductions. Medicaid is a joint federal and state program, and payment was on a fee-for-service basis for providers and on a cost-for-service basis for hospitals.

TYPES OF PREVENTION

One can think of three types of prevention: environmental, behavior, and clinical health. Funding for important environmental prevention programs comes from outside the health care field. Some examples of these programs include construction of safer highways, air and water pollution laws, violence prevention programs, air traffic control systems, car air bags and safety belts, and maintenance of a clean public drinking water supply. Some programs, such as pasteurization of milk and restaurant sanitary inspections, are under the direction of health departments.

Behavior prevention incorporates activities that individuals do or don't do, such as exercising, dieting, smoking, drinking to excess, taking part in high-risk sexual behavior, and using bicycle helmets. Advertisers try to influence individuals' behaviors by insinuating or promising that health and security accompany certain behaviors. These appeals have an effect on individuals' purchases.

Clinical health prevention includes activities such as disease screening and vaccinations, prenatal care, well-child visits, and periodic health check-ups. Two of these vaccination efforts, for smallpox and polio, have been so successful that smallpox does not exist in the open (outside the laboratory) and polio is no longer resident in all the Americas. At one time, these diseases had a massive effect on health care costs, morbidity, and mortality.

THE ROLE OF HEALTH INSURANCE

Traditionally, health insurance has paid for services covered under the insurance contract. Insurers controlled their costs by defining covered services. The economics of insurance worked best for coverage of acute hospital admissions, surgery, laboratory tests, emergency care, and expensive drugs. It did not work well, however, for coverage of preventive services, including regular preventive dental care; psychotherapy; and long-term nursing home care. Thus, the former were well covered and preventive services were underfunded. In addition, as the costs of the former rose, there was less money available for preventive services.

Medicare and Medicaid, which are available to the eligible poor and the elderly in nursing homes who cannot pay for their care, followed the payment methods of health insurance. These programs are now moving toward capitation payment. Capitation programs are those in which an organization is given a fixed amount of money for all services to a defined group of clients. Government-funded programs, however, have attempted to fill in gaps in coverage of preventive services. Special support has been provided for vaccines, mammography, influenza immunization for the elderly, prenatal care, and well-child visits. It is important to note that money is not the only barrier to the use of such preventive services. Clients may also face structural barriers (e.g., the availability and organization of services, ease of transportation) and personal barriers (e.g., acceptability of services, culture, language, attitudes toward and knowledge of services, competing time demands, levels of education, and income) (Institute of Medicine, 1993). These types of barriers discourage some from using such services, even when they are free.

As the cost of health insurance has gone up, more individuals have been left uninsured. The uninsured may seek out government-supported health services such as neighborhood health centers; the Veteran's Administration hospitals and clinics; or urban "hospitals of last resort," such as Bellvue in New York City, Cook County in Chicago, or Los Angeles General Hospital. Too often this care is provided in emergency departments, where care is expensive and without continuity.

President Clinton's health plan proposed to provide health insurance coverage for all. It was the latest in a long series of such plans dating back to the 1940s that have failed to become law. Because of this, attention has turned to the private sector and state initiatives of reform, particularly with respect to Medicaid. In the absence of a national health plan, marketplace economics are driving rapid and massive change.

THE NEW ECONOMIC CONTEXT OF HEALTH CARE

Forty years ago, a group of public health scholars and activists clearly distinguished the terms medical care and health care. *Medical care* was considered to be services received in hospitals, whereas *health care* was viewed as a broader range of activities, including the promotion of healthy life-styles, safe roads, sanitation, and air pollution control in addition to the services physicians and hospitals provided. Thus health care came to be regarded as a much larger set of activities. With time, however, this distinction has become blurred. For example, medical care research has been renamed health services research. In addition, there is now a federal agency, the Health Care Policy and Research (AHCPR) agency, that studies the organization and financing of medical care. Yet, for those in the health care industry who place high value on prevention, maintaining the distinction between health care and medical care is important. They point to examples such as the abstinence of smoking being the most effective "cure" for lung cancer. Furthermore, many nurses differentiate medical care (what physicians do) and nursing care or client care. In short, the terms medical care and health care, while apparently similar if not synonymous, imply for many persons subtle but significant differences in meaning.

As previously stated, American health services are undergoing very rapid change. The growth of large managed care systems competing for enrollees on the basis of price, quality, and acceptability is driving this change. These systems provide services based on capitation payment. As stated previously, for each enrolled member, the plan gets a fixed amount of money per month. Out of this amount, the plan provides a contracted range of medical and health services. To survive, the plan must satisfy its members; must satisfy the payors, whether it be the federal government for Medicare participants, state governments for Medicaid participants, or private companies for their employees and dependents; and must provide care within the amount of money available to it.

Capitation has reversed the economic incentives of providing services. Fee-for-service encourages more services, whereas capitation discourages use of services. Thus managed care systems, such as health maintenance organizations (HMOs), under capitation try to reduce the amount of hospital days and specialist services they will cover and therefore can charge lower premiums. Enrollment in such plans is steadily growing. Medicare participants can choose to join capitated plans. Many states are moving their Medicaid program members into capitation plans. As a result of these changes, the number of existing hospitals and medical specialists are no longer needed. Another result of capitation is a strong economic incentive for these plans to cover prevention measures and thus reduce the need for hospital and specialist services.

When fee-for-service plans were dominant, there was concern about "unnecessary surgery," too many laboratory tests, and too much cost. Under capitation, predictably, the concerns have shifted to areas such as rationing of care, denial of wanted services, and "drive-through deliveries."

WHO WILL PAY FOR PREVENTION?

As stated before, the funding for most prevention will come from outside of the medical care system, but now there are more reasons why managed care systems are becoming concerned about the costs of prevention, including the following (see also Chapter 3):

1. Payors are evaluating managed care plans on the basis of their prevention activities, such as the percent of appropriate members with influenza immunizations, Pap smears and mammograms, and well-child visits. Many plans are making great efforts

to measure these percentages and increase the rates. An example of an evaluation list is the Health Plan Employer Data and Information Set (HEDIS), a measurement tool designed to help give insurance consumers and purchasers the information they need to reliably compare the performance of managed care plans. HEDIS asks plans to report on preventive activities such as mammography and childhood immunization and the percent of appropriate enrollees who have received them.

2. Some prevention pays in the short run. Keeping persons with asthma out of the emergency room and out of the hospital can save the plan a lot of money. This can be done with client education, prevention, and self-care and at a lower cost than hospitalization.

3. Some persons choose plans because they like the plan's emphasis on prevention and health promotion. Attracting members who want to be healthy and who are willing to make the required effort may cost the plan less in medical care.

4. Because of membership turnover, some health promotion activities have a payoff so far into the future that the plan may never realize a benefit for coverage of these activities. Reducing teenage smoking to avoid lung cancer 30 years from now will, for example, be costly today and be of value many years later when most of these persons will no longer be plan members.

   In some areas, however, competing plans are getting together to promote and share the costs of preventive and public health programs. Thus several competing Medicaid plans may agree to share an effort to reduce the number of unplanned and unwanted teenage pregnancies for a city. They all gain, even though any one teenager may be in and out of Medicaid or shift plans several times. Partnerships between fiercely competing health plans and local health departments to help prevent costly illnesses may continue to grow; however, these plans will require positive results if they are to continue to support such efforts.

5. Given their fixed revenue, managed care plans have limited resources and must choose where to make their effort. Medical technology assessment, clinical decision analysis, cost-effectiveness analysis, and cost-benefit analysis play a part in what choices are made.

These methods are described in the following sections, and an example of their use in a large managed care plan is given as well.

GIVE VALUE FOR MONEY

For those who wish to advocate more preventive services within the U.S. medical care system, there is a new imperative. It is no longer adequate to just say that prevention is good and therefore support is justified; ideals and virtue alone will not be persuasive. It is necessary to demonstrate that the preventive program being advocated *really* works. It must give value for money. Louise B. Russell summarized her review of screening efficacy in 1986 as follows:

> A growing body of research indicate that the chronic, degenerative diseases of middle and old age can often be prevented or at least delayed many years.
>
> While prevention has great potential, it is neither riskless nor costless.
>
> The evidence also shows that, even after allowing for savings in treatment, prevention usually adds to medical expenditures, contrary to the popular view that it reduces them.
>
> Prevention cannot be assumed to be a better choice than cure in every case. Individual measures must be evaluated on their merits (pp. 109-110).

In her 1994 follow-up review, she stated:

> The issue of first importance for any screening test is whether it accomplishes anything. A test may detect the condition accurately, but does anything need to be done about the condition, and if something needs to be done, are any of the available therapies effective? Are they more effective when applied early? Unless early treatment makes a difference, screening is pointless.
>
> The high costs of screening are often ignored, indeed unrecognized, by those who develop recommendations (pp. 77, 81).

SHOW THAT IT WORKS

To show that a prevention effort works, one must do the following: Take two similar groups of persons who may benefit, and invite their participation. Involve one group in the prevention effort, and leave the other group alone. Then, look at the results for both groups and see whether the expected difference occurred.

Today, achieving similarity of groups is best assured by random assignment of persons to the groups. The study subjects should be similar to actual clients (generalizability) and numerous enough so that change can be observed (power). Participants are asked for informed consent, even though they may not know which group they are in (a blinded study). The intervention could be a screening test with follow-up treatment. The expected outcome should be clearly defined in advance (e.g., cancers found, years of life saved), well-measured, and posited to result from the preventive effort. The difference, if any, between the outcomes for the groups should be large enough so that they are unlikely to have occurred by chance (statistical tests of significance).

The U.S. Preventive Services Task Force used this approach to evaluate 169 clinical preventive services. The best evidence came from randomized controlled trials. Intermediate evidence came from other types of studies, and the lowest quality of evidence was based on expert opinion alone.

Even if something is known to work, is it worth doing? To answer this broader question, a new set of tools is needed. These include technology assessment; clinical decision analysis; and economic reasoning, including cost-benefit and cost-effectiveness analysis (Box 15-1). The U.S. Preventive Services Task Force recognized the difference between showing that an effort worked versus showing that it is worth doing. Adding in other information to its knowledge of efficacy (does it work), the task force developed an alphabetical summary score, which was based on the earlier work of the Canadian Preventive Services Task Force: *A* is good evidence for use, *B* is fair evidence for use, *C* is poor evidence for use, *D* is fair evidence to reject, and *E* is good evidence for exclusion from periodic health examinations.

These task forces paid particular attention to screening for disease. The following is a set of questions to ask to determine whether such tests are worth doing. These questions are associated with *clinical decision analysis.*

1. What are the alternative choices? The major clinical choices are to test or not test and treat or not treat.
2. Who makes the decision: the client, health care professional, health plan, or society? All have slightly different interests at stake. One reason for these differences are the economic consequences of the decision. For example, an individual with health insurance may pay only a small part of the cost for an examination, whereas the insurer would pay for most of the cost.

Box 15-1

Definitions of decision-making tools

Medical technology assessment is the broadest of these concepts. It is the total evaluation of the social impact of a medical technology, such as a surgical procedure, laboratory test, or early cancer detection.

Clinical decision analysis considers the choices; the consequences of those choices; the probability that those consequences will occur; how those consequences are valued; and given this information, how the right choice is made.

Cost-effectiveness analysis compares the costs of doing something and measures the outcomes in nonmonetary terms, such as years of life saved or cancers found. Cost per year of life saved is a typical outcome of such analysis.

Cost-benefit analysis compares the inputs measured in costs with the outputs (results or benefits), also in costs (or savings), to see whether the benefits are greater than the costs.

3. What is the prevalence or frequency of the disease among the population being tested or screened? The rarer the condition, the greater the costs per case. There is considerable agreement that mammography is appropriate for women older than 50 years and generally not appropriate for use as a screening tool among those younger than 40 years. There is a lively debate, however, about the appropriateness for all women ages 40 to 50 years. This debate is based in part on the prevalence of the condition, the predictive value of screenings, and where to draw the line for a policy recommendation and reimbursement.
4. How accurate is the test? There are two types of test errors—the test can be positive, but the client is healthy, or the test can be negative, but the client has the disease.
5. What is the probability of obtaining a positive result?
6. What is the next step if the test is positive?
7. If action to treat is taken, what are the assurances that the treatment will be beneficial? What are the expected outcomes of treatment?

After answering this set of questions, the next steps in clinical decision-making involve measuring the outcomes in a common metric (years of life saved, dollars spent or saved, cancers found) and comparing the choices according to their average expected outcomes. The one with the better average outcome is selected. This is the basic structure of clinical reasoning.

COST-EFFECTIVENESS ANALYSIS

Cost-effective analysis (CEA) relates the costs of the program (effort or inputs) to the outcomes (results or output) in the form of a ratio. Typical examples in health care are costs per cancer found, cost per auto accident avoided, cost per vaccination given, cost per life saved, cost per year of life saved, and cost per quality adjusted life year saved (QALYS).

Consider a study in which a large public awareness program aimed at reducing smoking is carried out in 11 communities (experimental) and not in 11 other similar (control) communities. The results are that 10% of moderate smokers quit because of the program. The cost of the program, including advertising and brochure costs, can be measured. The program lasted 3 years and cost $300,000 for each community. There were 5000 moderate smokers in the study, and 500 of those quit as a result of the program, according to the study results (1000 quit in the control communities, 1500 quit in the communities with the program, thus the 500 difference is presumed to be a result of the experimental program).

Are the costs appropriately measured? Was everything included? On the output side, the measure is the number of smokers who quit as a result of the program. The benefits derived from these individuals no longer smoking could be measured by transforming quitters into years of life saved. This could be estimated from epidemiologic studies relating smoking to mortality by age compared with the age-adjusted life expectancy of nonsmokers.

In this study, the cost in each community per quitter is $600 (500 quitters multiplied by $600 equals $300,000—the total cost of the program in each community). Should this preventive program be recommended? This question can only be answered by asking: How else can this money be spent? If the next best smoking cessation program has a cost effectiveness ratio of $1000 per quitter, then this program should be recommended. However, if another choice is to give the influenza immunization to the elderly at a cost of $50 per immunization, and only one choice can be selected, it is difficult to decide which one it should be.

It is necessary to transform the two different outcomes (quitters and immunizations) into a common metric, such as years of life saved, to make a comparison and a decision. One should note that after doing so, one group will benefit and the other will not. This is called the *distribution effect*. One way to decide which program to select is to calculate years of life saved for both programs and assume that 1 year of life is valued the same for all, and then choose the program with the lowest cost per year of life saved.

It is not necessary for health care professionals to engage in debates regarding the broader social, political, or economic outcomes of prevention choices (e.g., young smokers are productively employed, the elderly are revered for their age and wisdom); however, it is important to be aware of this issue of distributive justice.

In the last 15 years, there has been an explosion in the number of studies of the cost-effectiveness of preventive and medical treatments. These studies calculate program costs per year of life saved. Tammy Tengs and associates (1995) have summarized the results of 500 life saving interventions. In some examples, the analyses show that the intervention saves both money and lives. An example of this is the use of fire detectors in homes. The cost of the detectors was more than made up by reduced fire damage, and it saved lives. Some interventions showed a cost per year of life saved, but the cost was low, such as the chlorination of drinking water ($3100 per year of life saved). Some interventions are beyond our society's resources to fund. A sampling of health promotion and disease prevention program results based on estimated cost per year of life saved are listed in 15-1. Studies such as the one in Table 15-1 are conducted in specific settings and circumstances; applied elsewhere, the results could be different.

COST-BENEFIT ANALYSIS

Cost-benefit analysis (CBA) measures both inputs and outputs in dollar amounts. CBA allows decisions to be made in a way that is not possible using cost-effectiveness analysis. If the benefits of a program exceed the costs, it should be done. In the preceding example

Table 15-1

Examples of health related cost-effectiveness study results

PROGRAM STUDIED	ESTIMATED COST PER YEAR OF LIFE SAVED
Fire detectors in homes	Saved lives and money
Mandatory motor cycle helmet laws	Saved lives and money
Reduced lead content in gasoline	Saved lives and money
Sickle cell screening for African-American newborns	$240
Influenza vaccination for high-risk persons	$570
Mammography for women age 50 years	$810
Random motor vehicle inspection	$1500
Smoking cessation advice for women ages 45-49 years	$1900
Chlorination of drinking water	$3100
National speed limit of 55 miles per hour	$6600
Annual mammography versus current screening practices for women ages 40-49 years	$190,000
Preoperative chest x-rays to detect abnormalities in children	$360,000
Warning letters sent to problem drivers	$720,000
Asbestos ban in automatic transmission components	$66 million
Sickle cell screening for non-black low-risk newborns	$34 billion

Data from "Five-hundred life saving interventions and their cost effectiveness," by Tengs, T.O., Adams, M.E., Pliskin J.S. et al, 1995, Risk Analysis, 15, (3), pp. 369-390.

of a smoking cessation program, suppose the societal benefit of quitting smoking is $1000 per person in terms of treatment costs avoided and productive life prolonged. Five hundred smokers stopped as a result of this program, which cost $300,000 per community. In this example, the costs total $300,000, but the benefits total $500,000. (500 quitters multiplied by $1000 savings per quitter) Therefore this program should be implemented.

Cost-benefit analysis often requires translating years of human life into a dollar value. This is unnerving for many and the translation so imperfect that most analysts shy away from it.

Note that in the smoking cessation example, the costs and benefits are accrued to different persons or organizations. Taxpayers may have paid for the program; smokers benefited by a longer, better life; and their employers saved on the cost of health care benefits.

The practical use of cost-benefit analysis by a managed care plan in the example that follows is distinctive for several reasons: a series of clinical care improvements are listed, the costs of the programs are stated in advance, and the benefits to the plan and plan members are also stated in dollars. These benefits are the short term and directly accrue to the plan. If one $10,000 hospital admission can be avoided by one $2000 asthma education program, the plan can realize a rapid saving. Note that not all benefits are measured in this example. For instance, not measuring the dollar value of 25 asthmatic clients gaining the confidence to control their own asthma underestimates the benefits of this program. Further, the costs and benefits accrued to the health plan can result in savings that can be passed back to those who pay the premiums. The full academic scholarly analysis would be expected to include all these benefits. In the case of a real health plan, approximations suit the purpose.

....

Case Study

The following example is used to illustrate the process of determining the costs and benefits of health promotion programs in a managed care setting. The site is a middle-sized managed care organization (about 200,000 enrollees) committed to designing programs and services to improve quality while decreasing costs of health care for its members.

Many proposed health promotion projects are aimed at improving quality and reducing costs. Clinical projects can be submitted by health care professionals or any clinical department employee. A formal process has been developed to assist the organization in the selection and prioritization of projects. The projects are first considered by a quality project evaluation committee, which considers the value of the project and the ability to track project outcomes. An analysis is then conducted to determine the potential impact and applicability of each project to the managed care organization's population. The analysis has four stages: a review of the relevant literature, a review of available demographic databases, a determination of estimated cost savings, and a determination of each project's costs.

The initial stage in determining the feasibility of a project is a review of the relevant literature, including peer-reviewed published literature, as well as the recommendations from the U.S. Preventive Services Task Force. The literature is studied to determine the potential impact of an intervention. For example, a flu immunization program in an elderly population has been reported to reduce the hospitalization rates by 20% to 40% for pneumonia and influenza. Similarly, an education program involving the distribution of a self-care book and the integration of the book into medical care has been reported to decrease total medical visits and minor illness visits by 20%. Patient satisfaction surveys have also determined that the self-care program increases members' satisfaction with their health plan and allows health plan members to feel more confident in knowing how to take care of themselves.

The second stage includes a review of demographic databases to determine the potential impact of an intervention for the population of interest. Membership systems can be used to determine the number of members in a particular age or gender group. The number of senior or pediatric members or the number of members who receive care at a particular facility can be determined. A computerized client record system can be used to obtain the number of hospital admissions and/or ambulatory visits in the population of interest with a particular diagnosis. For example, the number of members admitted to hospitals with a myocardial infarction or the number of pediatric asthmatic office visits can be obtained. Information about the demographics of the membership can be used to target and tailor the project to the group or subgroup of interest.

The next step includes a determination of potential savings and the actual cost saving of a particular intervention. This involves obtaining data on the cost of a hospitalization, emergency room visit, or office visit for a particular diagnosis. Cost estimates can then be calculated. For example, the potential cost savings of a self-care program for pediatric members can be determined by multiplying the potential reduction in office visits resulting from the intervention, the number of pediatric members affected by the intervention, and the average cost of an office visit. Some benefits, such as increased member satisfaction resulting from the program, are less tangible and are hence more difficult to determine.

Table 15-2

Hypothetical cost savings table

Project	Description	Program Cost	Cost Savings	Net Savings	Area of Savings
Pediatric fever acute care	Use of fever education video and pamphlet for acute care	$1500	$400,000	$398,000	Office
Adult high utilizers	Serial questionnaires and educational feedback	$420,000	$1 million	$580,000	Office and hospital
Influenza immunization	Mailed and telephone reminders	$3000	$42,000	$39,000	Hospital
Smoking cessation	Education effort	$3000	$350,000	$347,000	Office and hospital
Hypertension medications	Conversion of clients to recommended medications; educational program	$10,000	$600,000	$590,000	Pharmacy
Asthma emergency department initiative	Identification of at-risk population; client and physician/staff education	$3000	$200,000	$197,000	Emergency room
Hyperlipidemia with known coronary artery disease	Integrated care and education	$250,000	$1.8 million	$1.5 million	Office and hospital
Diabetic amputation prevention	Identification of at-risk population; client education about foot care	$1500	$165,000	$163,500	Hospital
Self-care handbook	Self-care project, including handbook and reinforcement of self-care via integration into care	$110,000	$570,000	$460,000	Office, including phone calls

The final step is a determination of the fixed and variable costs of the program. The fixed costs include items such as materials. The variable costs are often difficult to estimate since they include the physician and the nurse educator time to deliver the intervention.

Table 15-2 illustrates how proposed projects can be ranked in terms of their potential cost savings. This table shows some hypothetical costs and potential cost savings from a variety of projects aimed at prevention of disease, improving members' care, and improving health outcomes. The program costs in the table include educational materials and variable personnel costs needed to implement them. The area of cost savings from the projects include office visit, hospitalization, and pharmacy costs.

One example of a project included in the table is the asthma emergency department initiative. This project is aimed at improving asthmatic client care and reducing emergency department costs. The program costs include the cost of materials for group classes and for educating clients, physicians, and nursing staff. The cost savings were calculated by determining the number of adult asthmatic clients in the managed care organization's population, the cost of an emergency department visit, and the potential reduction that could be accomplished through an intensive client and staff education program.

The process just described allows for the systematic evaluation and ranking of proposed health promotion projects. New projects are subjected to this process to determine where they rank relative to other ongoing projects. The program costs and their potential savings can then be compared.

Summary

The economics of medical care are rapidly changing. Large delivery systems that are reimbursed on a capitation basis will likely continue to compete for new membership. In this context, screening, prevention, and treatment will be reviewed to ensure that they are worth doing. Just as fee-for-services may have promoted excess utilization, capitation may discourage useful care. The expectation that preventive services must demonstrate value for money will continue. Managed care plans determine whether to cover a prevention program by calculating its costs and savings, ranking the priorities for the year, setting the program into place, and checking to see whether it has met expectations. The authors of this chapter believe this is the logic for choosing prevention activities that will be used in the future.

HELPFUL **RESOURCES**

American Association of Retired Persons. (1996). *Reforming the health care system: State profiles,* Washington, DC: Author.

Battista, R.N., & Laurence, R.S. (Eds.). (1988). *Implementing preventive services* [Supplement]. *American Journal of Preventive Medicine,* 4(4).

continued

HELPFUL **RESOURCES—cont'd**

Bernstein, P.L. (1996). *Against the gods: The remarkable story of risk,* New York: Wiley.

Canadian Task Force on the Periodic Health Examination. (1979). The periodic health examination. *Canadian Medical Association Journal, 121,* 1193-1254.

Elixhouser, A. (1993). Health care cost-benefit and cost-effectiveness analysis from 1979 to 1990, a bibliography [Supplement]. *Medical Care 31(7),* JS1-JS149.

Gold, M., Siegel, J. et al. (1996). *Cost effectiveness in health and medicine.* New York: Oxford University Press.

Johnson, H., & Broder, D. (1996). *The American way of politics at the breaking point.* Boston: Little, Brown.

Petitti, D. (1994). *Meta analysis, decision analysis and cost effectiveness analysis.* New York: Oxford University Press.

Reiser, S., & Anbar, M. (1984). *The machine at the bedside.* Cambridge, England: Cambridge University Press.

U.S. Preventive Services Task Force. (1996). *Guide to clinical preventive services* (2nd ed.). Baltimore: Williams & Wilkins.

U.S. Department of Health and Human Services, U.S. Public Health Service. (1990). *Healthy people 2000, National Health Promotion and Disease Prevention Objectives* Washington, DC: U.S. Government Printing Office.

U.S. Department of Health and Human Services, U.S. Public Health Service, Office of Disease Prevention and Health Promotion (ODPHP), Prevention report. Washington, DC: U.S. Government Printing Office. On-line: http://odphp.osophs.dhhs.gov

Weinstein, M., Fineberg, H. et al. (1980). *Clinical decision analysis.* Philadelphia: WB Saunders.

References

Institute of Medicine. (1993). *Access to health care in America.* Washington, DC: National Academy Press.

Russell, L.B. (1986). *Is prevention better than cure?* Washington, DC: The Brookings Institute.

Russell, L.B. (1994). *Educated guesses: Making policy about medical screening tests.* Berkeley, CA: University of California Press.

Tengs, T.O., Adams, M.E., Pliskin, J.S. et al. (1995). Five-hundred life saving interventions and their cost effectiveness. *Risk Analysis, 15*(3), 369-390.

CHAPTER

16

Future Directions for Health Promotion

Sherri Sheinfeld Gorin

The landscape for health promotion will no doubt change considerably as we enter the new millennium. Broad socio-demographic and economic changes have already occurred, including the growth in the aging population, transformations in the characteristics of the workforce, and alterations in the delivery of health care. These changes will probably broaden and deepen as the year 2000 approaches.

The population of the developed world is aging, thus straining health care systems throughout the world. In the United States alone, reform in the Medicare program has emerged as central to the political agenda, as well as more general changes in the Social Security system. Yet, the problems of a growing aging population have not been met by the political will necessary to address their solution.

A major piece of legislation, with prevention at its core, arose, gained national prominence, and died. The managed care area, designed to control costs and increase the quality of health care, has burgeoned and consolidated, alongside numerous attacks from consumers, health care professionals, the media, and governmental panels on the gap between its purported aims and its actions. Behavioral managed health care, in particular, is growing, as federally initiated programs such as the Community Mental Health Centers, with their community service orientation, continue to develop lucrative contracts with employer groups. Dental managed care, too, is emerging. Approximately 48% of those above the poverty line have private dental insurance; 90% of care is paid for either out-of-pocket or through this insurance (Oral Health Coordinating Committee, 1993). Public health agencies are privatizing by linking to managed care networks, with mixed outcomes for collective welfare and the costs of care. Community care networks are emerging as a means to enhance cooperation among health care, business, government, and community organizations to reduce the demand for services and to optimize resource use (American Hospital Association, 1994; Light, 1997). Additionally, U.S. consumers (an estimated 1 out of every 3 who speak English) (Eisenberg, Kessler, Foster et al, 1993) are increasingly using complementary and alternative medical therapies either instead of, or in addition to, conventional medicine. They are seeking more individualized care and longer health care professional-client interviews that they

401

often feel they receive from complementary and alternative medicine treatments (Joyce, 1994).

One may extend or extrapolate from existing trends and events for the purpose of forecasting. Predicting the future generally rests in the realm of the soothsayer (or the strategic planner), rather than the health care professional. Nonetheless, a guide to the most pronounced features likely to occur in health promotion in the near future follow.

DEMOGRAPHIC SHIFT TOWARD THE AGING

The aging processes are determined by and determine the societies in which one lives. Aging refers simultaneously to political, economic, physiologic, behavioral, social, religious, and chronologic events (Restrepo & Rozental, 1994). It is perceived differently in varied cultures, simultaneously as a loss and as a goal. In addition, dependency, often equated with aging, is socially created and may be diminished through increasing economic capabilities, enhancing opportunities for productive work, enriching social responsibilities, and decreasing the degree of deterioration experienced.

By the year 2150, the median age of the world's population will have risen to 42 years, up from 24 years in 1990 (University Center on Aging, 1993). During the next 2 decades, growth of the elderly will be moderate for most nations. After 2010, however, the number of elderly will increase rapidly (Tauber, 1993). Worldwide, the projected speed of relative increase in the world elderly population will be faster than that of the world child population. Among the elderly worldwide, the segment of those ages 80 and older is the fastest growing. Most of these octogenarians live in developed countries now; however, it is projected that by 2020 the majority will live in developing countries (Organización Pan Americana de la Salud, 1992).

In America, persons age 65 years and older constitute the fastest growing segment of the population. By 2020, more than 64 million Americans will be age 65 years or older, constituting nearly 22% of the U.S. population. Women will predominate; minorities, however, will be underrepresented in this age group (Koplan & Livengood, 1994). By the year 2000, 22% of elderly Americans will be 80 or older, very likely the largest proportion of the population in the world (Tauber, 1993).

By the year 2020, the dependency ratio (i.e., the proportion of persons not participating in the workforce to those who do participate) will increase because of the larger numbers of persons 65 and older. The ratio of working persons to those retired will be $3:1$, as opposed to $5:1$ at present (U.S. Senate Special Committee on Aging, 1991). This projection has obvious implications for changing health services and social support.

Policies designed to encourage health promotion among older persons are being proposed at present and will no doubt continue to emerge as lawmakers also age. Health promotion, which presently is mainly devoted to younger age groups—smoking cessation aimed at children and youths in schools and exercise programs for employees at work—will increasingly target programs for the elderly. To underpin that effort, the concept of "normality," in the sense of a common or prevalent finding (e.g., arthritis, root caries and peridontal disease, or an increase in blood pressure as a result of age) will require redefinition. Health care professionals will need to begin to view these "normalities" as risk factors for disease, rather than "immutable facts" of aging. For example, interventions designed to decrease blood pressure among the aged are critical to reducing the rates of stroke and coronary heart disease and thus must assume importance as public health goals.

Health promotion among older men and women will include functional independence and adding years of healthy life, rather than simply the elongation of life. Increasingly, older Americans will be living alone and may need special assistance to retain their independent functioning. This help will include assistance in performing activities of daily living (e.g., bathing, dressing, eating) so that they may remain residents in the community, rather than being placed in long-term nursing care. Social support thus is a critical factor in the older person being able to avoid institutionalization.

Chronic diseases are more common among the elderly than their younger counterparts. A considerable number of the major causes of death among persons age 65 and older—heart disease, cancer, stroke, chronic obstructive pulmonary disease, pneumonia, and influenza—are preventable or can be controlled. Changing certain health behaviors (e.g., stopping smoking, eating a balanced diet, reducing sodium, and losing weight) can reduce the risk of disease among older adults (Institute of Medicine [IOM] 1990). Physical activity is a central component of health promotion among the aging. Increasing levels of physical activity would reduce the incidence of coronary heart disease, hypertension, non-insulin–dependent diabetes mellitus, colon cancer, depression, and anxiety—the prominent diseases in older adults (Casperson, 1989).

Among older persons, increased immunizations against pneumococcal pneumonia, now generally administered only to the immunocompromised, would reduce its prevalence, which is 3 times more common among those older than 65 than younger persons and is responsible for restricted activity (National Center for Health Statistics, 1995). Immunizations against influenza are key among older adults, as death rates resulting from this disease are 34 to 104 times higher in this age group than in younger persons; only about 20% of persons age 65 and older receive such inoculations at present.

The appropriate use of medications, both prescribed and over-the-counter, are critical to health promotion among older persons. Adverse reactions may be exacerbated by decreased kidney and liver functions as individuals age; these physiologic alterations can change the way the body processes medications. Different drugs or lower doses may be used to offset these alterations.

Particularly among older individuals, health care professionals can monitor health status to detect early signs of health problems that can threaten independence, such as dementia or depression, as well as ensure an accurate distinction in diagnosis. Increased use of screening tools in primary care for the assessment of depression and early cognitive deficits, such as the deterioration of memory, orientation, general intellect, specific cognitive capacities, and social functioning—the clinical precursors to Alzheimer's disease and dementia—will become more important as the population ages. About 10% to 20% of these cases are treatable and may be caused by drug toxicity, metabolic disorders, depression, or hyperthyroidism (Clarfield, 1988; Larson, Reifler, Featherstone et al., 1984).

Health care professionals may counsel older women, in particular, about the benefits and risks of estrogen replacement therapy. Urinary incontinence is another condition that can affect functional independence because it increases with age, but it can generally be improved through pelvic muscle exercises and other behavioral treatments, drug therapy, and surgery (National Institute of Health, 1988).

Clearly, increased resources will need to be devoted to the elderly; given a declining workforce, however, from where will the resources come? An ethic of personal and family responsibility for health and the importance of life-style changes could again become an ideology to justify resource distributions. In contrast, an ideology that supports a fair, equitable distribution of bargaining power and resources among children, young, working adults and the old could be encouraged. Again, political will, as well as economic munificence, will be required to support these varied aims.

Concern for Social Justice

If one accepts the premise expressed in the World Health Organization Alma Alta Declaration, the task the health care field faces is to create social and economic conditions that allow *all* the world's citizens to achieve a state of health. Yet, many of the world's and, more locally, America's citizens—the poor, particularly poor children; the unemployed; and the economically marginal or exploited—face social situations that place them at high risk for disease and premature death, thus diminishing their health promotion. In fact, poverty—due in part to less education—leads to poorer health prospects overall (Marmot, Smith, Stansfeld et al, 1991; Tyroler, 1989; Salonen, 1982; Dayal, Power, & Chiu, 1982; Haan, Kaplan, & Camacho, 1987; Baquet, Horm, Gibbs, & Greenwald, 1991; Winkleby, Jatulis, Frank, & Fortmann, 1992; Guralink, Land, Blszer, Fillenbaum, & Branch, 1993; Charlton & White, 1995; Pappas, Queen, Hadden, & Fisher, 1993). The *Healthy People 2000 Midcourse Review* (1995) illustrates general movement forward toward health for most racial and ethnic minorities, who are overrepresented among the vulnerable in American society, relative to the population as a whole. African-Americans, however, have shown less movement toward health and are less likely to continue to move forward. This finding is of particular concern because, by the year 2000, African-Americans will comprise a larger proportion of the American populace than at present. This emphasizes the continued importance of targeting culturally relevant health promotion interventions to particular communities.

Increasingly, the poor and underserved will receive care through managed care organizations, Medicare, and Medicaid. This may result in increased continuity of care and integration of health care services, or it may result in less care for those most in need.

More and better insurance coverage for screening and counseling would encourage wider use of these services. Governments may encourage coverage for preventive services by commercial insurers and managed care entities by developing a market for such products and ensuring that they are financially viable. At present, many Americans have not received the clinical preventive services they need, in part due to financial barriers, thus contributing to the high levels of preventable morbidity and mortality in the population.

In addition, the number of individuals who are uninsured remains a problem and may be increasing, particularly among children (Employee Benefits Research Institute, 1997). Traditionally, the responsibility of caring for the uninsured has rested with local government agencies, such as health departments and public hospitals. Presently, these agencies are privatizing, particularly through mergers and contractual obligations with larger private health care companies, with mixed results for access and provision of services to vulnerable members of society.

Of course, access to preventive services depends on more than insurance coverage. Access also depends on the provision of enabling services, such as transportation and the reduction of language barriers. National health policies could encourage equity in access to health services. These policies could be implemented by local coordinating bodies, such as the public health department, and overseen by a federal agency, such as the Centers for Disease Control and Prevention (CDC) and/or the Health Care Financing Agency (US-DHHS, 1996; CDC, 1995). Continued advocacy from the health care field, coupled with federal legislation and strong federal public health leadership, will be necessary to promote health among society's most vulnerable members.

WORKSITES AS LOCI OF HEALTH PROMOTION

During the past 10 years, the workforce has been transforming. The number of women workers has increased, accounting for 46% of the total U.S. workforce in 1995, which is 6 out of every 10 women in the population. Women are projected to comprise 48% of the labor force in the year 2005 (U.S. Department of Labor, 1997). The number of older workers has increased also, and in certain areas of the country, such as the Southwest, the cultural and ethnic diversity of workers, too, has increased.

Meanwhile, the proportion of single-parent and dual-career families has grown in the United States. In 1992, 17.6% of all families were single-parent, primarily headed by women (U.S. Department of Labor, 1997); nearly one half (47%) of all African-American families were headed by women (U.S. Department of Labor, 1997). Women and minorities will comprise a large segment of tomorrow's labor force entrants. These changes in family structure due to labor force entrance have led to increased job pressures and constraints on discretionary, or leisure, time. The pressures are particularly acute among dual-career and single parents, particularly single mothers, who must balance child-care and occupational roles (Eckenrode & Gore, 1990; Gutek, Repetti, & Silver, 1988; Repetti, Matthews, & Waldron, 1989).

Economic recessions of the 1980s and 1990s have raised the unemployment rate among U.S. workers and prompted significant changes in the corporate culture, such as downsizing and rightsizing, and a shift from full-time to part-time employment in many sectors of the economy. For example, nearly 16% of the workforce lost at least one job during the recovery years of 1993-95, a rate that exceeds the 13% of the workforce that lost jobs during the *recession* of 1981-83 (Farber, 1997). These alterations have changed the social contract between employer and worker, and in many cases, have eroded the quality and scope of health insurance coverage and other employee benefits, especially among those shifted from permanent to contractual or temporary jobs. The proportion of nonelderly population with employer-sponsored health insurance has been declining since at least the late 1980s (Swartz, 1997). Employers are increasing the portion of health insurance premiums paid by employees, especially for dependent coverage, and increasing other cost-sharing expenses, to reduce labor costs. This drive to limit employer costs for employee health insurance benefits is causing more people with middle and low incomes either to lose their access to employer-sponsored insurance or to choose not to purchase insurance because their share of the premiums is beyond their means (Swartz, 1997). The costs of increased employer efficiency thus continues to be borne by individual workers and the effects felt by them, their families, and their communities.

These alterations have also placed increased psychosocial demands on those who remain in the workforce because they must do more work at the same level of compensation. Often, because of these labor uncertainties, workers stay in positions they dislike or perceive to be below their level of competence, thus leading to deleterious health consequences (Pelletier, 1994). Furthermore, employers, seeking better locations or economic conditions, may rearrange the physical space or location of the worksite, often requiring increased commuting, or they threaten workers with job elimination through automation. As a result of changed union protections, workers' concerns about job security and midlife career changes have increased (Stokols, Churchman, Scharf & Wright, 1990), often then leading to psychologic stress, elevated blood pressure, performance decrements, and increased illness symptoms (Novaco, Stokols, & Milanesi, 1990; Schaeffer, Street, Singer, & Baum, 1988).

Yet, worksites have the potential to serve as a center for community-based health promotion initiatives in the future. During the past 10 years, there has been a rapid rise in the growth of worksite health programs. For worksites to lead in community health promotion, however, the social changes that have occurred over the past 10 years, particularly the relationships among work organizations and the changes in technologies, family structures, and the larger community system, must be reflected in their programs.

Some comprehensive approaches to the creation of community health—through the development of a care continuum, systems of community accountability, and approaches to management with fixed resources—have been supported by the WK Kellogg Foundation, the Duke Endowment, Robert Wood Johnson Foundation, California Wellness Foundation, and the U.S. Public Health Service (American Hospital Association, 1998). Often, these involve collaboration among university researchers, corporate managers, insurance carriers, and primary care physicians (e.g., the Metropolitan Chicago Community Care Alliance, Healthcare 1999, the Stanford Coronary Risk Intervention Program (SCRIP) and corporate health programs at the Stanford University School of Medicine). These efforts could be expanded to include other sectors of the community (e.g., urban planners and television and news media) in an effort to establish "healthy cities" programs (Stokols, Pelletier, & Fielding, 1995). Collaborative links, including shared medical archives and databases, between corporate, community, and health care settings may foster similar comprehensive health programs in other communities.

Telecommunication technologies such as electronic mail, telefax, video, and computer interactive systems may increasingly be used in corporate settings to encourage employee participation in worksite health promotion programs. These technologies could be used to deliver programs on the healthy behaviors discussed in this text. Further, with the use of newer technologies, integrated systems designed to contain worksite health costs across the lifespan without compromising the quality of employees' medical care will continue to expand.

As the population ages and larger proportions of employees become retirees, industry will begin to consider the development of wellness programs for this group as well. Increasing retirees' quality of life could reduce health care expenditures under corporate plans, as well as enhance good will among former employees.

Further, partnerships are emerging among labor groups and public health organizations, as they begin to recognize many of their common interests. Labor's historically adversarial stance to management is beginning to change, with the continued growth of employee ownership and shared seats on boards of directors of major American corporations. Joint support for similar agendas concerning the health and welfare of working persons may continue to grow in the future.

GROWTH AND EXPANSION OF MANAGED CARE ORGANIZATIONS

Managed care will continue to grow as a result of increasing numbers of corporate mergers and evolution in the system's organization and role. Mergers among indemnity insurers and prepaid care plans, such as AETNA/USHealthcare, will continue, with mixed effects on corporate cultures, the collection of information on enrollees, and the provision of health promotive benefits.

Because of their clinical orientation, managed care organizations are likely to be active participants in the decisions regarding the provision of preventive services. These groups can partner with others, using their power to encourage education, legislation, and regulations to, for example, prevent the initiation of tobacco use or to encourage seat belt use among children and their parents. Alternatively, based upon the relative cost advantage of mortality for the most vulnerable, managed care companies may choose to fund fewer preventive services and thereby provide less care over an individual's shorter lifespan.

Many state-level public health agencies have dual roles with managed care organizations, as both partners and regulators; conflict between these roles may increase as managed care companies become more aggressive in their pursuit of cost savings. New mechanisms, such as legislation, for clarifying these relationships or resolving these conflicts may be warranted. In particular, state-level public health agencies, alongside community coalitions, may play a critical role in advocating for the continued provision of health promotion services, particularly to those most vulnerable, among whom savings may accrue over an extended period.

In addition, rigorous statewide longitudinal comparisons of clients receiving services in managed care settings versus those who are not are necessary to reveal clients' differing use of services as their health changes. Elderly clients, for example, may move in and out of the managed care arena as their health deteriorates (Morgan, Virnig, DeVito, & Persily, 1997). This movement may have important quality and fiscal ramifications.

Focus on the Health of the Community

As managed care organizations have become the primary providers of health care to large segments of the population, they have become more involved with the health of local communities. In part, this attention has grown to forestall regulatory interest in proscribing standards of consumer-oriented care for these companies. Yet, managed care organizations have also found that maintaining the health of populations is an important way to improve cost-effectiveness and to compete for new enrollees.

Collaboration among the business community, medical service providers, insurance carriers, government agencies, and universities will increase, as community rating becomes an important aspect of managed care. (To an insurer, community-rated premiums reflect the risk of the total community, including higher risk groups or individuals; experience-rated premiums, by contrast, reflect the risk of a delimited group, such as employees.) Further, coordinating bodies or agencies must emerge to ensure that a particular *catchment area* (a geographic area that defines a community to be enlisted) is well-served and that periodic appraisals of community health are monitored as a basis for health care decision-making. This could suggest a new role for the public health department.

Integration With Complementary and Alternative Medical Approaches

Managed care organizations are beginning to see an enrichment of community health through the integration of complementary and alternative medical (CAM) approaches with the more orthodox. This interest is generally borne of increased consumer use of CAM; its lower cost; and the personal experiences of several leaders of managed care organizations, such as the chief executive officer (CEO) of Oxford Health Plans, the CEO of Mutual of Omaha, Nebraska, and the CEO of Blue Cross of Washington and Alaska. The

CAM field has been legitimized by the formation of the National Institutes of Health Office of Alternative Medicine and the involvement of many noted scientific groups and universities in its study (e.g., more than 150 to 300 articles on research into complementary and alternative medicine are added each month to the British Library database, and Columbia University recently formed the Rosenthal Center for Alternative Medicine). As a result, efforts to integrate these two approaches to care will probably continue and expand.

At present, however, pilot efforts at integration have yielded limited results because managed care organizations generally have implemented a broad service benefit, with little client selection and few incentives to manage the care (Weeks, 1997). Further, the two approaches to health care—orthodox and complementary—reflect two different cultures, especially of science. Orthodox medical practice tends to view complementary approaches as placebos, or factors that are without specific activity for the condition being treated or evaluated (Shapiro, 1978). Orthodox medicine also views complementary and alternative medicine as using a less rigorous and a more qualitative approach to research. A recent scientific conference cited several methodologic difficulties in CAM, notably the difficulty of defining a control or comparison condition for study and the variability of care from client to client, thus making treatment comparisons difficult (Levin et al, 1997). Further, the two approaches speak different languages to describe their health promotive activities. Nonetheless, in the future, more contact between the two sets of approaches may yield more integration in effective health promotive interventions and more consonance in their conduct of scientific inquiry.

Accountability and Performance-based Care

Accountability to consumers, providers, and regulators is an important feature of managed care. Thus, managed care, health maintenance organizations (HMOs) in particular, has tremendous opportunities to influence the health of enrollees, as well as the communities from which they come. Health care purchasers, particularly large employers, have collaborated with HMOs to develop external systems to measure the quality of both preventive and treatment services in managed care and to hold HMOs accountable for their delivery. Employers have begun to review "report cards" from the Health Plan Employer Data and Information Set (HEDIS) and accreditation ratings from the Joint Commission on Accreditation of Health Care Organizations (JCAHO) when making decisions about the health care services they purchase. Purchasers are likely to continue to push for these evaluative mechanisms. If systems such as HEDIS continue to emphasize prevention, managed care entities will continue to view the provision of services, including preventive services, as competitive tools.

In a highly competitive environment, however, outcomes that are simpler to understand and more reliably measured, such as costs, must not displace quality (or quality of life) as desirable system aims. Therefore, Campbell's classic observation regarding quantitative indicators will remain pertinent to the measurement of health promotion within organizational contexts in the future

> "The more any quantitative indicator is used for social decision-making, the more it will be subject to corruption pressures, and the more apt it will be to distort and corrupt the social processes it is intended to monitor" (Campbell, 1974, p. 85).

The difficulty of retaining a sense of the overall performance of the organization, as reflected in its multiple activities and outcomes, is matched by the arduous task of choosing appropriate measures. As most health care organizations and networks adopt multiple performance criteria, health care professionals will continue to struggle with making sense of the whole or choosing the best index to reflect the quality of work performed. How will organizations judge whether increased effort in one criterion improves overall performance? Or, will an improvement in one criterion be offset by a reduction in another? In addition, will health promotion and, ultimately, health be included in these important criteria? At present, many industries are struggling with the issue of the "corporate scorecard" (Kurtzman, 1997, p. 128), particularly as different accreditors, trustees, administrators, staff, and clients prefer alternative weighing of criteria.

While organizations continue to merge and restructure to better negotiate for managed care contracts, the size of the resulting health care institutions will themselves encourage increased production of quantitative performance indicators. Both vertical and horizontal communication difficulties increase with growth; quantitative measures are easier to analyze and to verify. They better endure the rigors of extensive organizational travel, and they serve a symbolic function—they demonstrate that the organization is coming to grips with its problems in a rational manner (Sheinfeld Gorin, 1985).

More standardized and uniform measures of cost-effectiveness, cost-benefit, and productivity will be developed and used as increased attention is paid to quantitative measures of outcome. Extensive research on the cost-effectiveness of preventive interventions, particularly at multiple levels (e.g., policy, group, and individual) (e.g., Royce, Sheinfeld Gorin, Edelman, Rendino-Perrone, & Orlandi, 1990a, 1990b) should be supported by federal and foundation sources. A larger, more comprehensive consideration of the costs and benefits of preventive services, and their effects on longer-term behavioral change, also should be evaluated. Further, research on the conceptual and empirical links among diverse criteria of performance and their correlates in organizational effectiveness and client health will be necessary in the future.

On the micro-level, clients will become increasingly concerned about the ramifications of increased attention to performance measurement because the data are derived from their personal health records. Managed care companies develop risk profiles of their membership, and, through inducements as well as disincentives (e.g., dropping a provider from a managed care list) actively encourage providers to reduce risks among their clients. Clients may thus wonder about the limited protections to privacy of their own medical record. Insurance companies; employers; numerous managed care employees; and, oftentimes, colleagues, may review the results of risk screens or genetic tests, as well as act on them. Privacy will thus remain a critical issue in health promotion as the delivery system becomes increasingly performance-based.

GROWTH IN HEALTH CARE COSTS RESULTING FROM TECHNOLOGY

Genetic testing has emerged as one important new technology in which costs must be weighed against benefits. Interest in this technology will grow as we enter the next millenium. Since the end of World War II, the expansion of public and private health care insurance has provided considerable incentives to develop new technologies in health care. There has been a growing market for any new technology, however costly, that has the potential to enhance health (Shroder & Weisbrod, 1990). While new technologies have often brought improvements in quality, they have delivered these advances at substantial cost increases per episode of care. Overall, technology has helped to fuel the astounding growth in the cost of health care and is projected to be 16.4% of the gross national product by the end of the decade (USDHHS, 1995; Fuchs, 1972; Newhouse, 1993). (GNP is a measure of the value of all goods and services produced by the country.) Neither the proliferation of managed care organizations nor health policy changes have yet fully contained these costs.

Concomitant with the growth of medical care costs resulting from technology, the interest in medical technology assessment has grown. Technology assessment—the application of scientific methods to the evaluation of health practices—has expanded beyond safety and efficacy to encompass quality of life, client preferences, and the evaluation of costs and benefits (Office of Technology Assessment, 1980; Fuchs & Garber, 1993). This approach could be used to assess the impact of genetic testing, for example, a novel technology. At present, only two large companies analyze samples for the BRCA1, a mutant gene common among families in the population at high risk for breast cancer. The use of this technology is beginning to expand, yet if only 1% of the female population were tested, the cost of the test alone would be several billion dollars. Perhaps only 0.1% would test positive, predicting their lifetime risk for breast carcinoma. For others, the likelihood of locating the mutant gene is so low, and the probability of choosing testing so uncertain, that even the costs for implementing routine screening programs are prohibitive. Further, the potential psychologic, social, and ethical ramifications of routine testing are daunting.

Even among those who tested positive, however, the options would include genetic counseling, chemoprevention (e.g., with tamoxifen); more frequent screening; prophylactic treatment; or soon, gene therapy to manufacture proteins lacking the mutant gene. For prophylactic surgery alone, the cost might rise an additional $11 million (cf. Grann, Panegeas, Whang, Antman, & Neugut, in press). Even among those at high risk, who choose to know their status, the optimal preventive, surveillance, and treatment approaches for both long-term survival and quality of life are unknown. Further, without additional resources, monies spent on screening and treatment cannot be devoted to research on prevention.

In the near future, health care professionals will be increasingly challenged in working with clients regarding the decision to undergo genetic testing. Policy approaches to better characterize those most likely to benefit from novel technologies, such as genetic tests, as well as education, are strategies health care professionals must consider as they attend to both the cost and the benefits of new medical approaches.

VALUES FOR THE PRACTICE OF HEALTH PROMOTION

Because of the major changes in the sociodemographics of the American populace, delivery of health care, accountability, technology, and health promotion, ethical issues will emerge as critical to future practice. Some of the ethical questions to be answered in the near future are being posed now: Should women at high risk for breast cancer undergo genetic testing? Who should see the results? How should the results be protected? What kinds of decisions about insurance, work, and family life should be made on the basis of these results? Should risk appraisals inform employment decisions? Should decisions about the allocations of monies from federal and foundation sources be made on the basis of the health of a community? Should health promotion interventions be targeted to those most in need or those in largest number? Is is morally acceptable (good) to smoke, to remain overweight?

Core Values

To address these questions, health care professionals will need to clarify and better understand the value base of their work. Health care professionals require a set of moral values, or benefits that human beings provide to other individuals and communities (Baier, 1973; Kekes, 1993)—a compass to direct them in their work with clients. While some of the core values have been formalized as ethical guidelines (American Journal of Preventive Medicine, 1994), health care professionals working with clients toward health promotion must articulate their personal and collective vision of the "good life," "health," and the "good society." They should make clear the values, models, and ideals they wish for individuals and for societies. For example, do they hold an individualistic or a collectivist vision for society? They need "to explore and define what, very specifically, would be right. Toward what, stated as clearly as may be possible, should we aim?" (Galbraith, 1996, p. 1). This approach is consonant with teleological, or consequentialist, ethics, one of three major school of ethics (the other two are deontologic ethics and ethical skepticism). The teleological approach asserts that an individual's action may be deemed morally right or wrong only by judging the consequences of the action. The teleological approach requires that one act in a way as to produce "good" consequences, with good defined as pleasure, happiness, self-realization, and/or fulfillment. Utilitarian ethics, a unique type of teleological ethics best reflected in Jeremy Bentham's maxim, asserts that actions should produce the greatest good for the greatest number.

Deontological ethics maintain that there are rules, or principles, of action that have moral validity independent of the consequences of individual actions and that one must act in accordance with these rules, or principles. To the deontologist, acts are to be judged as moral or immoral through their comparison to some universal moral rule to which no exceptions can be made, such as those found in the Ten Commandments.

Ethical skepticism assumes that individual moral codes cannot be formulated and that there are many moral points of view.

In the United States, liberal philosophies of self-determination and rugged individualism generate fears of moralizing others' actions or intruding into someone else's moral space (Etzioni, 1993; Sandel, 1996). Yet, without moral direction, health care professionals' assumptions and practices may lead to abuses of power by their presuming to know best what clients need, stigmatizing clients with deficit-oriented labels, or neglecting to consider social injustices (Prilleltensky, 1997).

To assist professionals as they move into the future of health promotion, the field could carve a set of core social values. Although not comprehensive, these values would reflect both health promotion practice at present and may found the future, particularly as these values would be applicable to a variety of practice questions. The values include distributive justice, truth-seeking, human dignity, sharing, concern for the quality of life, and client loyalty (or advocacy) (cf., Sheinfeld, 1978; Sheinfeld & Lord, 1981). These values would operate as a whole in consort with one another. No one value should dominate another; the values should be regarded as complementary, rather than as mutually exclusive.

Distributive justice is based on Rawl's (1971) seminal work and refers to the ethical principle that the burdens and benefits of social institutions should be distributed in accord with standards of equality, need, or contract. It implies rules of nondiscrimination and of fairness in sharing and exchanging reciprocity and in restitution. Distributive justice promotes fair and equitable allocation of bargaining powers, resources, and obligations in society. Redistributing the power that rests in the hands of the health care professional is critical to achieve distributive justice for clients.

Concern for the quality of life often considers resource conservation, which leads to a prioritizing of the types of persons deserving of limited goods. In contrast to distributive justice, utilitarianism (the greatest good for the greatest number)—a foundation for much of current health policy—leaves important questions about access to resources for those in lesser numbers. Further, the concerns of the many may not always be apparent to health care professionals when they practice one person at a time.

As both scientist and practitioner, the health care professional, in the search for truth, must attempt as completely as possible to adopt Firth's (1952) stance of the "ideal observer"—an objective, impartial, omnipercipitent, and consistent judge of facts. To practice truth-seeking, the subsidiary values of personal competence, independence, and trust among the community of truth-seekers (or scientists) are critical. The epistemological (relating to the study of the foundations of knowledge) underpinnings of the truth-seeker are critical to understanding this value in practice. Epistemological underpinnings will determine the means by which client data are collected and thus their findings (Sheinfeld Gorin & Viswanathan, 1997).

Closely aligned to the concept of truth-seeking is that of protecting and respecting human dignity. Human dignity may be defined in terms of a person's ability to pursue alternative courses of action and to have available to him/her significant structural choices. The idea of alternatives, when so defined, emphasizes the individual's ability to control his/her own destiny, at least to some degree. Human dignity implies self-determination, in that clients may pursue their chosen goals without excessive frustration and in consideration of other person's needs or through reciprocal empowerment (Prilleltensky & Gonick, 1996).

Sharing is contained within the definitions of distributive justice (as reciprocity) and human dignity, (the right of each person to self-determine). Sharing is practiced by the health care professional and the client. It may promote a peaceful, respectful, and democratic process, whereby clients have meaningful input into decisions affecting their lives.

Advocacy, a manifestation of loyalty to the client, is generally exercised on behalf of one person or a group of clients to bring about changes that affect society as a whole. The health care professional may act as an advocate on behalf of clients when they have been deprived of their legal rights or have endured "public embarrassment or discourtesy . . . done them on the account of their age, race, incapacity, or status as recipients of assistance" (Keith-Lucas, 1971, p. 327). In this process, the ad-vocate may reflect caring and compassion, not only for the cause but for the client as well.

A Code of Ethics?

On these core value statements, strong in the face of changing political trends or narrow alignments of interest groups, an operational "code of ethics" might rest and a set of case study examples might be arranged.

While a code does not create virtue, it establishes certain regularities of procedure that elicit public confidence. The confidence elicited is fulfilled only in the personal relationship, a delicate alliance that may simultaneously encourage confidence and discourage dependence. A code may encourage the creation of their relationship or else the relationship—under the cold exigencies of scientific skill, technical expertise, harried services, lack of client choice, and other components of the new provision of health care—may "dehumanize" care (IOM, 1974). Yet, codes can tend to be reactive, considering present rather than future circumstances. They can be used by professionals to protect their own interests and many times are framed with little input from clients (Brown, 1994, 1997). Thus the commitment of the individual health care professional is required to pursue ethical practice.

A Dialogue on Values

Health care professionals working to promote health may benefit from strategies for translating these these core values into action. The aim is to generate a dialogue about the different conceptions of the good and how to arrive at them (Prilleltensky, 1997). Consensus is not sought, nor is a particular conception of the good life, health, or the good society.

It is particularly important for the health care professional to seek consistency in the application of values to ethical questions. This is a difficult undertaking. To assist in this process, a general problem strategy has long been developed and may be applied in a variety of health promotion ethical quandaries (Brody, 1976; Sheinfeld Gorin, 1981). The process begins with clarifying the values founding the responses to these questions. One would approach an ethical question by listing alternative responses. Alongside each possible response, one would frame an ethical statement, including the conditions under which it would apply, to whom, and to what. The long- and short-term consequences could be stated, and for each consequence, the values affected (for the individual, group, family, community, and society at large) would be clarified. Using a short test, the health care professional would ask: "Would I be satisfied to have this action taken upon me? My family? My friends? Others for whom I care? My community?" She/he could consider the representation of health, the good life, and the good society embodied in these alternative responses. The values for oneself and for others are compared with each consequence. If consistent, the ethical statement is valid. If inconsistent, the process begins again.

A cognizance of core values and the principles of action they imply would enable health care professionals to engage in ethical practice. This is critical to confronting the extraordinary questions that await.

COMMITMENT TO CHANGE

The ethical decisions health care professionals must continue to make emerge within a particular political context. At present, public policy for prevention is fragmented and fails to make use of the variety of strategies available to influence health promoting behaviors of individuals and institutions. The current array of community programs, funded largely through federal categorical or block grants to state and local public health agencies and community organizations, is also fragmented, uncoordinated, and insufficient to improve the health of communities.

The political environment, increasingly conservative, reflects a move away from "comprehensive" governmental solutions and toward incremental approaches in which a few problems are tackled at a time and a bipartisan consensus is built. Congress itself tends to enforce this practice. In addition, when popular bills are proposed, lawmakers and lobbyists add amendments, thus slowing the legislation. Further, seemingly small changes in health care can bring unintended effects. For example, many businesses and states fear a rise in premiums from any movement toward comprehensive efforts or an incremental federal derailing of state plans for health care reform. Finally, at present, little consensus exists regarding the direction of incremental changes. Some wish to move toward health insurance for all Americans, whereas others want to undercut the notion of shared insurance pools.

Further, movement toward increased health has been slower among the more vulnerable. Although of late, some political attention at both the national and many state levels has been turned to the problems of children's health, entirely new policies and programs designed to meet the needs of the most vulnerable members of society are few. Modifications of existing programs, such as increased access to managed care and expansion of the trial insurance programs for the poor who are uninsured, are more likely. In these cases, too, different political agendas challenge each proposal. The traditional policy debate over the most efficient way to provide health care to the poor emerges during each administration. On one hand, there are those who want to provide the poor with health insurance and leave it to them to obtain the care they need. On the other hand are advocates for special programs directly aimed at providing care for the poor (Fuchs, 1993). Comprehensive health care legislation is only successful under a unique set of historical forces, such as the push of the popularly rooted and widespread liberal Democratic groups of the 1960s for many of the Great Society legislative initiatives, including the Health Insurance for the Aged Act (Medicare Act) and the Medicaid Act, which were passed in 1965 (1994; Stocpol, 1996). In general, legislation attends to specialized aspects of health promotion, or narrow interests, such as nutrition or the health of older Americans.

Thus the leadership for comprehensive health promotion must arise from among those most interested in it. The health care professional must assess the impact of alterations in service delivery systems borne of particular policy choices on both the provision of care *and* its outcome for the most vulnerable members of society. The focus of health care professionals concerned with health promotion must continue to move society toward the broadest aims of social justice so that all may be healthy.

Leadership in defining requisite action and necessary resources is needed. In some other parts of the developed world, as well as in many U.S. cities, community life-style changes and multisectoral "healthy public policy" are burgeoning. For example, the Toronto Department of Public Health's "The Mandala of Health" (Department of Public Health, City of Toronto, 1983; Hancock & Perkins, 1985) has attempted to undergird its health promotion programs with premises specifying the enhancement of social justice, as well as ecological "sanity." Its efforts assume that persons can be healthy only in a healthy world. A concern with society's "forgotten" is coupled with a greater interest in the environment and a concomitant theoretical attention to environmental models of change, such as the ecological model.

A national health policy and appropriately funded programs are needed to achieve equity in access to health promotive care. Even more critical is an equitable sharing of basic health determinants for society—nutritious food, basic education, safe water, decent housing, secure employment, adequate income—and peace (McBeath, 1991). Leadership from all sectors—government, managed care organizations, and health care professionals in partnership with clients—are vital to ensuring fair allocation of these resources.

The Role of Government

Government may play an instrumental role in promoting health as a "public good" from which all benefit, rather than as a "commodity" to be bought and sold by self-interested entities (U.S. Senator D.P. Moynihan, personal communication, December 10, 1997). It may support the activities of other entities, such as worksites and managed care companies, as well as lead efforts of its own. In particular, the CDC may play an important role in building partnerships between managed care organizations, insurance purchasers, and public health agencies at all levels.

Partnership for Prevention, a nonprofit organization founded in 1991 to increase the priority of prevention in national policy and practice, has proposed a series of policy recommendations. The general guidelines deriving from these recommendations are found in the organization's monograph, *Prevention is Basic to Health Care Reform* (Partnership for Prevention, 1993). The role of government is seen as comprehensive and is stated in the following (Schauffler, 1994, p. 2):

1. Government provides the link between the science of prevention, policy for prevention, and the practice of prevention within the context of health care reform.
2. Government has a role in establishing national goals for health promotion and disease prevention, implementing public policy to accomplish these goals, and supporting an integrated and coordinated approach to health promotion and disease prevention at the national, state, and local levels.
3. Government has a role in defining uniform measures of health status for assessing system performance and for supporting the development of integrated and wholly compatible information systems at all levels in the health care system.
4. Government has a role in providing adequate funding to support the core public health functions in state and local health departments and health promotion programs provided by community organizations.
5. Government has a role in increasing the number of health professionals with the skills, competencies, and understanding necessary to prevent disease and promote the public's health.
6. Government has a role as an entrepreneur in funding new and innovative research to address the enormous gaps in our knowledge of how best to motivate individuals, organizations, and communities to engage in health-enhancing behaviors.
7. Government has a role in disseminating the findings of research in the form of practice guidelines to providers, health plans, communities, and states in a timely manner so that the prevention we practice is based on approaches that have been demonstrated to be most effective.

The Role of Managed Care Organizations

Managed care organizations are designed to address the medical needs of permanent employees and their families, rather than nonpermanent workers, unemployed individuals, and indigent groups. The future offers a challenge to these managed care entities to do the following:

1. Broaden their programs, particularly the HMOs, to encompass a wider variety of health promotive services.
2. Increase development of new managed care options for vulnerable groups in the population who currently lack access to adequate health care.
3. Grow employee assistance and community health programs to assist marginally employed and unemployed workers (Vinokur, Price, & Caplan, 1991).
4. Target programs to ethnic and racial minority populations. These groups will grow dramatically in the next century and will be highly represented among workforce entrants.

The growth in these practices, particularly within capitated systems (fixed reimbursement per enrollee), must be accompanied by additional incentives that favor investments in wellness, such as performance measures that are health-promotion oriented.

The Role of the Health Care Professional and the Health Promotion Matrix

Given these potent forces for change, the role of the health care professional, too, will alter. Emerging partnerships with clients will continue to demand a new approach to the provision of care and a strong sense of the moral values underpinning actions within these relationships. As health care organizations become larger and more diverse and complex, the professional will need to listen more closely to the often solitary and unique voice of the client.

The present picture of health care professional staffing portrays a general overabundance of physicians, particularly specialists, and an increase in training of nurse practitioners for the developing opportunities of independent practice. Government agencies, such as the Health Care Financing Administration, are currently implementing incentive programs to change the distribution pattern for physicians by offering inducements to academic medical institutions, many in major urban areas, to alter programs or to close. At present, many nursing programs are increasing their attention to wellness across the lifespan. The training of other health care professionals is moving toward the new managed care opportunities, or chronic care settings. These patterns are likely to continue into the future.

The Health Promotion Matrix (HPM) is offered as one means for assisting health care professionals to better listen to the client's voice in their clinical practice. Founded on robust theories of change and sound clinical principles, the HPM awaits empirical verification. The HPM may be implemented with any client system and its myriad experiences of health. Collaboration with clients in imagining their health will take precious time and skill to encourage active participation. Negotiating that time will require that health care professionals acquire more practical knowledge about managed care and how it works. Concretizing a client's image, by assessing its objective features, will require measures that continue to be developed and improved. Health care professionals must be trained to understand the meaning and use of measurement and be skilled in its application. Optimizing health supportive patterns and minimizing health depleting patterns will demand a recognition of the theoretical, empirical, and moral bases on which change rests. A deep understanding of the interrelatedness of the factors in the client's life—economic, social, political, psychologic, physiologic, and spiritual—as well as how the client uses those factors will dominate the health care professional's work. Proactive intervention to promote healthy client systems in healthy environments will demand a cognizance of both the complexity of client systems and an ability to simplify an approach. Finally, assisting the client to internalize an image will require extensive follow-up, in which the health care professional helps clients to "sell" themselves on the importance of the changes that they have begun.

The greatest potential for improving the health status of populations rests in policy change, community-based action, and research to improve effectiveness. These strategies will, however, require increased sophistication in their use, with health care professionals trained in community organization and group facilitation skills and skilled in collaborating with those from other disciplines. As health care professionals become more skilled in policy change, the adversaries to health promotion will become more tenacious (e.g., tobacco manufacturers or large agri-businesses that mount increasingly expensive and articulate legal campaigns to counter health promotive efforts). Health care professionals will need tenacity to pursue health promotive strategies in the face of this opposition and assistance in targeting them to appropriate behaviors and groups.

Summary

In this final chapter, the profound sociodemographic changes resulting from the aging of the population have been outlined. The growth of worksites as focii for health promotion and the size and power of managed care organizations have been detailed. Accountability for performance in the provision of services will remain a strong theme for future practice, as health care costs may continue to rise. These changes will require that health care professionals clarify the values upon which the field rests. Social justice—ensuring accessible and equitable care to society's most vulnerable—is proposed as one core value. To advance the value of social justice, change in the roles of government, managed care organizations, and health care professionals are essential. The Health Promotion Matrix, with its clinical orientation, is proffered as a means for guiding the change in health care professionals' roles.

The task of promoting health for all, therefore, remains a daunting one. We urge you to take the challenge.

References

American Hospital Association. (1994). *Transforming health care delivery: Toward community care networks.* Chicago: Author.

American Hospital Association. (1998). *The community care network demonstration program* [On-line]. Available: http://www.aha.org

Baier, K. (1973). The concept of value. In E. Laszlo & J.B. Wilbur (Eds.), *Value theory in philosophy and social science* (pp. 1-11). New York: Gordon & Breach Science Publishers.

Baquet, C.R., Horm, J.W. Gibbs, T., & Greenwald, P. (1991). Socioeconomic factors and cancer incidence among blacks and whites. *Journal of the American Cancer Institute, 83,* 553-557.

Brody, H. (1976). *Ethical decisions in medicine.* Boston: Little, Brown.

Brown, L.S. (1994). *Subversive dialogues: Theory in feminist therapy.* New York: Basic Books.

Brown, L.S. (1997). Ethics in psychology: Cui bono? In D. Fox & I. Prilleltensky (Eds.), *Critical psychology: An introduction* (pp. 51-67). London: Sage.

Campbell, D.T. (1974, September.). *Qualitative knowing in action research.* Kurt Lewin address, Society for the Psychological Study of Social Issues, Meeting with the American Psychological Association, New Orleans.

Casperson, C.J. (1989). Physical activity epidemiology: Concepts, methods and applications to exercise science. *Exercise and Sports Sciences Reviews, 17,* 423-73.

Centers for Disease Control and Prevention. (1995). Prevention and managed care: Opportunities for managed care organizations, purchasers of health care, and public health agencies. *Morbidity and Mortality Weekly Report, 44*(RR-14), 1-12.

Charlton, B.G., & White, M. (1995). Living on the margin: A salutogenic model for socioeconomic differentials in health. *Public Health, 109,* 235-243.

Clarfield, A.M. (1988). The reversible dementias: Do they reverse? *Annals of Internal Medicine, 109,* 476-486.

Dayal, H.H., Power, R.N., & Chiu, C. (1982). Race and socioeconomic status in survival from breast cancer. *Journal of Chronic Diseases, 35,* 675-683.

Department of Public Health, City of Toronto. (1983). *The unequal society: A challenge to public health.* Toronto: Author.

Eckenrode, J., & Gore, S. (1990). Stress and coping at the boundary of work and family. In J. Echenrode & S. Gore (Eds.), *Stress between work and family* (pp. 1-116). New York: Plenum Press.

Eisenberg, D.M., Kessler, R.C., Foster, C. et al. (1993). Unconventional medicine in the United States: Prevalence, costs and patterns of use. *New England Journal of Medicine, 328,* 246-252.

Employee Benefits Research Institute. (1997). *Over 149 million nonelderly Americans have employee-based health insurance, 41.4 million uninsured, according to March 1997 CPS (current population survey)* [On-line]. Available: http://www.ebri.org/notesx/1197note.htm

Ethical guidelines for health promotion. Medicine in the twenty first century: Challenges in personal and public health promotion. (1994). *American Journal of Preventive Medicine, 10*(3), 47.

Etzioni, A. (1993). *The spirit of community.* New York: Touchstone.

Farber, H. (1997). *The changing face of job loss in the United States.*[Working paper]. Princeton, NJ: Princeton University, Department of Economics.

Firth, R. (1952). Ethical absolutism and the ideal observer. *Philosophy and Phenomenological Research, 12,* 317-345.

Fuchs, V.R. (Ed). (1972). *Essays in the economics of health and medical care.* New York: National Bureau of Economic Research.

Fuchs, V.R. (1993). *The future of health policy.* Cambridge, MA: Harvard University Press.

Fuchs, V.R., & Garber, A.M. (1993). Technology assessment and health policy. In V.R. Fuchs, (Ed.), *The future of health policy* (pp. 192-203). Cambridge, MA: Harvard University Press.

Galbraith, J.K. (1996). *The good society.* New York: Houghton-Mifflin. June 6, 1997.

Grann, V.R., Panegeas, K.S., Whang, W., Antman, K.H., & Neugut, A.I. (in press). A decision analysis of prophylactic mastectomy and oophorectomy in BRCA1 or BRCA2 positive patients. *Journal of Clinical Oncology.*

Guralink, J.M., Land, K.C., Blszer, D., Fillenbaum, G.G., & Branch, L.G. (1993). Educational status and active life expectancy among older blacks and whites. *New England Journal of Medicine, 329,* 110-116.

Gutek, B.A., Repetti, R.L., & Silver, D.L. (1988). Nonwork roles and stress at work. In C.L. Cooper & R. Payne (Eds.), *Causes, coping, and consequences of stress at work* (pp. 141-174). Chichester, United Kingdom: John Wiley and Sons.

Haan, M., Kaplan, G.A., & Camacho, T. (1987). Poverty and health: Prospective evidence from the Alameda County study. *American Journal of Epidemiology, 125,* 989-999.

Hancock, T., & Perkins, F. (1985). The mandala of health: A conceptual model and teaching tool. *Health Education, 24*(1), 8-10.

Health Insurance for the Aged Act (Medicare Act), 42 U.S.C. § 301 *et seq.* (U.S. Government Printing Office 1994)

Institute of Medicine. (1974). *Ethics of health care. Papers of the Conference on Health Care and Changing Values, November 27-29, 1973.* Washington, DC: National Academy of Sciences.

Institute of Medicine. (1990). *The second fifty years: Promoting health and preventing disability.* Washington, DC: National Academy of Sciences.

Joyce, C.R.B. (1994, November 5). Placebo and complementary medicine. *The Lancet, 344,* 1279-1281.

Kekes, J. (1993). *The morality of pluralism.* Princeton, NJ: Princeton University Press.

Keith-Lucas, A. (1971). Ethics in social work. In R. Morris (Ed.), *Encyclopedia of social work* (vol 1, pp. 324-328). New York: National Association of Social Workers.

Koplan, J.P., & Livengood, J.R. (1994). The influence of changing demographic patterns on our health promotion priorities. *American Journal of Preventive Medicine, 10* (Suppl. 1), 42-44.

Kurtzman, J. (1997, February 17). Is your company off course? Now you can find out why. *Fortune,* 128-130.

Larson, E.B., Reifler, B.V., & Featherstone H.J., & English, D.R. (1984). Dementia in elderly outpatients: A prospective study. *Annals of Internal Medicine, 100,* 417-423.

Levin, J.S., Glass, T.A., Kushi, L.H., Schuck, J.R., Steele, L., & Jonas, W.B. (1997). Quantitative methods in research on complementary and alternative medicine: A methodological manifesto. *Medical Care, 35*(11), 1079-1094.

Light, D.W. (1997). From managed competition to managed cooperation: Theory and lessons from the British experience. *Milbank Memorial Quarterly, 75*(3), 297-341.

Marmot, M.G., Smith, G.D., & Stansfeld, S. et al. (1991). Health inequalities among British civil servants: The Whitehall II study. *Lancet, 337,* 1387-1393.

McBeath, W.H. (1991). Health for all: A public health vision. *American Journal of Public Health, 81*(12), 1560-1565.

Medicaid Act, 42 U.S.C. 1396 *et seq.* (U.S. Government Printing Office 1994).

Morgan, R.O., Virnig, B.A., DeVito, C.A., & Persily, N.A. (1997). The Medicare-HMO revolving door—The healthy go in and the sick go out. *New England Journal of Medicine, 337*(3), 169-175.

National Center for Health Statistics, Centers for Disease Control, U.S. Public Health Service, U.S. Department of Health and Human Services. (1995). *National health interview survey* Hyattsville, MD: Author.

National Institute of Health. (1988). *Consensus development conference statement: Urinary incontinence in adults, October 3-5, 1988.* Washington, DC: Author.

Newhouse, J.P. (1993). An iconoclastic view of health cost containment. *Health Affairs, 12,* (Suppl.) 152-171.

Novaco, R.W., Stokols, D., & Milanesi, L. (1990). Objective and subjective dimensions of travel impedance as determinants of commuting stress. *American Journal of Community Psychology, 18,* 231-257.

Office of Technology Assessment. (1980). The implications of cost-effective analysis of medical technology [On-line]. Available: http://www.wws.princeton.edu

Oral Health Coordinating Committee, U.S. Public Health Service. (1993). Toward improving the oral health of Americans: An overview of oral health status, resources, and care delivery. *Public Health* Reports, *108*(6), 657-672.

Organizición Pan Americana de la Salud. (1992). *Pronunciamiento de Consenso sobre politicas de atencion a los ancianos en America Latina* [Consensus statements about the policies regarding the elderly in Latin America]. Centro Latinoamericano de Demografia, Central Internacional del Envejecimiento. Santiago, Chile.

Pappas, G., Queen, S., Hadden, W., & Fisher, G. (1993). The increasing disparity in mortality between socioeconomic groups in the United States, 1960 to 1986. *New England Journal of Medicine, 329,* 103-109.

Partnership for Prevention. (1993). *Prevention is basic to health care reform.* A position paper from an expert panel. Washington, DC: Author.

Pelletier, K.R. (1994). *Sound mind—Sound body: A new model for lifelong health.* New York: Simon & Schuster.

Prilleltensky, I. (1997). Values, assumptions, and practices: Assessing the moral implications of psychological discourse and action. *American Psychologist, 52*(5), 517-535.

Prilleltensky, I., & Gonick, L. (1996). Politics change, oppression remains: On the psychology and politics of oppression. *Political Psychology, 17,* 127-147.

Rawls, J. (1971). *A theory of justice.* Cambridge, MA: Belknap Press.

Repetti, R.L., Matthews, K.A., & Waldron, I. (1989). Employment and women's health: Effects of paid employment on women's mental and physical health. *American Psychologist, 44,* 1394-1401.

Restrepo, H.E., & Rozental, M. (1994). The social impact of aging populations: Some major issues. *Social Science and Medicine, 39*(9), 1323-1338.

Royce, J., Sheinfeld Gorin, S., Edelman, B., Rendino-Perrone, R., & Orlandi, M. (1990a). Student nurses and smoking cessation. In P. F. Engstrom & B. Rimer (Eds.), *Advances in Cancer Control VII* (pp. 49-71). New York: Alan Liss.

Royce, J., Sheinfeld Gorin, S., Edelman, B., Rendino-Perrone, R., & Orlandi, M. (1990b). Student nurses and smoking cessation. *Progress in Clinical and Biological Research, 339,* 49-71.

Sandel, M.J. (1996). *Democracy's discontent: America in search of a public philosophy.* Cambridge, MA: Harvard University Press.

Salonen, J.T. (1982). Socioeconomic status and risk of cancer, cerebral stroke, and death due to coronary heart disease and any disease: A longitudinal study in eastern Finland. *Journal of Epidemiology and Community Health, 26,* 294-297.

Schaeffer, M.H., Street, S.W., Singer, J.E., & Baum, A. (1988). Effects of control on stress reactions of commuters. *Journal of Applied Social Psychology, 18,* 944-957.

Shapiro, A.K. (1978). The placebo effect. In W.G. Clark & J. DelGiudice (Eds.), *Principles of pharmacology* (2nd ed.). New York: Academic Press.

Schauffler, H.H. (1994). Introduction: Health promotion disease prevention in health care reform [Supplement]. *American Journal of Preventive Medicine, 10*(3), 1-3.

Sheinfeld, S.N. (1978). The evaluation profession in pursuit of value. *Evaluation and Program Planning, 1,* 113-115.

Sheinfeld, S., & Lord, G. (1981). The ethics of evaluation researchers: An exploration of value choices. *Evaluation Review, 5*(3), 377-391.

Sheinfeld, Gorin, S. (1985). Expect the unexpected: Consequences of the use of productivity indices. *Health Care Strategic Management, 3*(4), 12-15.

Sheinfeld Gorin, S., with Viswanathan, N. (1997). The integrative decision-making matrix: Models of decision making for social work. In D. Tucker, C. Garvin, & R. Sarri (Eds.), *Integration of social work and social science.* (pp. 116-125). Westport, CT: Greenwood Publishing Group.

Shroder, M., & Weisbrod, B.A. (1990). Medical malpractice, technological change, and learning-by-doing. In R.M. Scheffler & L. Rossiter (Eds.), *Advances in health economics and health services research* (pp. 195-200). Greenwich, CT: JAI Press.

Stocpol, T. (1996). *Boomerang*. New York: W.W. Norton.

Stokols, D., Pelletier, K.R., & Fielding, J.E. (1995). Toward an integration of medical care and worksite health promotion. *Journal of the American Medical Association, 273,* 1136-1142.

Stokols, D., Churchman, A., Scharf, T., & Wright, S. (1990). Workers' experiences of environmental change and transition at the office. In S. Fisher & C.L. Cooper (Eds.), *On the move: The psychology of change and transition* (pp. 231-49). Chichester, England: John Wiley and Sons.

Swartz, K. (1997, Fall). Where is efficiency leading our system of health insurance? *Inquiry, 34,* 193-195.

Tauber, C.M. (1993). *Sixty five plus in America*. Paris: Centres d'Études et de Recherches en Demographie (CICRED).

Tyroler, H.A. (1989). Socioeconomic status in the epidemiology and treatment of hypertension. *Hypertension, 13* (Suppl. 1), 194-197.

University Center on Aging. (1993). Demographic transition and aging. (pp. 69-84). In T.M. Schuman *Population aging: International perspectives*. Proceedings and recommendations of the international conference on population aging. San Diego, CA: 17-19 September 1992.

U.S. Department of Health and Human Services, Health Care Financing Administration. (1995). *Health care financing review*. Washington, DC: Superintendent of Documents.

U.S. Department of Health and Human Services, U.S. Public Health Service, Centers for Disease Control and Prevention. (1996). *Inventory of managed care projects for FY 1995-1996*. Atlanta, GA: Centers for Disease Control and Prevention.

U.S. Department of Health and Human Services, U.S. Public Health Service (1995). *Healthy people 2000: Midcourse review and 1995 revisions*. Washington, DC: U.S. Government Printing Office.

U.S. Department of Labor, Women's Bureau. (1997). *Facts on working women*. [On-line]. Available: http://www.dol.gov/dol/wb/public

U.S. Senate Special Committee on Aging. (1991). *Aging America: Trends and projections*. Washington, DC: U.S. Government Printing Office.

Vinokur, A.D., Price, R.H., & Caplan, R.D. (1991). From field experiments to program implementation: Assessing the potential outcomes of an experimental intervention program for unemployed persons. *American Journal of Community Psychology, 19,* 543-562.

Weeks, J. (1997). Managed care meets alternative medicine. *Alternative and Complementary Therapies, 3*(1), 37-41.

Winkleby, M.A., Jatulis, D.E., Frank, E., & Fortmann, S.P. (1992). Socioeconomic status and health: How education, income, and occupation contribute to risk factors for cardiovascular disease. *American Journal of Public Health, 82,* 816-820.

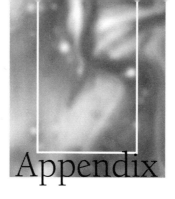

Appendix

The Health Promotion Matrix: Comprehensive Intervention Guide

The following instrument is designed to be used by the health care professional together with the client. It begins with a client description, then introduces the five dimensions of the Matrix, as described in Chapter 5 and detailed in Part Two. The dimensions are: image creation, image appraisal, minimize health depleting patterns, optimize health supportive patterns, and internalize idealized image. It will take several sessions to complete this comprehensive instrument because client change takes time and different health issues may emerge as the client begins to alter his/her behaviors. Further, changing behavior requires frequent practice and consistent positive feedback over time. The health care professional is a partner with the client in this extended change process.

In using the tool, introductory client data will provide background information. Image creation will help the client reveal his/her own personal image of health. During image appraisal, the health care professional guides the client through a detailed assessment of current patterns and practices in relation to the nine behaviors that define health in the Matrix (smoking cessation, eating well, physical activity, sexual awareness, injury prevention, substance safety, oral health, self-development, and productivity). The health care professional will also learn about the client's willingness to change. If the health care professional encounters clients who express resistance, she/he may want to consult the suggestions found in Part Two under the dimension of minimizing health depleting patterns. Numerous detailed assessment guides to supplement this instrument are also found in Part Two.

Recognizing that there are patterns that diminish health and affect the willingness to change, the health care professional moves with the client to minimizing health depleting patterns. Many approaches to reducing barriers to change are detailed in Part Two. Optimizing health supportive patterns enables the health care professional and client to identify concrete types of supports in the change process. Finally, as the client begins to internalize an idealized image of health, both the health care professional and the client move toward closure together. The client may then reflect on the behavioral changes that have been made, his/her own sense of accomplishment, and plans to maintain a healthier self.

THE HEALTH PROMOTION MATRIX: *A Comprehensive Script*

CLIENT HEALTH PROMOTION INFORMATION

Name _____

Address _____

Telephone number _____

Date of birth _____

Race/ethnicity _____

Present or former occupation(s) _____

   Is client working at present? _____

Hobbies/interests _____

Living arrangements _____

Type of housing (e.g., single family, shared, owned,

   rented) _____

Yearly household income (approximate) _____

Immunization status _____

Known allergies _____

Known client health problems/conditions _____

Known health problems or conditions in the client's family _____

Presenting health concerns _____

Date of last comprehensive physical examination _____

Date of last comprehensive oral examination _____

Date of last screening blood tests (e.g., cbc) _____

Date of last laboratory screening tests (e.g., PAP smear, fecal occult

   blood, PSA) _____

Height _____

Weight _____

Blood pressure, pulse, respiration _____

Health insurance policy number _____

Dental insurance policy number _____

Image Creation

Imagine yourself as a healthy person. What do you see if you try to picture yourself this way?

In this image of yourself, how do you feel? Physically? Emotionally? Spiritually?

Do you *smoke?* If so, how do you feel about being a cigarette smoker?

Do you visualize yourself as a nonsmoker?

When you imagine yourself *eating well,* what does it look like?

THE HEALTH PROMOTION MATRIX: *A Comprehensive Script—cont'd*

	What kinds of activities do you see yourself doing?
	If you could imagine yourself reaching your own personal ideal for *physical activity,* that is, the best level of physical activity for you, how would you see yourself?
	Is it becoming increasingly important for you to think about becoming physically active?
	Is *sexuality* a part of your image of yourself as healthy?
	What do you envision as a *healthy environment* at home?
	Do you visualize yourself as *drinking alcohol?* As someone who uses *drugs?*
	Do you picture yourself as having an *ideal smile?*
	Do you see yourself with *clean, healthy teeth and gums?* With *fresh breath?*
	Everyone experiences *loss.* Do you view yourself as living well with your losses?
	What do you envision when you see yourself as *productive?*
	When you imagine a productive environment for you, what does it look like?
	How closely does this image conform with your current health behaviors?
	How interested are you in becoming more like your own image of health?
	What changes would you like to make in yourself?
Image Appraisal	Have you ever made any changes in your behavior?
	When did you make those changes?
	Did you have any problems making those changes?

Smoking Cessation

Do you ever smoke cigarettes or cigars or chew tobacco?

Current smoking practice: (specify number of cigarettes/cigars/ amount of smokeless tobacco per week)

Smoking history: (specify when client stopped, how long smoked)

> *If the client smokes:*
> Have you ever stopped smoking?
>
> When was the last time? For how long did you stop?
>
> How did you stop?

continued

Would you like to stop smoking?

Do you think you could stop now?

What reasons would you have for stopping?

Would you be willing to develop a plan to stop smoking?

Can you agree to a stop date?

Would you be willing to cut down on your smoking?

Eating Well

How do you feel about eating?

Could you choose a typical day from this week or last and list what you ate?

What foods do you eat on a typical day?

Do you usually eat breakfast?

Where do you eat during the day?

Who prepares most of the foods that you really enjoy?

Are the foods you eat foods that you enjoy?

Would you be willing to change your diet at this time?

Would you be willing to fill out a food diary over the next week to record what you eat?

Physical Activity

On a scale measuring physical activity, are you "inactive," "moderately active," or "very active?" If you are "inactive" or "moderately active," can you imagine yourself participating in more physical activity, or are you interested in participating in more physical activity?

If you selected *inactive* as the level that describes you best, would you consider learning about how physical activity could benefit you?

If you selected *moderately active* as the level that describes you best, would you consider learning about a physical activity plan specifically designed for you?

If you selected *very active* as the level that describes you best, would you consider assistance in reviewing your current program for suggested changes, if needed?

Are you more than 90% confident that you can carry out your plan for physical activity?

THE HEALTH PROMOTION MATRIX: *A Comprehensive Script—cont'd*

Sexual Awareness

How satisfied are you with your sexual response?

Do you feel sexually fulfilled?

Do you engage in safe sex practices?

How many sexual partners have you had? Same sex? Opposite sex? Bisexual?

Injury Prevention

Do you use seat belts when you drive? About how often?

What have you heard about the role seat belts and not drinking play in reducing traffic accidents?

Do you use a designated driver or refuse to drive when you have drunk alcohol?

If client has a motorcycle: Do you use a helmet?

Do you have a smoke detector in your home?

Do you have fire extinguisher in your home?

How often do you test or check them?

Do you have a plan for a fire emergency (e.g., an evacuation plan, a meeting place)?

Is your hot water heater kept below 120°F?

Do you know cardiopulmonary resuscitation (CPR)? The Heimlich maneuver?

If the client has children:
Do you have a car seat for your babies and children? Do you use it every time you travel?

Have you heard about the importance of always placing children in the back seat of your car?

Do your children wear a helmet whenever they ride a bicycle?

Do you have gates or other devices to block access to stairs by children?

Do you keep poisons together, in labeled containers, in a place that is locked or latched [i.e., out of reach of children and pets]?

Do you keep all medications in labeled, child-proof containers and in a place that is locked or latched [i.e., out of reach of children and pets]?

continued

THE HEALTH PROMOTION MATRIX: *A Comprehensive Script—cont'd*

Do you have an emetic (such as 1 ounce of syrup of ipecac) in the home? Do you have the number of the local poison control center by the telephone?

Do your children sleep in fire-retardant clothing?

Do you store matches and lighters in child-resistant containers?

Do you watch your children when they swim in a pool or other body of water? Do you watch your children when they take a bath?

If the client lives in a high-rise and has children: Do you have window guards or locks to prevent falls?

If an older adult lives in the client's home:
Have you installed good lighting, hand railings, nonstick traction strips on floor surfaces to reduce falls? Have you removed rugs, electrical wires, and other items (such as toys) that promote tripping?

Have you padded sharp corners of furniture?

Does the older person wear sturdy shoes while at home?

Has the older person been evaluated for impaired hearing and/or vision? Has he/she been evaluated for changes in walking and balance?

Has adaptive equipment been added to the bathroom?

If the client has a pool:
Does a protective fence surround your pool and separate it from the house? Does it have a gate that is kept closed?

If the household lives or vacations near water:
Does everyone in your household know how to swim? Do they use life jackets if they go boating? Do they drink alcohol or use drugs while boating?

Substance Safety
Do you drink alcohol? If yes, about how many drinks do you have in a week?

On a day when you drink, how much do you drink?

How many days a month do you drink 4 or more drinks?

(Guidelines for adult men are drinking no more than 14 drinks/week; for adult women, no more than 7 drinks/week; and for adult men or women, at-risk drinking is a report of *any* single occasion when they have consumed more than 4 drinks in the past month. Guidelines for older adults recommend no more than 7 drinks/week, or 1 per day.)

The Health Promotion Matrix: *A Comprehensive Script—cont'd*

If drinking is above the guidelines:
How do you feel about drinking at a level that is considered risky?

If client's drinking is at risk:
Have you ever thought about cutting back on your alcohol use?

Have you ever tried to cut down on your drinking?

How do you feel about that level of alcohol use?

> Negotiate a drinking limit consonant with national guidelines. Complete the drinking agreement.

(Drug use is taking any prescription or over-the-counter drugs in excess of the directions and any use of nonmedical drugs.)

Do you use more than the recommended or prescribed amount of prescribed or over-the-counter medications?

Oral Health

Do you see yourself having your teeth cleaned regularly?

Have you been able to set aside time to complete thorough oral hygiene each day?

Do you examine the inside of your mouth every day?

Have you noticed any blood on your toothbrush or when you rinse your mouth?

Do you feel comfortable smiling and talking to people?

Do you sometimes have problems chewing food?

Do you feel as if you have a comfortable bite and can chew with ease?

Have you noticed a bad taste in your mouth?

Do you feel as if you have fresh breath?

When was your last dental visit? What was done?

Do you feel as if you have an acceptable smile?

Were you pleased with your smile after your dental visit?

Do you drink tap water or bottled water that is not flouridated?

Would you be willing to develop and to complete a plan to promote your oral health?

continued

THE HEALTH PROMOTION MATRIX: *A Comprehensive Script—cont'd*

Self-development

Everyone experiences losses. Some losses are never expressed. Can you remember a loss that you have experienced and perhaps never talked about?

How did this loss affect you?

Can you describe the feelings now?

Productivity

How productive are you with the work you do? (e.g., pay, benefits, promotions; the work itself in its level of challenge, routinization, autonomy, control, safety; relationships with supervisors, co-workers, clients, staff, suppliers, distributors; organizational decision-making structure, culture)

How is productivity measured in your present work environment?

How does your own work compare to the standards in place at this time?

Would you be willing to develop a plan to enhance your productivity?

Minimize Health Depleting Patterns

How successful do you feel you have been in making and sustaining personal change?

How committed are you to changing your current behaviors that are less healthy?

Can you identify ways to overcome barriers to changing these unhealthy behaviors?

How can you adjust your daily patterns to plan ahead so that these barriers do not limit your success?

Refer to the Helpful Resources sections found throughout Part Two.

What limits or prevents you from changing your current health behaviors in relation to the following:

- Smoking cessation (if appropriate)?
- Eating well?
- Physical activity?
- Sexual awareness?
- Injury prevention?
- Substance safety?

THE HEALTH PROMOTION MATRIX: *A Comprehensive Script—cont'd*

	· Oral health?
	· Self-development around losses in life?
	· Enhanced productivity?
Optimize Health Supportive Patterns	What are your health strengths?
	What are you most proud of about your health?
	What could you say to persons in your support network to help them learn about the kinds of things you would like them to do to further encourage your successfully carrying out your plan?
Internalize Idealized Image	In what ways has your idealized image of health become a reality to you?
	Do you feel you would be more successful if we further adjusted the goal?
	What aspects of your changed behaviors are the most satisfying? Least satisfying?
	What would you modify to make your practices more convenient? More enjoyable? Safer?
	How will you hold onto these changes?
	Establish a follow-up contact.

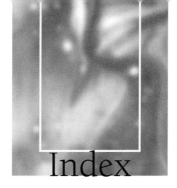

Index

Department
  of Agriculture, 47
  of Health and Human Services
    (DHHS), 47
  of Labor, 47
Dependence, substance abuse and,
  289-290
Development; *see* Self-development
DHHS; *see* Department of Health and
  Human Services
Diabetes, oral health and, 313, 314
Diary, food, 181
Diet; *see* Nutrition
Dietary Guidelines for Americans, 166
Dietary Supplement and Health
  Education Act of 1994, 278
Diphenhydramine 0.5%, mucositis and,
  318
Disability, adaptive behavior and, 7
Disability management, 372-373
Disease
  definition of, 5
  health as antithesis of, 4-5
Disease prevention
  versus health promotion and health
    protection, 20
  national policy and, 18-20
Distributive effect, cost-effectiveness
  analysis and, 395
Doctors Ought to Care (DOC), 53
Domestic violence, 249
Doshas, balance in health and, 6
DRI Wellness Center, 373-374
Drinking; *see* Alcohol
Drinking agreement, 297
Drug dependence, 289-290
Drugs
  over-the-counter, 277
  prescribed, 277
  social, 278
Dry mouth, oral health and, 312
Dyclonine 1, mucositis and, 318
Dysfunctional eating, 169

E

EAPs; *see* Employee assistance programs
Early childhood caries (ECC), 319
Eating well; *see* Nutrition
ECC; *see* Early childhood caries
Ecological model
  of health promotion, 21
  Health Promotion Matrix and, 93

Economic considerations
  cost-benefit analysis and, 395-399
  cost-effectiveness analysis and,
    394-395, 396
  health insurance and, 390
  in health promotion, 389-400
  helpful resources and, 399-400
  prevention in, 389-390, 391-393
Economic influences on health
  promotion, 56-66
Education
  continuing, therapeutic interaction
    and, 358
  injury prevention and, 256-257
Educational group, 107
Elderly
  oral health and, 321, 322-323
  physical activity counseling for,
    209
  sexual awareness in, 233-234
  smoking in, 125
  substance-related health promotion
    for, 289
Emergency rooms, health promotion
  and, 55-56
Employee assistance programs (EAPs),
  54, 65
Empowerment, health promotion and,
  10-11, 31, 77-79
Endocarditis, oral infection and, 312
Energy, acute exposure to, injury and,
  252
Engineering, injury prevention and, 258
English Towns Improvement Act of
  1847, 47
Environment, substance abuse and, 286
Environmental approaches to health
  promotion models, 20-23
Environmental prevention programs, 389
Environmental Protection Agency, 47
Environmental tobacco smoke (ETS),
  127
Epidemiologic Catchment Area Study,
  20, 279
Epidemiology, 5, 18
EPOs, managed care and, 64
ERT; *see* Estrogen replacement therapy
Erythematous type of oral candidiasis,
  HIV infection and, 317
Essential oils, antimicrobial rinses and,
  328
Estrogen replacement therapy (ERT),
  232